Exploring
Medical
Language

A Student-Directed Approach

Exploring Medical Language

A Student-Directed Approach

Sixth Edition

Myrna LaFleur Brooks, RN, BEd

Founding President
National Association of Health Unit Coordinators
Faculty Emeritus
Maricopa County Community College District
Phoenix, Arizona

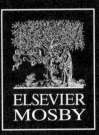

ELSEVIER
MOSBY

ELSEVIER
MOSBY

11830 Westline Industrial Drive
St. Louis, Missouri 63146

EXPLORING MEDICAL LANGUAGE
Copyright © 2005, Elsevier Inc.

All rights reserved. No part of this publication may be reproduced or transmitted in any form or by any means, electronic or mechanical, including photocopying, recording, or any information storage and retrieval system, without permission in writing from the publisher. Permissions may be sought directly from Elsevier's Health Sciences Rights Department in Philadelphia, PA, USA: phone: (+1) 215 239 3804, fax: (+1) 215 239 3805, email: healthpermissions@elsevier.com. You may also complete your request on-line via the Elsevier homepage (http://www.elsevier.com), by selecting 'Customer Support' and then 'Obtaining Permissions'.

Previous editions copyrighted 1985, 1989, 1994, 1998, 2002

ISBN-13: 978-0-323-02805-9
ISBN-10: 0-323-02805-5

Publishing Director: Andrew Allen
Executive Editor: Jeanne Wilke
Senior Developmental Editor: Linda Woodard
Publishing Services Manager: Linda McKinley
Senior Project Manager: Julie Eddy
Designer: Julia Dummitt

Printed in the United States of America

Last digit is the print number: 9   8   7   6   5   4   3   2

"The hardest construction to get into the mind of the beginner is that the education upon which he is engaged is not a college course, not a medical course, but a life course."

Sir William Osler (1849-1919),
often referred to as the most influential physician in history

REVIEWERS

Delena Austin, BTIS, CMA
Medical Assistant Program Coordinator
Macomb Community College
Clinton Township, Michigan

Gail Bicknell, HRT
Instructor
Health and Public Safety Department
Southern Alberta Institute of Technology
Calgary, Alberta, Canada

Linda Bray, BA, CMA-C
Instructor
San Bernadino Valley College
Colton, California

Christine Costa
Cardiac Monitor Technician
St. Luke's Medical Center
Phoenix, Arizona

Ann Ehrlich, RT(R)
Senior Instructor, Radiology
Western States Chiropractic College
Portland, Oregon

Marilyn Kachline, ASN, RN
Assistant Director of Education
Allied Medical and Technical Institute
Scranton, Pennsylvania

Linda Minnihan, RN, BSN
Instructor/Registered Nurse
Northcentral Technical College
Wausau, Wisconsin

Alice Noblin, MBA, RHIA
Visiting Instructor, HIM Program
University of Central Florida
Orlando, Florida

Judy A. Zimmerman, RN, BSN
Adjunct Faculty
Northcentral Technical College
Wausau, Wisconsin

Welcome to the sixth edition of *Exploring Medical Language*. Medical terminology, like any living language, is not static. It has become the common currency of not only those in medical professions but also insurers, lawyers, equipment suppliers, pharmaceutical representatives, and others who interact with health care providers and consumers. To keep apace of medical science and to communicate medical knowledge effectively, medical language must expand and change. The goal of this sixth edition is to reflect those changes with a presentation that is up to date, sound in its approach to language instruction, and visually supports the learning process.

New to This Edition

Some outstanding features have been added to the text to make it even more student and faculty friendly. Besides updating current material, deleting obsolete material, and adding new and interesting illustrations, the following are new to this edition.

CAM term boxes have been added as part of a holistic approach to promoting health and treating disease.

Clinical research terms and nutritional terms have been added to the Appendixes, reflecting development in these important fields.

Color photos have been added to more accurately depict the pathology being demonstrated.

Case studies are reformatted to look more like actual medical records. Exercises for reading medical documents aloud, for interacting with the documents, and for measuring comprehension of content are included.

Plural endings have been moved from the appendix into appropriate chapters accompanied by exercises and objectives.

Scoring function and audio pronunciation of the terms have been added to the extensively revised Student CD.

Lesson strategies, teaching opportunities, and PowerPoint Lecture Slides have been added to the Instructor's Curriculum Resource (ICR) to assist the instructor in the classroom. This will be a welcome addition for both new and seasoned faculty.

Questions in the computerized test bank, a part of the ICR, are now identified by objective, topic, and text page number. If objectives are omitted in a chapter by the faculty to fit the course outline, it is now equally as easy to omit the matching test questions.

Building Your Medical Vocabulary

Exploring Medical Language is designed to ensure your mastery of the language of medicine. This is accomplished by categorizing related terms into easily learned units and by introducing you to the structure of medical language. In this way you will be equipped to understand the terms included in this text as well as the new and unfamiliar terms you may encounter in a clinical setting.

Many medical terms are constructed from language elements known as *word parts*. The word parts, each with its own definition, combine to form specific medical terms. Retaining a proven aid to learning, this edition of *Exploring Medical Language* distinguishes medical terms that can be translated literally (or built) from word parts and provides a variety of exercises to help you learn the word parts and their meanings. Because the language of medicine is incomplete without them, terms not built from word parts are included in separate sections with their own exercises. These sections, if not part of your course of study, can easily be omitted.

Organization

Introductory Chapters

Chapters 1 through 3 provide a foundation for building medical vocabulary. Chapter 1 introduces the word part method of learning medical terminology and explains how prefixes, word roots, combining vowels, and suffixes are used to form terms. Chapter 2 establishes a base for the body system chapters that follow by providing information about body structure and by helping you build the terms related to color and oncology that apply to all body systems. Chapter 3 covers directional terms, anatomic planes, and regions and quadrants. All chapters are enhanced with many four-color illustrations, providing clarification of terms and procedures. Each chapter ends with a review, offering you, the student, an additional opportunity to evaluate your knowledge.

Body System Chapters

Chapters 4 through 16 present medical terms organized by body system. Each of these chapters opens by introducing the relevant anatomy. This section may either acquaint you with body structure and function or, if you have studied anatomy in a separate course, can serve as a review.

Body system word parts precede the medical terms. The medical term section is divided into four categories: disease and disorder terms, surgical terms, diagnostic terms, and complementary terms. Each category of terms is further divided into terms built from word parts and those not built from word parts. Considerable attention has been given in this edition to updating these terms, ensuring that they reflect current usage and include the newest techniques and procedures. Abbreviation exercises are included. Boxed information throughout the chapters amplifies definitions and describes the derivation of specific terms. Exercises follow each group of terms, giving you the opportunity to review and rehearse new vocabulary immediately after it is presented.

Appendixes

Helpful appendixes supplement the information provided in the chapters. Appendixes A and B list, in alphabetical order, all the combining forms, prefixes, and suffixes from the entire book by word part and by definition. Appendix C lists less commonly used word parts not presented in the chapters. Appendix D provides abbreviations to medical terms.

Appendixes E through J present medical terms that are not related to a particular body system but that are frequently used in the day-to-day health care environment. These terms that have a more general application fall into the categories of pharmacology, health care delivery/managed care, complementary and alternative medicine, behavioral health, clinical research, and nutrition.

Learning Aids

The sixth edition of *Exploring Medical Language* comes with a variety of learning aids intended to make your study of medical terminology as efficient and enjoyable as possible.

Student CD

Your copy of *Exploring Medical Language* includes a complimentary program on CD. It is not necessary to use the CD to complete your coursework, but it is a fun and easy way to reinforce your learning of the terms. It has a scoring function so you can measure what you know. Below is a list of exercises included in the CD.

- **Applied Vocabulary**—Features a case study related to the chapter content with medical terms highlighted and linked to the dictionary.
- **Picture It**—Match word parts with corresponding anatomic illustrations.
- **Define Word Parts**—Match word parts and combining forms with their definitions.
- **Build Medical Terms**—Type in word parts to complete a defined medical term built from word parts.
- **The Wordshop**—Build a new medical term from your knowledge of the meaning of word parts.
- **Define Medical Terms**—Match medical terms not built from word parts with their definitions.
- **Pronounce It**—Practice pronunciation by listening to medical terms. Medical terms are presented in correlation with the chapter content so that as you complete parts of the chapter, you may access the Pronounce It activity to practice.
- **Spell It**—Practice spelling by typing a medical term as it is read aloud.
- **Use It**—Type in a medical term that completes a sentence, which uses medical terminology in context.

Flash Cards

More than 480 flash cards come with *Exploring Medical Language*. Each flash card has a word part, combining form, suffix, or prefix on one side and the definition of the word part on the other side.

Mosby's Medical Terminology Online

Mosby's Medical Terminology Online to accompany *Exploring Medical Language* is a great resource to supplement your textbook. This web-delivered course supplement provides a range of visual, auditory, and interactive elements to reinforce your learning and synthesize concepts presented in the text. Interactive lesson reviews at the end of each module provide you with self-testing tools, but with a twist . . . they are fun! Not sure how to pronounce a term? Click on the term and hear it pronounced! In addition, related Internet resources may be accessed by links provided throughout the program. This online course supplement may be accessed if you have purchased the PIN code packaged with your book. If you did not purchase the book/PIN code package, ask your instructor for information or visit www.evolve.elsevier.com/LaFleur to purchase.

Audio CDs and Downloads with Pronunciations and Definitions

The audio program that accompanies *Exploring Medical Language* includes pronunciations and definitions. The program will help you to pronounce medical terms and to remember their definitions. The program is especially helpful when using your book is impractical, such as when you are driving in a car, walking, or doing daily chores. You may purchase the audio CDs separately or packaged with the book for a small additional cost. To purchase the downloadable version of the audio program, go to: iTerms.elsevier.com.

To the Instructor

Instructor's Curriculum Resource

The *Instructor's Curriculum Resource* (ICR) to accompany *Exploring Medical Language* is available as a CD, in print form, or on Evolve. You may request a copy by contacting your sales representative if you have adopted or are considering adopting *Exploring Medical Language.*

The ICR has been extensively revised and should be helpful to you in preparing for class and managing your classroom time:

Preparation for class: Lesson Strategies, Teaching Opportunities, and Course Objectives for each chapter will help prepare you to step into the classroom.

Class time: PowerPoint slides with lecture notes and embedded images from the text, which you can modify to suit your style, are included, as well as many exercises with answers that can be reproduced and used in the classroom. An exercise for using the medical dictionary is included. A complete version of the medical record that appears in each chapter of the text is here and can be used to support class discussion of the content.

Examination: Multiple choice examination questions, in print or computerized in Exam view, are identified by objective, topic, and text page number. If you omit objectives in a chapter to fit the course outline, it is now easy to omit the matching test questions. A recommended spelling list that may be used as part of the exam is included as well as test questions for the case study that appears on the Student CD.

Mosby's Medical Terminology Online

Connecting you and your students, *Mosby's Medical Terminology Online* to accompany *Exploring Medical Language* was developed with a creative approach to education in mind. The more resources available to facilitate learning and the more varied your presentation, the greater the likelihood your students will comprehend and retain the material you want them to learn. Rather than replacing the textbook, this unique course supplement, delivered in a web environment, provides a range of visual, auditory, and interactive elements to amplify text content, reinforce learning, synthesize concepts presented in the textbook, and demonstrate the practical application of medical language. More than 100 animations and slide shows convey difficult concepts that are impossible to demonstrate with static illustrations. A variety of communication options and administrative tools allow you to hold virtual office hours! See for yourself at www.evolve.elsevier.com/LaFleur. Then contact your sales representative for more information about how to adopt the online companion to supplement your course.

To the newcomer, the language of medicine is like a vast, uncharted frontier. *Exploring Medical Language* systematically guides you along a path of vocabulary development that is interesting and enjoyable and that thoroughly prepares you to communicate as a medical professional. While using this text, you will become familiar with the structure of medical language and with the most effective strategies for learning medical terms. A variety of learning activities will allow you the practice to grow confident in your use of the terminology. Follow the guidelines below to get the most from this textbook as you embark on your journey of acquiring a new language.

Understand the Content of Chapter 1 Before Moving on to Chapter 2.

Chapter 1 is the most important chapter in the text. Here you are introduced to word parts—word roots, prefixes, suffixes, and combining vowels—and the rules for combining them to build medical terms. You will use this information in each of the subsequent chapters to analyze, construct, define, and spell terms built from word parts.

Use Each Chapter Section Fully to Help You Master the Medical Terms Presented.

Objectives

1. *Read the objectives* before you begin the chapter. Objectives state what you can expect to learn as you progress through the chapter.
2. *Refer to the objectives when you have completed a chapter* to evaluate whether you have learned all the material presented.

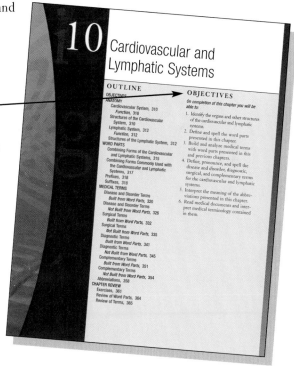

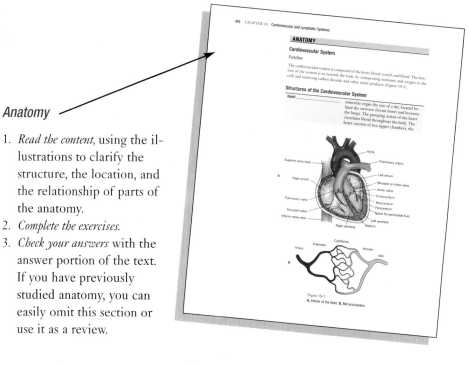

Anatomy

1. *Read the content*, using the illustrations to clarify the structure, the location, and the relationship of parts of the anatomy.
2. *Complete the exercises.*
3. *Check your answers* with the answer portion of the text. If you have previously studied anatomy, you can easily omit this section or use it as a review.

Word Parts

1. *Read each word part and its definition.*
2. *Complete the exercises.* Each list of words is followed by exercises that help you recall the definition of the word part and retrieve the word part when the definition is provided.
3. *Label the anatomic diagram* with the correct combining forms.
4. *Compare your answers* on both the diagram and the exercises with the answer portion of the text.
5. *Use the flash cards to help memorize the word parts.* Group the combining form flash cards separately for each body system. Gather the prefix and suffix flash cards from all the chapters because you will be using them throughout the text; keeping them together provides the opportunity for frequent review.
6. *Read the information boxes* to enrich your understanding about the derivation of the word parts.

Medical Terms

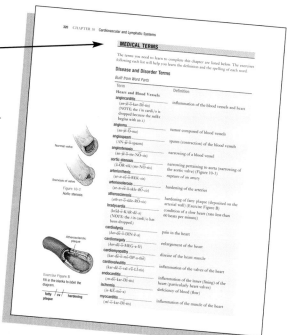

1. *Become familiar with the presentation of terms.* The medical terms are divided into four categories: *disease and disorder* terms, which are used to diagnose conditions; *surgical* terms, which are used to describe surgical procedures; *diagnostic* terms, which are used to describe diagnostic procedures and equipment; and *complementary* terms, which complete the vocabulary presented in a chapter by describing signs, symptoms, medical specialties, specialists, and related words. Understanding that the terms are categorized will assist you in the overall comprehension of medical language and how it is used. For example, you will soon learn that the suffix indicates whether a term is surgical, diagnostic, or procedural.

2. *Become familiar with the organization of terms* into those built from word parts and those not built from word parts. All the medical terms in the text are arranged into one of these two categories that determine the learning strategy you will use. Terms built from word parts are constructed from specific language elements through application of certain rules. Learning the rules for analyzing and combining word parts will help you master this set of terms. Terms not built from word parts may contain some of the word parts you know, but you cannot literally translate the term to arrive at its meaning; memorization is used to learn these terms.

3. *Read each of the terms and its definition.* If more information is necessary for comprehension of the term, it is included in parentheses following the definition.

4. *Use the pronunciation guide and the Pronounce It activity on the Student CD to practice pronouncing the medical terms.* Because it is impractical to use all the markings of an unabridged dictionary in a medical terminology book, the pronunciations provided in the text are approximate. In respelling for pronunciation, the words have been distorted minimally to indicate phonetic sound. Diacritical marks are used over vowels to show pronunciation. The macron (‾) is used to indicate long vowel sounds; unmarked vowels have a short vowel sound. An accent mark is the stress on a certain syllable. The primary accent is indicated in this text by capital letters, and the secondary accent (which is stressed, but not as strongly as the primary accent) is indicated by italics.

5. *Complete all the exercises for each word list.* The exercises may seem repetitive, but they are provided to allow the practice needed to master the terms.

6. *Read the information boxes;* they contain information on the origin of terms, the distinguishing features of the words, and complementary and alternative medicine terms.

7. *Use the appendixes* to assist you in building and defining terms built from word parts. Use Appendix A for a quick-reference, alphabetical listing of the meanings of word parts; use Appendix B to find the word part to match a definition.

8. *Label the diagrams* placed throughout this section by filling in the blanks with the correct word part. Check your answers against the Answers provided at the end of the text.

9. *Read the abbreviation list* and complete the exercises.

Chapter Review

1. *Complete the review exercises.* Use this as an opportunity to evaluate your comprehension of the content of the chapter. Some questions will require you to recall terms from previous chapters.
2. *Compare your answers* with the answers provided in the text.
3. *Review the lists of word parts and medical terms* presented in the chapter. Highlight terms that need more practice.
4. *Use the Pronounce It activity on the Student CD* with the review list to evaluate and practice your pronunciation.

Appendixes

Use the appendixes to quickly locate alphabetically listed word parts, definitions, and abbreviations. Additional appendixes have been provided to help you develop a familiarity with terms specific to the areas of pharmacology, health care delivery/managed care, complementary and alternative medicine, behavioral health, clinical research, and nutrition.

From the Author

After you've worked through a chapter, completing all the exercises and correcting errors, you will have met the chapter objectives and will feel confident and eager to move on to the next chapter. I wish you the best as you begin your discovery of the language of medicine.

APPENDIX J

Nutritional Terms

Term	Definition
amino acid	building block of protein that can be essential (must be consumed) or nonessential (made by the body); provides 4 calories per gram
body mass index (BMI)	a tool to measure the degree of undernutrition or overnutrition; equals weight in kilograms divided by height in meters squared
calorie	a measure of the energy contained in a food
carbohydrate	a simple or complex compound made up of carbon, oxygen, and hydrogen; provides 4 calories per gram
carbohydrate counting	a method used to control blood sugars by diet for those with diabetes; often used with patients on insulin pumps
cholesterol	waxy substance made in the body or taken in by diet; found only in animal products
diet technician	a nutrition professional who has an associate's degree and has completed formal training along with passing a national board exam
dietary reference intake (DRI)	a guide to the amount of nutrients needed to prevent disease and reduce the risk of diet-related diseases
enteral nutrition	provision of nutrients through a tube into the gastrointestinal tract
fat	glycerol molecule made up of carbon, oxygen, and hydrogen with fatty acids attached; provides 9 calories per gram
fiber	materials in food that cannot be digested by the body; found mainly in plants
glucose	simplest form of carbohydrate, commonly referred to as *blood sugar*; equivalent to dextrose
hydrogenation	process of changing a liquid fat to a solid fat
macronutrients	carbohydrate, fat, or protein
malnutrition	inadequacy or abundance of one or more nutrients leading to compromised health
metabolism	the sum of all chemical and physical changes in the body
micronutrients	vitamins or minerals
minerals	inorganic substances occurring in nature that are essential for normal function and development of body systems
monounsaturated fat	a fatty acid chain with one double bond, such as olive oil and canola oil; research has shown them to be a healthy type of fat
omega-3 fatty acids	unsaturated fatty acid found in fish that must be consumed (essential fatty acid); it is associated with decreased risk of heart disease and named for the position of the first double bond
parenteral nutrition	the provision of nutrients administered through the vein
phytochemical	plant-based food components that are nonnutritive (do not provide calories) and are linked to prevention of disease
pica	a craving or intake of nonfood substances such as dirt or laundry starch
polyunsaturated fat	a fatty acid chain that contains two or more double bonds; examples include corn oil and sunflower oil

ACKNOWLEDGMENTS

I am grateful to many who assisted in the preparation of the sixth edition of *Exploring Medical Language*. They shared their knowledge, imaginations, and precious time. With their help, I think we have captured the current medical climate in the written and spoken word.

My appreciation to William Bohnert, MD; Joyce Bohnert, RN; John Lampignano, MS, RT(R); Tony L. Rodriguez, EdD, RTT; Stanley R. Shorb, MD; and Charlene Theisen, CMT, FAAMT, who reviewed material in their areas of expertise and advised me on necessary changes.

Thanks to Elaine Gillingham, BA, CHUC, for reviewing the question and answer portion of the text.

Thanks to Linda A. Mottle, MSN-HAS, RN, for writing Appendix I, Clinical Research Terms; to Danielle LaFleur Brooks, MEd, MATLA, for updating Appendix G, Complementary and Alternative Medicine Therapies, and for writing the chapter CAM Term boxes; to Kelly Eiden, MS, LD, CSD, for writing Appendix J, Nutritional Terms; to Carolyn Ehrlich, MSN, Psy, NP, for updating Appendix H, Behavioral Health Terms; to Sharon Tomkins Luczu, RN, MA, MBA, for updating Appendix F, Health Care Delivery/Managed Care Terms; to Erinn Kao, PharmD, for updating Appendix D, Abbreviations and Appendix E, Pharmacology Terms; and to Marcia McCusker, BA, Ed, for reformatting the medical document series. With their expert contributions, I feel confident that these specialty areas are accurate and complete.

A special thanks to my family members who contributed to this work. My daughter, Danielle LaFleur Brooks, MEd, MATLA, extensively revised the *Instructor's Curriculum Resource* and the Student CD. Her combined expertise and dedication to quality have resulted in products that soundly support both learning and teaching. My husband, Richard K. Brooks, MD, critiqued the content of all chapters plus advised me on the most recent developments in the medical field.

Thanks to the Elsevier/Mosby staff; especially Jeanne Wilke, for her continued support of this text and especially for her vision of and drive to produce ancillary products to support this work; Linda Woodard, senior developmental editor, who was able to effortlessly, it appeared, monitor all the aspects of the revision of the text and who was always there with support and materials needed to get the job done; Julie Eddy, senior project manager, whom I have worked with on several projects and who continues her magic with this one; and Julia Dummitt, who dreams up the most beautiful designs. Thanks also to Billi Sharp for her work on *Mosby's Medical Terminology Online* and Jeanne Genz for her efforts with the *Instructor's Curriculum Resource*.

To the faculty who have adopted the text to use in their classrooms and online, and to those who took their time to give us feedback, I am forever grateful. And perhaps closest to my heart, I want to recognize the students who over the years have worn thin the pages of previous editions to acquire their own language of medicine.

Myrna LaFleur Brooks

CONTENTS

Exploring Medical Language

A Student-Directed Approach

1

Introduction to Word Parts

OBJECTIVES

On completion of this chapter you will be able to:

1. Identify and define the four word parts.
2. Identify and define a combining form.
3. Analyze and define medical terms.
4. Build medical terms for given definitions.

ORIGINS OF MEDICAL LANGUAGE

Medicine has a language of its own. Medical language, like the language of a people, also has a historic development. Current medical vocabulary includes terms built from *Greek and Latin word parts,* some of which were used by Hippocrates and Aristotle more than 2400 years ago, *eponyms, acronyms,* and terms from *modern language* (Figure 1-1). With the advancement of medical and scientific knowledge, medical language changes. Some words are discarded, the meanings of others are altered, and new words are added.

    Still, the majority of medical terms in current use are composed of Greek and Latin word parts. These terms can be learned by two ways: memorizing or learning word parts and how they fit together to form medical terms. Memorization can be monotonous;

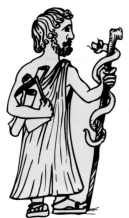

Greek and Latin terms
such as femur (L)
and hemorrhage (G)

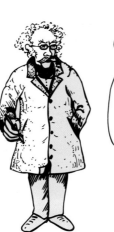

Eponyms
such as
Parkinson disease

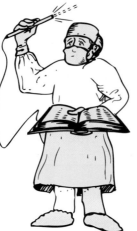

Acronyms such as laser
(*l*ight *a*mplification
by *s*timulated
*e*mission of *r*adiation)

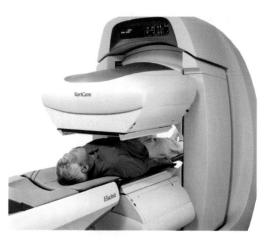

Modern language such as
nuclear medicine scanner

Figure 1-1

Origins of medical language.

Eponym

is a word based on the name of a person, such as Parkinson disease.

Acronym

is a word formed from the first letters of the words in a set phrase, such as SARS (*s*evere *a*cute *r*espiratory *s*yndrome).

learning word parts and how they fit together provides the key to learning scores of medical terms. Therefore the word part method is used to learn terms composed of word parts. The memorization method is used to learn other terms not built from word parts, such as *Alzheimer disease* or *coronary artery bypass graft*.

FOUR WORD PARTS

Most medical terms built from word parts consist of some or all of the following components:

1. Word roots
2. Suffixes
3. Prefixes
4. Combining vowels

Word Root

The word root is the word part that is the core of the word. The word root contains the fundamental meaning of the word.

Examples:	
In the word....................................	play/er, *play* is the word root.
In the medical term.............................	arthr/itis, *arthr* (which means *joint*) is the word root.
In the medical term.............................	hepat/itis, *hepat* (which means *liver*) is the word root.

 The word root is the core of the word; therefore each medical term contains one or more word roots.

Complete the following: A word root is _____

_____

Answer: the word part that is the core of the word

Suffix

The suffix is a word part attached to the end of the word root to modify its meaning.

Examples:	
In the word..	play/er,
	-er is the suffix.
In the medical term...........................	hepat/ic,
	-ic (which means *pertaining to*) is the suffix.
Hepat is the word root for *liver;* therefore *hepatic* means *pertaining to the liver.*	
In the medical term...........................	hepat/itis,
	-itis (which means *inflammation*) is the suffix.
The term *hepatitis* means *inflammation of the liver.*	

> The suffix is used to modify the meaning of a word. Most medical terms have a suffix.

Complete the following: The suffix is _____

_____

Answer: the word part attached to the end of the word root to modify its meaning

Prefix

The prefix is a word part attached to the beginning of a word root to modify its meaning.

Examples:	
In the word..	re/play,
	re- is the prefix.
In the medical term...........................	sub/hepat/ic,
	sub- (which means *under*) is the prefix.
Hepat is the word root for *liver,* and *-ic* is the suffix for *pertaining to.* The medical term *subhepatic* means *pertaining to under the liver.*	
In the medical term...........................	intra/ven/ous,
	intra- (which means *within*) is the prefix, *ven* (which means *vein*) is the word root, and *-ous* (which means *pertaining to*) is the suffix.
The word *intravenous* means *pertaining to within the vein.*	

> A prefix can be used to modify the meaning of a word. Many medical terms do not have a prefix.

Complete the following: The prefix is _____

_____

Answer: the word part attached to the beginning of a word root to modify its meaning

Suffixes
frequently indicate a *procedure,* such as **-scopy,** meaning visual examination, or **-tomy,** meaning surgical incision
a *condition,* such as **-itis,** meaning inflammation or a *disease,* such as **-oma,** meaning tumor.

Prefixes
often indicate a *number* such as **bi-,** meaning two
position, such as **sub-,** meaning under
direction, such as **intra-,** meaning within
time, such as **brady-,** meaning slow
or *negation,* such as **a-,** meaning without

Combining Vowel

Vowels
are speech sounds represented by the letters *a, e, i, o, u,* and sometimes *y.*

The combining vowel is a word part, usually an *o*, used to ease pronunciation.

Examples:	
In the word..	men/o/pause, *o* is the combining vowel used between two word roots.
In the medical term.............................	arthr/o/pathy, *o* is the combining vowel used between the word root *arthr* and the suffix *-pathy* (which means *disease*).
In the medical term.............................	sub/hepat/ic, the combining vowel is not used between the prefix *sub-* and the word root *hepat*.

The combining vowel is:

- **Used to connect two word roots**
- **Used to connect a word root and a suffix**
- **Not used to connect a prefix and a word root**

Guidelines For Using Combining Vowels

Guideline One

When connecting a word root and a suffix, a combining vowel is used if the suffix does not begin with a vowel.

Example:	
In the medical term.............................	arthr/o/pathy, the suffix *-pathy* does not begin with a vowel; therefore a combining vowel is used.

Guideline Two

When connecting a word root and a suffix, a combining vowel is usually not used if the suffix begins with a vowel.

Example:	
In the medical term.............................	hepat/ic, the suffix *-ic* begins with the vowel *i;* therefore a combining vowel is not used.

Guideline Three

When connecting two word roots, a combining vowel is usually used even if vowels are present at the junction.

Example:	
In the medical term.............................	oste/o/arthr/itis, *o* is the combining vowel used, even though the word root *oste* (which means *bone*) ends with the vowel *e*, and the word root *arthr* begins with the vowel *a*.

Guideline Four

When connecting a prefix and a word root, a combining vowel is not used.

Example:

In the medical term............................   sub/hepat/ic,
the combining vowel is not used between the
prefix *sub-* and the word root *hepat.*

> The combining vowel is used to ease pronunciation; therefore *not all medical terms have combining vowels*. Medical terms introduced throughout the text that have combining vowels other than *o* are highlighted at their introduction.

Complete the following: A combining vowel is _____

_____

Answer: a word part, usually an o, *used to ease pronunciation*

When connecting a word root and a suffix, a combining vowel is _____ if
the suffix does not begin with a vowel.

Answer: used

When connecting a word root and a suffix, a combining vowel is usually not used
if the suffix begins with a _____.

Answer: vowel

When connecting two _____ _____, a combining vowel is
usually used, even if vowels are present at the junction.

Answer: word roots

When connecting a prefix and a word root, a combining vowel is _____ used.

Answer: not

COMBINING FORM

**A combining form is a word root with the combining vowel attached, separated by
a vertical slash.**

> **Examples:**   arthr/o
> oste/o
> ven/o

The combining form is not a word part per se; rather it is the word root and the combining vowel. *For learning purposes word roots are presented together with their combining vowels as combining forms throughout the text.*

Complete the following: A combining form is _____

_____

Answer: a word root with the combining vowel attached, separated by a vertical slash

Learn word parts and combining forms by completing exercises 1 and 2.

EXERCISE 1

Match the phrases in the first column with the correct terms in the second column. Answers are located at the end of the book.

_____ 1. attached at the beginning of a word root

_____ 2. usually an *o*

_____ 3. all medical terms contain at least one

_____ 4. attached at the end of a word root

_____ 5. word root with combining vowel attached

a. combining vowel

b. prefix

c. combining form

d. word root

e. suffix

EXERCISE 2

Answer *T* for true and *F* for false.

_____ 1. There are always prefixes at the beginning of medical terms.

_____ 2. A combining vowel is always used when connecting a word root and a suffix that begins with the letter *o*.

_____ 3. A prefix modifies the meaning of the word.

_____ 4. A combining vowel is used to ease pronunciation.

_____ 5. *I* is the most commonly used combining vowel.

_____ 6. The word root is the core of a medical term.

_____ 7. A combining vowel is used between a prefix and a word root.

_____ 8. A combining form is a word part.

_____ 9. A combining vowel is used when connecting a word root and a suffix if the suffix begins with the letter *g*.

ANALYZING AND DEFINING MEDICAL TERMS

Analyzing

To analyze medical terms, divide them into word parts and label each word part and each combining form. Follow the procedure below:

1. **Divide the term** into word parts with vertical slashes.

   Example: oste/o/arthr/o/pathy

2. **Label each word part** by using the following abbreviations.

WR	WORD ROOT
P	PREFIX
S	SUFFIX
CV	COMBINING VOWEL

            WR   CV   WR   CV   S

Example: oste / o / arthr / o / pathy

3. **Label the combining forms.**

            WR   CV   WR   CV   S

Example: <u>oste / o</u> / <u>arthr / o</u> / pathy

            CF   CF

Analyze the following medical term:

osteopathy

         WR   CV   S

Answer: <u>oste / o</u> / *pathy*

        CF

Complete the following: To analyze medical terms, _____

_____

Answer: divide them into word parts and label each word part and each combining form

Defining

To define medical terms, apply the meaning of each word part contained in the term.

    Begin by defining the suffix, then move to the beginning of the term to complete the definition. (This method does not apply to all medical terms.)

    Apply this rule to find the definition of **oste/o/arthr/o/pathy.** Begin by defining the suffix *-pathy*, then move to the beginning of the term. Use the box below to find the meanings of the word parts. Oste/o/arthr/o/pathy means _____

_____

Answer: disease of the bone and joint

Word Roots	Definition	Suffixes	Definition
arthr	joint	-itis	inflammation
hepat	liver	-ic	pertaining to
ven	vein	-ous	pertaining to
oste	bone	-pathy	disease
Prefixes		**Combining Vowel**	
intra-	within	o	
sub-	under		

Complete the following: To define medical terms, _____

_____

Answer: apply the meaning of each word part contained in the term

Practice analyzing and defining medical terms by completing exercise 3.

EXERCISE 3

Using the box above to identify the word parts and their meanings, analyze and define the following terms.

              WR   CV   WR   CV   S

Example: oste / o / arthr / o / pathy   _disease of the bone and joint_
               CF   CF

1. arthritis _____

2. hepatitis _____

3. subhepatic _____

4. intravenous _____

5. arthropathy _____

6. osteitis _____

BUILDING MEDICAL TERMS

To build medical terms, place word parts together to form words.

Using the box on p. 7 as a reference, complete the following steps to build the medical term for _disease of a joint._

Step 1: Find the word part for _disease._ Write the word part in the correct space below.

Step 2: Find the word part for _joint._ Write the word part in the correct space below.

Step 3: The suffix does not begin with a vowel, so a combining vowel is needed. Insert the combining vowel _o_ in the correct space below.

_____ / _ / _____
           WR   CV   S

Answer: arthropathy

Complete the following: To build medical terms means _____

Answer: to place word parts together to form words

Practice building medical terms by completing exercise 4 and Exercise Figure A.

Keep in mind that the beginning of the definition usually indicates the suffix.

EXERCISE 4

Using the box on p. 7 as a reference, build medical terms for the following definitions and complete Exercise Figure A. Answers are located at the end of the book.

Example: disease of the joint   <u>arthr/ o /pathy</u>
                          WR /CV/ S

1. inflammation of the joint   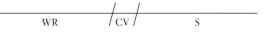
                           WR   S

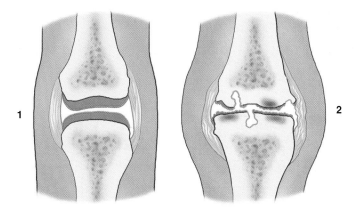

Exercise Figure A
Fill in the blanks to complete labeling of the diagram. **1,** Normal knee joint.
2, Knee joint showing _____ .
  bone   /   cv   /   joint   /   inflammation

2. pertaining to the liver   _____ / _____
                                    WR   S

3. pertaining to under the liver _____ / _____ / _____
                                    P   WR   S

4. pertaining to within the vein _____ / _____ / _____
                                    P   WR   S

5. inflammation of the bone   _____ / _____
                                    WR   S

6. inflammation of the liver   _____ / _____
                                    WR   S

7. disease of the bone and joint ____ / ____ / ____ / ____ / ____
                                    WR   CV   WR   CV   S

At this time do not be concerned about which word root goes first when building a term that contains two word roots. The order is usually dictated by common practice; for surgical or diagnostic terms, word roots are sometimes arranged by the order of function or by the order in which an instrument may encounter a structure. As you practice and learn you will become accustomed to the accepted order.

SUMMARY

Word Parts

Word root—core of a word; for example, **hepat**
Suffix—attached at the end of a word root to modify its meaning; for example, **-ic**
Prefix—attached at the beginning of a word to modify its meaning; for example, **sub-**
Combining vowel—usually an *o* used between two word roots or a word root and suffix to ease pronunciation; for example, hepat **o** pathy
Combining form—word root plus combining vowel separated by a vertical slash; for example, **hepat/o**

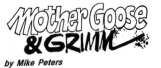
by Mike Peters

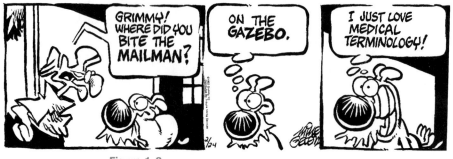

Figure 1-2
Reprinted by permission of Tribune Media Services.

Techniques for Learning Medical Terms Built from Word Parts

Analyzing—dividing medical terms into word parts, then labeling each word part and combining form

Defining—applying the meaning of each word part contained in the medical term to derive its meaning

Building—placing word parts together to form words

CHAPTER REVIEW

To complete this chapter successfully, you do not need to know what the word parts, such as *arthr,* mean. You will learn these in subsequent chapters. **It is important that you have met these objectives:**

1. Can you identify and define the four word parts?   yes ☐ no ☐
2. Can you identify and define combining forms?   yes ☐ no ☐
3. Can you use word parts to analyze and define medical terms?   yes ☐ no ☐
4. Can you use word parts to build medical terms for a given definition? yes ☐ no ☐

If you answered yes to these questions you need no further practice because you will be using these concepts repeatedly as you work your way through this text. Refer to this chapter to refresh your memory as needed. Move on to Chapter 2 and begin to build your medical vocabulary so that you will be better prepared than Grimm in Figure 1-2 to understand and use the language of medicine.

For further practice or to evaluate what you have learned, use the Student CD that accompanies this text.

2

Body Structure, Color, and Oncology

OUTLINE

OBJECTIVES

On completion of this chapter you will be able to:

1. Identify anatomic structures of the human body.
2. Define and spell the word parts presented in this chapter.
3. Build and analyze medical terms with word parts presented in this chapter.
4. Define, pronounce, and spell medical terms related to body structure, color, and oncology.
5. Interpret the meanings of the abbreviations presented in this chapter.
6. Read medical documents and interpret medical terminology contained in them.

ANATOMY

Organization of the Body

The structure of the human body falls into the following four categories: cells, tissues, organs, and systems. Each structure is a highly organized unit of smaller structures.

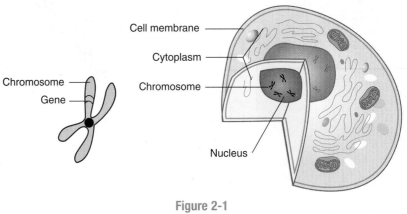

Figure 2-1
Body cell.

<table>
<tr><td>cell</td><td>basic unit of all living things (Figure 2-1). The human body is composed of trillions of cells, which vary in size and shape according to function.</td></tr>
<tr><td>cell membrane</td><td>forms the boundary of the cell</td></tr>
<tr><td>cytoplasm</td><td>gel-like fluid inside the cell</td></tr>
<tr><td>nucleus</td><td>largest structure within the cell, usually spherical and centrally located. It contains chromosomes for cellular reproduction and is the control center of the cell.</td></tr>
<tr><td>chromosomes</td><td>located in the nucleus of the cell. There are 46 chromosomes in all normal human cells, with the exception of mature sex cells, which have 23.</td></tr>
<tr><td>genes</td><td>regions within the chromosome. Each chromosome has several thousand genes that determine hereditary characteristics.</td></tr>
<tr><td>DNA (deoxyribonucleic acid)</td><td>comprises each gene; is a chemical that regulates the activities of the cell</td></tr>
<tr><td>tissue</td><td>group of similar cells that performs a specific task</td></tr>
<tr><td>muscle tissue</td><td>composed of cells that have a special ability to contract, usually producing movement</td></tr>
<tr><td>nervous tissue</td><td>found in the nerves, spinal cord, and brain. It is responsible for coordinating and controlling body activities.</td></tr>
<tr><td>connective tissue</td><td>connects, supports, penetrates, and encases various body structures. Adipose (fat) and osseous (bone) tissues and blood are types of connective tissue.</td></tr>
<tr><td>epithelial tissue</td><td>the major covering of the external surface of the body; forms membranes that line body cavities and organs and is the major tissue in glands</td></tr>
</table>

Cell

was named about 300 years ago by Robert Hooke. On seeing cells through a microscope, he named them **cells** because they reminded him of miniature prison cells.

Medical Genomics

A **genome** is the complete set of genes in a chromosome of each cell of a specific organism. **Genomics** is the study of the genome and its products and interactions. **Medical genomics** is the study of the genome and how it can be used in the cause, treatment, and prevention of disease. It is thought that it will alter twenty-first century medicine. **Gene therapy** is any therapeutic procedure in which genes are intentionally introduced into human body cells to achieve gene repair, gene suppression, or gene addition. Gene therapy is still in its infancy. The first human gene transfer was performed on a patient with malignant melanoma in 1989. Since then more than 30,000 patients have received gene therapy.

Refer to the Appendix I for a list of clinical research terms.

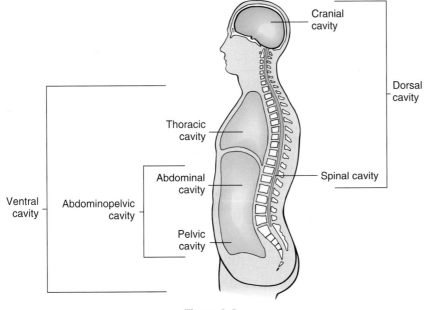

Figure 2-2
Body cavities.

organ	two or more kinds of tissues that together perform special body functions. For example, the skin is an organ composed of epithelial, connective, muscle, and nerve tissue.
system	group of organs that work together to perform complex body functions. For example, the cardiovascular system consists of the heart, blood vessels, and blood. Its function is to transport nutrients and oxygen to the cells and remove carbon dioxide and other waste products (Exercise Figure A, p. 15).

Body Cavities

The body is not a solid structure, as it appears on the outside, but has five cavities (Figure 2-2), each containing an orderly arrangement of the internal organs.

cranial cavity	space inside the skull (cranium) containing the brain
spinal cavity	space inside the spinal column containing the spinal cord
thoracic, or chest, cavity	space containing the heart, aorta, lungs, esophagus, trachea, and bronchi
abdominal cavity	space containing the stomach, intestines, kidneys, liver, gallbladder, pancreas, spleen, and ureters

| pelvic cavity | space containing the urinary bladder, certain reproductive organs, parts of the large intestine, and the rectum |
| abdominopelvic cavity | both the pelvic and abdominal cavities |

Learn the anatomic terms by completing exercises 1 and 2.

EXERCISE 1

Match the terms in the first column with the correct definitions in the second column.

_____ 1. chromosomes

_____ 2. nucleus

_____ 3. cytoplasm

_____ 4. cell

_____ 5. muscle

_____ 6. nerve

_____ 7. epithelial

_____ 8. bone

_____ 9. genes

_____ 10. DNA

a. type of connective tissue

b. regions within the chromosome

c. covers external body surface, lines body cavities and organs

d. gel-like fluid inside the cell

e. contains chromosomes

f. coordinates body activities

g. usually produces movement

h. contain genes

i. chest cavity

j. a chemical that regulates the activities of the cell

k. basic unit of all living things

EXERCISE 2

Match the terms in the first column with the correct definitions in the second column.

_____ 1. spinal cavity

_____ 2. thoracic cavity

_____ 3. organ

_____ 4. cranial cavity

_____ 5. pelvic cavity

_____ 6. system

_____ 7. abdominal cavity

a. group of organs functioning together

b. chest cavity

c. composed of two or more tissues

d. found in the skin

e. space inside the skull

f. contains the stomach

g. contains the urinary bladder

h. contains the spinal cord

WORD PARTS

Begin building your medical vocabulary by learning the word parts listed next. The list may appear long to you; however, the many exercises that follow are designed to help you understand and remember the word parts.

Reminder: the word root is the core of the word. The combining form is the word root with the combining vowel attached, separated by a vertical slash.

Combining Forms for Body Structure

Combining Form	Definition
aden/o	gland
cyt/o	cell
epitheli/o	epithelium
fibr/o	fiber
hist/o	tissue
kary/o	nucleus
lip/o	fat
my/o	muscle
neur/o	nerve
organ/o	organ
sarc/o	flesh, connective tissue
system/o	system
viscer/o	internal organs

Epithelium
originally meant **surface over the nipple. Epi** means **upon,** and **thela** means **nipple** (or projecting surfaces of many kinds).

Learn the anatomic locations and definitions of the combining forms by completing exercises 3 and 4 and Exercise Figures A and B.

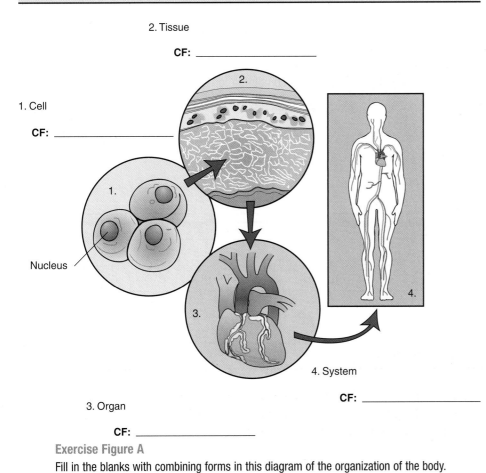

2. Tissue

CF: _____

1. Cell

CF: _____

Nucleus

3. Organ

CF: _____

4. System

CF: _____

Exercise Figure A
Fill in the blanks with combining forms in this diagram of the organization of the body.

Nerve

1. **CF:** _____

Epithelium

3. **CF:** _____

Connective

2. **CF:** _____

Muscle

4. **CF:** _____

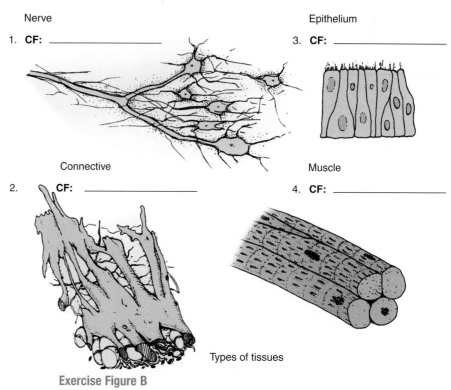

Types of tissues

Exercise Figure B
Fill in the blanks with combining forms in this diagram of types of tissues.

EXERCISE 3

Write the definitions of the following combining forms.

1. sarc/o _____

2. lip/o _____

3. kary/o _____

4. viscer/o _____

5. cyt/o _____

6. hist/o _____

7. my/o _____

8. neur/o _____

9. organ/o _____

10. system/o _____

11. epitheli/o _____

12. fibr/o _____

13. aden/o _____

EXERCISE 4

Write the combining form for each of the following.

1. internal organs _____

2. epithelium _____

3. organ _____

4. nucleus _____

5. cell _____

6. tissue _____

7. nerve _____

8. muscle _____

9. fat _____

10. system _____

11. connective tissue, flesh _____

12. fiber _____

13. gland _____

Combining Forms Commonly Used with Body Structure Terms

Combining Form	Definition
cancer/o, carcin/o	cancer (a disease characterized by the unregulated, abnormal growth of new cells)
eti/o	cause (of disease)
gno/o	knowledge
iatr/o	physician, medicine (also means treatment)
lei/o	smooth
onc/o	tumor, mass
path/o	disease
rhabd/o	rod-shaped, striated
somat/o	body

Learn the related combining forms by completing exercises 5 and 6.

Cancer
Carcin and **cancer** are derived from Latin and Greek words meaning **crab**. They originated before the nature of malignant growth was understood. One explanation was that the swollen veins around the diseased area looked like the claws of a crab.

EXERCISE 5

Write the definitions of the following combining forms.

1. onc/o _____

2. carcin/o _____

3. eti/o _____

4. path/o _____

5. somat/o _____

6. cancer/o _____

7. rhabd/o _____

8. lei/o _____

9. gno/o _____

10. iatr/o _____

EXERCISE 6

Write the combining form for each of the following.

1. disease _____

2. tumor, mass _____

3. cause (of disease) _____

4. cancer a. _____

   b. _____

5. body _____

6. smooth _____

7. rod-shaped, striated _____

8. knowledge _____

9. physician, medicine _____

Combining Forms for Terms that Describe Color

Combining Form	Definition
chlor/o	green
chrom/o	color
cyan/o	blue
erythr/o	red
leuk/o	white
melan/o	black
xanth/o	yellow

Learn the color combining forms by completing exercises 7 and 8.

Erythro
Aristotle noted "two colors of blood" and applied the term **erythro** to the dark red blood.

EXERCISE 7

Write the definitions of the following combining forms.

1. cyan/o _____

2. erythr/o _____

3. leuk/o _____

4. xanth/o _____

5. chrom/o_____

6. melan/o _____

7. chlor/o _____

EXERCISE 8

Write the combining form for each of the following.

1. blue _____

2. red _____

3. white _____

4. black _____

5. yellow _____

6. color _____

7. green _____

> Reminder: prefixes are placed at the beginning of word roots to modify their meanings.

Prefixes

Prefix	Definition
dia-	through, complete
dys-	painful, abnormal, difficult, labored
hyper-	above, excessive
hypo-	below, incomplete, deficient
meta-	after, beyond, change
neo-	new
pro-	before

Learn the prefixes by completing exercises 9 and 10.

EXERCISE 9

Write the definitions of the following prefixes.

1. neo- _____

2. hyper- _____

3. meta- _____

4. hypo- _____

5. dys- _____

6. dia- _____

7. pro- _____

EXERCISE 10

Write the prefix for each of the following.

1. new _____

2. above, excessive _____

3. below, incomplete, deficient _____

4. beyond, after, change _____

5. abnormal, painful, labored, difficult _____

6. through, complete _____

7. before _____

> Reminder: suffixes are placed at the end of word roots to modify their meanings.

Suffixes

Suffix	Definition
-al, -ic, -ous	pertaining to
-cyte	cell
(NOTE: *cyte* ends in an *e* when used as a suffix.)	
-gen	substance or agent that produces or causes
-genesis	origin, cause
-genic	producing, originating, causing
-logist	one who studies and treats (specialist, physician)
-logy	study of
-oid	resembling
-oma	tumor, swelling
-osis	abnormal condition (means *increase* when used with blood cell word roots)
-pathy	disease
-plasia	condition of formation, development, growth
-plasm	growth, substance, formation
-sarcoma	malignant tumor

> Some suffixes are made of a word root plus a suffix; they are presented as suffixes for ease of learning. For example, **-pathy** is made up of the word root **path** and the suffix **-y.** When analyzing a word, divide the suffixes as learned. For example, a word such as **somatopathy** should be divided somat/o/pathy and **not** somat/o/path/y.

| -sis | state of |
| -stasis | control, stop, standing |

Refer to Appendix A and Appendix B for alphabetized lists of word parts and their meanings.

Learn the suffixes by completing exercises 11 and 12.

EXERCISE 11

Match the suffixes in the first column with their correct definitions in the second column.

_____ 1. -logy

_____ 2. -osis

_____ 3. -pathy

_____ 4. -plasm

_____ 5. -al, -ic, -ous

_____ 6. -stasis

_____ 7. -oid

_____ 8. -cyte

_____ 9. -genesis

_____ 10. -logist

_____ 11. -oma

_____ 12. -gen

_____ 13. -sarcoma

_____ 14. -plasia

_____ 15. -genic

_____ 16. -sis

a. producing, originating, causing

b. cell

c. specialist, physician

d. new

e. disease

f. substance, growth, formation

g. pertaining to

h. resembling

i. study of

j. control, stop, standing

k. substance that produces

l. abnormal condition

m. condition of formation, development, growth

n. tumor, swelling

o. state of

p. origin, cause

q. malignant tumor

Sarcoma has been used since the time of ancient Greece to describe any fleshy tumor. Since the introduction of cellular pathology, the meaning was restricted to mean a **malignant connective tissue tumor.**

EXERCISE 12

Write the definitions of the following suffixes.

1. -logist _____

2. -pathy _____

3. -logy _____

4. -ic _____

5. -stasis _____

6. -cyte _____

7. -osis _____

8. -ous _____

9. -plasm _____

10. -al _____

11. -plasia _____

12. -oid _____

13. -gen _____

14. -genic _____

15. -oma _____

16. -genesis _____

17. -sarcoma _____

18. -sis _____

MEDICAL TERMS

Oncology

Oncology is the study of tumors. Tumors develop from excessive growth of cells from a body part. Tumors, or masses, are benign (noncancerous) or malignant (cancerous). The names of tumors are often made of the word root for the body part and the suffix **-oma,** as in the term *my/oma.*

Oncology terms are introduced in this chapter because of their relation to cells and cell abnormalities. This is an introductory list only. More oncology terms appear in subsequent chapters and are presented with the introduction of the related body parts.

Oncology Terms

Built from Word Parts

> Practice two things in your dealings with disease: either help or do not harm the patient.
> **Hippocrates**   460-375 BC

The medical terms listed below are built from the word parts you have already learned. Using this knowledge, you will analyze, define, and build medical terms in the following exercises. At first the list of terms may seem long to you; however, many of the word parts are repeated in many of the words. You will soon find that knowing parts of the terms makes learning the words easy. **Further explanation of terms beyond definition of their word parts, if needed, is included in parentheses.**

Term	Definition
adenocarcinoma (*ad*-e-nō-*kar*-si-NŌ-ma)	cancerous tumor composed of glandular tissue
adenoma (ad-e-NŌ-ma)	tumor composed of glandular tissue (benign)
carcinoma (Ca) (*kar*-si-NŌ-ma)	cancerous tumor (malignant) (Exercise Figure C)
chloroma (klo-RŌ-ma)	tumor of green color (malignant, arising from myeloid tissue)
epithelioma (ep-i-*thē*-lē-O-ma)	tumor composed of epithelium
fibroma (fī-BRŌ-ma)	tumor composed of fiber (fibrous tissue)

fibrosarcoma.............................. malignant tumor composed of fiber (fibrous
(fī-brō-sar-KŌ-ma)   tissue)

leiomyoma.................................. tumor of smooth muscle (benign)
(lī-ō-mī-Ō-ma)

leiomyosarcoma .... malignant tumor of smooth muscle
(*lī-ō-mī*-ō-sar-KŌ-ma)

lipoma .... tumor composed of fat (benign tumor)
(li-PŌ-ma)

liposarcoma............................... malignant tumor composed of fat
(lip-ō-sar-KŌ-ma)

melanocarcinoma..................... cancerous black tumor (malignant)
(*mel*-a-nō-*kar*-si-NŌ-ma)

melanoma.................................. black tumor (primarily of the skin)
(mel-a-NŌ-ma)   (Exercise Figure C)

myoma.. tumor composed of muscle (benign)
(mī-Ō-ma)

neoplasm................................... new growth (of abnormal tissue or tumor)
(NĒ-ō-plazm)

neuroma..................................... tumor composed of nerve (benign)
(nū-RŌ-ma)

rhabdomyoma........................... tumor of striated muscle (benign)
(*rab*-dō-mī-Ō-ma)

rhabdomyosarcoma .... malignant tumor of striated muscle
(*rab*-dō-mī-ō-sar-KŌ-ma)   (Exercise Figure C)

sarcoma..................................... tumor composed of connective tissue (such
(sar-KŌ-ma)   as bone or cartilage) (highly malignant)
(NOTE: sarc/o also is   (Exercise Figure C)
presented in this chapter as
a word root.)

Practice saying each of these terms aloud. Refer to the Pronunciation Guide on page 25 for explanation of the pronunciation key. To hear the terms, access the **PRONOUNCE IT** activity for this chapter on the Student CD that accompanies this text. Or, to hear the terms and their definitions with a CD player or computer, obtain the Pronunciation CD designed for use with this text.

Learn the definitions and spellings of the oncology terms built from word parts by completing exercises 13, 14, and 15.

EXERCISE 13

Analyze and define the following terms. Refer to Chapter 1, p. 6, to review analyzing and defining techniques. **This is an important exercise; do not skip any portion of it.**

WR CV WR CV   S
Example: lei/o/my/o/sarcoma *malignant tumor of smooth muscle*
CF   CF

1. sarcoma _____

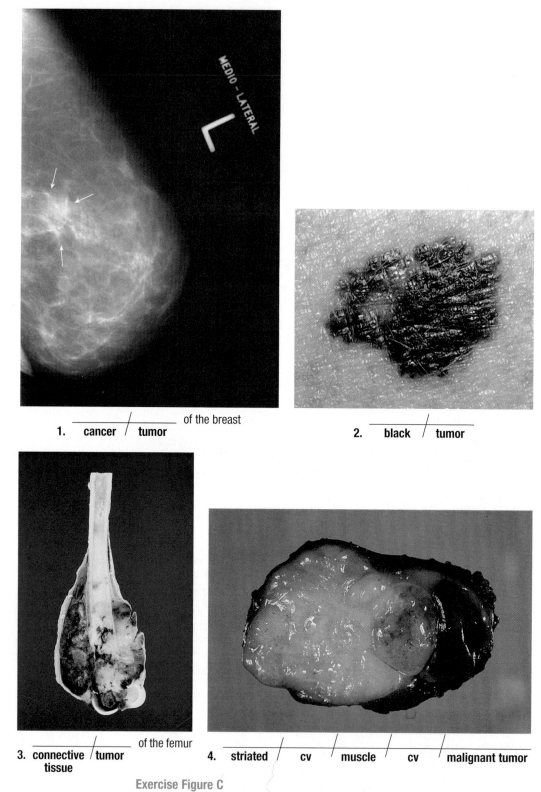

1. _____ / _____ of the breast
      cancer   /   tumor

2. _____ / _____
      black   /   tumor

3. _____ / tumor of the femur
   connective /
   tissue

4. _____ / cv / _____ / cv / _____
     striated /   /   muscle   /   / malignant tumor

Exercise Figure C

Fill in the blanks to complete labeling of these diagrams of types of cancers.

TABLE 2-1

PRONUNCIATION GUIDE

The following is a simple guide to use for practicing pronunciation of the medical terms. The pronunciations are only approximate; however, they are adequate to meet the needs of the beginning student.

In respelling for pronunciation, words are minimally distorted to indicate phonetic sound.

Example: doctor (dok-tor)
gastric (gas-trik)

Diacritical marks are used over vowels to indicate pronunciation. The macron (̄) is used to indicate the *long* vowel sounds.

Example: donate (dō-nāte)
hepatoma (hep-a-tō-ma)
ā as in *ate, say*
ē as in *eat, beet, see*
ī as in *I, mine, sky*
ō as in *oats, so*
ū as in *unit, mute*

Vowels with no markings have the short sound.

Example: discuss (dis-kus)
medical (med-i-kal)
a as in *at, lad*
e as in *edge, bet*
i as in *itch, wish*
o as in *ox, top*
u as in *sun, come*

An accent mark indicates the stress on a certain syllable. The primary accent is indicated by capital letters, and the secondary accent (which is stressed, but not as strongly as the primary accent) is indicated by italics.

Example: altogether (*all*-tū-GETH-er)
pancreatitis (*pan*-krē-a-TĪ-tis)

When analyzing terms that have a suffix containing a word root, it may appear, as in the word **neoplasm,** that the word is composed of only a prefix and a suffix. Keep in mind that the word does have a word root but that it is embedded in the suffix. S(WR) indicates that the word root is embedded in the suffix.

2. melanoma _____

3. epithelioma _____

4. lipoma _____

5. neoplasm _____

6. myoma _____

7. neuroma _____

8. carcinoma _____

9. melanocarcinoma _____

10. rhabdomyosarcoma _____

11. leiomyoma _____

12. rhabdomyoma _____

13. fibroma _____

14. liposarcoma _____

15. fibrosarcoma _____

16. adenoma _____

17. adenocarcinoma _____

18. chloroma _____

EXERCISE 14

Build medical terms for the following definitions by using the word parts you have learned. If you need help, refer to p. 8 to review word-building techniques. **Once again, this is an integral part of the learning process; do not skip any part of this exercise.**

Example: a tumor composed of fat $\underline{\text{lip}}$ / $\underline{\text{oma}}$
　　　　　　　　　　　　　　　　　　WR 　 S

1. black tumor

    _____ / _____
    　　WR 　　　　　　 S

2. cancerous tumor

    _____ / _____
    　　WR 　　　　　　 S

3. new growth

    _____ / _____
    　　P 　　　　　　 S(WR)

4. tumor composed of epithelium

    _____ / _____
    　　WR 　　　　　　 S

5. tumor composed of connective tissue

    _____ / _____
    　　WR 　　　　　　 S

6. cancerous black tumor

    _____ / CV / _____ / S
    　WR 　　　　　　 WR

7. tumor composed of nerve

    _____ / _____
    　　WR 　　　　　　 S

8. tumor composed of muscle

    WR   /   S

9. malignant tumor of striated
   muscle

    WR   / CV / WR / CV /   S

10. tumor of smooth muscle

    WR   / CV / WR /   S

11. tumor of striated muscle

    WR   / CV / WR /   S

12. malignant tumor of smooth
    muscle

    WR   / CV / WR / CV /   S

13. malignant tumor composed
    of fat

    WR   / CV /   S

14. tumor composed of fiber
    (fibrous tissue)

    WR   /   S

15. malignant tumor composed
    of fiber (fibrous tissue)

    WR   / CV /   S

16. tumor composed of glandular
    tissue

    WR   /   S

17. cancerous tumor composed
    of glandular tissue

    WR   / CV / WR /   S

18. tumor of green color

    WR   /   S

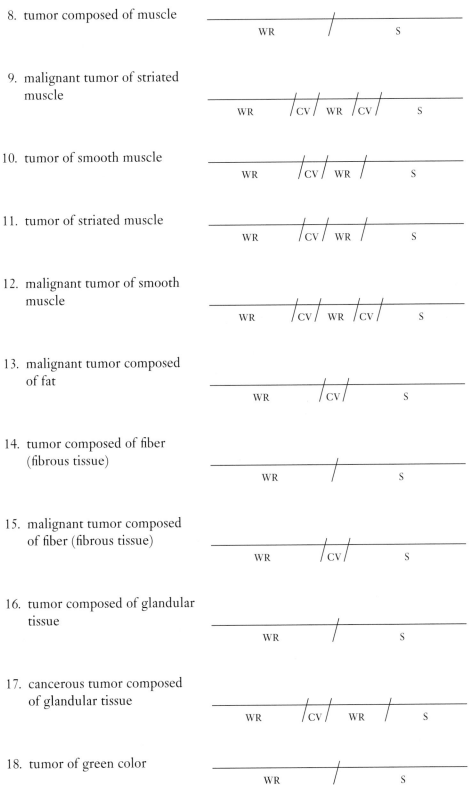

EXERCISE   15

Spell each of the oncology terms built from word parts. Have someone dictate the terms on pp. 22-23 to you. Think about the word parts before attempting to write the word. Study any words you have spelled incorrectly.

1. _____   11. _____

2. _____   12. _____

3. _____   13. _____

4. _____   14. _____

5. _____   15. _____

6. _____   16. _____

7. _____   17. _____

8. _____   18. _____

9. _____   19. _____

10. _____

Oncology Terms

Not Built from Word Parts

> **Medical terms not built from word parts** cannot be correctly defined by applying the meanings of the word parts. *The terms are learned by memorizing the whole word* by using recall and spelling exercises.

The oncology terms in this list are not built from word parts. The terms are commonly used in the medical world and you will need to know them. *In some of the words, you may recognize a word part; however, these terms cannot be literally translated to find the meaning.* New knowledge may have changed the meanings of the terms since they were coined; some terms are eponyms, some are acronyms, and some have no apparent explanation for their names. Memorization is used in the following exercises to learn the terms.

Benign
is derived from the Latin word root **bene,** meaning **well** or **good,** as used in **benefit** or **benefactor.**

Situ
is from the Latin term **situs,** which means **position** or **place.** Think of **in situ** as meaning "in place" or "not wandering around."

Term	Definition
benign .... (bē-NĪN)	not malignant, nonrecurrent, favorable for recovery (Figure 2-3)
carcinoma in situ .... (in-SĪ-too)	cancer in the early stage before invading surrounding tissue (Figure 2-4)
chemotherapy (chemo) .... (kē-mō-THER-a-pē)	treatment of cancer with drugs

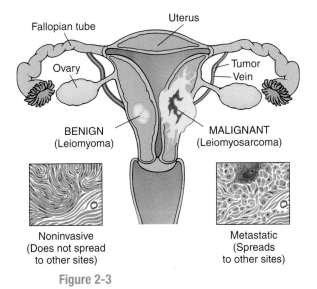

Fallopian tube

Uterus

Ovary

Tumor

Vein

BENIGN
(Leiomyoma)

MALIGNANT
(Leiomyosarcoma)

Noninvasive
(Does not spread
to other sites)

Metastatic
(Spreads
to other sites)

Figure 2-3

Examples of benign and malignant tumors.

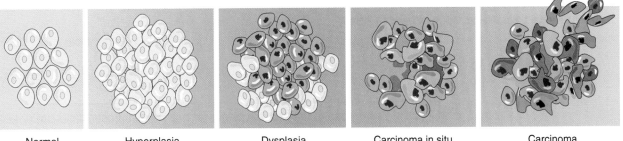

Normal

Hyperplasia

Dysplasia

Carcinoma in situ
(severe dysplasia)

Carcinoma
(invasive)

Figure 2-4

Progression of cell growth.

encapsulated (en-KAP-sū-lā-ted)	enclosed in a capsule, as with benign tumors (Figure 2-6)
exacerbation (eg-*zas*-er-BĀ-shun)	increase in the severity of a disease or its symptoms
idiopathic (id-ē-ō-PATH-ik)	pertaining to disease of unknown origin
inflammation (in-fla-MĀ-shun)	response to injury or destruction of tissue characterized by redness, swelling, heat, and pain
in vitro (in VĒ-trō)	within a glass, observable within a test tube
in vivo (in VĒ-vō)	within the living body
malignant (ma-LIG-nant)	tending to become progressively worse and to cause death, as in cancer (see Figure 2-3)
radiation therapy (XRT) (rā-dē-Ā-shun THER-a-pē)	treatment of cancer with a radioactive substance, x-ray, or radiation (also called *radiation oncology* and *radiotherapy*) (Figure 2-5)

Idiopathic
is derived from the Greek word **idios** meaning **one's own** and **path** or **disease**. The term probably originated from the idea that disease of unknown origin comes from within oneself and is not acquired from without.

Inflammatory and Inflammation
are spelled with two *m*'s. *Inflame* and *inflamed* have one *m*.

Malignant
is derived from the Latin word root **mal** meaning **bad**, as used in **malicious, malaise, malady,** and **malign.**

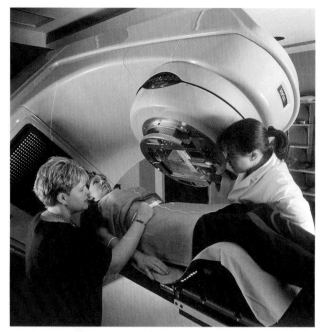

Figure 2-5
Radiation therapist preparing the patient for radiation therapy.

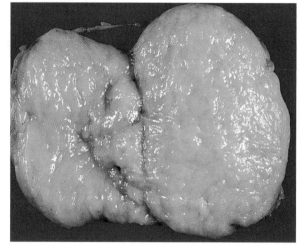

Figure 2-6
An encapsulated benign tumor.

remission... (rē-MISH-un)	improvement or absence of signs of disease

Practice saying each of these terms aloud. To assist you in pronunciation, refer to the Pronunciation Guide on p. 25. To hear the terms, access the **PRONOUNCE IT** activity for this chapter on the Student CD that accompanies this text. Or, to hear the terms and their definitions with a CD player or computer, obtain the Pronunciation CD designed for use with this text.

Learn the definitions and spellings of the oncology terms not built from word parts by completing exercises 16 and 17.

EXERCISE 16

Write the definitions for the following terms.

1. benign _____

2. malignant _____

3. remission _____

4. idiopathic _____

5. inflammation _____

6. chemotherapy _____

7. radiation therapy _____

8. encapsulated _____

9. in vitro _____

10. in vivo _____

11. carcinoma in situ _____

12. exacerbation _____

EXERCISE 17

Spell each of the oncology terms not built from word parts. Have someone dictate the terms on pp. 28-30 to you. Study any words you have spelled incorrectly.

1. _____   7. _____

2. _____   8. _____

3. _____   9. _____

4. _____   10. _____

5. _____   11. _____

6. _____   12. _____

Body Structure Terms

Built from Word Parts

The following terms are built from the word parts you have already learned. By analyzing, defining, and building the terms in the exercises that follow, you will come to know the terms.

Term	Definition
cancerous (KAN-ser-us)	pertaining to cancer
carcinogen (kar-SIN-ō-jen)	substance that causes cancer
carcinogenic (*kar*-sin-ō-JEN-ik)	producing cancer
cyanosis (sī-a-NO-sis)	abnormal condition of blue (bluish discoloration of the skin caused by inadequate supply of oxygen in the blood)
cytogenic (sī-tō-JEN-ik)	producing cells
cytoid (SĪ-toid)	resembling a cell
cytology (sī-TOL-ō-jē)	study of cells

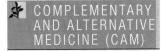

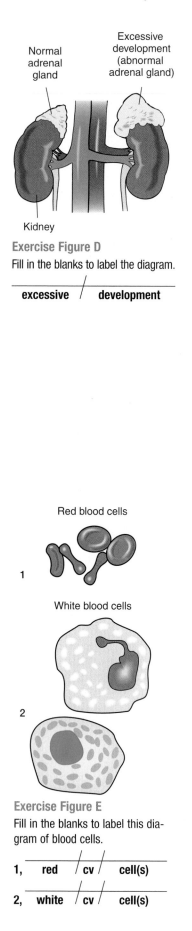

Normal adrenal gland

Excessive development (abnormal adrenal gland)

Kidney

Exercise Figure D

Fill in the blanks to label the diagram.

_____ / _____
excessive / **development**

Red blood cells

1

White blood cells

2

Exercise Figure E

Fill in the blanks to label this diagram of blood cells.

1, _**red**_ / **cv** / **cell(s)**

2, _**white**_ / **cv** / **cell(s)**

> 💡 An essential part of a word, such as the word root for **blood,** may be omitted from a medical term, as in **erythrocyte,** which means **red** *blood* **cell,** by common consent. The practice is called **ellipsis.**

cytoplasm .... (SĪ-tō-plazm)	cell substance
diagnosis (Dx) .... (dī-ag-NŌ-sis)	state of complete knowledge (identifying a disease)
dysplasia .... (dis-PLĀ-zhē-a)	abnormal development (see Figure 2-4)
epithelial .... (ep-i-THĒ-lē-al)	pertaining to epithelium
erythrocyte (RBC) .... (e-RITH-rō-sīt)	red (blood) cell (see Exercise Figure E)
erythrocytosis .... (e-rith-rō-sī-TŌ-sis)	increase in the number of red (blood) cells
etiology .... (ē-tē-OL-ō-jē)	study of causes (of diseases)
histology .... (his-TOL-ō-jē)	study of tissue
hyperplasia .... (hī-per-PLĀ-zhē-a)	excessive development (number of cells) (Exercise Figure D) (see Figure 2-4)
hypoplasia .... (hī-pō-PLĀ-zhē-a)	incomplete development (of an organ or tissues)
iatrogenic .... (ī-at-rō-JEN-ik)	produced by a physician (the unexpected results from a treatment prescribed by a physician)
iatrology .... (ī-a-TROL-ō-jē)	study of medicine
karyocyte .... (KAR-ē-ō-sīt)	cell with a nucleus
karyoplasm .... (KAR-ē-ō-plazm)	substance of a nucleus
leukocyte (WBC) .... (LU-kō-sīt)	white (blood) cell (Exercise Figure E)
leukocytosis .... (lu-kō-sī-TŌ-sis)	increase in the number of white (blood) cells
lipoid .... (LIP-oid)	resembling fat
metastasis (pl. metastases) (mets) .... (me-TAS-ta-sis)	beyond control (transfer of disease from one organ to another, as in the transfer of malignant tumors) (Figure 2-7)
myopathy .... (mī-OP-a-thē)	disease of the muscle

neopathy .... new disease
    (nē-OP-a-thē)

neuroid .... resembling a nerve
    (NŪ-royd)

oncogenic .... causing tumors
    (*ong*-kō-JEN-ik)

oncologist .... a physician who studies and treats tumors
    (ong-KOL-ō-jist)

oncology .... study of tumors (a branch of medicine
    (ong-KOL-ō-jē)   concerned with the study of malignant
                                tumors)

pathogenic .... producing disease
    (path-ō-JEN-ik)

pathologist .... a physician who studies diseases (examines
    (pa-THOL-ō-jist)   biopsies and performs autopsies to determine
                                the cause of disease or death)

pathology .... study of disease (a branch of medicine deal-
    (pa-THOL-ō-jē)   ing with the study of the causes of disease
                                and death)

prognosis (Px) .... state of before knowledge (prediction of the
    (prog-NŌ-sis)   outcome of disease)

somatic .... pertaining to the body
    (sō-MAT-ik)

somatogenic .... originating in the body (organic as opposed
    (sō-ma-tō-JEN-ik)   to psychologic)

somatopathy .... disease of the body
    (sō-ma-TOP-a-thē)

somatoplasm .... body substance
    (sō-MAT-ō-plazm)

Oncology and Oncologic
are used to name the medical specialty and hospital nursing units devoted to the treatment and care of cancer patients.

Prognosis
was used by Hippocrates to mean the same then as now: **to foretell the course of a disease.**

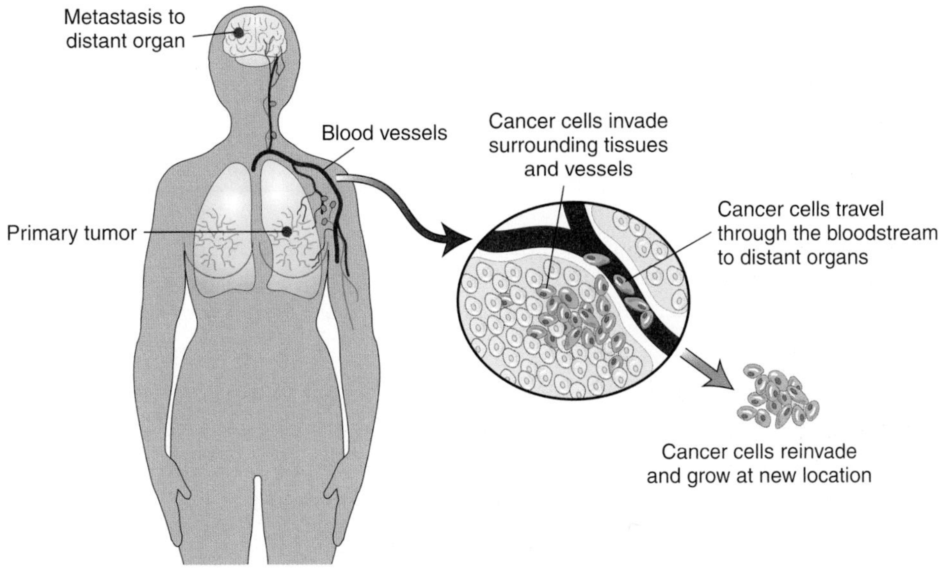

Figure 2-7
Metastasis.

systemic.. (sis-TEM-ik)	pertaining to a (body) system (or the body as a whole)
visceral.. (VIS-er-al)	pertaining to the internal organs
xanthochromic................................... (*zan*-thō-KRŌ-mik)	pertaining to yellow color
xanthosis.. (zan-THŌ-sis)	abnormal condition of yellow (discoloration)

Practice saying each of these terms aloud. Refer to the Pronunciation Guide on p. 25 for an explanation of the pronunciation key. To hear the terms, access the **PRONOUNCE IT** activity for this chapter on the Student CD that accompanies this text. Or, to hear the terms and their definitions with a CD player or computer, obtain the Pronunciation CD designed for use with this text.

Learn the definitions and spellings of the complementary terms by completing exercises 18, 19, and 20.

EXERCISE 18

Analyze and define the following complementary terms.

> WR CV S
> **Example:** path/o/genic *producing disease*
> CF

1. cytology _____

2. histology _____

3. pathology _____

4. pathologist _____

5. visceral _____

6. metastasis _____

7. oncogenic _____

8. oncology _____

9. karyocyte _____

10. neopathy _____

11. karyoplasm _____

12. cytogenic _____

13. systemic _____

14. cancerous _____

15. cytoplasm _____

16. carcinogenic _____

17. somatic _____

18. somatogenic _____

19. somatoplasm _____

20. somatopathy _____

21. neuroid _____

22. myopathy _____

23. erythrocyte _____

24. leukocyte _____

25. cyanosis _____

26. epithelial _____

27. lipoid _____

28. etiology _____

29. xanthosis _____

30. xanthochromic _____

31. hyperplasia _____

32. erythrocytosis _____

33. leukocytosis _____

34. carcinogen _____

35. hypoplasia _____

36. cytoid _____

37. oncologist _____

38. dysplasia _____

39. pathogenic _____

40. prognosis _____

41. diagnosis _____

42. iatrogenic _____

43. iatrology _____

EXERCISE **19**

Build medical terms for the following definitions by using the word parts you have learned.

Example: producing cells $\dfrac{cyt \;/\; o \;/\; genic}{WR \;/\; CV \;/\; S}$

1. cell substance

$\dfrac{ \;/\; \;/\; }{WR \;/\; CV \;/\; S}$

2. pertaining to yellow color

$\dfrac{ \;/\; \;\; \;/\; }{WR \;/\; CV \;/\; WR \;/\; S}$

3. beyond control

$\dfrac{ \;/\; }{P \;/\; S(WR)}$

4. new disease

$\dfrac{ \;/\; }{P \;/\; S(WR)}$

5. study of the cause (of disease)

$\dfrac{ \;/\; \;/\; }{WR \;/\; CV \;/\; S}$

6. substance of a nucleus

$\dfrac{ \;/\; \;/\; }{WR \;/\; CV \;/\; S}$

7. study of tumors

$\dfrac{ \;/\; \;/\; }{WR \;/\; CV \;/\; S}$

8. study of diseases

$\dfrac{ \;/\; \;/\; }{WR \;/\; CV \;/\; S}$

9. pertaining to the body

$\dfrac{ \;/\; }{WR \;/\; S}$

10. a physician who studies diseases

$\dfrac{ \;/\; \;/\; }{WR \;/\; CV \;/\; S}$

11. disease of the muscle

$\dfrac{ \;/\; \;/\; }{WR \;/\; CV \;/\; S}$

12. body substance

$\dfrac{ \;/\; \;/\; }{WR \;/\; CV \;/\; S}$

13. abnormal condition of yellow

_____ / _____
WR   S

14. pertaining to the internal organs

_____ / _____
WR   S

15. causing tumors

_____ /CV/ _____
WR   S

16. originating in the body

_____ /CV/ _____
WR   S

17. disease of the body

_____ /CV/ _____
WR   S

18. red (blood) cell

_____ /CV/ _____
WR   S

19. resembling a nerve

_____ / _____
WR   S

20. pertaining to a (body) system

_____ / _____
WR   S

21. white (blood) cell

_____ /CV/ _____
WR   S

22. cell with a nucleus

_____ /CV/ _____
WR   S

23. resembling fat

_____ / _____
WR   S

24. pertaining to cancer

_____ / _____
WR   S

25. study of cells

_____ /CV/ _____
WR   S

26. excessive development (of cells)

_____ / _____
P   S(WR)

27. resembling a cell

      WR   /   S

28. pertaining to epithelium

      WR   /   S

29. abnormal condition of blue

      WR   /   S

30. producing cancer

      WR   / CV /   S

31. producing disease

      WR   / CV /   S

32. study of tissue

      WR   / CV /   S

33. increase in the number of
    red (blood) cells

      WR / CV / WR / S

34. incomplete development
    (of an organ or tissue)

      P   /   S(WR)

35. increase in the number of
    white (blood) cells

      WR / CV / WR / S

36. substance that causes cancer

      WR   / CV /   S

37. physician who studies and
    treats tumors

      WR   / CV /   S

38. abnormal development

      P   /   S(WR)

39. study of medicine

      WR   / CV /   S

40. state of complete knowledge

      P   / WR /   S

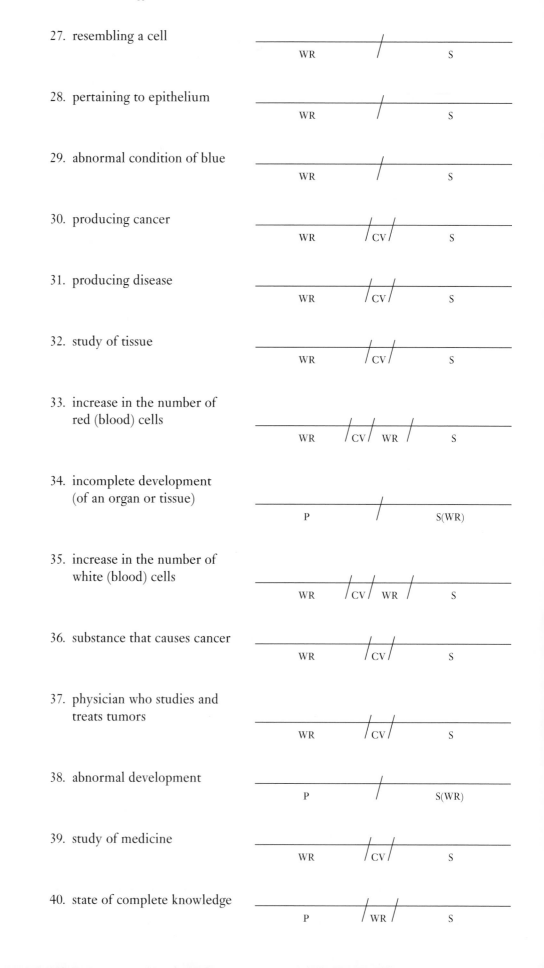

41. produced by a physician

    ————————— / ———— / —————
    WR   CV   S

42. state of before knowledge

    ————————— / ———— / —————
    P   WR   S

EXERCISE 20

Spell each of the complementary terms. Have someone dictate the terms on pp. 31-33
to you. Remember to think about the word parts before attempting to write the word.
Study any words you have spelled incorrectly.

1. _____   20. _____

2. _____   21. _____

3. _____   22. _____

4. _____   23. _____

5. _____   24. _____

6. _____   25. _____

7. _____   26. _____

8. _____   27. _____

9. _____   28. _____

10. _____   29. _____

11. _____   30. _____

12. _____   31. _____

13. _____   32. _____

14. _____   33. _____

15. _____   34. _____

16. _____   35. _____

17. _____   36. _____

18. _____   37. _____

19. _____   38. _____

39. _____   42. _____

40. _____   43. _____

41. _____

Abbreviations

Ca	carcinoma
chemo	chemotherapy
Dx	diagnosis
mets	metastasis
Px	prognosis
RBC	red blood cell
RXT	radiation therapy
WBC	white blood cell

Refer to Appendix D for a complete list of abbreviations.

EXERCISE 21

Write the term for each of the abbreviations in the following paragraph.

A 55-year-old white woman was admitted to the oncology unit with a **Dx** _____ of **Ca** _____ of the breast, **mets** _____ to the lung. Her **Px** _____ was tentative. Laboratory tests, including **RBC** _____ _____ _____ and **WBC** _____ _____ _____ counts, were ordered. She will receive both **chemo** _____ and **XRT** _____ _____.

CHAPTER REVIEW

EXERCISE 22 *Interact with Medical Records*

Below is a physician's progress note. Complete the record by writing the medical terms in the blanks that correspond to the numbered definitions.

University Hospital and Medical Center
4700 North Main Street • Wellness, Arizona 54321 • (987) 555-3210

PATIENT NAME: Morris Greeley   **CASE NUMBER:**   830293-ONC
DATE OF BIRTH: 08/03/xx   **DATE:**   02/12/xx

PROGRESS NOTE

SUBJECTIVE: Mr. Greeley arrives today for a 1. _____ treatment for 2. _____ of the sigmoid colon.

He had an anterior sigmoid resection in October. 3. _____ study revealed 4. _____ tumor cells in two of six lymph nodes.

The 5FU/Leucovorin protocol is being administered weekly for 6 weeks. Today is his sixth infusion. We plan to start
5. _____ _____ after a 2-week hiatus from the chemotherapy.

The patient continues to do well and is receiving significant support from his family. He has had no hair loss, oral ulcerations, abdominal pain, nausea, or diarrhea.

OBJECTIVE: Vital signs show a temperature of 98. Pulse is 60. Respirations 20. Blood pressure is 152/65. His current weight is 183 pounds. HEENT: Tongue and pharynx are normal. PULMONARY: Clear to auscultation. HEART: Regular rate and rhythm without a murmur, rub, or gallop. ABDOMEN: Soft and nontender. No masses or organomegaly. EXTREMITIES: No edema or
6. _____ .

ASSESSMENT:
1. Adenocarcinoma of the sigmoid colon with 7. _____ to regional lymph nodes.

PLAN:
1. 5FU/Leucovorin protocol as outlined above, treatment six of six today, followed by radiation therapy after 2-week period of rest.

_____

Brian Smith, MD

BS/mcm

---

1. treatment of cancer by using drugs
2. cancerous tumor composed of glandular tissue
3. study of disease
4. tending to become progressively worse
5. treatment of cancer by using radioactive substance, x-rays, or radiation
6. abnormal condition of blue
7. beyond control

EXERCISE 23 *Interpret Medical Terms*

To test your understanding of the terms introduced in this chapter, circle the words that correctly complete each sentence. The italicized words refer to the correct answer.

1. Mr. Roberts was diagnosed as having a cancerous *tumor composed of connective tissue,* or (sarcoma, melanoma, lipoma). The doctor said the tumor was *becoming progressively worse;* that is, it was (benign, malignant, pathogenic).
2. The blood test showed an *increased amount of red blood cells,* or (erythrocytosis, leukocytosis, cyanosis).
3. (Organic, Visceral, Systemic) means *pertaining to internal organs.*
4. *A tumor composed of fat,* or (neuroma, carcinoma, lipoma), is *benign,* or (recurrent, nonrecurrent, cancerous).
5. Many substances are thought to be *cancer producing,* or (carcinogenic, carcinogen, cancerous).
6. *Etiology* is the study of (the causes of disease, tissue disease, the causes of tumors).
7. A *tumor* may be called a (cytoplasm, neoplasm, karyoplasm).
8. The pain *originated in the body,* or was (somatogenic, oncogenic, pathogenic).
9. Any *disease of a muscle* is called (myoma, myopathy, somatopathy).
10. The term for *abnormal development* is (hypoplasia, dysplasia, hyperplasia).
11. The term that means *produced by a physician* is (diagnosis, iatrogenic, prognosis).
12. The incidence of malignant *black tumor* (fibrosarcoma, fibroma, melanoma) is increasing in the white population. One *study of disease* (pathology, pathogenic, liposarcoma) finding influencing *state of before knowledge* (cancer in situ, in vitro, prognosis) may be tumor thickness.
13. The term that means *within the living organism* is (in vitro, in vivo, encapsulated).
14. A (liposarcoma, fibroma, myoma) is a *malignant tumor.*
15. (DNA, RBC, WBC) regulates the *activities of a cell.*

EXERCISE 24 *Read Medical Terms in Use*

Practice pronunciation of terms by reading aloud the following medical document. Use the pronunciation key after each medical term to assist you in saying the words. The script contains medical terms not yet presented. Treat them as information only; you will learn more about them as you continue to study. Or, if desired, look for their meanings in your medical dictionary.

A 54-year-old woman presented to the office with a 3-week history of bloody diarrhea. She had been diagnosed with ulcerative colitis at age 25 years. She was referred for a colonoscopy. The examination revealed a suspicious lesion in the transverse colon. A biopsy was performed and a **cytology** (sī-TOL-ō-jē) specimen was obtained. The **pathologist** (pa-THOL-ō-jist) made a **diagnosis** (*dī*-ag-NŌ-sis) of **carcinoma** (*kar*-si-NŌ-ma) of the colon. Advanced **dysplasia** (dis-PLĀ-zhē-a) and **inflammation** (in-fla-MĀ-shun) existed in the specimen. The patient underwent surgery and was found to have no evidence of **metastasis** (me-TAS-ta-sis). Her entire colon was removed because of a high risk for developing a **malignant** (ma-LIG-nant) lesion in the remaining colon. She made an uneventful recovery and was referred to an **oncologist** (ong-kol-ō-jist) for consideration of **chemotherapy** (kē-mō-THER-a-pē). Her **prognosis** (prog-NŌ-sis) is generally positive. **Radiation therapy** (rā-dē-Ā-shun) (THER-a-pē) is not indicated in this case.

EXERCISE 25   *Comprehend Medical Terms in Use*

Test your comprehension of terms in the previous medical document by answering *T* for true and *F* for false.

_____ 1. The cancer has spread from the colon to other surrounding organs.

_____ 2. The specimen is described as having abnormal development.

_____ 3. The patient's prognosis is carcinoma of the colon.

_____ 4. The patient's colon was removed to avoid development of a malignant lesion in the remaining colon.

_____ 5. The patient was referred to a pathologist for consideration of treatment for the cancer with drugs.

> For additional information on cancer visit the National Cancer Institute at www.nic.nih.gov

For further practice or to evaluate what you have learned, use the Student CD that accompanies this text.

COMBINING FORMS CROSSWORD PUZZLE

Across Clues	Down Clues
2. tissue	1. organ
4. nerve	3. flesh, connective tissue
7. red	5. system
8. nucleus	6. cell
9. tumor	7. cause (of disease)
12. epithelium	10. internal organs
16. disease	11. cancer
17. cancer	13. fat
19. body	14. white
20. muscle	15. color
21. blue	18. yellow
22. black	

REVIEW OF WORD PARTS

Can you define and spell the following word parts?

Combining Forms

aden/o	erythr/o	leuk/o	rhabd/o
cancer/o	eti/o	lip/o	sarc/o
carcin/o	fibr/o	melan/o	somat/o
chlor/o	gno/o	my/o	system/o
chrom/o	hist/o	neur/o	viscer/o
cyan/o	iatr/o	onc/o	xanth/o
cyt/o	kary/o	organ/o	
epitheli/o	lei/o	path/o	

Prefixes   Suffixes

Prefixes	Suffixes		
dia-	-al	-logist	-pathy
dys-	-cyte	-logy	-plasia
hyper-	-gen	-oid	-plasm
hypo-	-genesis	-oma	-sarcoma
meta-	-genic	-osis	-sis
neo-	-ic	-ous	-stasis
pro-			

REVIEW OF TERMS

Can you build, analyze, define, spell, and pronounce the following terms *built from word parts?*

Oncology   Body Structure

Oncology	Body Structure		
adenocarcinoma	cancerous	hyperplasia	oncologist
adenoma	carcinogen	hypoplasia	oncology
carcinoma (Ca)	carcinogenic	iatrogenic	pathogenic
chloroma	cyanosis	iatrology	pathologist
epithelioma	cytogenic	karyocyte	pathology
fibroma	cytoid	karyoplasm	prognosis (Px)
fibrosarcoma	cytology	leukocyte (WBC)	somatic
leiomyoma	cytoplasm	leukocytosis	somatogenic
leiomyosarcoma	diagnosis (Dx)	lipoid	somatopathy
lipoma	dysplasia	metastasis (mets)	somatoplasm
liposarcoma	epithelial	myopathy	systemic
melanocarcinoma	erythrocyte (RBC)	neopathy	visceral
melanoma	erythrocytosis	neuroid	xanthochromic
myoma	etiology	oncogenic	xanthosis
neoplasm	histology		
neuroma			
rhabdomyoma			
rhabdomyosarcoma			
sarcoma			

Can you define, pronounce, and spell the following terms *not built from word parts?*

Oncology

benign	encapsulated	inflammation	malignant
carcinoma in situ	exacerbation	in vitro	radiation therapy (XRT)
chemotherapy (chemo)	idiopathic	in vivo	remission

3

Directional Terms, Anatomic Planes, Regions, and Quadrants

OUTLINE

OBJECTIVES

On completion of this chapter you will be able to:

1. Write the definitions of the word parts included in this chapter.
2. Build, analyze, define, pronounce, and spell the terms used to describe directions with respect to the body.
3. Define, pronounce, and spell the terms used to describe the anatomic planes.
4. Define, pronounce, and spell the terms used to describe the abdominopelvic regions.
5. Identify and spell the four abdominopelvic quadrants.
6. Interpret the meanings of the abbreviations presented in this chapter.
7. Read medical documents and interpret medical terminology contained in them.

ANATOMIC POSITION

In the description of body directions and planes, a position of reference is used. In the *anatomic position* the body is viewed as erect, arms at the side, with palms of the hands facing forward and feet placed side by side (Figure 3-1). Whether the patient is standing or lying down face up, the directional terms are the same.

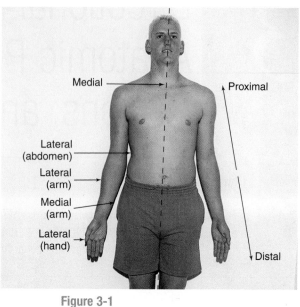

Figure 3-1
Medial and lateral, proximal and distal.

WORD PARTS FOR DIRECTIONAL TERMS

Study the following word parts and their definitions.

Combining Forms for Directional Terms

Combining Form	Definition
anter/o	front
caud/o	tail (downward)
cephal/o	head (upward)
dist/o	away (from the point of attachment of a body part)
dors/o	back
infer/o	below
later/o	side
medi/o	middle
poster/o	back, behind
proxim/o	near (the point of attachment of a body part)
super/o	above
ventr/o	belly (front)

Learn the directional term combining forms by completing exercises 1 and 2 and Exercise Figure A.

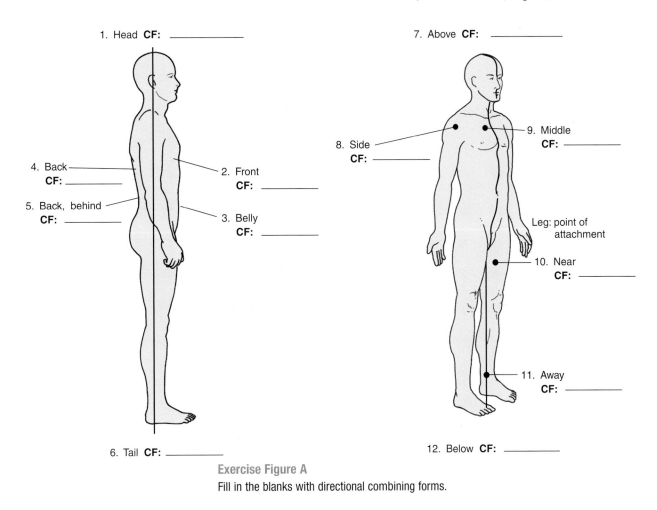

1. Head **CF:** _____

4. Back _____
   CF: _____

5. Back, behind _____
   CF: _____

2. Front
   CF: _____

3. Belly
   CF: _____

6. Tail **CF:** _____

7. Above **CF:** _____

8. Side _____
   CF: _____

9. Middle
   CF: _____

Leg: point of attachment

10. Near
    CF: _____

11. Away
    CF: _____

12. Below **CF:** _____

Exercise Figure A
Fill in the blanks with directional combining forms.

EXERCISE 1

Write the definitions for the following combining forms.

1. ventr/o _____

2. cephal/o _____

3. later/o _____

4. medi/o _____

5. infer/o _____

6. proxim/o _____

7. super/o _____

8. dist/o _____

9. dors/o _____

10. caud/o _____

11. anter/o _____

12. poster/o _____

EXERCISE 2

Write the combining form for each of the following.

1. side _____

2. above _____

3. head _____

4. away (from the point of
   attachment of a body part) _____

5. front _____

6. middle _____

7. back _____

8. belly _____

9. tail _____

10. below _____

11. back, behind _____

12. near (the point of attach-
    ment of a body part) _____

Prefixes

bi-..	two
uni-..	one

Suffixes

-ad..	toward
-ior..	pertaining to

Refer to Appendix A and Appendix B for alphabetized lists of word parts and their meanings.

 Many suffixes mean **"pertaining to."** You have already learned three of them in Chapter 2: **-al, -ic,** and **-ous.** You will learn more in subsequent chapters. With practice, you will learn which suffix is most commonly used with a particular word root or combining form.

EXERCISE 3

Match the prefixes and suffixes in the first column with their correct definitions in the second column.

_____ 1. -ad   a. one

_____ 2. -ior   b. pertaining to

_____ 3. bi-   c. toward

_____ 4. uni-   d. two

EXERCISE 4

Write the definitions of the following prefixes and suffixes.

1. -ior _____

2. -ad _____

3. bi- _____

4. uni- _____

DIRECTIONAL TERMS

The following list of terms is built from word parts you have already learned. You will learn the terms by completing the analyzing, defining, and word-building exercises (Figure 3-2).

Term	Definition
anterior (ant) .... (an-TĒR-ē-or)	pertaining to the front
posterior .... (pos-TĒR-ē-or)	pertaining to the back

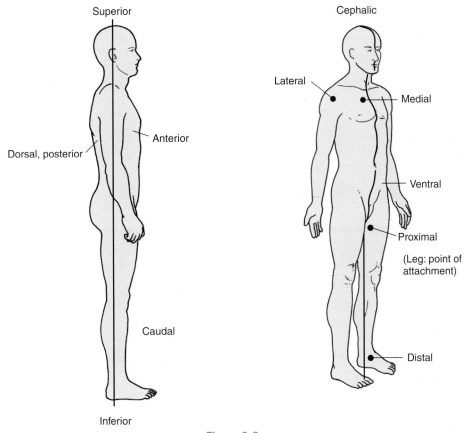

Figure 3-2
Directional terms.

inferior (inf) .... (in-FĒR-ē-or)	pertaining to below
superior (sup) .... (sū-PER-ē-or)	pertaining to above
distal... (DIS-tal)	pertaining to away (from the point of attachment of a body part)
proximal .... (PROK-si-mal)	pertaining to near (to the point of attachment of a body part)
dorsal .... (DOR-sal)	pertaining to the back
ventral .... (VEN-tral)	pertaining to the belly (front)
caudal.. (KAW-dal)	pertaining to the tail
cephalic... (se-FAL-ik)	pertaining to the head
anteroposterior (AP) .... (*an*-ter-ō-pos-TĒR-ē-or)	pertaining to the front and to the back
posteroanterior (PA) .... (*pos*-ter-ō-an-TĒR-ē-or)	pertaining to the back and to the front
lateral (lat).. (LAT-e-ral)	pertaining to a side
medial (med) .... (MĒ-dē-al)	pertaining to the middle
unilateral .... (ū-ni-LAT-er-al)	pertaining to one side (only)
bilateral .... (bī-LAT-er-al)	pertaining to two sides
mediolateral .... (*mē*-dē-ō-LAT-er-al)	pertaining to the middle and to the side
mediad .... (MĒ-dē-ad)	toward the middle
cephalad... (SEF-a-lad)	toward the head

Practice saying each of these terms aloud. To hear the terms, access the **PRONOUNCE IT** activity for this chapter on the Student CD that accompanies this text. Or, to hear the terms and their definitions with a CD player or computer, obtain the Pronunciation CD designed for use with this text. Refer to the Pronunciation Guide on p. 25 as needed.

Learn the definitions and spelling of the terms used to describe body directions by completing exercises 5, 6, and 7.

EXERCISE 5

Analyze and define the following directional terms.

1. cephalad _____

2. cephalic _____

3. caudal _____

4. anterior _____

5. posterior _____

6. dorsal _____

7. superior _____

8. inferior _____

9. proximal _____

10. distal _____

11. lateral _____

12. medial _____

13. mediad _____

14. ventral _____

15. posteroanterior _____

16. unilateral _____

17. mediolateral _____

18. anteroposterior _____

19. bilateral _____

EXERCISE 6

Build directional terms for the following definitions by using the word parts you have learned. Also label the diagram in Exercise Figure B.

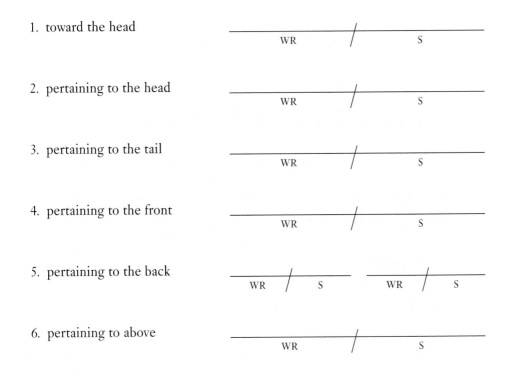

1. toward the head
   _____ / _____
   WR   S

2. pertaining to the head
   _____ / _____
   WR   S

3. pertaining to the tail
   _____ / _____
   WR   S

4. pertaining to the front
   _____ / _____
   WR   S

5. pertaining to the back
   _____ / _____   _____ / _____
   WR   S   WR   S

6. pertaining to above
   _____ / _____
   WR   S

7. pertaining to below

_____ / _____
        WR   S

8. pertaining to near

_____ / _____
        WR   S

9. pertaining to away

_____ / _____
        WR   S

10. pertaining to a side

_____ / _____
        WR   S

11. pertaining to the middle

_____ / _____
        WR   S

12. toward the middle

_____ / _____
        WR   S

13. pertaining to the belly

_____ / _____
        WR   S

14. pertaining to the back and
    to the front

_____ / ___ / _____ / _____
   WR   CV   WR   S

15. pertaining to the middle
    and to the side

_____ / ___ / _____ / _____
   WR   CV   WR   S

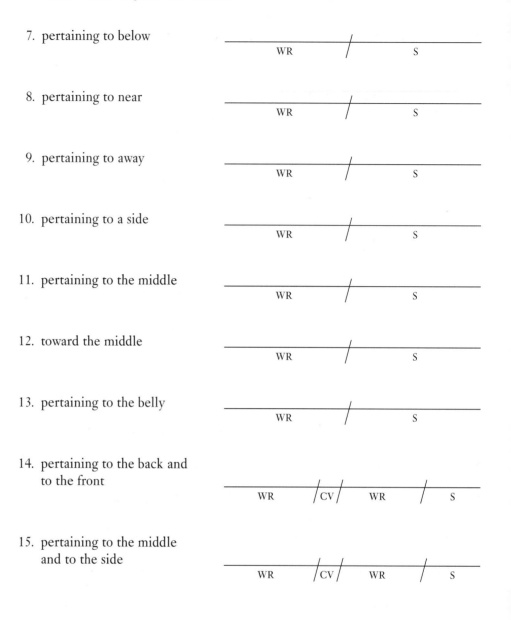

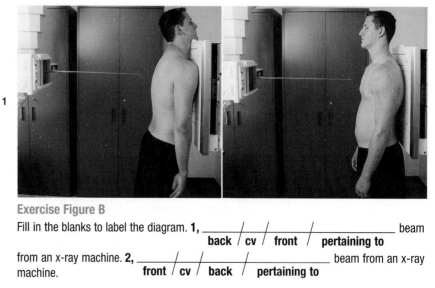

Exercise Figure B

Fill in the blanks to label the diagram. **1,** _____ / __ / _____ / _____ beam
                                             back / cv / front / pertaining to
from an x-ray machine. **2,** _____ / __ / _____ / _____ beam from an x-ray
machine.   **front / cv / back / pertaining to**

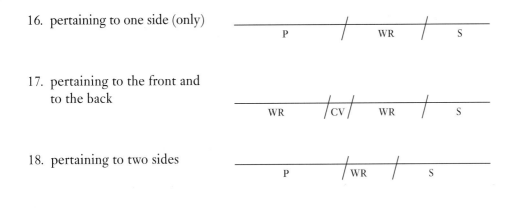

16. pertaining to one side (only)

P / WR / S

17. pertaining to the front and
    to the back

WR /CV/ WR / S

18. pertaining to two sides

P /WR / S

EXERCISE   7

Have someone dictate the terms on pp. 49-50 to you. Think about the word parts before attempting to write the word. Study any words you have spelled incorrectly.

1. _____

2. _____

3. _____

4. _____

5. _____

6. _____

7. _____

8. _____

9. _____

10. _____

11. _____

12. _____

13. _____

14. _____

15. _____

16. _____

17. _____

18. _____

19. _____

ANATOMIC PLANES

Planes are imaginary flat fields used as points of reference to identify the position of parts of the body (Figure 3-3). These terms are not built from word parts. Memorization is the learning method used in the exercises that follow.

Term	Definition
frontal or coronal.......................... (FRON-tl) (ko-RŌN-al)	vertical field passing through the body from side to side, dividing the body into anterior and posterior portions (Figure 3-4)
sagittal .... (SAJ-i-tal)	vertical field running through the body from front to back, dividing the body into right and left sides (Figure 3-5)

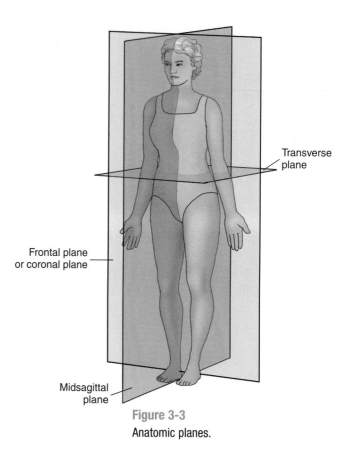

Transverse plane

Frontal plane or coronal plane

Midsagittal plane

Figure 3-3
Anatomic planes.

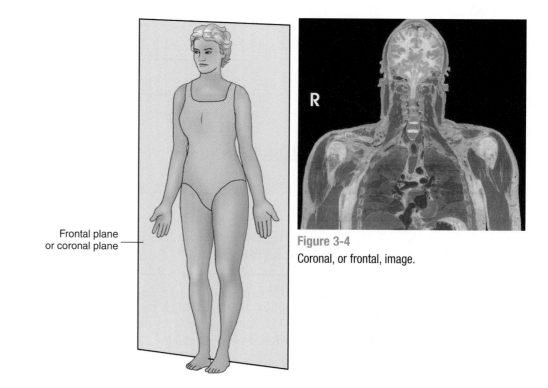

Frontal plane or coronal plane

Figure 3-4
Coronal, or frontal, image.

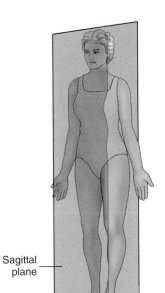

Sagittal
plane

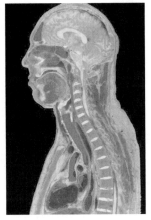

Figure 3-5
Sagittal image.

midsagittal .... (mid-SAJ-i-tal)	divides the body into right and left halves (Figure 3-3)
transverse .... (trans-VERS)	horizontal field dividing the body into upper and lower portions (Figure 3-6)

Practice saying each of the terms aloud. To hear the terms, access the **PRONOUNCE IT** activity for this chapter on the Student CD that accompanies this text. Or, to hear the terms and their definitions with a CD player or computer, obtain the Pronunciation CD designed for use with this text.

Learn the definitions and spellings of the terms used to describe the anatomic planes by completing exercises 8 and 9 and Exercise Figure C.

EXERCISE   8

Fill in the blanks with the correct terms.

1. The plane that divides the body into upper and lower portions is the
   _____ plane.

2. The plane that divides the body into right and left halves is the
   _____ plane.

3. The plane that divides the body into anterior and posterior portions is the
   _____ or _____ plane.

4. The plane that divides the body into right and left sides is the
   _____ plane.

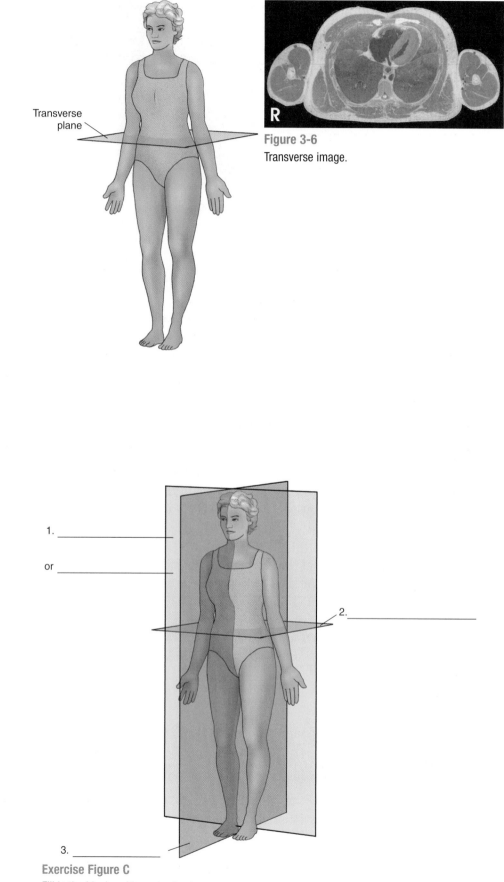

Transverse plane

Figure 3-6
Transverse image.

1. _____

or _____

2. _____

3. _____

Exercise Figure C
Fill in the blanks with anatomic planes.

EXERCISE 9

Spell each of the terms used to describe the anatomic planes. Have someone dictate the terms on pp. 53 and 55 to you. Study any words you have spelled incorrectly.

1. _____   4. _____

2. _____   5. _____

3. _____

ABDOMINOPELVIC REGIONS

To assist medical personnel in locating medical problems with greater accuracy and for identification purposes, the abdomen and pelvis are divided into nine regions (Figure 3-7). Although these terms are made up of word parts, most of the word parts are presented in later chapters; therefore memorization is the learning method used in the exercises that follow. The number indicates the number of regions.

Term	Definition
umbilical region (1) .... (um-BIL-i-kal)	around the navel (umbilicus)
epigastric region (1) .... (*ep*-i-GAS-trik)	directly above the umbilical region
hypogastric region (1) .... (*hī*-pō-GAS-trik)	directly below the umbilical region

Umbilicus
is a term derived from the Latin **umbo,** which denoted the boss, or protuberant part, of a shield. Around the first century the term was used to designate either a raised or a depressed spot in the middle of anything.

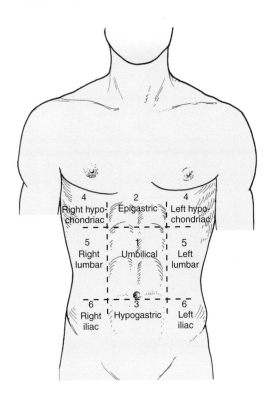

Figure 3-7
Abdominopelvic regions.

Hypochondriac
is derived from the Greek **hypo,** meaning **under,** and **chondros,** meaning **cartilage.** This ancient term was used by Hippocrates to refer to the region just below the cartilages of the ribs. In 1765 the term was first used to refer to people who experienced discomfort or painful sensations in this area but had no organic findings. Now, a person who falsely believes he or she has an illness is referred to as a **hypochondriac.**

hypochondriac regions (2)............	to the right and left of the epigastric region
(*hī-pō*-KON-*drē*-ak)	
lumbar regions (2)........................	to the right and left of the umbilical region
(LUM-bar)	
iliac regions (2)............................	to the right and left of the hypogastric region
(IL-*ē*-ak)	

Practice saying each of these words aloud. To hear the terms, access the **PRONOUNCE IT** activity for this chapter on the Student CD that accompanies this text. Or, to hear the terms and their definitions with a CD player or computer, obtain the Pronunciation CD designed for use with this text.

Learn the definitions and spellings of the terms used to describe the abdominopelvic regions by completing exercises 10, 11, and 12 and Exercise Figure D.

EXERCISE 10

Fill in the blanks with the correct terms.

1. The regions to the right and left of the hypogastric region are the _____ regions.

2. The _____ region is directly above the umbilical region.

3. Inferior to the umbilical region is the _____ region.

4. The _____ are the regions to the right and left of the epigastric region.

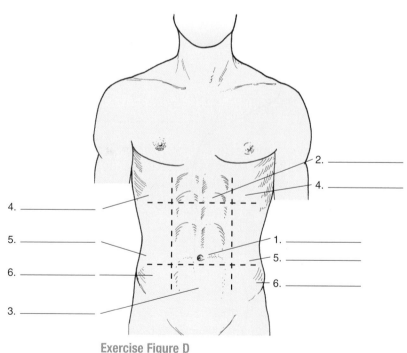

Exercise Figure D
Fill in the blanks with abdominopelvic regions.

5. Superior to the hypogastric region is the _____ region.

6. To the right and the left of the umbilical region are the _____ regions.

EXERCISE 11

Match the terms in the first column with the correct definitions in the second column.

_____ 1. epigastric

_____ 2. hypochondriac

_____ 3. hypogastric

_____ 4. iliac

_____ 5. lumbar

_____ 6. umbilical

a. inferior to the umbilical region

b. superior to the umbilical region

c. right and left of the umbilical region

d. right and left of the epigastric region

e. right and left of the hypogastric region

f. below the hypogastric region

g. inferior to the epigastric region

EXERCISE 12

Spell each of the terms used to describe the abdominopelvic regions. Have someone dictate the terms on pp. 57-58 to you. Study any words you have spelled incorrectly.

1. _____

2. _____

3. _____

4. _____

5. _____

6. _____

ABDOMINOPELVIC QUADRANTS

The abdominopelvic area can also be divided into four quadrants by using imaginary vertical and horizontal lines that intersect at the umbilicus. These divisions are used by health professionals to locate an anatomic position to describe pain, incisions, markings, lesions, and so forth (Figure 3-8). The four divisions are the following:

1. right upper quadrant (RUQ)
2. left upper quadrant (LUQ)
3. right lower quadrant (RLQ)
4. left lower quadrant (LLQ)

EXERCISE 13

Learn the abdominopelvic quadrants by completing Exercise Figure E.

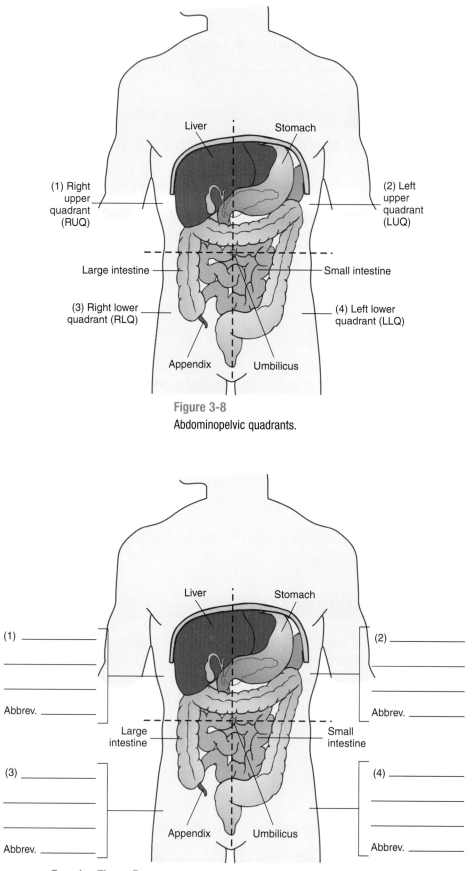

Figure 3-8
Abdominopelvic quadrants.

Exercise Figure E
Fill in the blanks with abdominopelvic quadrants and the abbreviations for each.

EXERCISE 14

Spell each of the terms used to describe the abdominopelvic quadrants. Have someone dictate the terms on p. 59 to you. Study any words you have spelled incorrectly.

1. _____   3. _____

2. _____   4. _____

Abbreviations

ant	anterior
AP	anteroposterior
inf	inferior
lat	lateral
LLQ	left lower quadrant
LUQ	left upper quadrant
med	medial
PA	posteroanterior
RLQ	right lower quadrant
RUQ	right upper quadrant
sup	superior

Refer to Appendix D for a complete list of abbreviations.

EXERCISE 15

Write the meaning of each abbreviation in the space provided.

1. sup _____

2. ant _____

3. inf _____

4. PA _____

5. AP _____

6. med _____

7. lat _____

CHAPTER REVIEW

EXERCISE 16 *Interact with Medical Documents*

Complete the physician's progress note by writing the medical terms in the blanks. Use the list of definitions with corresponding numbers.

University Hospital and Medical Center
4700 North Main Street • Wellness, Arizona 54321 • (987) 555-3210

PATIENT NAME: Zoe Parker   **CASE NUMBER:** 817254-DPQ
DATE OF BIRTH: 03/27/xx   **DATE:** 11/24/xx

PROGRESS NOTE

Mrs. Parker is here today for follow-up for degenerative joint disease of both knees. She arrived ambulatory with the assistance of a cane, walking slowly with a fairly steady gait.

On examination of the knees, there is marked crepitus that is palpable with pressure applied to the kneecaps with the knees flexed and extended, right greater than left. She has a range of motion from 11 degrees to 106 degrees in the right knee. Pain is evident at the end of extension at 11 degrees. The right knee is stable when stressed in an 1. _____, valgus, and varus manner.

On examination of the right ankle, there is some mild tenderness on palpation above the right ankle. The right ankle moves from 0 degrees of dorsiflexion to 25 degrees of plantar flexion. From the 2. _____ joint line at the knee to the malleolus at the ankle, the right tib/fib is 1.5 cm shorter than the left. There is pigment change mainly on the 3. _____ and 4. _____ aspect of the right lower leg. There is a slight bony deformity over the 5. _____ aspect of the mid-tibial area.

IMPRESSION:
1. Degenerative joint disease of both knees, stable.

PLAN:
1. Patient is to continue on current medications unchanged.

Robert Means MD

RM/mcm

---

1. pertaining to the front and to the back
2. pertaining to the side
3. pertaining to the back

4. pertaining to the middle
5. pertaining to the front

EXERCISE 17 *Interpret Medical Terms*

To test your understanding of the terms introduced in this chapter, complete the sentence by filling in the blank with the term that corresponds to the definition provided.

1. A polyp was found in the colon _____ to the splenic flexure. (pertaining to away from the point of attachment of a body part)

2. The drainage catheter is placed over the right _____ pelvis. (pertaining to the front)

3. The incision was made at the _____ pole of the lesion. (pertaining to above)

4. A(n) _____ chest film is taken in the _____ plane. (pertaining to the front and to the back) (dividing the body into anterior and posterior portions)

5. The patient complained of _____ pain. (directly above the umbilical region)

6. A _____ chest x-ray displays the anatomy in the _____ plane. (pertaining to a side) (divides the body into right and left sides)

7. The patient was scheduled for an ultrasound-guided _____ thoracentesis. (pertaining to two [both] sides)

EXERCISE 18 *Read Medical Terms in Use*

Practice pronunciation of terms by reading aloud the following medical document. Use the pronunciation key following the medical term to assist you in saying the word. The script contains medical terms not yet presented. Treat them as information only; you will learn more about them as you continue to study. Or, if desired, look for their meanings in your medical dictionary.

> The patient presented to her physician with pain in the right **lumbar** (LUM-bar) region and right **unilateral** (ū-ni-LAT-er-al) leg pain. The pain was felt in the **posterior** (pos-TER-ē-or) portion of the leg and radiated to the **distal** (DIS-tal) **lateral** (LAT-e-ral) portion of the extremity. There was some **proximal** (PROK-si-mal) muscle weakness reported of the affected leg. A lumbar spine radiograph was normal. If the pain does not respond to antiinflammatory medication, she will be referred to an orthopedist.

EXERCISE 19 *Comprehend Medical Terms in Use*

Test your comprehension of terms in the previous medical document by answering *T* for true and *F* for false.

_____ 1. The patient had pain on both sides of her leg and to the right of the hypogastric region.

_____ 2. The pain was felt at the back of the leg and radiated away from this point to the side of the extremity.

_____ 3. The muscle weakness was felt near the point of attachment.

For further practice or to evaluate what you have learned, use the Student CD that accompanies this text.

DIRECTIONAL TERMS CROSSWORD PUZZLE

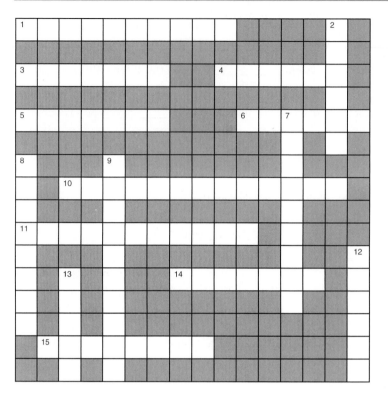

Across Clues

1. plane that divides the body into upper and lower portions
3. pertaining to the belly
4. regions to the right and left of the umbilical region
5. pertaining to a side
6. pertaining to the tail
10. regions to the right and left of the epigastric region
11. region directly below the umbilical region
14. plane dividing the body into anterior and posterior portions
15. plane dividing the body into right and left sides

Down Clues

2. pertaining to the back of the body
7. region around the navel
8. pertaining to the head
9. region directly above the umbilical region
12. toward the midline or middle
13. regions to the right and left of the hypogastric region

REVIEW OF WORD PARTS

Can you define and spell the following word parts?

Combining Forms		Prefixes	Suffixes
anter/o	medi/o	bi-	-ad
caud/o	poster/o	uni-	-ior
cephal/o	proxim/o		
dist/o	super/o		
dors/o	ventr/o		
infer/o			
later/o			

REVIEW OF TERMS

Can you define, pronounce, and spell the following terms?

Body Directional Terms	Anatomic Planes	Abdominopelvic Regions	Abdominopelvic Quadrants
anterior (ant)	frontal or coronal	epigastric	left lower quadrant (LLQ)
anteroposterior (AP)	midsagittal	hypochondriac	left upper quadrant (LUQ)
bilateral	sagittal	hypogastric	right lower quadrant (RLQ)
caudal	transverse	iliac	right upper quadrant (RUQ)
cephalad		lumbar	
cephalic		umbilical	
distal			
dorsal			
inferior (inf)			
lateral (lat)			
mediad			
medial (med)			
mediolateral			
posterior			
posteroanterior (PA)			
proximal			
superior (sup)			
unilateral			
ventral			

Integumentary System

The remaining chapters are organized according to body systems; therefore they present material in a consistent format. The better you understand the format, the quicker and easier you will learn the material. Take time now to review How To Use This Text in the Front Matter to reacquaint yourself with the finer points of using this textbook to its ultimate potential.

OBJECTIVES

On completion of this chapter you will be able to:

1. Identify organs and structures of the integumentary system.
2. Define and spell the word parts presented in this chapter.
3. Build and analyze medical terms with word parts presented in this and previous chapters.
4. Define, pronounce, and spell the disease and disorder, surgical, and complementary terms for the integumentary system.
5. Interpret the meanings of the abbreviations presented in this chapter.
6. Read medical documents and interpret medical terminology contained in them.

ANATOMY

Function

The integumentary system is composed of the skin, nails, and glands. The skin forms a protective covering for the body that, when unbroken, prevents entry of bacteria and other invading organisms. The skin also protects the body from water loss and the damaging effects of ultraviolet light. Other functions include regulation of body temperature and synthesis of vitamin D (Figure 4-1).

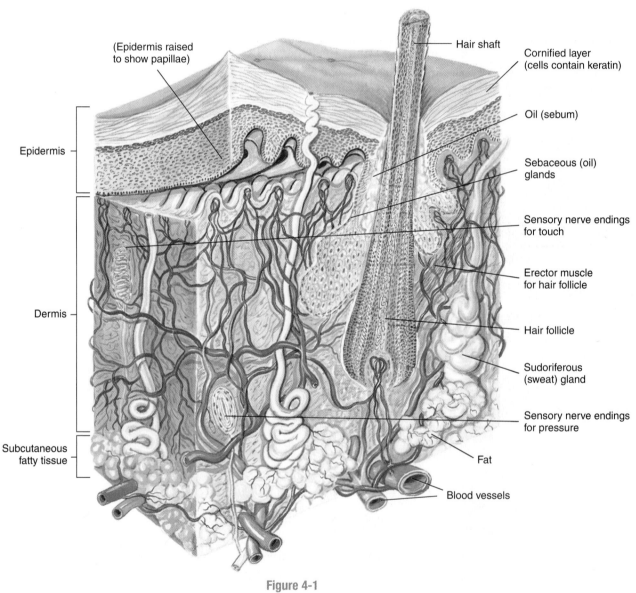

(Epidermis raised to show papillae)

Hair shaft

Cornified layer (cells contain keratin)

Oil (sebum)

Epidermis

Sebaceous (oil) glands

Sensory nerve endings for touch

Erector muscle for hair follicle

Dermis

Hair follicle

Sudoriferous (sweat) gland

Sensory nerve endings for pressure

Subcutaneous fatty tissue

Fat

Blood vessels

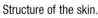

Figure 4-1
Structure of the skin.

The Skin

epidermis	outer layer of skin
keratin	horny, or cornified, layer composed of protein. It is contained in the hair, skin, and nails.
melanin	color, or pigmentation, of the skin
dermis	inner layer of skin (also called the *true skin*)
sudoriferous (sweat) glands	tiny, coiled, tubular structures that emerge through pores on the skin's surface and secrete sweat
sebaceous glands	secrete sebum (oil) into the hair follicles where the hair shafts pass through the dermis

> **Integumentary**
> is derived from the Latin word **teqere,** meaning **to cover.**

Accessory Structures of the Skin

hair	compressed, keratinized cells that arise from hair follicles; the sacs that enclose the hair fibers
nails	originate in the epidermis. Nails are found on the upper surface of the ends of the fingers and toes. The white area at the base of the nail is called the *lunula,* or *moon.*

Learn the anatomic structures by completing exercise 1.

EXERCISE 1

Match the terms in the first column with the correct definitions in the second column.

_____ 1. dermis

_____ 2. epidermis

_____ 3. hair

_____ 4. melanin

_____ 5. nail

_____ 6. sebaceous glands

_____ 7. sudoriferous glands

a. coiled, tubular structures

b. responsible for skin color

c. true skin

d. outermost layer of the skin

e. white area at the nail's base

f. originates in the epidermis

g. composed of compressed, keratinized cells

h. secrete sebum

WORD PARTS

Combining Forms for the Integumentary System

Study the word parts and their definitions listed below. Learning will be made easier by completing the exercises that follow.

Combining Form	Definition
cutane/o, derm/o, dermat/o..............	skin
hidr/o..	sweat
kerat/o..	horny tissue, hard
(NOTE: *kerat/o* is also used to refer to the cornea of the eye; see Chapter 12.)	
onych/o, ungu/o.....................................	nail
seb/o..	sebum (oil)
trich/o...	hair

Learn the anatomic locations and meanings of these combining forms by completing exercises 2 and 3 and Exercise Figures A and B.

Do not be concerned about which word root to use for skin or nail. As you continue to study and use medical terms, you will become familiar with common usage of each word part.

EXERCISE 2

Write the definitions of the following combining forms.

1. hidr/o _____

2. derm/o _____

3. onych/o _____

4. trich/o _____

5. kerat/o _____

6. dermat/o _____

7. seb/o _____

8. ungu/o _____

9. cutane/o _____

EXERCISE 3

Write the combining form for each of the following.

1. hair _____

2. sweat _____

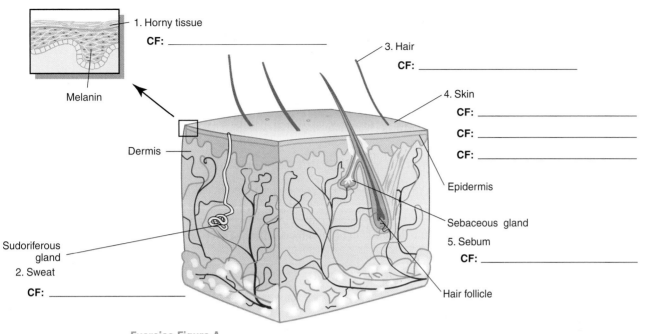

Exercise Figure A

Fill in the blanks with combining forms in this diagram of a cross section of the skin.

Labels in figure:
1. Horny tissue   CF: _____
Melanin
3. Hair   CF: _____
4. Skin   CF: _____
CF: _____
CF: _____
Epidermis
Sebaceous gland
5. Sebum   CF: _____
Dermis
Sudoriferous gland
2. Sweat   CF: _____
Hair follicle

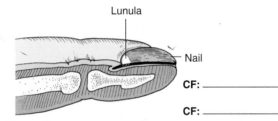

Labels in figure:
Lunula
Nail   CF: _____
CF: _____

Exercise Figure B

Fill in the blanks with combining forms in this cross section of the finger with nail.

3. nail   a. _____

                 b. _____

4. sebum   _____

5. skin   a. _____

                 b. _____

                 c. _____

6. hard, horny tissue   _____

Combining Forms Commonly Used with Integumentary System Terms

Combining Form	Definition
aut/o	self
bi/o	life

coni/o	dust
crypt/o	hidden
heter/o	other
myc/o	fungus
necr/o	death (cells, body)
pachy/o	thick
rhytid/o	wrinkles
staphyl/o	grapelike clusters
strept/o	twisted chain
xer/o	dry

Learn the combining forms by completing exercises 4 and 5.

 The prefix **bi-,** which means **two,** was presented in Chapter 3. The word root **bi** means **life.**

EXERCISE 4

Write the definitions of the following combining forms.

1. necr/o _____

2. staphyl/o _____

3. crypt/o _____

4. pachy/o _____

5. coni/o _____

6. myc/o _____

7. bi/o _____

8. heter/o _____

9. strept/o _____

10. xer/o _____

11. aut/o _____

12. rhytid/o _____

EXERCISE 5

Write the combining form for each of the following.

1. fungus _____

2. death (cells, body) _____

3. other _____

4. dry _____

5. thick _____

6. twisted chains _____

7. wrinkles _____

8. grapelike clusters _____

9. self _____

10. hidden _____

11. dust _____

12. life _____

Prefixes

Prefix	Definition
epi-	on, upon, over
intra-	within
para-	beside, beyond, around
per-	through
sub-	under, below

Learn the prefixes by completing exercises 6 and 7.

EXERCISE   6

Write the definitions of the following prefixes.

1. sub- _____

2. para- _____

3. epi- _____

4. intra- _____

5. per- _____

EXERCISE   7

Write the prefix for each of the following.

1. within _____

2. under, below _____

3. on, upon, over _____

4. beside, beyond, around _____

5. through _____

Suffixes

Suffix	Definition
-a	noun suffix, no meaning
-coccus (*pl.* -cocci)	berry-shaped (form of bacterium)
-ectomy	excision or surgical removal
-ia	diseased or abnormal state, condition of
-itis	inflammation
-malacia	softening
-opsy	view of, viewing
-phagia	eating or swallowing
-plasty	surgical repair
-rrhea	flow, excessive discharge
-tome	instrument used to cut

Refer to Appendix A and Appendix B for alphabetical lists of word parts and their meanings. Learn the suffixes by completing exercises 8 and 9.

EXERCISE 8

Match the suffixes in the first column with the correct definitions in the second column.

_____ 1. -coccus   a. inflammation

_____ 2. -ectomy   b. surgical repair

_____ 3. -itis   c. berry-shaped

_____ 4. -malacia   d. eating or swallowing

_____ 5. -opsy   e. excision or surgical removal

_____ 6. -rrhea   f. instrument used to cut

_____ 7. -phagia   g. thick

_____ 8. -plasty   h. flow, excessive discharge

_____ 9. -tome   i. view of, viewing

_____ 10. -ia   j. softening

      k. diseased or abnormal state, condition of

EXERCISE 9

Write the definitions of the following suffixes.

1. -plasty _____

2. -ectomy _____

3. -malacia _____

4. -itis _____

5. -tome _____

6. -phagia _____

7. -rrhea _____

8. -coccus _____

9. -opsy _____

10. -ia _____

MEDICAL TERMS

The terms you need to learn to complete this chapter are listed on the following pages. The exercises at the end of each list will help you learn each word well enough to add it to your vocabulary.

Disease and Disorder Terms

Built from Word Parts

Term	Definition
dermatitis (*der*-ma-TĪ-tis)	inflammation of the skin (Figure 4-2, *E*)
dermatoconiosis (*der*-ma-tō-kō-nē-Ō-sis)	abnormal condition of the skin caused by dust
dermatofibroma (*der*-ma-tō-fī-BRŌ-ma)	fibrous tumor of the skin
hidradenitis (*hī*-drad-e-NĪ-tis)	inflammation of a sweat gland
leiodermia (lī-ō-DER-mē-a)	condition of smooth skin
onychocryptosis (*on*-i-kō-krip-TŌ-sis)	abnormal condition of a hidden nail (also called *ingrown nail*)
onychomalacia (*on*-i-kō-ma-LĀ-shē-a)	softening of the nails
onychomycosis (*on*-i-kō-mī-KŌ-sis)	abnormal condition of a fungus in the nails (see Figure 4-2, *B*)
onychophagia (*on*-i-kō-FĀ-jē-a)	eating the nails (nail biting)
pachyderma (pak-i-DER-ma) (NOTE: the *a* ending is a noun suffix and has no meaning.)	thickening of the skin

★ CAM TERM

Hypnotherapy is using the power of suggestion and a state of altered consciousness involving focused attention to promote wellness. Hypnotherapy may be used to modulate stress associated with the exacerbation of dermatitis and eczema.

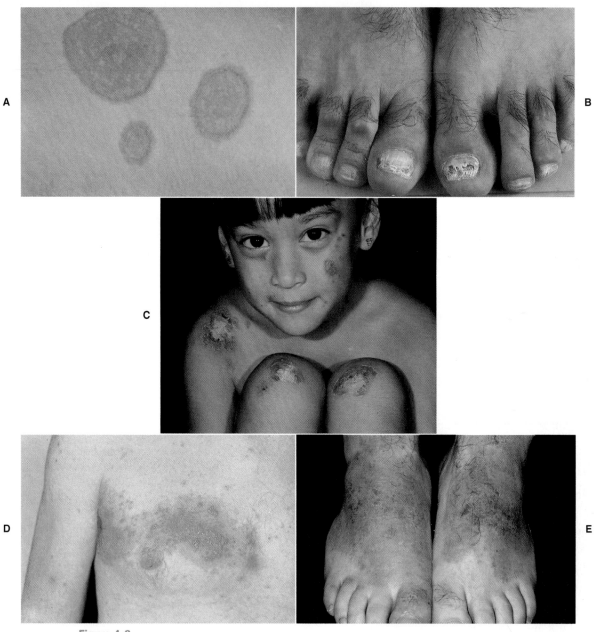

Figure 4-2
Common skin disorders: **A,** tinea; **B,** onychomycosis; **C,** impetigo; **D,** herpes zoster; **E,** dermatitis.

paronychia..
(par-ō-NIK-ē-a)
(NOTE: the *a* from para-
has been dropped. The final
vowel in a prefix may be
dropped when the word to
which it is added begins
with a vowel.)

diseased state around the nail (Exercise
Figure C)

seborrhea..
(*seb*-ōr-Ē-a)

excessive discharge of sebum

trichomycosis..
(*trik*-ō-mī-KŌ-sis)

abnormal condition of a fungus in the hair

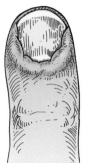

Exercise Figure C
Fill in the blanks to label the diagram.

—————— / ———— / ——————
around / **nail** / **diseased state**

xeroderma... dry skin
   (zē-rō-DER-ma)
   (NOTE: the *a* ending is a
   noun suffix and has no
   meaning.)

Practice saying each of these terms aloud. To hear the terms, access the **PRONOUNCE IT** activity for this chapter on the Student CD that accompanies this text. Or, to hear the terms and their definitions with a CD player or computer, obtain the Pronunciation CD designed for use with this text. Refer to the Pronunciation Guide on p. 25 as needed.

Learn the definitions and spellings of the terms used to describe diseases and disorders of the integumentary system by completing exercises 10, 11, and 12.

EXERCISE 10

Analyze and define the following terms used to describe integumentary system diseases and disorders. If you need to, refer to p. 6 for a review.

         WR   CV WR   S
Example: onych/o/myc/osis *abnormal condition of a fungus in the nails*
         CF

1. dermatoconiosis _____

2. hidradenitis _____

3. dermatitis _____

4. pachyderma _____

5. onychomalacia _____

6. trichomycosis _____

7. dermatofibroma _____

8. paronychia _____

9. onychocryptosis _____

10. seborrhea _____

11. onychophagia _____

12. xeroderma _____

13. leiodermia _____

EXERCISE 11

Build disease and disorder terms for the following definitions by using the word parts you have learned. If you need help, refer to p. 8 to review word-building techniques.

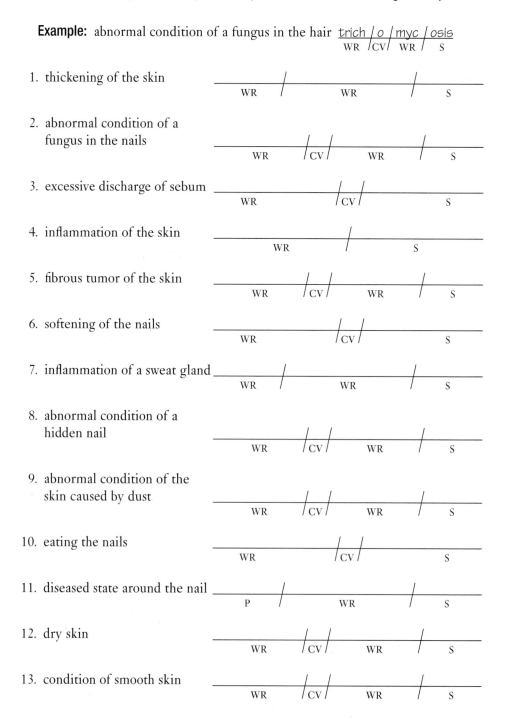

Example: abnormal condition of a fungus in the hair $\underline{\text{trich}}$ / $\underline{\text{o}}$ / $\underline{\text{myc}}$ / $\underline{\text{osis}}$
WR /CV/ WR / S

1. thickening of the skin
   _____ / _____ / _____
   WR   WR   S

2. abnormal condition of a
   fungus in the nails
   _____ /CV/ _____ / _____
   WR   WR   S

3. excessive discharge of sebum
   _____ /CV/ _____
   WR   S

4. inflammation of the skin
   _____ / _____
   WR   S

5. fibrous tumor of the skin
   _____ /CV/ _____ / _____
   WR   WR   S

6. softening of the nails
   _____ /CV/ _____
   WR   S

7. inflammation of a sweat gland
   _____ / _____ / _____
   WR   WR   S

8. abnormal condition of a
   hidden nail
   _____ /CV/ _____ / _____
   WR   WR   S

9. abnormal condition of the
   skin caused by dust
   _____ /CV/ _____ / _____
   WR   WR   S

10. eating the nails
    _____ /CV/ _____
    WR   S

11. diseased state around the nail
    _____ / _____ / _____
    P   WR   S

12. dry skin
    _____ /CV/ _____ / _____
    WR   WR   S

13. condition of smooth skin
    _____ /CV/ _____ / _____
    WR   WR   S

EXERCISE 12

Spell each of the terms used to describe integumentary diseases and disorders. Have someone dictate the terms on pp. 75-77 to you. **Think about the word parts before attempting to write the word.** Study any words you have spelled incorrectly.

1. _____   8. _____

2. _____   9. _____

3. _____   10. _____

4. _____   11. _____

5. _____   12. _____

6. _____   13. _____

7. _____   14. _____

Disease and Disorder Terms

Not Built from Word Parts

Term	Definition
abrasion (a-BRĀ-zhun)	scraping away of the skin by mechanical process or injury
abscess (AB-ses)	localized collection of pus
acne (AK-nē)	inflammatory disease of the skin involving the sebaceous glands and hair follicles
actinic keratosis (ack-TIN-ik) (ker-a-TŌ-sis)	a precancerous skin condition of horny tissue formation that results from excessive exposure to sunlight. It may evolve into a squamous cell carcinoma (Figure 4-3, *A*).
basal cell carcinoma (BCC) (BĀ-sal) (sel) (kar-si-NŌ-ma)	epithelial tumor arising from the epidermis. It seldom metastasizes but invades local tissue (Figure 4-3, *B*). Common in individuals who have had excessive sun exposure.
candidiasis (kan-di-DĪ-a-sis)	an infection of the skin, mouth (thrush), or vagina caused by the yeast-type fungus *Candida albicans. Candida* is normally present in the mucous membranes; overgrowth causes an infection. Esophageal candidiasis is often seen in patients with AIDS (acquired immunodeficiency syndrome).
carbuncle (KAR-bung-kl)	skin infection composed of a cluster of boils caused by staphylococcal bacteria
cellulitis (sel-ū-LĪ-tis)	inflammation of the skin and subcutaneous tissue caused by infection, leading to redness, swelling, and fever

Abscess
is derived from the Latin **ab**, meaning **from,** and **cedo,** meaning **to go.** The tissue dies and goes away, with the pus replacing it.

Acne
may be derived from **akme,** meaning **point.** Thus it was named for the point on a pimple.

Candida
comes from the Latin **candidus,** meaning **gleaming white;** albicans is from the Latin verb **albicare,** meaning **to make white.** The growth of the fungus is white, and the infection produces a white discharge.

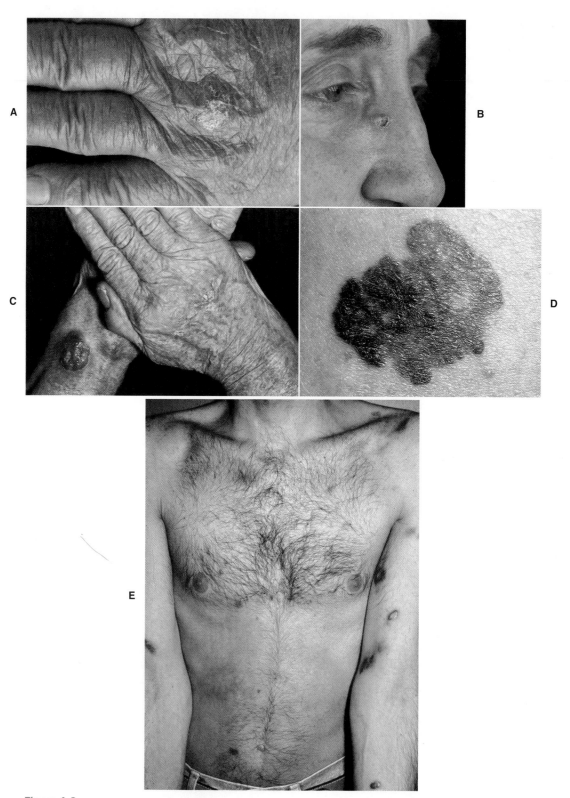

Figure 4-3

Percutaneous lesion and cancers of the skin. **A,** Actinic keratosis; **B,** basal cell carcinoma; **C,** squamous cell carcinoma; **D,** melanoma; **E,** Kaposi sarcoma.

contusion

(kon-TŪ-zhun)

injury with no break in the skin, characterized by pain, swelling, and discoloration (also called a *bruise*)

eczema

(EK-ze-ma)

noninfectious, inflammatory skin disease characterized by redness, blisters, scabs, and itching

fissure

(FISH-ūr)

slit or cracklike sore in the skin

furuncle

(FER-ung-kl)

painful skin node caused by staphylococcal bacteria in a hair follicle (also called a *boil*)

gangrene

(GANG-grēn)

death of tissue caused by loss of blood supply followed by bacterial invasion

herpes

(HER-pēz)

inflammatory skin disease caused by herpes virus characterized by small blisters in clusters. Many types of herpes exist. *Herpes simplex*, for example, causes fever blisters; *herpes zoster*, also called *shingles*, is characterized by painful skin eruptions that follow nerves inflamed by the virus (see Figure 4-2, *D*).

Herpes
is derived from the Greek **herpo**, meaning to **creep along.** It is descriptive of the course and type of skin lesion.

impetigo

(im-pe-TĪ-gō)

superficial skin infection characterized by pustules and caused by either staphylococci or streptococci (see Figure 4-2, *C*)

Kaposi sarcoma

(KAP-ō-sē) (sar-KŌ-ma)

a cancerous condition starting as purple or brown papules on the lower extremities that spreads through the skin to the lymph nodes and internal organs. Frequently seen with AIDS.

laceration

(*las*-er-A-shun)

torn, ragged-edged wound

lesion

(LĒ-zhun)

any visible change in tissue resulting from injury or disease. It is a broad term that includes sores, wounds, ulcers, and tumors.

pediculosis

(pe-*dik*-ū-LŌ-sis)

invasion into the skin and hair by lice

psoriasis

(so-RĪ-a-sis)

chronic skin condition producing red lesions covered with silvery scales

scabies

(SKĀ-bēz)

skin infection caused by the itch mite, characterized by papule eruptions that are caused by the female burrowing in the outer layer of the skin and laying eggs. This condition is accompanied by severe itching (Figure 4-4).

scleroderma

(skle-rō-DER-ma)

a disease characterized by chronic hardening (induration) of the connective tissue of the skin and other body organs

shingles

(SHIN-gls)

development of painful, inflamed blisters that follow the nerve routes. Caused by the same virus that causes chickenpox (see Figure 4-2, *D*) (also called *herpes zoster*).

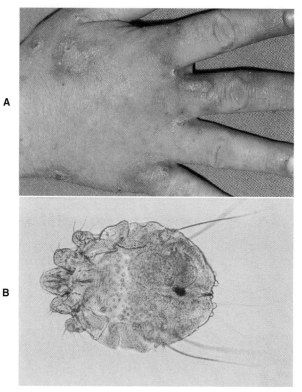

Figure 4-4
A, Scabies; **B,** scabies mite.

squamous cell carcinoma (SqCCa) ....
(SQWĀ-mus) (sel)
(kar-si-NŌ-ma)

a malignant growth that develops from scale-like epithelial tissue. On the skin it appears as a firm, red, painless bump. The most frequent cause is chronic exposure to sunlight (see Figure 4-3, *C*).

systemic lupus erythematosus (SLE) ....
(sis-TEM-ik) (LŪ-pus)
(e-rith-ma-TŌ-sus)

a chronic inflammatory disease involving the skin, joints, kidneys, and nervous system. This autoimmune disease is characterized by periods of remission and exacerbations. It also may affect other organs.

tinea ....
(TIN-ē-a)

fungus infection of the skin (see Figure 4-2) (also called *ringworm*)

urticaria ....
(ūr-ti-KA-rē-a)

an itching skin eruption composed of wheals of varying size and shape. It is usually related to an allergy (also called *hives*).

Practice saying each of these terms aloud. To hear the terms, access the **PRONOUNCE IT** activity for this chapter on the Student CD that accompanies this text. Or, to hear the terms and their definitions with a CD player or computer, obtain the Pronunciation CD designed for use with this text.

Learn the definitions and spellings of the terms by completing exercises 13, 14, 15, and 16.

EXERCISE 13

Fill in the blanks with the correct disease and disorder terms.

1. A chronic inflammatory disease affecting the skin, joints, and other organs is
_____ _____ _____.

2. A(n) _____ is a localized collection of pus.

3. A cracklike sore in the skin is called a(n) _____.

4. The scraping away of the skin by mechanical process or injury is called a(n)
_____.

5. _____ is a chronic skin condition characterized by red lesions
covered with silvery scales.

6. An inflammatory skin disease characterized by small blisters in clusters is
called _____.

7. _____ is the name given to the invasion of the skin and hair by
lice.

8. A fungus infection of the skin, also known as *ringworm,* is called
_____.

9. An injury with no break in the skin and characterized by pain, swelling, and
discoloration is called a(n) _____.

10. _____ is the name given to tissue death caused by a loss of blood
supply followed by bacterial invasion.

11. Any visible change in tissue resulting from injury or disease is called a
_____.

12. _____ _____ is a cancerous condition starting as purple or brown papules on the lower extremities.

13. A horny tissue formation that results from excessive exposure to sunlight and
is precancerous is called _____ _____.

14. A cluster of boils caused by staphylococcal bacteria is a _____.

15. An inflammatory skin disease that involves the oil glands and hair follicles is
called _____.

16. _____ is the name given to a torn, ragged-edged wound.

17. A painful skin node caused by staphylococcal bacteria in a hair follicle is
called a(n) _____.

18. A malignant growth that develops from scalelike epithelial tissue is known as
_____ _____ carcinoma.

19. Inflammation of the skin and subcutaneous tissue caused by infection and
creating redness, swelling, and fever is called _____.

20. _____ is the name given to a superficial skin infection characterized by pustules and caused by either staphylococci or streptococci.

21. _____ is a noninfectious inflammatory skin disease characterized by redness, blisters, scabs, and itching.

22. A skin inflammation caused by the itch mite is called _____.

23. _____ is an itching skin eruption composed of wheals.

24. An epithelial tumor commonly found on the face of individuals who have had excessive sun exposure is _____ _____ carcinoma.

25. _____ is a disease characterized by induration of the connective tissue.

26. _____ is an infection of the mouth, skin, or vagina caused by *Candida albicans.*

27. A condition of painful, inflamed blisters that follow nerve routes is called _____.

EXERCISE 14

Match the words in the first column with their correct definitions in the second column.

_____ 1. abrasion

_____ 2. abscess

_____ 3. acne

_____ 4. actinic keratosis

_____ 5. basal cell carcinoma

_____ 6. carbuncle

_____ 7. cellulitis

_____ 8. contusion

_____ 9. eczema

_____ 10. fissure

_____ 11. furuncle

_____ 12. gangrene

_____ 13. scleroderma

a. death of tissue caused by loss of blood supply and entry of bacteria

b. cracklike sore in the skin

c. cluster of boils

d. induration of connective tissue

e. noninfectious inflammatory skin disease having redness, blisters, scabs, and itching

f. scraped-away skin

g. involves sebaceous glands and hair follicles

h. painful skin node caused by staphylococci in a hair follicle

i. inflammation of skin and subcutaneous tissue with redness, swelling, and fever

j. localized collection of pus

k. injury characterized by pain, swelling, and discoloration

l. precancerous skin condition caused by excessive exposure to sunlight

m. epithelial tumor commonly found in individuals who have had excessive sun exposure

n. red lesions with silvery scales

EXERCISE   15

Match the words in the first column with the correct definitions in the second column.

_____ 1. herpes

_____ 2. impetigo

_____ 3. Kaposi sarcoma

_____ 4. laceration

_____ 5. lesion

_____ 6. pediculosis

_____ 7. psoriasis

_____ 8. scabies

_____ 9. squamous cell carcinoma

_____ 10. systemic lupus erythematosus

_____ 11. tinea

_____ 12. urticaria

_____ 13. candidiasis

_____ 14. shingles

a. skin inflammation caused by the itch mite

b. fungus infection of the skin

c. red lesions covered by silvery scales

d. inflammatory skin disease having clusters of blisters

e. chronic inflammatory disease involving the skin, joints, kidney, and nervous system

f. a cancerous condition that starts as brown or purple papules on the lower extremities

g. composed of wheals

h. torn, ragged-edged wound

i. superficial skin condition having pustules and caused by staphylococci or streptococci

j. infection of the skin, mouth, or vagina caused by a yeast-type fungus

k. invasion of the hair and skin by lice

l. visible change in tissue resulting from injury or disease

m. a malignant growth that develops from scalelike epithelial tissue

n. lesions caused by herpes zoster virus

o. cracklike sore in the skin

EXERCISE   16

Spell each of the terms not built from word parts that are used to describe integumentary diseases and disorders. Have someone dictate the terms on pp. 79 and 81-82 to you. Study any words you have spelled incorrectly.

1. _____

2. _____

3. _____

4. _____

5. _____

6. _____

7. _____

8. _____

9. _____ 18. _____

10. _____ 19. _____

11. _____ 20. _____

12. _____ 21. _____

13. _____ 22. _____

14. _____ 23. _____

15. _____ 24. _____

16. _____ 25. _____

17. _____ 26. _____

27. _____

Surgical Terms

Built from Word Parts

Term	Definition
biopsy (bx) (BĪ-op-sē)	view of life (the removal of living tissue from the body to be viewed under the microscope)
dermatoautoplasty (*der*-ma-tō-AW-tō-*plas*-tē)	surgical repair using one's own skin (skin graft) (also called *autograft*)
dermatoheteroplasty (*der*-ma-tō-HET-er-ō-*plas*-tē)	surgical repair using skin from others (skin graft) (also called *allograft*)
dermatoplasty (DER-ma-tō-*plas*-tē)	surgical repair of the skin
onychectomy (on-i-KEK-tō-mē)	excision of a nail
rhytidectomy (rit-i-DEK-tō-mē)	excision of wrinkles (also called *facelift*)
rhytidoplasty (RIT-i-dō-*plas*-tē)	surgical repair of wrinkles

Practice saying each of these terms aloud. To hear the terms, access the **PRONOUNCE IT** activity for this chapter on the Student CD that accompanies this text. Or, to hear the terms and their definitions with a CD player or computer, obtain the Pronunciation CD designed for use with this text.

Learn the definitions and spellings of the surgical terms by completing exercises 17, 18, and 19.

Mohs Surgery
allows for complete tumor removal while sparing surrounding normal tissue. It includes removing layers of tissue and examining them for tumor cells. If found, more tissue is removed until the margins are cancer free.
It is used to treat recurrent skin cancers, especially lesions on the nose and ears, or areas that need tissue sparing. It is named after **Dr Fredric Mohs,** Wisconsin, who first used the concept in 1936. The technique has evolved since that time.

EXERCISE 17

Analyze and define the following surgical terms.

　　　　　　WR　　CV　　S
Example: dermat/o/plasty　*surgical repair of the skin*
　　　　　　　　CF

1. rhytidectomy _____

2. biopsy _____

3. dermatoautoplasty _____

4. onychectomy _____

5. rhytidoplasty _____

6. dermatoheteroplasty _____

EXERCISE 18

Build surgical terms for the following definitions by using the word parts you have learned.

Example: surgical repair using one's own skin　dermat / o / aut / o / plasty
　　　　　　　　　　　　　　　　　　　　　　　WR　 /CV/ WR /CV/　 S

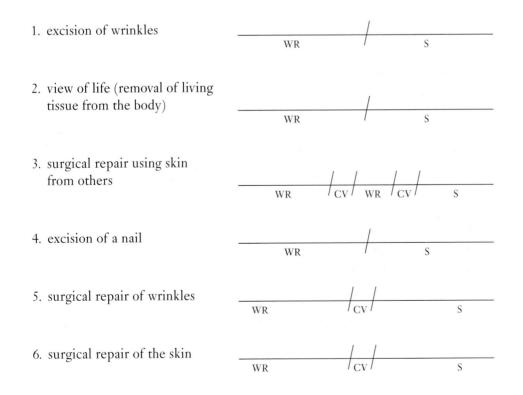

1. excision of wrinkles

　　WR　　　　　S

2. view of life (removal of living tissue from the body)

　　WR　　　　　S

3. surgical repair using skin from others

　　WR　　CV　WR　CV　　S

4. excision of a nail

　　WR　　　　　S

5. surgical repair of wrinkles

　　WR　　CV　　　S

6. surgical repair of the skin

　　WR　　CV　　　S

EXERCISE 19

Spell each of the surgical terms. Have someone dictate the terms on p. 86 to you. Think about the word parts before attempting to write each word. Study any words you have spelled incorrectly.

1. _____   5. _____

2. _____   6. _____

3. _____   7. _____

4. _____

Complementary Terms

Built from Word Parts

Term	Definition
dermatologist............................ (*der*-ma-TOL-ō-jist)	a physician who studies and treats skin (diseases)
dermatology .... (der-ma-TOL-ō-jē)	study of the skin (a branch of medicine that deals with the diagnosis and treatment of skin diseases)
dermatome................................ (DER-ma-tōm) (NOTE: when two consonants of the same letter come together, one is sometimes dropped.)	instrument used to cut skin
epidermal.................................. (*ep*-i-DER-mal)	pertaining to upon the skin
erythroderma............................. (e-rith-rō-DER-ma) (NOTE: the *a* ending is a noun suffix and has no meaning.)	red skin (abnormal redness of the skin)
hypodermic................................ (*hī*-pō-DER-mik)	pertaining to under the skin
intradermal .... (*in*-tra-DER-mal)	pertaining to within the skin
keratogenic............................... (ker-a-tō-JEN-ik)	originating in horny tissue
leukoderma................................ (lū-kō-DER-ma) (NOTE: the *a* ending is a noun suffix and has no meaning.)	white skin (less color than normal)
necrosis.................................... (ne-KRŌ-sis)	abnormal condition of death (cells and tissue die because of disease)

percutaneous .... (per-kū-TĀ-nē-us)	pertaining to through the skin
staphylococcus (*pl.* **staphylococci**) **(staph)** .... (*staf*-il-ō-KOK-us, *staf*-il-ō-KOK-si)	berry-shaped (bacteria) in grapelike clusters (these bacteria cause many skin diseases) (Exercise Figure D)

Refer to Table 13-1, Plural Endings.

streptococcus (*pl.* **streptococci**) **(strep)** .... (*strep*-tō-KOK-us, *strep*-tō-KOK-si)	berry-shaped (bacteria) in twisted chains (Exercise Figure E)
subcutaneous (subQ) .... (sub-kū-TĀ-nē-us)	pertaining to under the skin
ungual .... (UNG-gwal)	pertaining to the nail
xanthoderma .... (zan-thō-DER-ma) (NOTE: the *a* ending is a noun suffix and has no meaning.)	yellow skin (also called *jaundice*)

Practice saying each of these terms aloud. To hear the terms, access the **PRONOUNCE IT** activity for this chapter on the Student CD that accompanies this text. Or, to hear the terms and their definitions with a CD player or computer, obtain the Pronunciation CD designed for use with this text.

Learn the definitions and spellings of the complementary terms by completing exercises 20, 21, and 22.

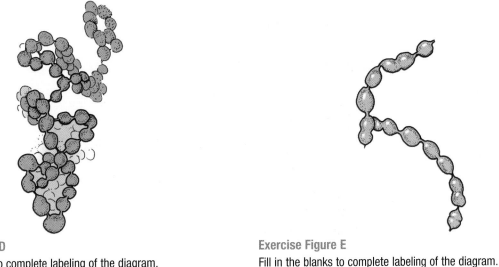

Exercise Figure D
Fill in the blanks to complete labeling of the diagram.

_____ bacteria
grapelike clusters / **cv** / **berry-shaped (plural)**

Exercise Figure E
Fill in the blanks to complete labeling of the diagram.

_____ bacteria
twisted chains / **cv** / **berry-shaped (plural)**

EXERCISE 20

Analyze and define the following complementary terms.

Example: $\overset{P}{\text{intra}}/\overset{WR}{\text{derm}}/\overset{S}{\text{al}}$ _pertaining to within the skin_

1. ungual _____

2. dermatome _____

3. streptococcus _____

4. hypodermic _____

5. dermatology _____

6. subcutaneous _____

7. staphylococcus _____

8. keratogenic _____

9. dermatologist _____

10. necrosis _____

11. epidermal _____

12. xanthoderma _____

13. erythroderma _____

14. leukoderma _____

15. percutaneous _____

EXERCISE 21

Build complementary terms for the integumentary system by using the word parts you have learned.

Example: pertaining to under the skin $\underset{\text{P}}{\text{hypo}}/\underset{\text{WR}}{\text{derm}}/\underset{\text{S}}{\text{ic}}$

1. study of the skin

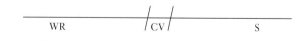

2. abnormal condition of death
   (of cells and tissue)

3. instrument used to cut skin _____/_____
                                   WR   S

4. pertaining to the nail _____/_____
                              WR   S

5. berry-shaped bacteria in
   grapelike clusters _____/__/_____
                          WR   CV   S

6. a physician who studies and
   treats skin (diseases) _____/__/_____
                             WR   CV   S

7. pertaining to within the skin _____/_____/_____
                                     P   WR   S

8. pertaining to upon the skin _____/_____/_____
                                   P   WR   S

9. pertaining to under the skin _____/_____/_____
                                    P   WR   S

   _____/_____/_____
      P   WR   S

10. berry-shaped bacteria in
    twisted chains _____/__/_____
                       WR   CV   S

11. originating in the horny tissue _____/__/_____
                                        WR   CV   S

12. white skin _____/__/_____/_____
                   WR   CV   WR   S

13. red skin _____/__/_____/_____
                 WR   CV   WR   S

14. yellow skin _____/__/_____/_____
                    WR   CV   WR   S

15. pertaining to through the skin _____/_____/_____
                                       P   WR   S

EXERCISE 22

Spell each of the complementary terms. Have someone dictate the terms on pp. 88-89 to you. Think about the word parts before attempting to write the word. Study any words you have spelled incorrectly.

1. _____   9. _____

2. _____   10. _____

3. _____   11. _____

4. _____   12. _____

5. _____   13. _____

6. _____   14. _____

7. _____   15. _____

8. _____   16. _____

Adipose

contains the Latin word root **adip** meaning **fat**. Adipose tissue is composed of fat cells arranged in lobules. **Lip** is the Greek word root for **fat.**

Albino

contains the Latin word root **alb** meaning **white. Leuk** is the Greek word root meaning **white.**

Complementary Terms

Not Built from Word Parts

Term	Definition
adipose .... (AD-i-pōs)	fat, fatty
albino .... (al-BĪ-nō)	an individual with pigment deficiency in the eyes, hair, and skin. A hereditary disorder (Figure 4-5).
allergy .... (AL-er-jē)	hypersensitivity to a substance

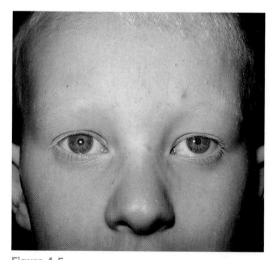

Figure 4-5
White hair and pale skin of albino.

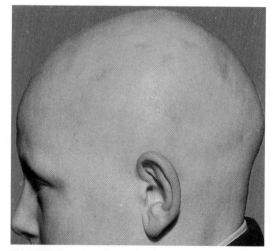

Figure 4-6
Alopecia totalis (loss of hair from the scalp) with absence of eyelashes.

alopecia .... loss of hair (Figure 4-6)
 (al-ō-PĒ-shē-a)

Alopecia
is derived from the Greek **alopex,** meaning **fox.** One was thought to bald like a mangy fox.

cicatrix .... scar
 (SIK-a-triks)

cyst .... a closed sac containing fluid or semisolid
 (sist)   material (Table 4-1)

cytomegalovirus (CMV) .... a herpes-type virus that usually causes disease
 (sī-tō-meg-a-lō-VĪ-rus)   when the immune system is compromised

debridement .... removal of contaminated or dead tissue and
 (da-BRĒD-mon)   foreign matter from an open wound

dermabrasion .... procedure to remove skin scars with abrasive
 (*derm*-a-BRĀ-zhun)   material, such as sandpaper

diaphoresis .... profuse sweating
 (dī-a-fō-RĒ-sis)

Diaphoresis
is derived from Greek **dia,** meaning **through,** and **phoreo,** meaning **I carry.** Translated, it means the carrying through of perspiration.

ecchymosis .... escape of blood into the tissues, causing super-
 (ek-i-MŌ-sis)   ficial discoloration; a "black and blue" mark

edema .... puffy swelling of tissue from the accumulation
 (e-DĒ-ma)   of fluid

emollient .... agent that softens or soothes the skin
 (e-MOL-yent)

erythema .... redness
 (er-i-THĒ-ma)

induration .... abnormal hard spot(s)
 (in-dū-RĀ-shun)

jaundice .... condition characterized by a yellow tinge to
 (JAWN-dis)   the skin (xanthoderma)

keloid .... overgrowth of scar tissue (Figure 4-7)
 (KĒ-loyd)

leukoplakia .... condition characterized by white spots or
 (lū-kō-PLĀ-kē-a)   patches on mucous membrane, which may be
                                              precancerous

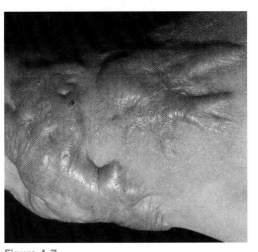

Figure 4-7
Burn keloid.

TABLE 4-1

Common Skin Lesions

Lesion	Definition	Cutaway Sections	Example
Macule	flat, colored spot on the skin		freckle
Papule	small solid skin elevation		skin tag basal cell carcinoma
Nodule	a small knotlike mass		lipoma metastatic carcinoma rheumatoid nodule
Wheal	round, itchy elevation of the skin		urticaria (hive)
Vesicle	small elevation of epidermis containing liquid		shingles *(Herpes zoster)* Herpes simplex contact dermatitis
Pustule	elevation of the skin containing pus		impetigo acne
Cyst	a closed sac containing fluid or semisolid material		acne

macule (MAK-ūl)	flat, colored spot on the skin (see Table 4-1)
nevus (*pl.* nevi) (NĒ-vus, NĒ-vī)	circumscribed malformation of the skin, usually brown, black, or flesh colored. A congenital nevus is present at birth and is referred to as a birthmark (see Figure 4-9, *A*) (also called a *mole*).
nodule (NOD-ūl)	a small knotlike mass that can be felt by touch (see Table 4-1)
pallor (PAL-ōr)	paleness
papule (PAP-ūl)	small, solid skin elevation (Table 4-1) (also called *pimple*)
petechia (*pl.* petechiae) (pe-TĒ-kē-a, pe-TĒ-kē-ē)	pinpoint skin hemorrhages
pruritus (prū-RĪ-tus)	severe itching
purpura (PER-pū-ra)	disorder characterized by hemorrhages into the tissue, giving the skin a purple-red discoloration
pustule (PUS-tūl)	elevation of skin containing pus (see Table 4-1)
ulcer (UL-ser)	eroded sore on the skin or mucous membrane (Figure 4-8)
verruca (ver-RŪ-ka)	circumscribed cutaneous elevation caused by a virus (see Figure 4-9, *A*) (also called *wart*)
vesicle (VES-i-kl)	small elevation of the epidermis containing liquid (see Table 4-1) (also called *blister*)
virus (VĪ-ras)	an infectious agent
wheal (hwēl)	transitory, itchy elevation of the skin with a white center and a red surrounding area; a wheal is an individual urticaria (hive) lesion (see Table 4-1)

Macule
is probably derived from the ancient Sanskrit word **mala,** meaning **dirt.**

Petechia
is originally from the Italian **petechio,** meaning **flea bite.** The small hemorrhagic spot resembles the mark made by a flea.

Pressure Ulcer
is an open skin area that often occurs in bedridden patients. Also known as a **decubitus ulcer** or **bed sore.**

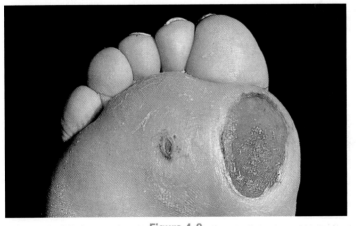

Figure 4-8
Skin ulcer.

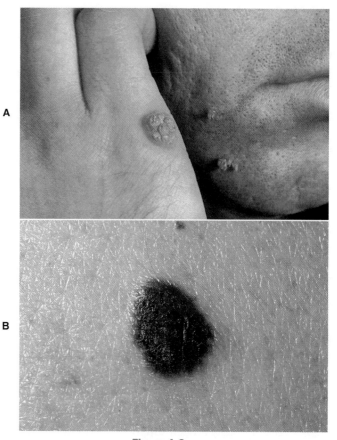

Figure 4-9
A, Verruca (wart); **B,** nevus (mole).

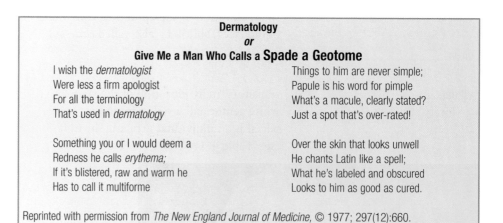

Dermatology
or
Give Me a Man Who Calls a Spade a Geotome

I wish the *dermatologist*
Were less a firm apologist
For all the terminology
That's used in *dermatology*

Something you or I would deem a
Redness he calls *erythema;*
If it's blistered, raw and warm he
Has to call it multiforme

Things to him are never simple;
Papule is his word for pimple
What's a macule, clearly stated?
Just a spot that's over-rated!

Over the skin that looks unwell
He chants Latin like a spell;
What he's labeled and obscured
Looks to him as good as cured.

Reprinted with permission from *The New England Journal of Medicine,* © 1977; 297(12):660.

Practice saying each of these terms aloud. To hear the terms, access the **PRONOUNCE IT** activity for this chapter on the Student CD that accompanies this text. Or, to hear the terms and their definitions with a CD player or computer, obtain the Pronunciation CD designed for use with this text.

Learn the definitions and spellings of the terms by completing exercises 23 through 26.

EXERCISE 23

Fill in the blanks with the correct terms.

1. Another name for *scar* is _____.

2. Profuse sweating is called _____.

3. The term for an agent that softens or soothes the skin is _____.

4. The medical term for *wart* is _____.

5. _____ is the name for a flat, colored skin spot.

6. A yellow skin condition is known as _____.

7. The condition of white spots or patches on mucous membrane is called _____.

8. _____ are pinpoint hemorrhages of the skin.

9. An eroded sore is called a(n) _____.

10. A(n) _____ is an overgrowth of scar tissue.

11. Another name for paleness is _____.

12. Superficial skin discoloration caused by escaping blood is referred to as _____.

13. An individual with pigment deficiency is called a(n) _____.

14. A small knotlike mass that can be felt by touch is called a(n) _____.

15. Another term for fat is _____.

16. A closed sac containing fluid or semisolid material is called a(n) _____.

17. Severe itching is called _____.

18. Another name for redness is _____.

19. The condition of tissue hemorrhages giving the skin a purple-red discoloration is known as _____.

20. _____ is another name for mole.

21. The removal of dead or contaminated tissue from an open wound is called _____.

22. The term for loss of hair is _____.

23. Hypersensitivity to a substance is called a(n) _____.

24. A small, solid skin elevation is called a(n) _____.

25. A transitory skin elevation with a white center and a red surrounding area is a(n) _____.

26. A(n) _____ is a skin elevation containing pus.

27. A blister is also called a(n) _____.

28. _____ is the procedure that uses abrasive material to remove scars.

29. A(n) _____ is an infectious agent.

30. An abnormal hard spot(s) is called _____.

31. _____ is the swelling of tissue.

32. _____ is a herpes-type virus.

EXERCISE 24

Match the words in the first column with their correct definitions in the second column.

_____ 1. adipose

_____ 2. albino

_____ 3. allergy

_____ 4. alopecia

_____ 5. cicatrix

_____ 6. debridement

_____ 7. nodule

_____ 8. dermabrasion

_____ 9. diaphoresis

_____ 10. cyst

_____ 11. ecchymosis

_____ 12. emollient

_____ 13. erythema

_____ 14. jaundice

_____ 15. edema

_____ 16. induration

a. loss of hair

b. superficial discoloration caused by blood escaping into the tissues

c. yellow color to the skin

d. closed sac containing fluid

e. removal of dead tissue from an open wound

f. agent that softens or soothes the skin

g. profuse sweating

h. hypersensitivity to a substance

i. hard spot(s)

j. scar

k. redness

l. procedure to remove skin scars by using abrasive material

m. fat

n. small knot

o. an individual with pigment deficiency

p. patches

q. swelling of tissue

EXERCISE 25

Match the terms in the first column with their correct definitions in the second column.

_____ 1. keloid

_____ 2. leukoplakia

_____ 3. macule

_____ 4. nevus

_____ 5. pallor

_____ 6. papule

_____ 7. petechiae

_____ 8. pruritus

_____ 9. purpura

_____ 10. pustule

_____ 11. ulcer

_____ 12. verruca

_____ 13. vesicle

_____ 14. wheal

_____ 15. virus

_____ 16. cytomegalovirus

a. mole

b. severe itching

c. wart

d. condition of white spots or patches on mucous membranes

e. hemorrhages in tissue giving skin a red-purple color

f. skin elevation containing pus

g. overgrowth of scar tissue

h. small elevation of epidermis containing liquid

i. individual urticaria lesion

j. flat, colored spot on skin

k. small, solid skin elevation

l. paleness

m. an infectious agent

n. pinpoint skin hemorrhages

o. eroded sore on the skin or mucous membrane

p. profuse sweating

q. herpes-type virus

EXERCISE 26

Spell each of the complementary terms. Have someone dictate the terms on pp. 92, 93, and 95 to you. Study any words you have spelled incorrectly.

1. _____

2. _____

3. _____

4. _____

5. _____

6. _____

7. _____

8. _____

9. _____

10. _____

11. _____

12. _____

13. _____

14. _____

15. _____

16. _____

17. _____   25. _____

18. _____   26. _____

19. _____   27. _____

20. _____   28. _____

21. _____   29. _____

22. _____   30. _____

23. _____   31. _____

24. _____   32. _____

Abbreviations

BCC	basal cell carcinoma
bx	biopsy
CMV	cytomegalovirus
SLE	systemic lupus erythematosus
SqCCA	squamous cell carcinoma
staph	staphylococcus
strep	streptococcus
subQ	subcutaneous

Refer to Appendix D for a complete list of abbreviations.

EXERCISE 27

Write the meaning for each of the abbreviations in the following sentences.

1. The most common form of skin cancer is **BCC** _____
   _____ _____.

2. It is rare to see cutaneous **CMV** _____ infections.

3. **SLE** _____ _____ _____ is a
   chronic relapsing disease, often with long periods of remission.

4. Long-term exposure to sunlight is by far the most frequent cause of **SqCCA**
   _____ _____ _____.

5. The **bx** _____ results were negative.

6. The medication was administered by **subQ**_____
   injection.

7. **Staph** _____ bacterium was cultured from the abscess.

8. The culture confirmed a **strep** _____ infection of the throat.

CHAPTER REVIEW

EXERCISE 28   *Interact with Medical Records*

Below is a written operative report. Complete the report by writing the medical terms in the blanks that correspond to the numbered definitions.

University Hospital and Medical Center
4700 North Main Street • Wellness, Arizona 54321 • (987) 555-3210

PATIENT NAME: Sandra Wharton   **CASE NUMBER:** 76548-INT
DATE OF BIRTH: 10/03/xx   **DATE:** 07/27/xx

OPERATIVE REPORT

CASE HISTORY: Mrs. Wharton is a 50-year-old white woman presenting to the 1. _____ clinic for follow-up of a 2. _____ located at the 3. _____ aspect of her left eyebrow.

Patient's medical history is also significant for 4. _____ _____, primarily of the scalp and ears, as well as chronic 5. _____, primarily of the forearms bilaterally.

INDICATIONS FOR PROCEDURE: Comparing today's exam with past medical records and photos from 10/20/xx, the nevus shows changes that include hair loss, "crusty" surface, and some enlargement of a 6. _____. The nevus has been present for approximately 3 years. Risks, benefits, indications, and expectations were discussed with the patient regarding excision and biopsy, and she has agreed to proceed.

PREOPERATIVE DIAGNOSIS: Dysplastic nevus, left eyebrow.

ANESTHESIA: Xylocaine 1% with Epinephrine.

PROCEDURE: After written consent was obtained, the site was prepped and draped in the usual sterile fashion with Betadine. The skin was incised at the 7. _____ pole of lesion. The lesion was then excised as diagnosed, including a margin of clinically normal dermis. Specimen was submitted to 8. _____. The superior pole was sutured. Hemostasis was achieved with electrocautery. Two A-T flaps were then constructed on superior aspect of upper left eyelid. Flaps and upper left eyelid undermined 2 to 3 mm. Flaps sutured with 6-0 Vicryl, followed by 6-0 nylon for closure. Pressure dressing was applied.

Patient tolerated the procedure well.

POSTOPERATIVE DIAGNOSIS: 9. _____ revealed 10. _____ _____ _____, nodular, transected at base.

William Hickman, MD (surgeon)

WH/mcm

---

1. study of skin
2. mole
3. pertaining to the middle
4. precancerous skin condition
5. noninfectious, inflammatory skin disease with redness, blisters, scabs, and itching
6. changes in tissue resulting from injury or disease
7. pertaining to above
8. study of disease
9. view of life
10. epithelial tumor arising from epidermis

EXERCISE 29 *Interpret Medical Terms*

To test your understanding of the terms introduced in this chapter, circle the words that correctly complete the sentences. The italicized words refer to the correct answer.

1. The physician called *the injury with pain, swelling, and discoloration with no break in the skin* a (fissure, contusion, laceration).
2. *Berry-shaped bacteria in grapelike clusters* are (streptococci, staphylococci, pediculosis).
3. The physician ordered lotions applied to the patient's *skin* to alleviate *dryness,* or (pachyderma, dermatoconiosis, xeroderma).
4. The injection given *within the skin* is called a(n) (intradermal, epidermal, hypodermic) injection.
5. The diagnosis of *onychomalacia* was given by the physician for (ingrown nails, nail biting, softening of the nails).
6. The *pinpoint hemorrhages,* or (nevi, verrucae, petechiae), were distributed over the patient's entire body.
7. The primary symptom of the disease was *profuse sweating,* or (diaphoresis, ecchymosis, pruritus).
8. The patient had an *abnormal condition of fungus in the hair;* therefore the doctor recorded the diagnosis as (onychocryptosis, trichomycosis, onychomycosis).
9. The student nurse learned that the medical name for a *blister* was (verruca, keloid, vesicle).
10. The patient was to receive a *skin graft from her mother,* so the operation was listed as a (dermatoplasty, dermatoautoplasty, dermatoheteroplasty).
11. An *abnormal hard spot* is called (edema, induration, virus).
12. Another word for *jaundice* is (erythroderma, leukoderma, xanthoderma).
13. *Leiodermia* is a condition of (striated, smooth, sweaty) skin.

EXERCISE 30 *Read Medical Terms in Use*

Practice pronunciation of terms by reading aloud the following medical document. Use the pronunciation key following the medical term to assist you in saying the word.

> Emily visited the **dermatology** (der-ma-TOL-ō-jē) clinic because of **pruritus** (prū-RĪ-tus) secondary to **dermatitis** (*der*-ma-TĪ-tis) involving her scalp, arms, and legs. A diagnosis of **psoriasis** (so-RĪ-a-sis) was made. **Eczema** (EK-ze-ma), **scabies** (SKĀ-bēz), and **tinea** (TIN-ē-a) were considered in the differential diagnosis. An **emollient** (e-MOL-yent) cream was prescribed. In addition the patient showed the **dermatologist** (*der*-ma-TOL-ō-jist) the tender, discolored, thickened nail of her right great toe. Emily learned she had **onychomycosis** (*on*-i-kō-mī-KŌ-sis), for which she was given an additional prescription for an oral antifungal drug.

EXERCISE 31 *Comprehend Medical Terms in Use*

Test your comprehension of terms in the above medical document by circling the correct answer.

1. Emily sought medical attention because of:
   a. an eroded sore and inflammation of the skin
   b. severe itching and inflammation of the skin
   c. severe itching and thickness of the skin
   d. an eroded sore and thickening of the skin

2. T F An inflammatory disease of the skin involving sebaceous glands and hair follicles was considered in the differential diagnosis.
3. Emily was given an additional prescription for an abnormal condition of fungus in the:
   a. sudoriferous glands
   b. hair follicles
   c. sebaceous glands
   d. nails

For further practice or to evaluate what you have learned, use the Student CD that accompanies this text.

COMBINING FORMS CROSSWORD PUZZLE

Across Clues
 4. dust
 5. skin
 7. hair
11. grapelike clusters
13. death (cells, body)
17. wrinkles
18. self
19. other

Down Clues
 1. horny tissue, hard
 2. sweat
 3. dry
 6. sebum
 8. skin
 9. fungus
10. thick
12. twisted chains
14. hidden
15. nail
16. life

REVIEW OF WORD PARTS

Can you define and spell the following word parts?

Combining Forms

aut/o	myc/o
bi/o	necr/o
coni/o	onych/o
crypt/o	pachy/o
cutane/o	rhytid/o
dermat/o	seb/o
derm/o	staphyl/o
heter/o	strept/o
hidr/o	trich/o
kerat/o	ungu/o
	xer/o

Prefixes

epi-
intra-
para-
per-
sub-

Suffixes

-coccus (*pl.* -cocci)
-ectomy
-ia
-itis
-malacia
-opsy
-phagia
-plasty
-rrhea
-tome

REVIEW OF TERMS

Can you build, analyze, define, pronounce, and spell the following terms *built from word parts?*

Diseases and Disorders

dermatitis	onychomycosis
dermatoconiosis	onychophagia
dermatofibroma	pachyderma
hidradenitis	paronychia
leiodermia	seborrhea
onychocryptosis	trichomycosis
onychomalacia	xeroderma

Surgical

biopsy (bx)
dermatoautoplasty
dermatoheteroplasty
dermatoplasty
onychectomy
rhytidectomy
rhytidoplasty

Complementary

dermatologist	necrosis
dermatology	percutaneous
dermatome	staphylococcus (staph)
epidermal	(*pl.* staphylococci)
erythroderma	streptococcus (strep)
hypodermic	(*pl.* streptococci)
intradermal	subcutaneous (subQ)
keratogenic	ungual
leukoderma	xanthoderma

Can you define, pronounce, and spell the following terms *not built from word parts?*

Diseases and Disorders

abrasion	herpes
abscess	impetigo
acne	Kaposi sarcoma
actinic keratosis	laceration
basal cell carcinoma (BCC)	lesion
candidiasis	pediculosis
carbuncle	psoriasis
cellulitis	scabies
contusion	scleroderma
eczema	shingles
fissure	squamous cell carcinoma (SqCCA)
furuncle	systemic lupus erythematosus (SLE)
gangrene	tinea
	urticaria

Complementary

adipose	jaundice
albino	keloid
allergy	leukoplakia
alopecia	macule
cicatrix	nevus (*pl.* nevi)
cyst	nodule
cytomegalovirus (CMV)	pallor
debridement	papule
dermabrasion	petechia (*pl.* petechiae)
diaphoresis	pruritus
ecchymosis	purpura
edema	pustule
emollient	ulcer
erythema	verruca
induration	vesicle
	virus
	wheal

5

Respiratory System

OUTLINE

OBJECTIVES

On completion of this chapter you will be able to:

1. Identify the organs and other structures of the respiratory system.
2. Define and spell the word parts presented in this chapter.
3. Build and analyze medical terms with word parts presented in this and previous chapters.
4. Define, pronounce, and spell the disease and disorder, diagnostic, surgical, and complementary terms for the respiratory system.
5. Interpret the meanings of the abbreviations presented in this chapter.
6. Read medical documents and interpret medical terminology contained in them.

ANATOMY

Function

The function of the respiratory system is the exchange of oxygen (O_2) and carbon dioxide (CO_2) between the atmosphere and body cells. The process is called *respiration*. During external respiration, or breathing, oxygen passes from the lungs to the blood in the capillaries. Carbon dioxide also passes from the capillaries back into the lungs to be expelled. During internal respiration the body cells take on oxygen from the blood and give back carbon dioxide, which is transported back to the lungs. The process of inhalation brings air into the lungs. Exhalation expels air from the lungs. Respirations, or breathing, normally occur every 3 to 5 seconds (Figure 5-1).

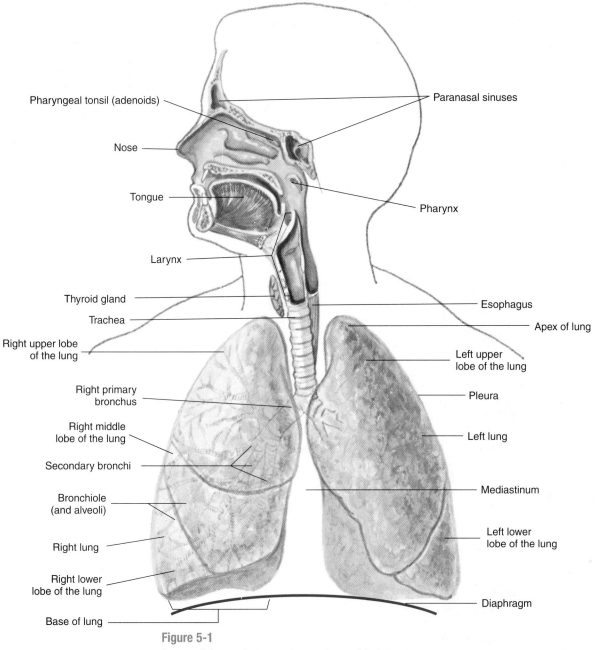

Figure 5-1

Organs of the respiratory system and associated structures.

Organs of the Respiratory System

nose	lined with mucous membrane and fine hairs. It acts as a filter to moisten and warm the entering air (Figure 5-2).
nasal septum	partition separating the right and left nasal cavities (see Figure 5-2)
paranasal sinuses	air cavities within the cranial bones that open into the nasal cavities
pharynx (also called the *throat*)	serves as a food and air passageway. Air enters from the nasal cavities and passes through the pharynx to the larynx. Food enters the pharynx from the mouth and passes into the esophagus.
adenoids	lymphoid tissue located behind the nasal cavity (see Figure 5-1)
tonsils	lymphoid tissue located behind the mouth (see Figure 5-2)
larynx (also called the *voice box*)	location of the vocal cords. Air enters from the pharynx (see Figure 5-1).
epiglottis	flap of cartilage that automatically covers the opening of and keeps food from entering the larynx during swallowing (see Figure 5-2)
trachea (also called the *windpipe*)	passageway for air to the bronchi (see Figure 5-1)

Adam's Apple
is the largest ring of cartilage in the larynx and is also known as the **thyroid cartilage.** The name came from the belief that Adam, realizing he had sinned when he ate the forbidden fruit, was unable to swallow the apple lodged in his throat.

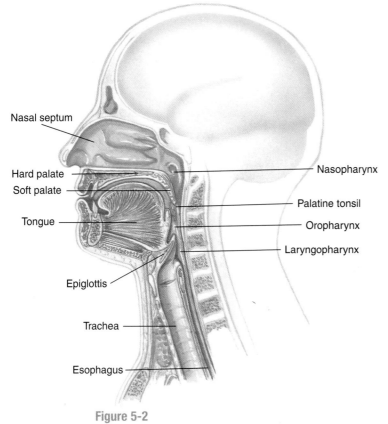

Nasal septum

Hard palate
Soft palate
Tongue

Nasopharynx
Palatine tonsil
Oropharynx
Laryngopharynx

Epiglottis

Trachea

Esophagus

Figure 5-2
Structures of the nasal passages and throat.

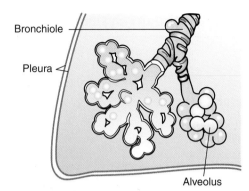

Figure 5-3
Bronchioles and alveoli.

Bronchi
originated from the Greek **brecho**, meaning **to pour** or **wet**. An ancient belief was that the esophagus carried solid food to the stomach and the bronchi carried liquids.

bronchus (*pl.* bronchi)........................ one of two branches from the trachea that conducts air into the lungs, where it divides and subdivides. The branchings resemble a tree; therefore they are referred to as a *bronchial tree*.

bronchioles.. smallest subdivision of the bronchial tree

alveolus (*pl.* alveoli)........................ air sacs at the end of the bronchioles. Oxygen and carbon dioxide are exchanged through the alveolar walls and the capillaries (Figure 5-3).

lungs.. two spongelike organs in the thoracic cavity. The right lung consists of three lobes, and the left lung has two lobes (see Figure 5-1).

pleura.. serous membrane covering each lung and lining the thoracic cavity

diaphragm... muscular partition that separates the thoracic cavity from the abdominal cavity. It aids in the breathing process.

Mediastinum
literally means **to stand in the middle** because it is derived from the Latin **medius**, meaning **middle**, and **stare**, meaning **to stand.**

mediastinum...................................... space between the lungs. It contains the heart, esophagus, trachea, great blood vessels, and other structures.

Learn the above terms by completing exercises 1 and 2.

EXERCISE   1

Match the terms in the first column with the correct definitions in the second column.

_____ 1. alveoli

_____ 2. bronchi

_____ 3. larynx

_____ 4. lungs

_____ 5. pharynx

_____ 6. pleura

_____ 7. adenoids

_____ 8. trachea

a. tubes carrying air between the trachea and lungs

b. passageway for air to the bronchi

c. located in the thoracic cavity

d. membrane covering the lung

e. lymphoid tissue behind the nasal cavity

f. acts as food and air passageway

g. location of the vocal cords

h. air sacs at the end of the bronchioles

i. keeps food out of the trachea and larynx

EXERCISE   2

Fill in the blanks with the correct terms.

1. The partition that separates the right and left nasal cavities is called the

   _____ _____.

2. The _____ is a flap of cartilage that prevents food from entering the larynx.

3. The smallest subdivisions of the bronchial tree are the _____.

4. The _____ serves as a filter to moisten and warm air entering the body.

5. The thoracic cavity is separated from the abdominal cavity by the

   _____.

6. The space between the lungs is called the _____.

7. The lymphoid tissues located in the pharynx behind the mouth are called the

   _____.

> Do not be concerned about which word root to use for lung or nose at this time. As you continue to study and use medical terms you will become familiar with common usage of each word part.

WORD PARTS

Combining Forms of the Respiratory System

Study the word parts and their definitions listed below. Completing the exercises that follow will help you learn the terms.

Combining Form	Definition
adenoid/o	adenoids
alveol/o	alveolus
bronch/i, bronch/o	bronchus
(NOTE: both *i* and *o* combining vowels are used with the word root *bronch*.)	
diaphragmat/o	diaphragm
epiglott/o	epiglottis
laryng/o	larynx
lob/o	lobe
nas/o,	
rhin/o	nose
pharyng/o	pharynx
pleur/o	pleura
pneum/o,	
pneumat/o,	
pneumon/o	lung, air

Adenoid
is derived from the Greek **aden,** meaning **gland,** and **eidos,** meaning **like.** The word was once used for the prostate gland. The first adenoid surgery was performed in 1868.

Lobe
literally means **the part that hangs down,** although it comes from the Greek **lobos,** meaning **capsule** or **pod.** Also applied to the lobe of an ear, liver, or brain.

pulmon/o...	lung
sept/o...	septum (wall off, fence)
sinus/o...	sinus
thorac/o...	thorax (chest)
tonsill/o...	tonsil
(NOTE: tonsil has one *l*, and the combining form has two *l*s.)	
trache/o...	trachea

Learn the anatomic locations and meanings of the combining forms by completing Exercise Figure A and exercises 3 and 4.

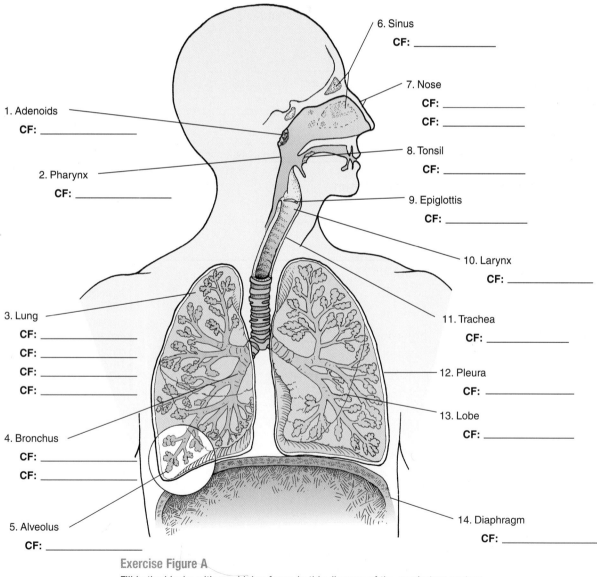

6. Sinus

CF: _____

7. Nose

CF: _____

CF: _____

1. Adenoids

CF: _____

8. Tonsil

CF: _____

2. Pharynx

CF: _____

9. Epiglottis

CF: _____

10. Larynx

CF: _____

3. Lung

CF: _____

CF: _____

CF: _____

CF: _____

11. Trachea

CF: _____

12. Pleura

CF: _____

13. Lobe

CF: _____

4. Bronchus

CF: _____

CF: _____

14. Diaphragm

CF: _____

5. Alveolus

CF: _____

Exercise Figure A

Fill in the blanks with combining forms in this diagram of the respiratory system.

EXERCISE   3

Write the definitions of the following combining forms.

1. laryng/o _____

2. bronch/o, bronch/i _____

3. pleur/o _____

4. pneum/o _____

5. tonsill/o _____

6. pulmon/o _____

7. diaphragmat/o _____

8. trache/o _____

9. alveol/o _____

10. pneumon/o _____

11. thorac/o _____

12. adenoid/o _____

13. pharyng/o _____

14. rhin/o _____

15. sinus/o _____

16. lob/o _____

17. epiglott/o _____

18. pneumat/o _____

19. nas/o _____

20. sept/o _____

EXERCISE   4

Write the combining form for each of the following terms.

1. nose   a. _____

                   b. _____

2. larynx   _____

3. lung, air

a. _____

b. _____

c. _____

4. lung   _____

5. tonsils   _____

6. trachea   _____

7. adenoids   _____

8. pleura   _____

9. diaphragm   _____

10. sinus   _____

11. thorax   _____

12. alveolus   _____

13. pharynx   _____

14. bronchus

a. _____

b. _____

15. lobe   _____

16. epiglottis   _____

17. septum   _____

Combining Forms Commonly Used with Respiratory System Terms

Combining Form	Definition
atel/o	imperfect, incomplete
capn/o	carbon dioxide
hem/o, hemat/o	blood
muc/o	mucus
orth/o	straight
ox/o, ox/i	oxygen
(NOTE: the combining vowels *o* and *i* are used with the word root *ox*.)	
py/o	pus
somn/o	sleep
spir/o	breathe, breathing

Learn the combining forms by completing exercises 5 and 6.

Oxygen
was discovered in 1774 by Joseph Priestley. In 1775 Antoine-Laurent Lavoisier, a French chemist, noted that all the acids he knew contained oxygen. Because he thought it was an acid producer, he named it using the Greek **oxys,** meaning **sour,** and the suffix **gen,** meaning **to produce.**

EXERCISE 5

Write the definition of the following combining forms.

1. ox/o, ox/i _____

2. spir/o _____

3. muc/o _____

4. atel/o _____

5. orth/o _____

6. py/o _____

7. hem/o, hemat/o _____

8. somn/o _____

9. capn/o _____

EXERCISE 6

Write the combining form for each of the following.

1. breathe, breathing   _____

2. oxygen   a. _____

          b. _____

3. imperfect, incomplete   _____

4. straight   _____

5. pus   _____

6. mucus   _____

7. blood   a. _____

          b. _____

8. sleep   _____

Prefixes

Prefix	Definition
a-, an-	without or absence of
(NOTE: *an-* is used when the word root begins with a vowel.)	

endo-	within
(NOTE: the prefix *intra-*, introduced in Chapter 4, also means *within*.)	
eu-	normal, good
pan-	all, total
poly-	many, much

Learn the prefixes by completing exercises 7 and 8.

EXERCISE 7

Write the definitions of the following prefixes.

1. endo- _____

2. a-, an- _____

3. pan- _____

4. eu- _____

5. poly- _____

EXERCISE 8

Write the prefix for each of the following.

1. within _____

2. normal, good _____

3. without or absence of   a. _____

                  b. _____

4. all, total _____

5. many, much _____

Suffixes

Suffix	Definition
-algia	pain
-ar, -ary, -eal	pertaining to
-cele	hernia or protrusion

-centesis	surgical puncture to aspirate fluid (with a sterile needle)
-ectasis	stretching out, dilatation, expansion
-emia	blood condition
-gram	record, x-ray image
-graphy	process of recording, x-ray imaging
-meter	instrument used to measure
-metry	measurement
-oxia	oxygen
-pexy	surgical fixation, suspension
-phonia	sound or voice
-pnea	breathing
-rrhagia	rapid flow of blood
-scope	instrument used for visual examination
-scopic	pertaining to visual examination
-scopy	visual examination
-spasm	sudden, involuntary muscle contraction (spasmodic contraction)
-stenosis	constriction or narrowing
-stomy	creation of an artificial opening
-thorax	chest
-tomy	cut into or incision

Learn the suffixes by completing exercises 9, 10, and 11. Refer to Appendix A and Appendix B for alphabetical lists of word parts and their meanings.

EXERCISE 9

Match the suffixes in the first column with their correct definitions in the second column.

_____ 1. -algia

_____ 2. -ar, -ary, -eal

_____ 3. -cele

_____ 4. -centesis

_____ 5. -ectasis

_____ 6. -emia

_____ 7. -gram

_____ 8. -graphy

_____ 9. -meter

_____ 10. -metry

_____ 11. -scopic

a. record, x-ray image

b. stretching out, dilatation, expansion

c. surgical puncture to aspirate fluid

d. measurement

e. pertaining to visual examination

f. pertaining to

g. hernia or protrusion

h. instrument used to measure

i. rapid flow of blood

j. blood condition

k. pain

l. process of recording, x-ray imaging

EXERCISE **10**

Match the suffixes in the first column with their correct definitions in the second column.

_____ 1. -rrhagia
_____ 2. -stomy
_____ 3. -tomy
_____ 4. -oxia
_____ 5. -pexy
_____ 6. -phonia
_____ 7. -pnea
_____ 8. -scope
_____ 9. -scopy
_____ 10. -spasm
_____ 11. -stenosis
_____ 12. -thorax

a. cut into or incision
b. instrument used for visual examination
c. rapid flow of blood
d. constriction, narrowing
e. sound or voice
f. creation of an artificial opening
g. sudden, involuntary muscle contraction
h. chest
i. oxygen
j. breathing
k. surgical fixation, suspension
l. visual examination

EXERCISE **11**

Write the definitions of the following suffixes.

1. -thorax _____

2. -ar, -ary, -eal _____

3. -stenosis _____

4. -cele _____

5. -stomy _____

6. -pexy _____

7. -meter _____

8. -spasm _____

9. -algia _____

10. -scopy _____

11. -centesis _____

12. -tomy _____

13. -scope _____

14. -rrhagia _____

15. -ectasis _____

16. -gram _____

17. -pnea _____

18. -graphy _____

19. -metry _____

20. -emia _____

21. -oxia _____

22. -phonia _____

23. -scopic _____

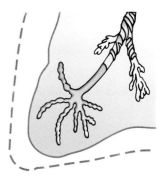

Figure 5-4
Atelectasis showing the collapsed alveoli.

MEDICAL TERMS

The terms you need to learn to complete this chapter are listed below. The exercises following each list will help you learn the definition and the spelling of each word.

Disease and Disorder Terms

Built from Word Parts

Term	Definition
adenoiditis .... (*ad*-e-noyd-Ī-tis)	inflammation of the adenoids
atelectasis .... (at-e-LEK-ta-sis)	incomplete expansion (of the lung of a new-born or collapsed lung) (Figure 5-4)
bronchiectasis .... (*bron*-ki-EK-ta-sis)	dilation of the bronchi (Exercise Figure B)
bronchitis .... (bron-KĪ-tis)	inflammation of the bronchi
bronchogenic carcinoma .... (bron-kō-JEN-ik) (kar-si-NŌ-ma)	cancerous tumor originating in the bronchus
bronchopneumonia .... (*bron*-kō-nū-MŌ-nē-a)	diseased state of the bronchi and lungs
diaphragmatocele .... (*dī*-a-frag-MAT-ō-sēl)	hernia of the diaphragm
epiglottitis .... (*ep*-i-glot-Ī-tis)	inflammation of the epiglottis
hemothorax .... (hē-mō-THŌ-raks)	blood in the chest (pleural space)
laryngitis .... (*lar*-in-JĪ-tis)	inflammation of the larynx
laryngotracheobronchitis (LTB) .... (lar-*ing*-gō-*trā*-kē-ō-bron-KĪ-tis)	inflammation of the larynx, trachea, and bronchi (the acute form is called *croup*)

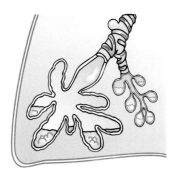

Exercise Figure B
Fill in the blanks to complete labeling of the diagram.

_____ / _____ / _____
bronchus / **cv** / **dilation**
showing the alveoli

Atelectasis
is derived from the Greek **ateles**, meaning **not perfect**, and **ektasis**, meaning **expansion**. It denotes an incomplete expansion of the lungs, especially at birth.

lobar pneumonia .... (LŌ-bar) (nū-MŌ-nē-a)	pertaining to the lobe(s); diseased state of the lung (infection of one or more lobes of the lung)
nasopharyngitis .... (nā-zō-far-in-JĪ-tis)	inflammation of the nose and pharynx
pansinusitis .... (*pan*-sī-nū-SĪ-tis)	inflammation of all sinuses
pharyngitis .... (far-in-JĪ-tis)	inflammation of the pharynx
pleuritis .... (plū-RĪ-tis)	inflammation of the pleura (also called *pleurisy*)
pneumatocele .... (nū-MAT-ō-sēl)	hernia of the lung (lung tissue protrudes through an opening in the chest)
pneumoconiosis .... (nū-mō-*kō*-nē-Ō-sis)	abnormal condition of dust in the lungs
pneumonia .... (nū-MŌ-nē-a)	diseased state of the lung (the infection and inflammation are caused by bacteria such as *Pneumococcus, Staphylococcus, Streptococcus,* and *Haemophilus;* viruses; and fungi)
pneumonitis .... (*nū*-mō-NĪ-tis)	inflammation of the lung
pneumothorax .... (*nū*-mō-THŌ-raks)	air in the chest (pleural space), which causes collapse of the lung (Exercise Figure C)
pulmonary neoplasm .... (PUL-mō-nar-ē) (NĒ-ō-plazm)	pertaining to (in) the lung, new growth (tumor)
pyothorax .... (pī-ō-THŌ-raks)	pus in the chest (pleural space) (also called *empyema*)

Pneumoconiosis
is the general name given for chronic inflammatory disease of the lung caused by excessive inhalation of mineral dust. When the disease is caused by a specific dust, it is named for the dust. For example, the disease caused by silica dust is called **silicosis**.

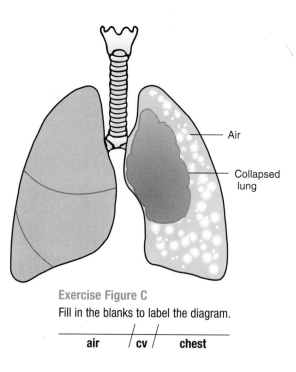

— Air

— Collapsed lung

Exercise Figure C
Fill in the blanks to label the diagram.

_____ / ____ / _____
   air   cv   chest

rhinitis	inflammation of the (mucous membranes) nose
(rī-NĪ-tis)	
rhinomycosis	abnormal condition of fungus in the nose
(rī-nō-mī-KŌ-sis)	
rhinorrhagia	rapid flow of blood from the nose (also called *epistaxis*)
(rī-nō-RĀ-jē-a)	
thoracalgia	pain in the chest
(thō-rak-AL-jē-a)	
tonsillitis	inflammation of the tonsils
(*ton*-sil-Ī-tis)	
tracheitis	inflammation of the trachea
(trā-kē-Ī-tis)	
tracheostenosis	narrowing of the trachea
(trā-kē-ō-sten-Ō-sis)	

Epistaxis
and rhinorrhagia are both medical terms for **nosebleed.**

Practice saying each of the terms aloud. To hear the terms, access the **PRONOUNCE IT** activity for this chapter on the Student CD that accompanies this text. Or, to hear the terms and their definitions with a CD player or computer, obtain the Pronunciation CD designed for use with this text.

Learn the definitions and spellings of the disease and disorder terms by completing exercises 12, 13, and 14.

EXERCISE   12

Analyze and define the following terms.

Example: $\underset{CF}{\underbrace{\overset{WR}{diaphragmat}/\overset{CV}{o}/\overset{S}{cele}}}$ *hernia of the diaphragm*

1. pleuritis _____

2. nasopharyngitis _____

3. pneumothorax _____

4. pansinusitis _____

5. atelectasis _____

6. rhinomycosis _____

7. tracheostenosis _____

8. epiglottitis _____

9. thoracalgia _____

10. pulmonary neoplasm _____

11. bronchiectasis _____

12. tonsillitis _____

13. pneumoconiosis _____

14. bronchopneumonia _____

15. pneumonitis _____

16. laryngitis _____

17. pneumatocele _____

18. pyothorax _____

19. rhinorrhagia _____

20. bronchitis _____

21. pharyngitis _____

22. tracheitis _____

23. laryngotracheobronchitis _____

24. adenoiditis _____

25. hemothorax _____

26. lobar pneumonia _____

27. rhinitis _____

28. bronchogenic carcinoma _____

29. pneumonia _____

EXERCISE 13

Build disease and disorder terms for the following definitions with the word parts you have learned.

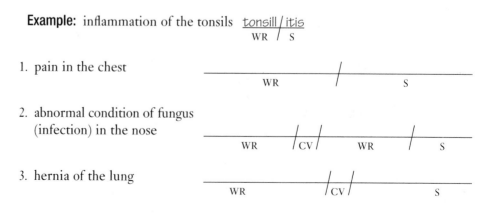

Example: inflammation of the tonsils   tonsill / itis
                                              WR / S

1. pain in the chest

    _____ / _____
         WR   /   S

2. abnormal condition of fungus
   (infection) in the nose

    _____ / ___ / _____ / ___
      WR   / CV /   WR   / S

3. hernia of the lung

    _____ / ___ / _____
         WR   / CV /   S

4. pertaining to the lung; new growth (tumor)

_____ / _____   _____ / _____
WR   S   P   S(WR)

5. inflammation of the larynx

_____ / _____
      WR   S

6. incomplete expansion (of the lung)

_____ / _____
      WR   S

7. inflammation of the adenoids

_____ / _____
      WR   S

8. inflammation of the larynx, trachea, and bronchi

____ / __ / ____ / __ / ____ / __
WR   CV   WR   CV   WR   S

9. dilation of the bronchi

_____ / __ / _____
   WR   CV   S

10. inflammation of the pleura

_____ / _____
      WR   S

11. abnormal condition of dust in the lung

_____ / __ / _____ / _____
  WR   CV   WR   S

12. inflammation of the lung

_____ / _____
      WR   S

13. inflammation of all sinuses

____ / ____ / ____ / ____
 P   WR   S

14. narrowing of the trachea

_____ / __ / _____
   WR   CV   S

15. inflammation of the nose and pharynx

_____ / __ / _____ / _____
  WR   CV   WR   S

16. pus in the chest (pleural space)

_____ / __ / _____
   WR   CV   S

17. inflammation of the epiglottis

_____ / _____
      WR   S

18. hernia of the diaphragm

_____ / __ / _____
   WR   CV   S

19. air in the chest (pleural space)

_____ / __ / _____
   WR   CV   S

20. diseased state of the bronchi and the lungs

_____ / __ / _____ / _____
  WR   CV   WR   S

21. rapid flow of blood from the nose

	/ /	
WR	CV	S

22. inflammation of the pharynx

	/	
WR		S

23. blood in the chest (pleural space)

	/ /	
WR	CV	S

24. inflammation of the trachea

	/	
WR		S

25. inflammation of the bronchi

	/	
WR		S

26. pertaining to the lobe(s); diseased state of the lung(s)

	/			/	
WR		S		WR	S

27. inflammation of the (mucous membranes) nose

	/	
WR		S

28. cancerous tumor originating in a bronchus

	/ /	
WR	CV	S

	/	
WR		S

29. diseased state of the lung

	/	
WR		S

EXERCISE   14

Spell each of the disease and disorder terms. Have someone dictate the terms on pp. 117-119 to you. Think about the word parts before attempting to write the word. Study any words you have spelled incorrectly.

1. _____   8. _____

2. _____   9. _____

3. _____   10. _____

4. _____   11. _____

5. _____   12. _____

6. _____   13. _____

7. _____   14. _____

15. _____   23. _____

16. _____   24. _____

17. _____   25. _____

18. _____   26. _____

19. _____   27. _____

20. _____   28. _____

21. _____   29. _____

22. _____   30. _____

Disease and Disorder Terms

Not Built from Word Parts

Term	Definition
adult respiratory distress syndrome (ARDS) .... (a-DULT) (RES-pir-a-*tor*-ē) (di-STRES) (SIN-drŏm)	respiratory failure in an adult as a result of disease or injury. Symptoms include dyspnea, rapid breathing, and cyanosis. (It is also called *acute respiratory distress syndrome*.)
asthma.. (AZ-ma)	respiratory disease characterized by paroxysms of coughing, wheezing, and shortness of breath
chronic obstructive pulmonary disease (COPD).................................... (KRON-ik) (ob-STRUK-tiv) (PUL-mō-nar-ē) (di-ZEZ)	a group of disorders that are almost always a result of smoking that obstructs bronchial flow. One or more of the following is present in COPD in varying degrees: emphysema, chronic bronchitis, bronchospasm, and bronchiolitis.
coccidioidomycosis............................ (kok-*sid*-ē-oyd-ō-mī-KO-sis)	fungal disease affecting the lungs and sometimes other organs of the body (also called *valley fever* or *cocci*)
cor pulmonale............................... (kōr) (pul-mō-NAL-ē)	serious cardiac disease associated with chronic lung disorders, such as emphysema
croup... (krŭp)	condition resulting from acute obstruction of the larynx, characterized by a barking cough, hoarseness, and stridor. It may be caused by viral or bacterial infection, allergy, or foreign body. Occurs mainly in children.
cystic fibrosis (CF)............................. (SIS-tik) (fī-BRO-sis)	hereditary disorder of the endocrine glands characterized by excess mucus production in the respiratory tract, pancreatic deficiency, and other symptoms.
deviated septum.............................. (SEP-tum)	one part of the nasal cavity is smaller because of malformation or injury

Adult Respiratory Distress Syndrome (ARDS)
is respiratory failure in an adult. In newborns the condition is referred to as **respiratory distress syndrome of newborn (RDS)** or **hyaline membrane disease**.

Asthma
is derived from the Greek **astma**, meaning **to pant**.

☘ CAM TERM
Biofeedback is learned self-control of physiologic responses by using electronic devices to demonstrate signals from the body. Biofeedback could be used to address symptoms of asthma.

Cystic Fibrosis
affects approximately 30,000 people in the United States. The median survival age is 33.4 years.

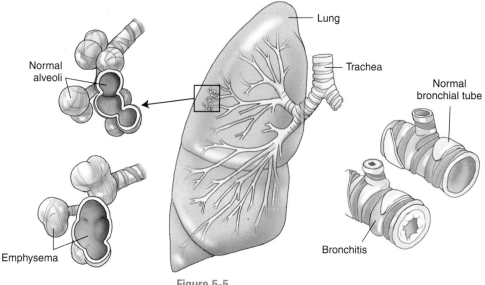

Figure 5-5
Emphysema and bronchitis.

emphysema ....
(em-fi-SĒ-ma)
stretching of lung tissue caused by the alveoli becoming distended and losing elasticity (Figure 5-5)

epistaxis ....
(ep-i-STAK-sis)
nosebleed (synonymous with *rhinorrhagia*)

influenza ....
(in-flū-EN-za)
highly infectious respiratory disease caused by a virus (also called *flu*)

Legionnaire disease ....
(lē-je-NAR) (di-ZĒZ)
a lobar pneumonia caused by the bacterium *Legionella pneumophila*

obstructive sleep apnea (OSA) ....
(AP-nē-a)
repetitive pharyngeal collapse during sleep, which leads to absence of breathing (Figure 5-6)

pertussis ....
(per-TUS-sis)
respiratory disease characterized by an acute crowing inspiration, or whoop (synonymous with *whooping cough*)

pleural effusion ....
(PLŪ-ral) (e-FŪ-zhun)
escape of fluid into the pleural space as a result of inflammation

***Pneumocystis carinii (P. carinii)*
pneumonia (PCP)** ....
(nū-mō-SIS-tis) (car-i-NĒ-ī)
a pneumonia caused by *P. carinii,* a fungus. Common disease in patients with AIDS (Figure 5-7).

pulmonary edema ....
(PUL-mō-nar-ē) (e-DĒ-ma)
fluid accumulation in the alveoli and bronchioles

**pulmonary embolism
(*pl.* emboli) (PE)** ....
(PUL-mō-nar-ē)
(EM-bō-lizm)
foreign matter, such as a blood clot, air, or fat clot, carried in the circulation to the pulmonary artery, where it blocks circulation (Figure 5-8)

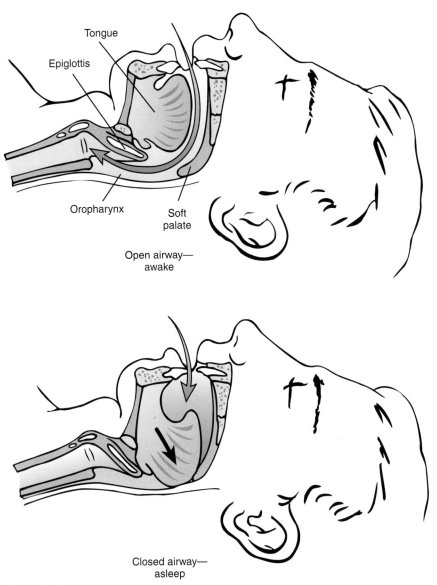

Tongue
Epiglottis
Oropharynx
Soft palate
Open airway—awake
Closed airway—asleep

Figure 5-6
Obstructive sleep apnea. During sleep the absence of activity of the pharyngeal muscle structure allows the airway to close.

tuberculosis (TB) .... an infectious disease, caused by an acid-fast bacillus, most commonly spread by inhalation of small particles and usually affecting the lungs
(tū-ber-kū-LO-sis)

upper respiratory infection (URI)......... infection of the nasal cavity, pharynx, or larynx.
(UP-er) (RE-spi-ra-tō-rē) (in-FEK-shun)

Tuberculosis
is considered the deadliest infectious disease known to human beings and has a high mortality rate.

Practice saying each of these terms aloud. To hear the terms, access the **PRONOUNCE IT** activity for this chapter on the Student CD that accompanies this text. Or, to hear the terms and their definitions with a CD player or computer, obtain the Pronunciation CD designed for use with this text.

Learn the definitions and spellings of the diagnostic terms by completing exercises 15, 16, and 17.

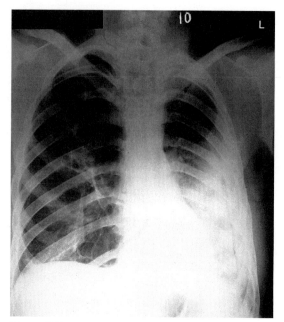

Figure 5-7
Chest radiograph of a patient with pneumonia.

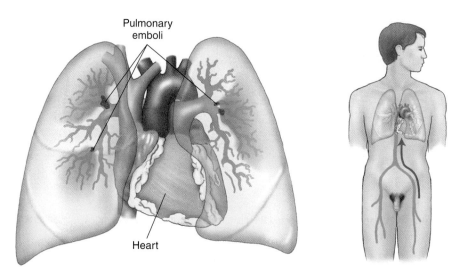

Figure 5-8
Pulmonary embolism.

EXERCISE 15

Fill in the blanks with the correct terms.

1. A disease characterized by lung tissue stretching that results from the alveoli losing elasticity and becoming distended is called _____.

2. _____ _____ is the name given to the escape of fluid into the pleural space as a result of inflammation.

3. A cardiac condition that is associated with chronic lung disorders is called_____ _____.

4. A fungal disease affecting the lungs is called _____.

5. _____ _____ is a hereditary disorder characterized by excess mucus production in the respiratory tract.

6. The medical name of the infectious respiratory disease commonly referred to as *flu* is _____.

7. A group of disorders that obstruct the bronchial airflow is known as

_____ _____ _____ _____.

8. The medical name for the disease characterized by an acute crowing inspiration is _____.

9. _____ is a condition resulting from an acute obstruction of the larynx.

10. A chronic respiratory disease characterized by shortness of breath, wheezing, and paroxysmal coughing is called _____.

11. A condition in which fluid accumulates in the alveoli and bronchioles is

_____ _____.

12. A(n) _____ _____ _____ generally refers to an infection involving the nasal cavity, pharynx, or larynx.

13. Foreign matter, such as a clot, air, or fat carried in the circulation to the pulmonary artery, where it blocks circulation, is called a(n) _____

_____.

14. _____ is another name for nosebleed.

15. A lobar pneumonia caused by the *Legionella pneumophila* bacterium is commonly called _____ _____.

16. A pneumonia most commonly found in patients with AIDS is called

_____ _____ _____.

17. _____ _____ is one part of the nasal cavity that is smaller than the other because of malformation or injury.

18. The diagnosis for repetitive pharyngeal collapse is _____

_____.

19. An infectious disease usually affecting the lungs and caused by inhaling infected small particles is _____.

20. _____ _____ _____ _____ occurs in adults as a result of disease or injury.

EXERCISE 16

Match the terms in the first column with the correct definitions in the second column.

_____ 1. asthma

_____ 2. chronic obstructive pulmonary disease

_____ 3. coccidioidomycosis

a. alveoli become distended and lose elasticity

b. caused by a virus (commonly called *flu*)

c. hereditary disorder characterized by excess mucus in the respiratory system

_____ 4. cor pulmonale

_____ 5. croup

_____ 6. cystic fibrosis

_____ 7. emphysema

_____ 8. epistaxis

_____ 9. influenza

_____ 10. Legionnaire disease

d. characterized by wheezing, paroxysmal coughing, and shortness of breath

e. nosebleed

f. cardiac disease associated with chronic lung disorders

g. condition resulting from obstruction of the larynx

h. also called *valley fever*

i. lobar pneumonia caused by the bacterium *Legionella pneumophila*

j. lung disorder that obstructs the bronchial airflow

EXERCISE 17

Match the terms in the first column with the correct definitions in the second column.

_____ 1. pertussis

_____ 2. pleural effusion

_____ 3. pulmonary edema

_____ 4. pulmonary embolism

_____ 5. upper respiratory infection

_____ 6. deviated septum

_____ 7. obstructive sleep apnea

_____ 8. *P. carinii* pneumonia

_____ 9. tuberculosis

_____ 10. adult respiratory distress syndrome

a. respiratory failure in an adult

b. escape of fluid into pleural cavity

c. fluid accumulation in alveoli and bronchioles

d. whooping cough

e. foreign material, moved by circulation, that blocks the pulmonary artery

f. infection of the nasal cavity, pharynx, or larynx

g. common in patients with AIDS

h. unequal size of nasal cavities

i. repetitive pharyngeal collapse

j. an infectious disease usually affecting the lungs

EXERCISE 18

Spell the disease and disorder terms. Have someone dictate the terms on pp. 123-125 to you. Study any words you have spelled incorrectly.

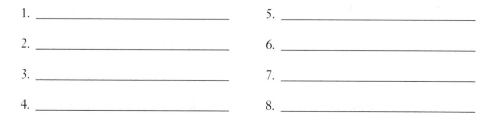

1. _____   5. _____

2. _____   6. _____

3. _____   7. _____

4. _____   8. _____

9. _____   15. _____

10. _____   16. _____

11. _____   17. _____

12. _____   18. _____

13. _____   19. _____

14. _____   20. _____

Surgical Terms

Built from Word Parts

Term	Definition
adenoidectomy................................. (*ad*-e-noyd-EK-tō-mē)	excision of the adenoids (Exercise Figure D)
adenotome....................................... (AD-e-nō-tōm) (NOTE: the *oid* is missing from the word root *adenoid* in this term.)	surgical instrument used to cut the adenoids (see Exercise Figure D)
bronchoplasty................................ (BRON-kō-plas-tē)	surgical repair of a bronchus
laryngectomy................................. (lār-in-JEK-tō-mē)	excision of the larynx
laryngoplasty................................. (lar-IN-gō-*plas*-tē)	surgical repair of the larynx
laryngostomy................................. (lar-in-GOS-tō-mē)	creation of an artificial opening into the larynx
laryngotracheotomy......................... (lar-in-gō-*trā*-kē-OT-ō-mē)	incision of the larynx and trachea
lobectomy....................................... (lō-BEK-tō-mē)	excision of a lobe (of the lung) (Figure 5-9)

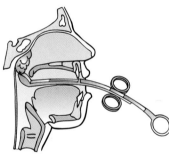

Exercise Figure D
Fill in the blanks to complete
labeling of the diagram.

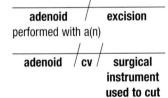

_____ / _____
adenoid   **excision**
performed with a(n)

_____ / ___ / _____
adenoid   **cv**   **surgical**
                     instrument
                     used to cut

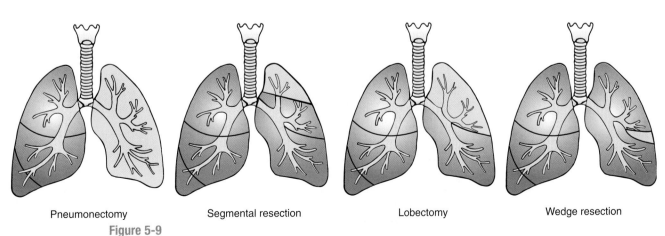

Pneumonectomy   Segmental resection   Lobectomy   Wedge resection

Figure 5-9
Types of lung resection. The amount of lung tissue removed with each type of surgery is illustrated.

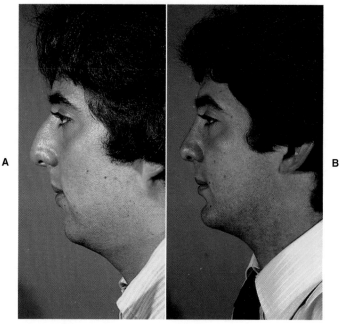

A

B

Figure 5-10
Side view of patient before **(A)** and after **(B)** rhinoplasty and chin augmentation.

pleuropexy.......................... (plū-rō-PEK-sē)	surgical fixation of the pleura
pneumobronchotomy .... (nū-mō-bron-KOT-ō-mē)	incision of lung and bronchus
pneumonectomy.................................. (nū-mō-NEK-tō-mē)	excision of a lung (see Figure 5-7)
rhinoplasty .... (RĪ-nō-plast-ē)	surgical repair of the nose (Figure 5-10)
septoplasty.................................. (sep-tō-PLAS-tē)	surgical repair of the (nasal) septum
septotomy.. (sep-TOT-ō-mē)	incision into the (nasal) septum
sinusotomy.................................... (sī-nū-SOT-ō-mē)	incision of a sinus
thoracocentesis .... (thō-rak-ō-sen-TĒ-sis)	surgical puncture to aspirate fluid from the chest cavity (also called *thoracentesis*) (Exercise Figure E)
thoracotomy .... (thō-ra-KOT-ō-mē)	incision into the chest cavity
tonsillectomy.................................. (ton-sil-EK-tō-mē)	excision of the tonsils
tracheoplasty .... (TRĀ-kē-ō-*plas*-tē)	surgical repair of the trachea
tracheostomy.................................... (trā-kē-OS-tō-mē)	creation of an artificial opening into the trachea (Exercise Figure F)

Video-Assisted Thoracic Surgery (VATS)
is the use of a thoracoscope and video equipment for an endoscopic approach to diagnose and treat thoracic conditions. It replaces the traditional thoracotomy, which required a large incision and greater recovery time.

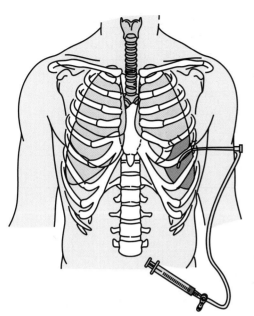

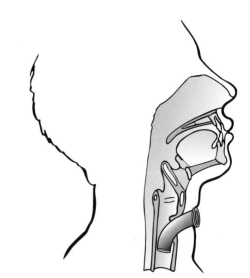

Exercise Figure E

Fill in the blanks to complete labeling of the diagram.

_____ / cv / surgical puncture to remove fluid
       chest

is used for both diagnosis and treatment.

Exercise Figure F

Fill in the blanks to complete labeling of the diagram.

_____ / cv / creation of an artificial opening ,
       trachea

with tube in place.

tracheotomy .... incision of the trachea
   (trā-kē-OT-ō-mē)

Practice saying each of the terms aloud. To hear the terms, access the **PRONOUNCE IT** activity for this chapter on the Student CD that accompanies this text. Or, to hear the terms and their definitions with a CD player or computer, obtain the Pronunciation CD designed for use with this text.

Learn the definitions and spellings of the surgical terms by completing exercises 19, 20, and 21.

EXERCISE 19

Analyze and define the following surgical terms.

             WR   S
  Example: pneumon/ectomy *excision of lung* _____

1. tracheotomy _____

2. laryngostomy _____

3. adenoidectomy _____

4. rhinoplasty _____

5. adenotome _____

6. tracheostomy _____

7. sinusotomy _____

8. laryngoplasty _____

9. pneumobronchotomy _____

10. bronchoplasty _____

11. lobectomy _____

12. laryngotracheotomy _____

13. tracheoplasty _____

14. thoracotomy _____

15. laryngectomy _____

16. thoracocentesis _____

17. tonsillectomy _____

18. pleuropexy _____

19. septoplasty _____

20. septotomy _____

EXERCISE 20

Build surgical terms for the following definitions by using the word parts you have learned.

Example: surgical fixation of the pleura <u>pleur / o / pexy</u>
                                              WR /CV/   S

1. surgical repair of the trachea _____ / ____ / _____
                                      WR   / CV /   S

2. incision of larynx and trachea _____ / ___ / _____ / ___ / ____
                                     WR   / CV /   WR   / CV /   S

3. surgical instrument used to
   cut the adenoids   _____ / ____ / _____
                                      WR   / CV /   S

4. incision into the chest cavity _____ / ____ / _____
                                      WR   / CV /   S

5. creation of an artificial
   opening into the trachea   _____ / ____ / _____
                                      WR   / CV /   S

6. excision of the tonsils   _____ / _____
                                      WR   /   S

7. incision of the trachea

    WR   / CV /   S

8. surgical repair of a bronchus

    WR   / CV /   S

9. excision of the larynx

    WR   /   S

10. surgical repair of the nose

    WR   / CV /   S

11. incision of a sinus

    WR   / CV /   S

12. surgical puncture to aspirate
fluid from the chest cavity

    WR   / CV /   S

or

    WR   /   S

13. excision of the adenoids

    WR   /   S

14. surgical repair of the larynx

    WR   / CV /   S

15. excision of a lobe (of the lung)

    WR   /   S

16. incision of a lung and
bronchus

    WR   / CV /   WR   / CV /   S

17. creation of an artificial
opening into the larynx

    WR   / CV /   S

18. excision of a lung

    WR   /   S

19. incision into the septum

    WR   / CV /   S

20. surgical repair of the septum

    WR   / CV /   S

EXERCISE 21

Spell each of the surgical terms. Have someone dictate the terms on pp. 129-130 to you. Think about the word parts before attempting to write the word. Study any words you have spelled incorrectly.

1. _____   3. _____

2. _____   4. _____

5. _____

6. _____

7. _____

8. _____

9. _____

10. _____

11. _____

12. _____

13. _____

14. _____

15. _____

16. _____

17. _____

18. _____

19. _____

20. _____

21. _____

Diagnostic Terms

Built from Word Parts

Term	Definition
Endoscopy	
bronchoscope (BRON-kō-skōp)	instrument used for visual examination of the bronchi (Table 5-1, Figure 5-11, and Exercise Figure G)
bronchoscopy (bron-KOS-kō-pē)	visual examination of the bronchi (see Exercise Figure G)
endoscope (EN-dō-skōp)	instrument used for visual examination within (a hollow organ or body cavity). (Current trend is to use endoscopes for surgical procedures as well as for viewing.)
endoscopic (en-dō-SKOP-ic)	pertaining to visual examination within (a hollow organ or body cavity) (used to describe the practice of performing surgeries that use endoscopes)
endoscopy (en-DOS-kō-pē)	visual examination within (a hollow organ or body cavity)
laryngoscope (*lar*-IN-gō-skōp)	instrument used for visual examination of the larynx (Exercise Figure H)
laryngoscopy (lar-in-GOS-kō-pē)	visual examination of the larynx
thoracoscope (tho-RAK-ō-skōp)	instrument used for visual examination of the thorax
thoracoscopy (tho-ra-KOS-kō-pē)	visual examination of the thorax
Pulmonary Function	
capnometer (kap-NOM-e-ter)	instrument used to measure carbon dioxide (levels in expired gas) (Figure 5-12, *A*)

Scope
is taken from the Greek **skopein,** which means to **see** or to **view.** It also means **observing for a purpose.** To the ancient Greeks it meant "to look out for, to monitor, or to examine."

Today the suffix **-scope** is used to describe the **instrument used to view or to examine,** such as in the term **endoscope** (means **instrument used for visual examination within** a hollow organ or body cavity). **-Scopy** is the suffix, which means **visual examination,** such as in the term **endoscopy** (**visual examination within** a hollow organ or body cavity). **-Scopic** is the adjectival suffix, which means **pertaining to visual examination,** such as in the term **endoscopic** (**pertaining to visual examination within** a hollow organ or body cavity). **Endoscopic surgery** is now a common term used to describe modern surgery performed with the use of endoscopes. Most often the suffixes **-scope, -scopy,** and **-scopic** mean **to examine visually,** and that is the definition given in this text. However, a term included in a subsequent chapter, **stethoscope,** is an **instrument used for monitoring** and not for viewing.

TABLE   5-1

Types of Diagnostic Procedures

The following table includes the types of diagnostic procedures included for study in the diagnostic category of this text.

Diagnostic Imaging

Radiography produces images of internal organs by using ionizing radiation.

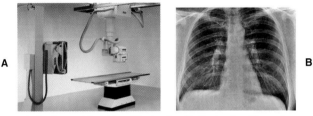

A, Radiographic table with chest unit; **B,** chest radiograph.

Nuclear medicine produces scans by using radioactive material.

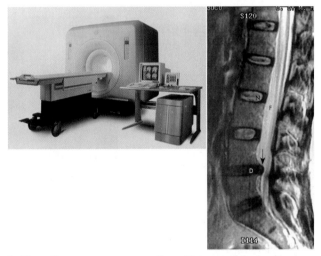

Posterior   RPO   Rt. lateral   LPO

Perfusion lung scan

Hx: 46-year-old female; history of shortness of breath

Diacam
Matrix: 128×128
Dose: 3mCi 99mTc-MPA
Counts: 500K/view

Dx: Normal lung study

Lt. lateral   Anterior

A, Nuclear medicine scanner; **B,** lung scan.

Computed tomography produces scans of computerized images of body organs in transverse slices.

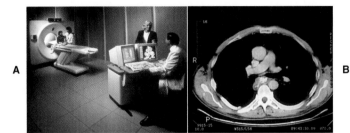

A, Computed tomography scanner; **B,** scan of the chest with intravenous contrast medium.

Magnetic resonance imaging produces scans that give information about the body's biochemistry by placing the patient in a magnetic field.

A, Magnetic resonance scanner; **B,** sagittal scan of the lumbar spine with herniated disk *(arrow).*

Ultrasound produces scans by using high-frequency sound waves.

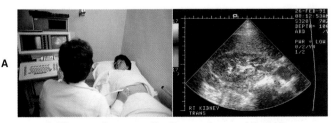

A, Ultrasound scanner; **B,** ultrasound scan of the kidney.

Continued

TABLE 5-1

Types of Diagnostic Procedures—cont'd

Endoscopy

Endoscopy uses endoscopes, which are lighted, flexible instruments, to visually examine a hollow organ or body cavity, such as the bronchus.

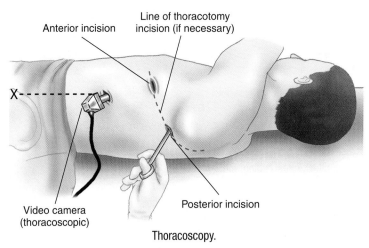

Thoracoscopy.

Laboratory

Laboratory procedures are performed on specimens such as blood, tissue, and urine.

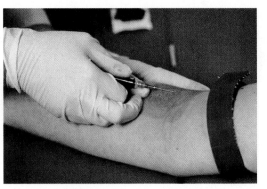

Drawing blood for laboratory test.

Pulmonary Function

Pulmonary function tests are performed in a variety of methods to determine lung function.

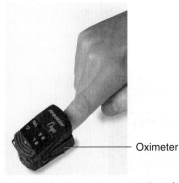

Pulse oximetry measures oxygen saturation of the blood.

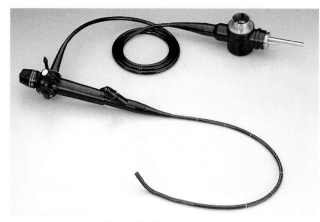

Figure 5-11
Fibroscopic bronchoscope.

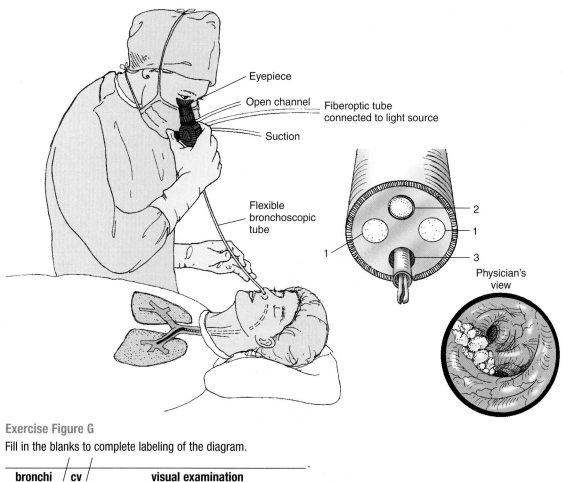

Eyepiece

Open channel — Fiberoptic tube
connected to light source

Suction

Flexible
bronchoscopic
tube

2

1

3

Physician's
view

Exercise Figure G

Fill in the blanks to complete labeling of the diagram.

_____ .
bronchi / cv /   visual examination

The _____ is inserted through the nostril into the
bronchi / cv /   instrument used for visual examination

bronchi. The tube has four channels: *1,* two light sources; *2,* viewing channel; *3,* channel to hold biopsy forceps and other
instruments.

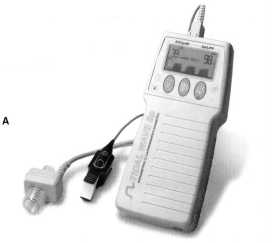

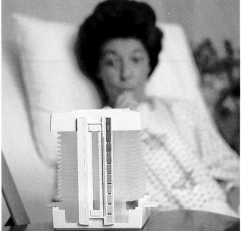

Figure 5-12
A, Capnometer; **B,** spirometer.

oximeter .... (ok-SIM-e-ter) (NOTE: the combining vowel is *i*.)	instrument used to measure oxygen (saturation in the blood) (see Table 5-1)
spirometer .... (spī-ROM-e-ter)	instrument used to measure breathing (or lung volumes) (Figure 5-12, *B*)
spirometry .... (spī-ROM-e-trē)	a measurement of breathing (or lung volumes)

Sleep Studies

polysomnography (PSG) .... (*pol*-ē-som-NOG-rah-f ē)	process of recording many (tests) during sleep (performed to diagnose obstructive sleep apnea [see Figures 5-5 and 5-6]). Tests include electrocardiography, electromyography, electroencephalography, air flow monitoring, and oximetry.

Practice saying each of these words aloud. To hear the terms, access the **PRONOUNCE IT** activity for this chapter on the Student CD that accompanies this text. Or, to hear the terms and their definitions with a CD player or computer, obtain the Pronunciation CD designed for use with this text.

Learn the definition and spelling of the diagnostic terms by completing exercises 22, 23, and 24.

EXERCISE 22

Analyze and define the following procedural terms.

WR CV S
Example: bronch/o/scopy *visual examination of the bronchi* _____
CF

1. spirometer _____

2. laryngoscope _____

3. capnometer _____

4. spirometry _____

5. oximeter _____

6. laryngoscopy _____

7. bronchoscope _____

8. thoracoscope _____

9. endoscope _____

10. thoracoscopy _____

11. endoscopic _____

12. endoscopy _____

13. polysomnography _____

EXERCISE 23

Build procedural terms that correspond to the following definitions by using the word parts you have learned.

Example: instrument used to measure oxygen   <u>ox / i / meter</u>
WR/CV   S

1. visual examination of the
   larynx
   _____ / __ / _____
   WR   CV   S

2. instrument used to measure
   breathing
   _____ / __ / _____
   WR   CV   S

3. instrument used to measure
   carbon dioxide
   _____ / __ / _____
   WR   CV   S

4. instrument used for visual
   examination of the larynx
   _____ / __ / _____
   WR   CV   S

5. visual examination of the
   bronchi
   _____ / __ / _____
   WR   CV   S

6. measurement of breathing
   _____ / __ / _____
   WR   CV   S

7. instrument used for visual
   examination of the bronchi
   _____ / __ / _____
   WR   CV   S

8. visual examination of a
   hollow organ or body cavity

   _____ / _____
        P   S(WR)

9. instrument used for visual
   examination of the thorax

   _____ / CV / _____
        WR   S

10. instrument used for visual
    examination of a hollow
    organ or body cavity

    _____ / _____
         P   S(WR)

11. visual examination of the
    thorax

    _____ / CV / _____
         WR   S

12. pertaining to visual exami-
    nation of a hollow organ or
    body cavity

    _____ / _____
         P   S(WR)

13. process of recording of
    many (tests) during sleep

    _____ / WR / CV / _____
         P   S

EXERCISE   24

Spell each of the diagnostic terms. Have someone dictate the terms on pp. 134 and
138 to you. Think about the word parts before attempting to write the word. Study any
you have spelled incorrectly.

1. _____   8. _____

2. _____   9. _____

3. _____   10. _____

4. _____   11. _____

5. _____   12. _____

6. _____   13. _____

7. _____   14. _____

Diagnostic Terms

Not Built from Word Parts

Term	Definition
Diagnostic Imaging	
chest computed tomography (CT) scan	computerized images of the chest created in sections sliced from front to back. Used to
(tō-MOG-ra-fē)	

diagnose tumors, abscesses, and pleural effusion. Computed tomography is used to visualize other body parts such as the abdomen and the brain (see Table 5-1).

chest x-ray (CXR) .... an x-ray image of the chest used to evaluate the lungs and the heart (also called a *chest radiograph*) (see Table 5-1).

ventilation-perfusion scanning (VPS) .... a nuclear medicine procedure used to
(ven-ti-LA-shun) diagnose pulmonary embolism and other
(per-FU-zhun) conditions (also called a *lung scan*) (see Table 5-1)

Laboratory

acid-fast bacilli (AFB) smear............ a test performed on sputum to determine the
(AS-id-fast) (bah-SIL-ī) presence of acid-fast bacilli, which cause tuberculosis

Pulmonary Function

arterial blood gases (ABGs).............. a test performed on arterial blood to deter-
(ar-TE-rē-al) mine levels of oxygen, carbon dioxide, and other gases present

pulmonary function tests (PFTs)....... a group of tests performed to measure
(PUL-mō-ner-ē) breathing, which is used to determine respiratory function or abnormalities

pulse oximetry.................................... a noninvasive method of measuring oxygen
(ok-SIM-e-trē) in the blood by using a device that attaches to the fingertip (see Table 5-1)

Other

**purified protein derivative (PPD)
skin test**.. a test performed on individuals who have recently been exposed to tuberculosis. PPD of the tuberculin bacillus is injected intradermally. Positive tests indicate previous exposure, not necessarily active tuberculosis.

> **Helical Computed Tomography (CT) Scan**
> of the chest, also called **spiral scan**, is an improvement over standard CT and is the preferred study to identify pulmonary embolism. Images are continually obtained as the patient passes through the gantry, which is part of the scanner. It produces a more accurate and faster image, which can be performed with one breath hold.

EXERCISE 25

Fill in the blanks with the correct terms.

1. _____ _____ _____ is a nuclear medicine procedure used to diagnose pulmonary embolism and other conditions.

2. Computerized images of the chest, created in sections sliced from front to back, are called a(n) _____ _____ _____ scan.

3. _____ _____ is used to evaluate the lungs and the heart.

4. The test performed on arterial blood to determine levels of oxygen, carbon dioxide, and other gases present is called _____ _____ _____.

5. A noninvasive test to measure oxygen in the blood is called _____
_____.

6. A test performed on sputum to diagnose tuberculosis is called

_____ _____ _____ _____.

7. _____ _____ _____ is the name of a
group of tests performed on breathing to determine respiratory function or
abnormalities.

8. _____ _____ _____ is a test that, when posi-
tive, indicates an individual has been exposed to tuberculosis.

EXERCISE 26

Match the terms in the first column with their correct definitions in the second column.

_____ 1. ventilation-perfusion scanning

_____ 2. chest x-ray

_____ 3. chest CT scan

_____ 4. acid-fast bacilli smear

_____ 5. pulse oximetry

_____ 6. arterial blood gases

_____ 7. pulmonary function tests

_____ 8. PPD skin test

a. computerized images of the chest

b. a noninvasive method used to measure oxygen in the blood

c. a blood test used to determine oxygen and other gases in the blood

d. a test for tuberculosis

e. chest radiograph

f. a nuclear medicine procedure used to diagnose pulmonary conditions

g. injected intradermally

h. tests performed on breathing

i. an instrument to measure pulse waves

EXERCISE 27

Spell each of the diagnostic terms. Have someone dictate the terms on pp. 140-141 to you. Study any words you have spelled incorrectly.

1. _____

2. _____

3. _____

4. _____

5. _____

6. _____

7. _____

8. _____

Complementary Terms

Built from Word Parts

Term	Definition
acapnia (a-CAP-nē-a)	condition of absence (less than normal level) of carbon dioxide (in the blood)

anoxia.. absence (deficiency) of oxygen
    (a-NOK-sē-a)

aphonia... absence of voice
    (ā-FŌ-nē-a)

apnea.. absence of breathing
    (AP-nē-a)

bronchoalveolar............................ pertaining to the bronchi and alveoli
    (*bron*-kō-al-VĒ-ō-lar)

bronchospasm............................... spasmodic contraction in the bronchi
    (BRON-kō-spazm)

diaphragmatic................................ pertaining to the diaphragm
    (*dī*-a-frag-MAT-ik)

dysphonia...................................... difficult speaking (voice)
    (dis-FŌ-nē-a)

dyspnea... difficult breathing
    (DISP-nē-a)

endotracheal.................................. pertaining to within the trachea (see Exercise
    (*en*-dō-TRĀ-kē-al)   Figure H)

eupnea... normal breathing
    (ŪP-nē-a)

hypercapnia................................... condition of excessive carbon dioxide (in the
    (hī-per-KAP-nē-a)   blood)

> **Anoxia**
> literally means **without oxygen** or **absence of oxygen.** The term actually denotes an oxygen deficiency in the body tissues.

Exercise Figure H

Fill in the blanks to complete labeling of the diagram. The physician is inserting a(n)

_____ / _____ / _____ tube with a(n)
  within / **trachea** / **pertaining to**

_____ / _____ / _____.
  larynx / **cv** / **instrument used for visual examination**

hyperpnea................................... (hī-perp-NĒ-a)	excessive breathing
hypocapnia................................ (hī-pō-KAP-nē-a)	condition of deficient carbon dioxide (in the blood)
hypopnea................................... (hī-pop-NĒ-a)	deficient breathing
hypoxemia................................. (hī-pok-SĒ-mē-a) (NOTE: the *o* from *hypo* has been dropped. The final vowel in a prefix may be dropped when the word to which it is added begins with a vowel.)	deficient oxygen in the blood
hypoxia..................................... (hī-POK-sē-a) (NOTE: see note for hypoxemia.)	deficient oxygen (to the tissues)
intrapleural............................... (in-tra-PLUR-al)	pertaining to within the pleura (space between the two pleural membranes)
laryngeal.................................. (lar-IN-jē-al)	pertaining to the larynx
laryngospasm............................. (lar-ING-gō-spazm)	spasmodic contraction of the larynx
mucoid..................................... (MŪ-koyd)	resembling mucus
mucous.................................... (MŪ-kus)	pertaining to mucus
nasopharyngeal......................... (*nā*-zō-fa-RIN-jē-al)	pertaining to the nose and pharynx
orthopnea................................. (or-THOP-nē-a)	able to breathe only in an upright position
pulmonary................................ (PUL-mō-ner-ē)	pertaining to the lungs
rhinorrhea................................ (rī-nō-RĒ-a)	discharge from the nose (as in a cold)
thoracic................................... (tho-RAS-ik)	pertaining to the chest

 Mucus is the noun that means the slimy fluid secreted by the mucous membrane. **Mucous** is the adjective that means pertaining to the mucous membrane. Pronunciation is the same for both terms.

Practice saying each of the terms aloud. To hear the terms, access the **PRONOUNCE IT** activity for this chapter on the Student CD that accompanies this text. Or, to hear the terms and their definitions with a CD player or computer, obtain the Pronunciation CD designed for use with this text.

Learn the definitions and spellings of the complementary terms related to the respiratory system by completing exercises 28, 29, and 30.

EXERCISE 28

Analyze and define the following complementary terms.

          P   WR S

Example: hyper/capn/ia *condition of excessive carbon dioxide (in the blood)*

1. laryngeal _____

2. eupnea _____

3. mucoid _____

4. apnea _____

5. hypoxia _____

6. laryngospasm _____

7. endotracheal _____

8. anoxia _____

9. dysphonia _____

10. bronchoalveolar _____

11. dyspnea _____

12. hypocapnia _____

13. bronchospasm _____

14. orthopnea _____

15. hyperpnea _____

16. acapnia _____

17. hypopnea _____

18. hypoxemia _____

19. aphonia _____

20. rhinorrhea _____

21. thoracic _____

22. mucous _____

23. nasopharyngeal _____

24. diaphragmatic _____

25. intrapleural _____

26. pulmonary _____

EXERCISE 29

Build the complementary terms for the following definitions by using the word parts you have learned.

Example: pertaining to bronchi and alveoli <u>bronch</u> / <u>o</u> / <u>alveol</u> / <u>ar</u>
WR /CV/ WR / S

1. deficient oxygen

———————————— / ————————————
P   S(WR)

2. resembling mucus

———————————— / ————————————
WR   S

3. able to breathe only in an upright position

———————————— /CV/ ————————————
WR   S

4. pertaining to within the trachea

———————————— / ———————————— / ————————————
P   WR   S

5. absence of oxygen

———————————— / ————————————
P   S(WR)

6. difficult breathing

———————————— / ————————————
P   S(WR)

7. pertaining to the larynx

———————————— / ————————————
WR   S

8. excessive carbon dioxide in the blood

———————————— / ———————————— / ————————————
P   WR   S

9. normal breathing

———————————— / ————————————
P   S(WR)

10. absence of voice

———————————— / ————————————
P   S(WR)

11. spasmodic contraction of the larynx

———————————— /CV/ ————————————
WR   S

12. deficient carbon dioxide in the blood

———————————— / ———————————— / ————————————
P   WR   S

13. pertaining to the nose and pharynx

———————————— /CV/ ———————————— / ————————————
WR   WR   S

14. pertaining to the diaphragm

———————————— / ————————————
WR   S

15. absence of breathing

———————————— / ————————————
P   S(WR)

16. deficient oxygen in the blood

_____ / _____ / _____
P   WR   S

17. excessive breathing

_____ / _____
P   S(WR)

18. spasmodic contraction in the bronchi

_____ / _____ / _____
WR   CV   S

19. deficient breathing

_____ / _____
P   S(WR)

20. condition of absence of carbon dioxide (in the blood)

_____ / _____ / _____
P   WR   S

21. difficulty in speaking (voice)

_____ / _____
P   S(WR)

22. discharge from the nose

_____ / _____ / _____
WR   CV   S

23. pertaining to mucus

_____ / _____
WR   S

24. pertaining to the chest

_____ / _____
WR   S

25. pertaining to within the pleura

_____ / _____ / _____
P   WR   S

26. pertaining to the lungs

_____ / _____
WR   S

EXERCISE 30

Spell each of the complementary terms. Have someone dictate the terms on pp. 142-144 to you. Think about the word parts before attempting to write the word. Study any words you have spelled incorrectly.

1. _____   10. _____

2. _____   11. _____

3. _____   12. _____

4. _____   13. _____

5. _____   14. _____

6. _____   15. _____

7. _____   16. _____

8. _____   17. _____

9. _____   18. _____

19. _____   23. _____

20. _____   24. _____

21. _____   25. _____

22. _____   26. _____

Complementary Terms

Not Built from Word Parts

Term	Definition
airway (AR-wā)	passageway by which air enters and leaves the lungs as well as a mechanical device used to keep the air passageway unobstructed
asphyxia (as-FIK-sē-a)	deprivation of oxygen for tissue use; suffocation
aspirate (AS-per-āt)	to withdraw fluid or to suction as well as to draw foreign material into the respiratory tract
bronchoconstrictor (*bron*-kō-kon-STRIK-tor)	agent causing narrowing of the bronchi
bronchodilator (*bron*-kō-dī-LĀ-tor)	agent causing the bronchi to widen
cough (kawf)	sudden, noisy expulsion of air from the lungs
hiccup (HIK-up)	sudden catching of breath with a spasmodic contraction of the diaphragm (also called *hiccough*)
hyperventilation (*hī*-per-ven-ti-LĀ-shun)	ventilation of the lungs beyond normal body needs
hypoventilation (*hī*-pō-ven-ti-LĀ-shun)	ventilation of the lungs that does not fulfill the body's gas exchange needs
mucopurulent (*mū*-kō-PŪR-ū-lent)	containing both mucus and pus
mucus (MŪ-kus)	slimy fluid secreted by the mucous membranes
nebulizer (*neb*-ū-LĪZ-er)	device that creates a mist used to deliver medication for giving respiratory treatment (Figure 5-13)
nosocomial infection (nos-ō-KŌ-mē-al)	an infection acquired during hospitalization
paroxysm (PAR-ok-sizm)	periodic, sudden attack
patent (PĀ-tent)	open (an airway must be patent)
sputum (SPŪ-tum)	mucous secretion from the lungs, bronchi, and trachea expelled through the mouth

Continuous Positive Airway Pressure (CPAP) is a type of ventilator used for patients who can initiate their own breathing. It is often used in the treatment of obstructive sleep apnea (OSA).

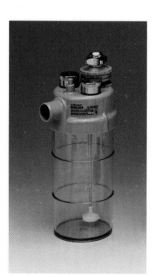

Figure 5-13
Nebulizer.

Sputum is derived from the Latin **spuere**, meaning **to spit.** In a 1693 dictionary it is defined as a "secretion thicker than ordinary spittle."

| ventilator................................. | mechanical device used to assist with or substitute for breathing when patient cannot breathe unassisted (Figure 5-14) |
| (VEN-ti-lā-tor) | |

Practice saying each of these terms aloud. To hear the terms, access the **PRONOUNCE IT** activity for this chapter on the Student CD that accompanies this text. Or, to hear the terms and their definitions with a CD player or computer, obtain the Pronunciation CD designed for use with this text.

Learn the definitions and spellings of the complementary terms by completing exercises 31, 32, and 33.

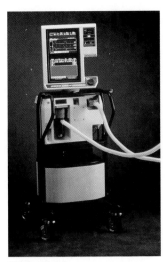

Figure 5-14
Positive pressure ventilator.

EXERCISE 31

Fill in the blanks with the correct terms.

1. Another term for ventilation of the lungs beyond normal body needs is

   _____.

2. A device that creates a mist used to deliver medication for giving respiratory treatment is a(n) _____.

3. A(n) _____ is an agent that causes the air passages to widen.

4. A patient who has difficulty breathing can be attached to a mechanical breathing device called a(n) _____.

5. Another term for suffocation is _____.

6. Material made up of mucous secretions from the lungs, bronchi, and trachea is called _____.

7. To suction or withdraw fluid is to _____.

8. A(n) _____ is a mechanical device that keeps the air passageway unobstructed.

9. A sudden catching of breath with spasmodic contraction of the diaphragm is called a(n) _____.

10. A sudden, noisy expulsion of air from the lung is a(n) _____.

11. Material containing both mucus and pus is referred to as being

    _____.

12. _____ is the name given to ventilation of the lungs that does not fulfill the body's gas exchange needs.

13. An infection acquired during hospitalization is called _____.

14. The term that applies to a periodic sudden attack is _____.

15. An airway must be kept _____ (open) for the patient to breathe.

16. An agent that causes bronchi to narrow is called a(n) _____.

17. _____ is the name given to the slimy fluid secreted by the mucous membranes.

EXERCISE 32

Match the terms in the first column with their correct definitions in the second column.

_____ 1. airway

_____ 2. aspirate

_____ 3. bronchoconstrictor

_____ 4. bronchodilator

_____ 5. cough

_____ 6. hiccup

_____ 7. hyperventilation

_____ 8. asphyxia

a. sudden, noisy expulsion of air from the lungs

b. mechanical device used to keep the air passageway unobstructed

c. agent that narrows the bronchi

d. catching of breath with spasmodic contraction of diaphragm

e. mucus from throat and lungs

f. suffocation

g. ventilation of the lungs beyond normal body needs

h. to draw foreign material into the respiratory tract

i. agent that widens the bronchi

EXERCISE 33

Match the terms in the first column with their correct definitions in the second column.

_____ 1. hypoventilation

_____ 2. mucopurulent

_____ 3. mucus

_____ 4. nebulizer

_____ 5. nosocomial

_____ 6. patent

_____ 7. sputum

_____ 8. ventilator

_____ 9. paroxysm

a. open

b. mucous secretion from lungs, bronchi, and trachea, expelled through the mouth

c. respiratory treatment device that sends a mist

d. mechanical breathing device

e. ventilation of the lungs that does not fulfill the body's gas exchange needs

f. periodic, sudden attack

g. agent that widens air passages

h. containing both mucus and pus

i. slimy fluid secreted by mucous membranes

j. hospital-acquired infection

EXERCISE 34

Spell each of the complementary terms. Have someone dictate the terms on pp. 148-149 to you. Study any words you have spelled incorrectly.

1. _____

2. _____

3. _____

4. _____

5. _____

6. _____

7. _____

8. _____

9. _____

10. _____

11. _____

12. _____

13. _____

14. _____

15. _____

16. _____

17. _____

Abbreviations

ABGs	arterial blood gases
AFB	acid-fast bacilli
ARDS	adult respiratory distress syndrome
CF	cystic fibrosis
CO_2	carbon dioxide
COPD	chronic obstructive pulmonary disease
CT	computed tomography
CXR	chest x-ray
flu	influenza
LLL	left lower lobe
LTB	laryngotracheobronchitis
LUL	left upper lobe
O_2	oxygen
OSA	obstructive sleep apnea
PCP	*Pneumocystis carinii* pneumonia
PE	pulmonary embolism
PFTs	pulmonary function tests
PSG	polysomnography
RLL	right lower lobe
RML	right middle lobe
RUL	right upper lobe
TB	tuberculosis
URI	upper respiratory infection
VPS	ventilation-perfusion scanning

EXERCISE 35

Write the meaning of the abbreviations in the following sentences.

1. A variety of tests are used to diagnose **COPD** _____ _____ _____ _____, including **PFTs** _____ _____ _____, **CXR** _____ _____, **ABGs** _____ _____ _____, and chest **CT** _____ _____ scan.

2. **VPS** _____ _____ _____ is very helpful in diagnosing **PE** _____ _____.

3. The lobes of the left lung are **LUL** _____ _____ _____ and **LLL** _____ _____ _____; the lobes of the right lung are **RUL** _____ _____ _____ _____, **RML** _____ _____ _____, and **RLL** _____ _____ _____.

4. **AFB** _____ _____ _____ smear is used to support the diagnosis of **TB** _____.

5. **PSG** _____ is used to confirm the diagnosis of OSA _____ _____ _____.

6. **PCP** _____ _____ _____ is a fungally in- duced pneumonia commonly seen as an opportunistic infection attributable to AIDS.

7. Respiration is the exchange of **O₂** _____ and **CO₂** _____ _____ between the atmosphere and body cells.

EXERCISE 36

Write the definition for the following abbreviations.

1. ARDS _____ _____ _____ _____

2. CF _____ _____

3. flu _____

4. LTB _____

5. URI _____ _____ _____

CHAPTER REVIEW

EXERCISE 37 *Interact with Medical Records*

Complete the medical consultation report by writing the medical terms in the blanks. Use the list of definitions with the corresponding numbers.

University Hospital and Medical Center
4700 North Main Street • Wellness, Arizona 54321 • (987) 555-3210

PATIENT NAME: Victor Marquez   **CASE NUMBER:** 516987-RSP
DATE OF BIRTH: 02/01/xx   **DATE:** 02/16/xx

MEDICAL CONSULT REPORT

HISTORY: Victor Marquez is a 55-year-old Mexican-American man who came to the Emergency Department on 02/16/xx because of recent onset of 1. _____ and 2. _____ . He has also had weight loss and cough for the past 6 months. He denies hemoptysis, chest pain, fever, or night sweats. He has a history of smoking two packs of cigarettes a day for 40 years. It was decided that he should be admitted and scheduled for a 3. _____ consultation.

PHYSICAL EXAMINATION: VITAL SIGNS: Temperature, 98.2. Pulse, 60. Respirations, 18. The chest is clear except for scattered rhonchi over left posterior lung. Blood pressure, 148/82. The heart is regular rhythm without murmur. He is in no acute distress. Pulses are full and equal throughout. There is mild clubbing of fingers.

PULMONARY EXAM: 4. _____ _____ reveals a suspicious lesion in the left upper lobe of the lung with diffuse interstitial fibrotic lesions. Fiberoptic 5. _____ shows edematous vocal cords with no obvious nodules. However, at the entry of the left bronchus, a lesion is observed that partially obstructs the opening. A biopsy and brush cytology of the specimen were obtained. 6. _____ _____ _____ shows mild 7. _____ .

IMPRESSION: It is my impression that the patient has 8. _____ _____.

DISPOSITION:
1. Obtain 9. _____ _____ _____ to include lung volumes and diffusing capacity.
2. Obtain a CT scan of the chest and a 10. _____ surgery consultation.

_____
Miguel Valdez, MD

MV/mcm

---

1. sudden noisy expulsion of air from the lungs
2. difficult breathing
3. pertaining to the lungs
4. x-ray image used to evaluate the lungs and heart
5. visual examination of the bronchi
6. test performed on arterial blood to determine the presence of oxygen, carbon dioxide, and other gases
7. deficient oxygen in the blood
8. cancerous tumor originating in the bronchus
9. a group of tests performed on breathing
10. pertaining to the chest

EXERCISE 38 *Interpret Medical Terms*

To test your understanding of the terms introduced in this chapter, circle the words that correctly complete the sentences. The italicized words refer to the correct answer.

1. The patient in the emergency room was admitted with a *severe nosebleed,* or (rhinomycosis, epistaxis, nasopharyngitis).
2. The accident caused damage to the larynx, necessitating *a surgical repair,* or a (laryngectomy, laryngostomy, laryngoplasty).
3. Mr. Prince was *able to breathe only in an upright position,* so the nurse recorded that he had (orthopnea, eupnea, dyspnea).
4. The *test on arterial blood to determine oxygen and carbon dioxide levels* (pulse oximetry, pulmonary function tests, arterial blood gases) indicated that the patient was *deficient in oxygen,* or had (dysphonia, hypoxia, hypocapnia).
5. The physician informed the patient that a heart attack was not the cause of the *chest pain,* or (thoracalgia, pneumothorax, thoracentesis).
6. The patient reported dizziness brought on by *ventilation of the lungs beyond normal body needs,* or (hyperventilation, hypoventilation, dysphonia).
7. The physician wished the patient to have the medication given by *a device that delivers mist,* so he ordered that the treatment be given by (airway, nebulizer, ventilator).
8. The patient with *blood in the chest* was diagnosed as having a (pneumothorax, pleuritis, hemothorax).
9. After surgery, the patient had *a block in the circulation to the pulmonary artery* or (pleural effusion, pulmonary edema, pulmonary embolism).
10. The patient was diagnosed as having *a fungal disease affecting the lung,* or (obstructive sleep apnea, *P. carinii* pneumonia, coccidioidomycosis).
11. The physician ordered an *x-ray image of the chest* (chest x-ray, chest CT scan, bronchogram) because she suspected *an infection acquired during hospitalization,* or (patent, nosocomial, paroxysm) pneumonia.
12. The patient received an *intradermal injection to determine if she had been exposed to TB* or (AFB, ABGs, PPD skin test).

EXERCISE 39 *Read Medical Terms in Use*

Practice pronouncing the terms by reading the following medical document. Use the pronunciation key following the medical terms to assist you in saying the word.

A 24-year-old man visited the emergency department because of **dyspnea** (DISP-nē-a), **hyperpnea** (hī-perp-NĒ-a), **paroxysms** (PAR-ok-sizms) of **cough** (kawf), and the presence of thick, tenacious **mucus** (MŪ-kus). He had a history of **asthma** (AZ-ma) since the age of 12 years. A chest x-ray was negative for **pneumonia** (nū-MŌ-nē-a). **Arterial** (ar-TĒ-rē-al) **blood gases** showed **hypoxemia** (hī-pok-SĒ-mē-a) but no **hypercapnia** (hī-per-KAP-nē-a). **Pulmonary** (PUL-mō-ner-ē) **function tests** disclosed bronchoconstriction, which was corrected by a **bronchodilator** (*bron-kō-dī-LĀ-tor*). The physician prescribed a **nebulizer** (neb-ū-LĪZ-er) treatment. The asthma attack was probably precipitated by an episode of **bronchitis** (bron-KĪ-tis).

EXERCISE 40   *Comprehend Medical Terms in Use*

For additional information on diseases of the lung, visit the American Lung Association at www.lungusa.org.

Test your comprehension of terms in the previous medical document by answering *T* for true and *F* for false.

_____ 1. The patient visited the emergency department because of many symptoms, one of which was sudden, periodic coughing.

_____ 2. Diagnostic procedures were performed to assist with the diagnosis. ABGs showed increased O_2 and decreased CO_2.

_____ 3. An agent that causes the bronchi to widen was used to treat the condition diagnosed with the PFTs.

_____ 4. The asthma attack was precipitated by narrowing of the bronchi.

COMBINING FORMS CROSSWORD PUZZLE

Across Clues
1. pleura
3. tonsil
5. mucus
6. sinus
7. pus
8. nose
10. pharynx
12. trachea
14. alveolus
16. straight
17. nose

Down Clues
1. lung
2. lung, air
4. larynx
9. lobe
11. adenoids
13. breathe
15. oxygen

REVIEW OF WORD PARTS

Can you define and spell the following word parts?

Combining Forms

adenoid/o	hemat/o	ox/o	rhin/o
alveol/o	hem/o	pharyng/o	sept/o
atel/o	laryng/o	pleur/o	sinus/o
bronch/i	lob/o	pneumat/o	somn/o
bronch/o	muc/o	pneum/o	spir/o
capn/o	nas/o	pneumon/o	thorac/o
diaphragmat/o	orth/o	pulmon/o	tonsill/o
epiglott/o	ox/i	py/o	trache/o

Prefixes

a-
an-
endo-
eu-
pan-
poly-

Suffixes

-algia
-ar
-ary
-cele
-centesis
-eal
-ectasis
-emia

-gram
-graphy
-meter
-metry
-oxia
-pexy
-phonia
-pnea
-rrhagia

-scope
-scopic
-scopy
-spasm
-stenosis
-stomy
-thorax
-tomy

REVIEW OF TERMS

Can you build, analyze, define, pronounce, and spell the following terms *built from word parts?*

Diseases and Disorders

adenoiditis
atelectasis
bronchiectasis
bronchitis
bronchogenic carcinoma
bronchopneumonia
diaphragmatocele
epiglottitis
hemothorax
laryngitis
laryngotracheobronchitis
   (LTB)
lobar pneumonia
nasopharyngitis
pansinusitis
pharyngitis
pleuritis
pneumatocele
pneumoconiosis
pneumonia
pneumonitis
pneumothorax
pulmonary neoplasm
pyothorax
rhinitis
rhinomycosis
rhinorrhagia
thoracalgia
tonsillitis
tracheitis
tracheostenosis

Surgical

adenoidectomy
adenotome
bronchoplasty
laryngectomy
laryngoplasty
laryngostomy
laryngotracheotomy
lobectomy
pleuropexy
pneumobronchotomy
pneumonectomy
rhinoplasty
septoplasty
septotomy
sinusotomy
thoracocentesis
thoracotomy
tonsillectomy
tracheoplasty
tracheostomy
tracheotomy

Diagnostic

bronchoscope
bronchoscopy
capnometer
endoscope
endoscopic
endoscopy
laryngoscope
laryngoscopy
oximeter
polysomnography (PSG)
spirometer
spirometry
thoracoscope
thoracoscopy

Complementary

acapnia
anoxia
aphonia
apnea
bronchoalveolar
bronchospasm
diaphragmatic
dysphonia
dyspnea
endotracheal
eupnea
hypercapnia
hyperpnea
hypocapnia
hypopnea
hypoxemia
hypoxia
intrapleural
laryngeal
laryngospasm
mucoid
mucous
nasopharyngeal
orthopnea
pulmonary
rhinorrhea
thoracic

Can you define, pronounce, and spell the following terms *not built from word parts?*

Diseases and Disorders

adult respiratory distress
   syndrome (ARDS)
asthma
chronic obstructive pulmonary
   disease (COPD)
coccidioidomycosis
cor pulmonale
croup
cystic fibrosis (CF)
deviated septum
emphysema
epistaxis
influenza (flu)
Legionnaire disease
obstructive sleep apnea (OSA)
pertussis
pleural effusion
Pneumocystis carinii
   pneumonia (PCP)
pulmonary edema
pulmonary embolism (PE)
tuberculosis (TB)
upper respiratory infection
   (URI)

Diagnostic

acid-fast bacilli smear (AFB)
arterial blood gases (ABGs)
chest computed tomography
   (CT) scan
chest x-ray (CXR)
PPD skin test
pulmonary function tests
   (PFTs)
pulse oximetry
ventilation-perfusion scanning
   (VPS)

Complementary

airway
asphyxia
aspirate
bronchoconstrictor
bronchodilator
cough
hiccup
hyperventilation
hypoventilation
mucopurulent
mucus
nebulizer
nosocomial infection
paroxysm
patent
sputum
ventilator

6

Urinary System

OUTLINE

OBJECTIVES

On completion of this chapter you will be able to:

1. Identify the organs and other structures of the urinary system.
2. Define and spell the word parts presented in this chapter.
3. Build and analyze medical terms with word parts presented in this and previous chapters.
4. Define, pronounce, and spell the disease and disorder, diagnostic, surgical, and complementary terms for the urinary system.
5. Interpret the meanings of the abbreviations presented in this chapter.
6. Read medical documents and interpret medical terminology contained in them.

ANATOMY

Function

The urinary system removes waste material from the body, regulates fluid volume, and maintains electrolyte concentration in the body fluid. Organs of the urinary system are the kidneys, ureters, bladder, and urethra (Figures 6-1 and 6-2).

Organs of the Urinary System

kidneys	two bean-shaped organs located on each side of the vertebral column on the posterior wall of the abdominal cavity behind the parietal peritoneum. Their function is to remove waste products from the blood and to aid in maintaining water and electrolyte balances (see Figure 6-2).
nephron	urine-producing microscopic structure. Approximately 1 million nephrons are located in each kidney.

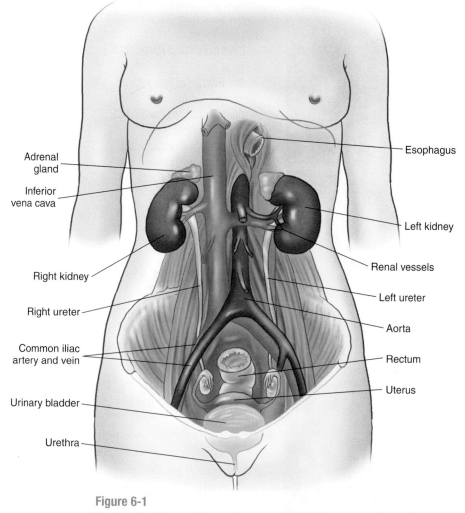

Figure 6-1

The female urinary system and some associated structures.

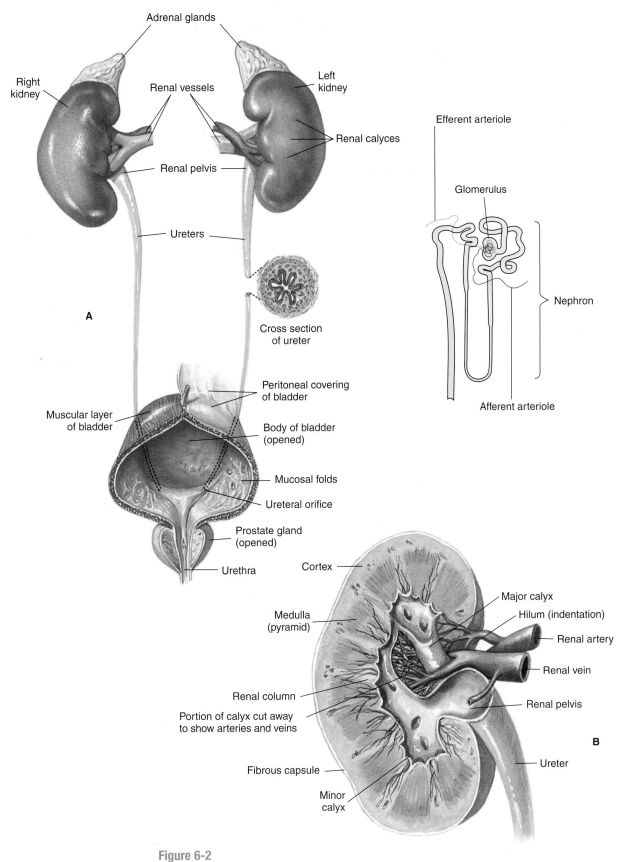

Figure 6-2
A, Anatomy of the male urinary tract; **B,** frontal section of the kidney.

glomerulus (*pl.* glomeruli)............ cluster of capillaries at the entrance of the nephron. The process of filtering the blood, thereby forming urine, begins here.

renal pelvis.................................... funnel-shaped reservoir that collects the urine and passes it to the ureter

hilum .... indentation on the medial side of the kidney where the ureter leaves the kidney

ureters.. two slender tubes, approximately 10 to 13 inches (26 to 33 cm) long, that receive the urine from the kidneys and carry it to the posterior portion of the bladder (see Figure 6-2)

urinary bladder.............................. muscular, hollow organ that temporarily holds the urine. As it fills, the thick, muscular wall becomes thinner, and the organ increases in size.

urethra .... lowest part of the urinary tract, through which the urine passes from the urinary bladder to the outside of the body. This narrow tube varies in length by sex. It is 1.5 inches (3.8 cm) long in the female and 8 inches (20 cm) in the male, in whom it is also part of the reproductive system. It carries seminal fluid (semen) at the time of ejaculation (see Figure 6-2).

urinary meatus............................... opening through which the urine passes to the outside

---

Learn the anatomic terms by completing exercise 1.

Bladder
is a derivative of the Anglo-Saxon **blaeddre,** meaning a **blister** or **windbag.**

EXERCISE 1

Match the anatomic terms in the first column with the correct definitions in the second column.

_____ 1. kidney(s)

_____ 2. glomerulus

_____ 3. nephron

_____ 4. ureters

_____ 5. urinary bladder

_____ 6. urinary meatus

_____ 7. urethra

a. stores urine

b. outside opening through which the urine passes

c. carry urine from the kidney to the urinary bladder

d. cluster of capillaries in the kidney where the urine begins to form

e. carries urine from the bladder to the urinary meatus

f. kidney's urine-producing unit

g. organs that remove waste products from the blood

WORD PARTS

Combining Forms of the Urinary System

Study the word parts and their definitions listed below. Completing exercises 2 and 3 and Exercise Figures A and B will help you learn the terms.

Combining Form	Definition
cyst/o, vesic/o	bladder, sac
(NOTE: these refer to the *urinary bladder* unless otherwise identified.)	
glomerul/o	glomerulus
meat/o	meatus (opening)
nephr/o, ren/o	kidney
pyel/o	renal pelvis
ureter/o	ureter
urethr/o	urethra

Glomerulus
is derived from the Latin **glomus**, which means **ball of thread.** It was thought that the rounded cluster of capillary loops at the nephron's entrance resembled thread in a ball.

Meatus
is derived from the Latin **meare**, meaning **to pass** or **to go.** Other anatomic passages share the same name, such as the auditory meatus.

Pyelos
is the Greek word for **tub-shaped vessel,** which describes the kidney's shape.

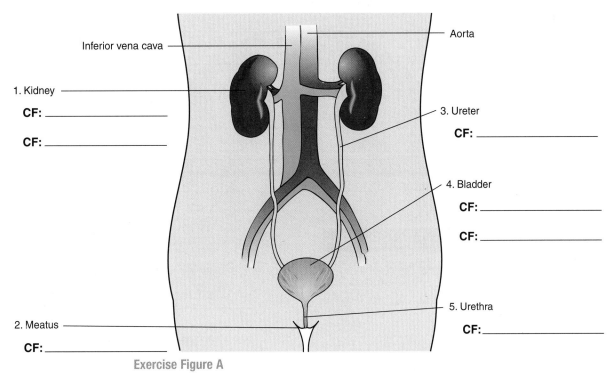

1. Kidney
   CF: _____
   CF: _____

2. Meatus
   CF: _____

3. Ureter
   CF: _____

4. Bladder
   CF: _____
   CF: _____

5. Urethra
   CF: _____

Inferior vena cava
Aorta

Exercise Figure A
Fill in the blanks with combining forms for the diagram of the urinary system.

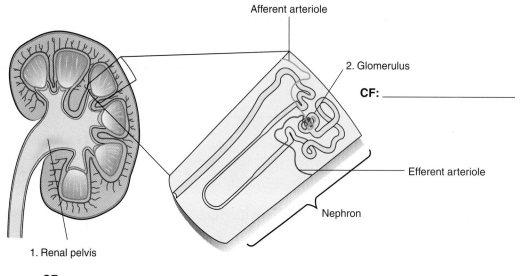

Afferent arteriole

2. Glomerulus

CF: _____

Efferent arteriole

Nephron

1. Renal pelvis

CF: _____

Exercise Figure B

Fill in the blanks to label the diagram of the internal kidney structure.

EXERCISE 2

Write the definitions of the following combining forms.

1. glomerul/o _____

2. vesic/o _____

3. nephr/o _____

4. pyel/o _____

5. ureter/o _____

6. cyst/o _____

7. urethr/o _____

8. ren/o _____

9. meat/o _____

EXERCISE 3

Write the combining form for each of the following terms.

1. kidney   a. _____

                         b. _____

2. bladder, sac   a. _____

                         b. _____

3. ureter _____

4. renal pelvis _____

5. glomerulus _____

6. urethra _____

7. meatus _____

Combining Forms Commonly Used with Urinary System Terms

Combining Form	Definition
albumin/o	albumin
azot/o	urea, nitrogen
blast/o	developing cell, germ cell
glyc/o, glycos/o	sugar
hydr/o	water
lith/o	stone, calculus
noct/i (NOTE: the combining vowel is i.)	night
olig/o	scanty, few
son/o	sound
tom/o	cut, section
urin/o, ur/o	urine, urinary tract

Learn the combining forms by completing exercises 4 and 5.

EXERCISE   4

Write the definitions of the following combining forms.

1. hydr/o _____

2. azot/o _____

3. noct/i _____

4. lith/o _____

5. tom/o _____

6. albumin/o _____

7. urin/o _____

8. son/o _____

9. glyc/o _____

10. blast/o _____

11. olig/o _____

12. ur/o _____

13. glycos/o _____

EXERCISE 5

Write the combining form for each of the following.

1. sugar
   a. _____
   b. _____

2. sound
   _____

3. urine, urinary tract
   a. _____
   b. _____

4. water
   _____

5. developing cell, germ cell
   _____

6. cut, section
   _____

7. albumin
   _____

8. night
   _____

9. urea, nitrogen
   _____

10. stone, calculus
    _____

11. scanty
    _____

Suffixes

Suffix	Definition
-iasis, -esis	condition
-lysis	loosening, dissolution, separating
-megaly	enlargement
-ptosis	drooping, sagging, prolapse
-rrhaphy	suturing, repairing

-tripsy.............................	surgical crushing
-trophy.............................	nourishment, development
-uria.................................	urine, urination

Refer to Appendix A and Appendix B for alphabetized lists of word parts and their meanings.

Learn the suffixes by completing exercises 6 and 7.

EXERCISE 6

Match the suffixes in the first column with their correct definitions in the second column.

_____ 1. -iasis, -esis		a. nourishment, development
_____ 2. -lysis		b. urine, urination
_____ 3. -megaly		c. condition
_____ 4. -rrhaphy		d. enlargement
_____ 5. -ptosis		e. surgical crushing
_____ 6. -tripsy		f. suturing, repairing
_____ 7. -trophy		g. drooping, sagging, prolapse
_____ 8. -uria		h. stretching out
		i. loosening, dissolution, separating

EXERCISE 7

Write the definitions of the following suffixes.

1. -rrhaphy _____

2. -lysis _____

3. -iasis, -esis _____

4. -trophy _____

5. -uria _____

6. -megaly _____

7. -ptosis _____

8. -tripsy _____

MEDICAL TERMS

The terms you need to learn to complete this chapter are listed next. The exercises following each list will help you learn the definition and the spelling of each word.

Disease and Disorder Terms

Built from Word Parts

Term	Definition
cystitis (sis-TĪ-tis)	inflammation of the bladder
cystocele (SIS-tō-sēl)	protrusion of the bladder
cystolith (SIS-tō-lith)	stone in the bladder (Exercise Figure C)
glomerulonephritis (glō-*mer*-ū-lō-ne-FRĪ-tis)	inflammation of the glomeruli of the kidney
hydronephrosis (*hī*-drō-ne-FRŌ-sis)	abnormal condition of water in the kidney (distension of the renal pelvis with urine because of an obstruction)
nephritis (ne-FRĪ-tis)	inflammation of a kidney
nephroblastoma (nef-rō-blas-TŌ-ma)	kidney tumor containing developing cell (malignant tumor) (also called Wilms tumor)
nephrohypertrophy (*nef*-rō-hī-PER-trō-fē) (NOTE: the prefix *hyper-* appears in the middle of this term.)	excessive development (increase in size) of the kidney
nephrolithiasis (*nef*-rō-lith-Ī-a-sis)	condition of stone(s) in the kidney
nephroma (nef-RŌ-ma)	tumor of the kidney
nephromegaly (*nef*-rō-MEG-a-lē)	enlargement of a kidney

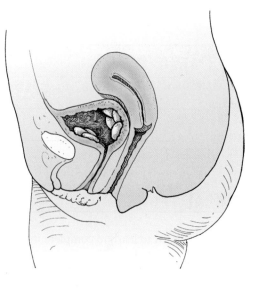

Exercise Figure C

Fill in the blanks to label the diagram.

——————— / —— / ———
bladder / cv / stone

nephroptosis............................. (*nef*-rop-TŌ-sis)	drooping kidney
pyelitis..................................... (pī-e-LĪ-tis)	inflammation of the renal pelvis
pyelonephritis .... (pī-e-lō-ne-FRĪ-tis)	inflammation of the renal pelvis and the kidney
uremia..................................... (ū-RĒ-mē-a)	condition of urine (urea) in the blood (toxic condition resulting from retention of by-products of the kidney in the blood)
ureteritis................................ (ū-rē-ter-Ī-tis)	inflammation of a ureter
ureterocele............................. (ū-RĒ-ter-ō-sēl)	protrusion of a ureter
ureterolithiasis .... (ū-rē-ter-ō-lith-Ī-a-sis)	condition of stones in the ureters
ureterostenosis .... (ū-rē-ter-ō-sten-Ō-sis)	narrowing of the ureter
urethrocystitis........................ (ū-*rē*-thrō-sis-TĪ-tis)	inflammation of the urethra and the bladder

 Nephroptosis is also known as a **floating kidney** and occurs when the kidney is no longer held in place and drops out of its normal position. The kidney is normally held in position by connective and adipose tissue, so it is prone to injury and also may cause the ureter to twist. Truck drivers and horseback riders are prone to this condition.

Practice saying each of these terms aloud. To hear the terms, access the **PRONOUNCE IT** activity for this chapter on the Student CD that accompanies this text. Or, to hear the terms and their definitions with a CD player or computer, obtain the Pronunciation CD designed for use with this text.

Learn the definitions and spellings of the disease and disorder terms by completing exercises 8, 9, and 10.

EXERCISE 8

Analyze and define the following terms.

             WR   CV WR S
Example: glomerul/o/nephr/itis *inflammation of the glomeruli of the kidney*
                CF

1. nephroma _____

2. cystolith _____

3. nephrolithiasis _____

4. uremia _____

5. nephroptosis _____

6. cystocele _____

7. nephrohypertrophy _____

8. cystitis _____

9. pyelitis _____

10. ureterocele _____

11. hydronephrosis _____

12. nephromegaly _____

13. ureterolithiasis _____

14. pyelonephritis _____

15. ureteritis _____

16. nephritis _____

17. urethrocystitis _____

18. ureterostenosis _____

19. nephroblastoma _____

EXERCISE 9

Build disease and disorder terms for the following definitions with the word parts you have learned.

Example: inflammation of the ureter <u>ureter</u> / <u>itis</u>
　　　　　　　　　　　　　　　　　　 WR　 /　 S

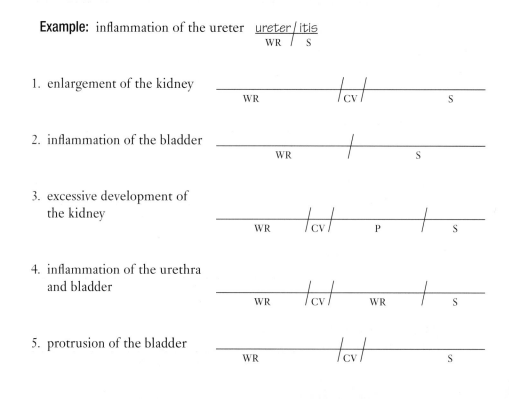

1. enlargement of the kidney

　　　　　　　　　　　WR　　　　 CV　　　　　　　 S

2. inflammation of the bladder

　　　　　　　　　　　WR　　　　　 S

3. excessive development of the kidney

　　　　　　　　　　　WR　　 CV　　　 P　　　　 S

4. inflammation of the urethra and bladder

　　　　　　　　　　　WR　　 CV　　 WR　　　 S

5. protrusion of the bladder

　　　　　　　　　　　WR　　　　 CV　　　　　 S

6. abnormal condition of
   water in the kidney

   —————— /CV/ —————— / ——————
   WR   CV   WR   S

7. stone in the bladder

   —————————— /CV/ ——————
   WR   CV   WR

8. inflammation of the
   glomeruli of the kidney

   —————— /CV/ —————— / ——————
   WR   CV   WR   S

9. tumor of the kidney

   —————————— / ——————
   WR   S

10. a drooping kidney

    —————— /CV/ ——————
    WR   CV   S

11. inflammation of a kidney

    —————————— / ——————
    WR   S

12. condition of stones in the
    kidney

    —————— /CV/ —————— / ——————
    WR   CV   WR   S

13. protrusion of a ureter

    —————————— /CV/ ——————
    WR   CV   S

14. inflammation of the renal
    pelvis

    —————————— / ——————
    WR   S

15. condition of urine (urea) in
    the blood

    —————————— / ——————
    WR   S

16. narrowing of the ureter

    —————————— /CV/ ——————
    WR   CV   S

17. inflammation of the renal
    pelvis and the kidney

    —————— /CV/ —————— / ——————
    WR   CV   WR   S

18. condition of stones in the
    ureters

    —————— /CV/ —————— / ——————
    WR   CV   WR   S

19. kidney tumor containing
    developing cell tissue

    —————— /CV/ —————— / ——————
    WR   CV   WR   S

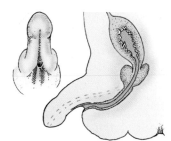

Figure 6-3
Hypospadias.

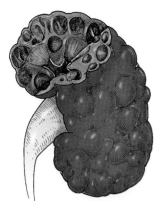

Figure 6-4
Polycystic kidney.

EXERCISE 10

Spell each of the disease and disorder terms. Have someone dictate the terms on pp. 168-169 to you. Think about the word parts before attempting to write the word. Study any words you have spelled incorrectly.

1. _____
2. _____
3. _____
4. _____
5. _____
6. _____
7. _____
8. _____
9. _____
10. _____

11. _____
12. _____
13. _____
14. _____
15. _____
16. _____
17. _____
18. _____
19. _____
20. _____

Disease and Disorder Terms

Not Built from Word Parts

Term	Definition
epispadias .... (*ep*-i-SPĀ-dē-as)	congenital defect in which the urinary meatus is located on the upper surface of the penis
hypospadias .... (hī-pō-SPĀ-dē-as)	congenital defect in which the urinary meatus is located on the underside of the penis; a similar defect can occur in the female (Figure 6-3)
polycystic kidney disease .... (*pol*-i-SIS-tik) (KID-nē) (di-ZĒZ)	condition in which the kidney contains many cysts and is enlarged (Figure 6-4)
renal calculi .... (RĒ-nal) (KAL-kū-lī)	stones in the kidney
renal hypertension .... (RĒ-nal) (hī-per-TEN-shun)	elevated blood pressure resulting from kidney disease
sepsis .... (SEP-sis)	a condition in which pathogenic microorganisms, usually bacteria, enter the bloodstream, causing a systemic inflammatory response to the infection (also called *septicemia*)
urinary retention .... (Ū-rin-*ā*-rē) (rē-TEN-shun)	abnormal accumulation of urine in the bladder because of an inability to urinate

urinary suppression	sudden stoppage of urine formation
(Ū-rin-ā-rē) (sū-PRESH-un)	
urinary tract infection (UTI)	infection of one or more organs of the
(Ū-rin-ā-rē) (trakt)	urinary tract

Practice saying each of these terms aloud. To hear the terms, access the **PRONOUNCE IT** activity for this chapter on the Student CD that accompanies this text. Or, to hear the terms and their definitions with a CD player or computer, obtain the Pronunciation CD designed for use with this text.

Learn the definitions and spellings of the disease and disorder terms by completing exercises 11, 12, and 13.

> **CAM TERM**
>
> **Kegel exercises** are the tightening and release of vaginopelvic muscles in intervals to improve muscular tone. Kegel exercises can be used to prevent urinary tract infections and to strengthen pelvic floor muscles to improve bladder control.

EXERCISE 11

Fill in the blanks with the correct terms.

1. Stones in the kidney are also called _____ _____.

2. The inability to urinate, which results in an abnormal amount of urine in the bladder, is known as _____ _____.

3. The name given to a condition in which a kidney is enlarged and contains many cysts is _____ _____ _____.

4. The condition in which the urinary meatus is located on the underside of the penis is called _____.

5. Elevated blood pressure resulting from kidney disease is _____ _____.

6. Sudden stoppage of urine formation is referred to as _____ _____.

7. _____ is a condition in which the urinary meatus is located on the upper surface of the penis.

8. Infection of one or more organs of the urinary system is called _____ _____ _____.

9. _____ is a condition in which pathogenic microorganisms enter the bloodstream.

EXERCISE 12

Match the terms in the first column with the correct definitions in the second column.

_____ 1. epispadias

_____ 2. hypospadias

_____ 3. renal calculi

_____ 4. renal hypertension

_____ 5. polycystic kidney disease

a. enlarged kidney with many cysts

b. sudden stoppage of urine formation

c. urinary meatus on the upper surface of the penis

d. kidney stones

_____ 6. urinary retention   e. inability to urinate

_____ 7. urinary suppression   f. urinary meatus on the underside of the penis

_____ 8. urinary tract infection   g. infection of one or more organs of the urinary system

_____ 9. sepsis

h. characterized by elevated blood pressure

i. causes a systemic inflammatory response to infection

j. excessive amount of urine

EXERCISE 13

Spell the disease and disorder terms. Have someone dictate the terms on pp. 172-173 to you. Study any words you have spelled incorrectly.

1. _____   6. _____

2. _____   7. _____

3. _____   8. _____

4. _____   9. _____

5. _____

Surgical Terms

Built from Word Parts

Term	Definition
cystectomy (sis-TEK-tō-mē)	excision of the bladder
cystolithotomy (*sis*-tō-li-THOT-ō-mē)	incision of the bladder to remove a stone
cystorrhaphy (sist-OR-a-fē)	suturing the bladder
cystostomy (sis-TOS-tō-mē)	creating an artificial opening into the bladder (Exercise Figure D)
cystotomy (sis-TOT-ō-mē)	
or vesicotomy (*ves*-i-KOT-ō-mē)	incision of the bladder
lithotripsy (LITH-ō-trip-sē)	surgical crushing of a stone (Exercise Figure E)
meatotomy (*mē*-a-TOT-ō-mē)	incision of the meatus
nephrectomy (ne-FREK-tō-mē)	excision of a kidney

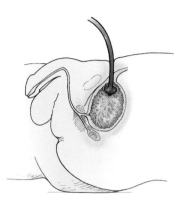

Exercise Figure D

Fill in the blanks to label the diagram.

_____ / ___ / _____
   bladder / **cv** / **creation of an artificial opening**

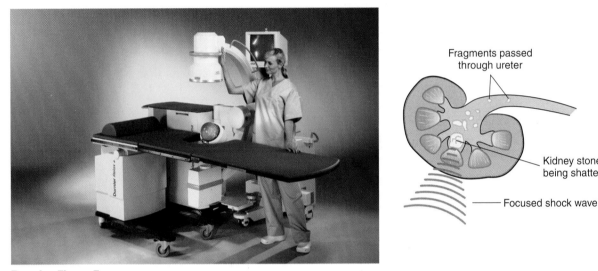

Fragments passed through ureter

Kidney stone being shattered

Focused shock wave

Exercise Figure E

Fill in the blanks to complete the labeling of the diagram.

Extracorporeal shock wave _____ / ___ / _____ .
   stone / **cv** / **surgical crushing**

ESWL breaks down the kidney stone into fragments by shock waves from outside the body. The broken fragments are eliminated from the body with the passing of urine.

nephrolysis.............................. (ne-FROL-i-sis)	separating the kidney (from other body structures)
nephropexy.............................. (NEF-rō-*peks*-ē)	surgical fixation of the kidney
nephropyelolithotomy...................... (*nef*-rō-pī-e-lō-THOT-ō-mē)	incision through the kidney to the renal pelvis to remove a stone
nephrostomy.............................. (nef-ROS-tō-mē)	creation of an artificial opening into the kidney (Exercise Figure F)
pyelolithotomy...................... (*pī*-el-ō-lith-OT-ō-mē)	incision of the renal pelvis to remove a stone (Exercise Figure G)
pyeloplasty.............................. (PĪ-el-ō-*plas*-tē)	surgical repair of the renal pelvis
ureterectomy.............................. (ū-*re*-ter-EK-tō-mē)	excision of a ureter

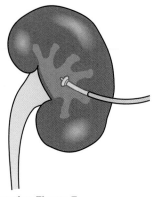

Exercise Figure F
Fill in the blanks to label the diagram.

_____ / ____ / _____
kidney / cv / creation of an
              artificial opening

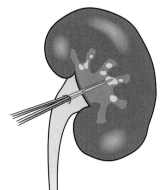

Exercise Figure G
Fill in the blanks to label the diagram.

_____ / ____ / _____ / ____ / _____
renal / cv / stone / cv / incision
pelvis

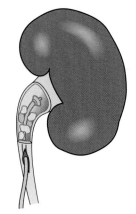

Exercise Figure H
Fill in the blanks to label the diagram.

_____ / ____ / _____
ureter / cv / creation of an
              artificial opening

ureterostomy............................ (ū-*rē*-ter-OS-tō-mē)	creation of an artificial opening into the ureter (Exercise Figure H)
urethroplasty............................ (ū-RĒ-thrō-*plas*-tē)	surgical repair of the urethra
vesicourethral suspension............... (ves-i-kō-ū-RĒ-thral)	suspension pertaining to the bladder and urethra

Practice saying each of these terms aloud. To hear the terms, access the **PRONOUNCE IT** activity for this chapter on the Student CD that accompanies this text. Or, to hear the terms and their definitions with a CD player or computer, obtain the Pronunciation CD designed for use with this text.

Learn the definitions and spellings of the surgical terms by completing exercises 14, 15, and 16.

Stress Incontinence
is the involuntary intermittent leakage of urine as a result of pressure, from a cough or a sneeze, on the weakened area around the urethra and bladder. The Marshall-Marchetti Krantz technique, or **vesicourethral suspension,** is a bladder suspension surgery performed on patients with stress incontinence.

EXERCISE 14

Analyze and define the following surgical terms.

1. vesicotomy _____

2. cystotomy _____

3. nephrostomy _____

4. nephrolysis _____

5. cystectomy _____

6. pyelolithotomy _____

7. nephropexy _____

8. cystolithotomy _____

9. nephrectomy _____

10. ureterectomy _____

11. cystostomy _____

12. pyeloplasty _____

13. cystorrhaphy _____

14. meatotomy _____

15. lithotripsy _____

16. urethroplasty _____

17. vesicourethral suspension _____

18. nephropyelolithotomy _____

EXERCISE 15

Build surgical terms for the following definitions by using the word parts you have learned.

1. incision of the urethra

   _____ / ___ / _____
   WR   CV   S

2. excision of a kidney

   _____ / _____
   WR   S

3. incision of the renal pelvis
   to remove a stone

   _____ / CV / WR / CV / _____
   WR   CV   WR   CV   S

4. suturing of the bladder

   _____ / CV / _____
   WR   CV   S

5. separating the kidney
   (from other structures)

   _____ / CV / _____
   WR   CV   S

6. creation of an artificial
   opening into the kidney

   _____ / CV / _____
   WR   CV   S

7. surgical repair of the
   urethra

   _____ / CV / _____
   WR   CV   S

8. excision of the bladder

   _____ / _____
   WR   S

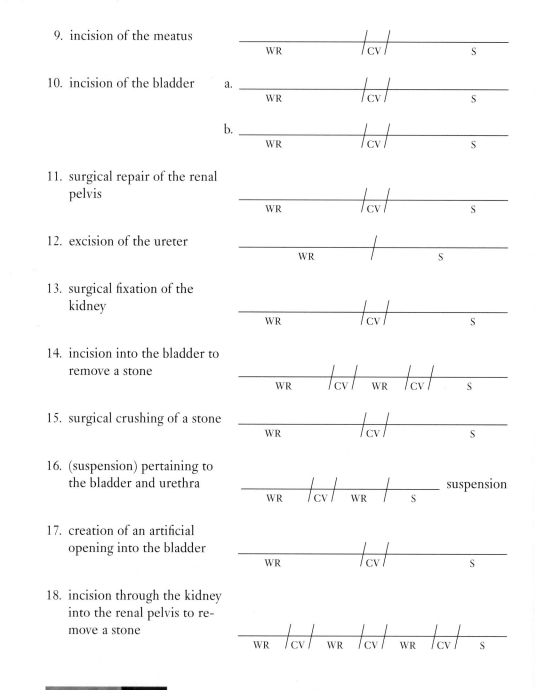

9. incision of the meatus

_____ / _ / _____
WR   CV   S

10. incision of the bladder   a. _____ / _ / _____
WR   CV   S

           b. _____ / _ / _____
WR   CV   S

11. surgical repair of the renal pelvis

_____ / _ / _____
WR   CV   S

12. excision of the ureter

_____ / _____
WR   S

13. surgical fixation of the kidney

_____ / _ / _____
WR   CV   S

14. incision into the bladder to remove a stone

_____ / _ / _____ / _ / _____
WR   CV   WR   CV   S

15. surgical crushing of a stone

_____ / _ / _____
WR   CV   S

16. (suspension) pertaining to the bladder and urethra

_____ / _ / _____ / _____ suspension
WR   CV   WR   S

17. creation of an artificial opening into the bladder

_____ / _ / _____
WR   CV   S

18. incision through the kidney into the renal pelvis to remove a stone

_____ / _ / _____ / _ / _____ / _ / _____
WR   CV   WR   CV   WR   CV   S

EXERCISE 16

Spell each of the surgical terms. Have someone dictate the terms on pp. 174-176 to you. Think about the word parts before attempting to write the word. Study any words you have spelled incorrectly.

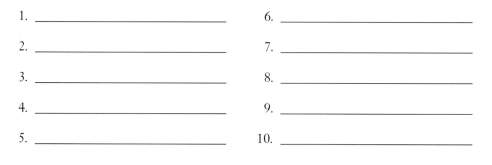

1. _____   6. _____

2. _____   7. _____

3. _____   8. _____

4. _____   9. _____

5. _____   10. _____

11. _____   15. _____

12. _____   16. _____

13. _____   17. _____

14. _____   18. _____

Surgical Terms

Not Built from Word Parts

Term	Definition
extracorporeal shock wave lithotripsy (ESWL).................... (ek-stra-kor-POR-ē-al) (LITH-ō-trip-sē)	a noninvasive treatment for removal of kidney or ureteral stone(s). By using ultrasound and fluoroscopic imaging, the stone is positioned at a focal point. Repeated firing of shock waves renders the stone into fragments that pass from the body in the urine (also called *shock wave lithotripsy [SWL]*) (see Exercise Figure E).
fulguration... (ful-gū-RA-shun)	destruction of living tissue with an electric spark (a method commonly used to remove bladder growths) (Figure 6-5)
renal transplant.................................... (RĒ-nal) (*trans*-plant)	surgical implantation of a donor kidney to replace a nonfunctioning kidney (Figure 6-6)

Extracorporeal means occurring **outside the body.**

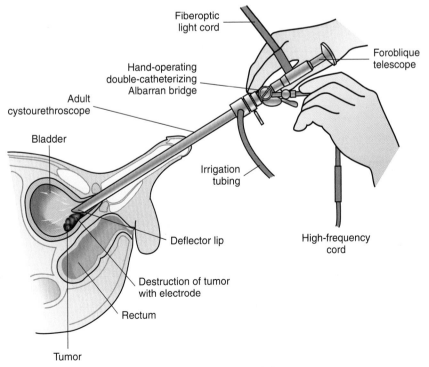

Figure 6-5
Bladder fulguration.

Labels: Fiberoptic light cord; Foroblique telescope; Hand-operating double-catheterizing Albarran bridge; Adult cystourethroscope; Bladder; Irrigation tubing; Deflector lip; High-frequency cord; Destruction of tumor with electrode; Rectum; Tumor

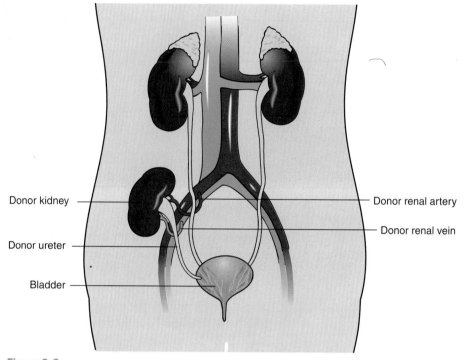

Donor kidney

Donor ureter

Bladder

Donor renal artery

Donor renal vein

Figure 6-6
Renal transplant showing donor kidney and blood vessels in place. Recipient's kidney is not always removed unless it is infected, is a cause of hypertension, or contains a malignant tumor.

EXERCISE 17

1. The surgical implantation of a donor kidney to replace a nonfunctioning kidney is called _____ _____.

2. The destruction of living tissue with an electric spark is _____.

3. _____ _____ _____ _____ is a noninvasive treatment for removal of kidney or ureteral stones.

EXERCISE 18

Match the terms in the first column with their correct definitions in the second column.

_____ 1. fulguration

_____ 2. renal transplant

_____ 3. ESWL

a. used to replace a nonfunctioning kidney

b. used to remove bladder growths

c. used to remove tumors

d. also called *shock wave lithotripsy*

EXERCISE 19

Spell each of the surgical terms. Have someone dictate the terms on this page to you. Study any words you have spelled incorrectly.

1. _____

2. _____

3. _____

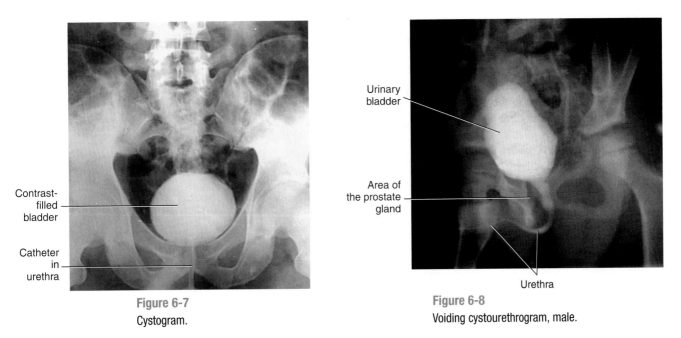

Figure 6-7
Cystogram.

Figure 6-8
Voiding cystourethrogram, male.

Diagnostic Terms

Built from Word Parts

Review Table 5-1, Types of Diagnostic Procedures, pp. 135-136 before proceeding.

Term	Definition
Diagnostic Imaging	
cystogram .... (SIS-tō-gram)	x-ray image of the bladder (Figure 6-7)
cystography .... (sis-TOG-ra-fē)	x-ray imaging of the bladder
intravenous urogram (IVU) .... (in-tra-VĒ-nus) (Ū-rō-gram)	x-ray image of the urinary tract (with contrast medium injected intravenously) (also called *intravenous pyelogram*)
nephrogram .... (NEF-rō-gram)	x-ray image of the kidney
nephrography .... (ne-FROG-ra-fē)	x-ray imaging of the kidney
nephrosonography .... (*nef*-rō-so-NOG-ra-fē)	process of recording the kidney using sound (an ultrasound test) (Figure 6-9)
nephrotomogram .... (*nef*-rō-TŌ-mō-gram)	(sectional) x-ray image of the kidney (Figure 6-10)
renogram .... (RĒ-nō-gram)	(graphic) record of the kidney (produced by radioactivity after injecting a radiopharmaceutical, or radioactive material, into the blood) (a nuclear medicine test)
retrograde urogram .... (RET-rō-grād) (Ū-ro-gram)	x-ray image of the urinary tract (retrograde means to move in a direction opposite from normal) with contrast medium instilled through urethral catheters by a cystoscope (Exercise Figure I)

Spiral CT
scans are replacing intravenous urograms to detect urinary tract stones and perirenal infections.

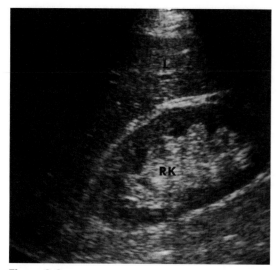

Figure 6-9
Ultrasound (nephrosonogram) of the right kidney, sagittal view.

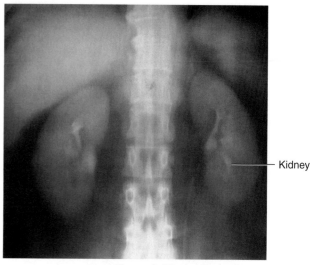

Kidney

Figure 6-10
Nephrotomogram.

> **Ultrasonography, computed tomography (CT),** and **magnetic resonance imaging (MRI)** can be used in evaluating structure and function of the urinary system organs. See Table 5-1.

voiding cystourethrography............. (VOID-ing) (*sis*-tō-ū-rē-THROG-rō-fe)	x-ray imaging of the bladder and the urethra (Figure 6-8). Radiopaque dye is instilled in the bladder. X-ray images are taken of the bladder and during urination of the dye.

Endoscopy

cystoscope... (SIS-tō-skōp)	instrument used for visual examination of the bladder
cystoscopy... (sis-TOS-kō-pē)	visual examination of the bladder
meatoscope... (mē-AT-ō-skōp)	instrument used for visual examination of the meatus
meatoscopy... (mē-ā-TOS-kō-pē)	visual examination of the meatus
nephroscopy....................................... (ne-FROS-kō-pē)	visual examination of the kidney (Figure 6-11)
urethroscope...................................... (ū-RE-thrō-skōp)	instrument used for visual examination of the urethra

Other

urinometer.. (ū-ri-NOM-e-ter)	instrument used to measure (the specific gravity of) urine (Exercise Figure J)

Practice saying each of these words aloud. To hear the terms, access the **PRONOUNCE IT** activity for this chapter on the Student CD that accompanies this text. Or, to hear the

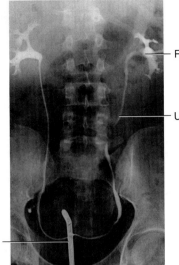

Renal pelvis

Ureter

Cystoscope

Exercise Figure I
Fill in the blanks to complete labeling of the diagram.
Retrograde _____ / _____ / _____ . A urethral

  urinary tract / **cv** / **x-ray image**

catheter is passed by a cystoscope, and contrast material is injected to show urinary system structures.

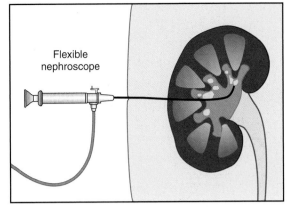

Figure 6-11
Nephroscopy.

Flexible
nephroscope

terms and their definitions with a CD player or computer, obtain the Pronunciation CD designed for use with this text.

Learn the definitions and spellings of the diagnostic terms by completing exercises 20, 21, and 22.

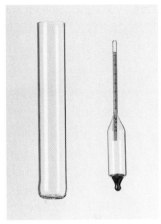

Exercise Figure J
Fill in the blanks to label the diagram.

_____ / _____ / **instrument**
  urine / **cv** / **used to**
measure

EXERCISE 20

Analyze and define the following diagnostic terms.

1. voiding cystourethrography _____

2. meatoscope _____

3. cystography _____

4. urethroscope _____

5. nephrosonography _____

6. cystoscope _____

7. nephrotomogram _____

8. cystogram _____

9. meatoscopy _____

10. nephrogram _____

11. cystoscopy _____

12. nephrography _____

13. urinometer _____

14. (intravenous) urogram _____

15. retrograde urogram _____

16. renogram _____

17. nephroscopy _____

EXERCISE 21

Build diagnostic terms that correspond to the following definitions by using the word parts you have learned.

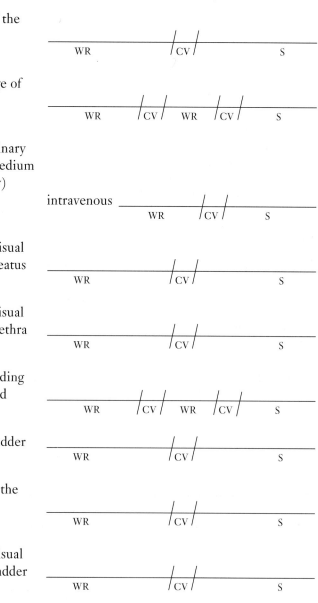

1. visual examination of the bladder

    _____ / ___ / ___ _____
    WR   CV   S

2. (sectional) x-ray image of the kidney

    _____ / ___ / ___ / ___ / ___ _____
    WR   CV   WR   CV   S

3. x-ray image of the urinary tract (with contrast medium injected intravenously)

    intravenous _____ / ___ / ___ _____
                 WR   CV   S

4. instrument used for visual examination of the meatus

    _____ / ___ / ___ _____
    WR   CV   S

5. instrument used for visual examination of the urethra

    _____ / ___ / ___ _____
    WR   CV   S

6. process of x-ray recording the kidney using sound

    _____ / ___ / ___ / ___ / ___ _____
    WR   CV   WR   CV   S

7. x-ray image of the bladder

    _____ / ___ / ___ _____
    WR   CV   S

8. visual examination of the meatus

    _____ / ___ / ___ _____
    WR   CV   S

9. instrument used for visual examination of the bladder

    _____ / ___ / ___ _____
    WR   CV   S

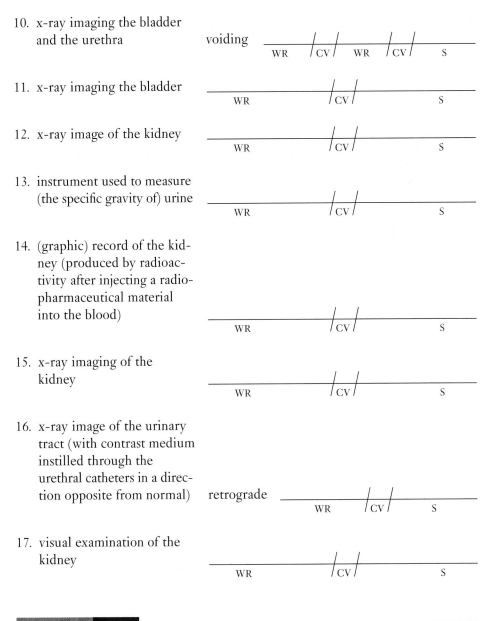

10. x-ray imaging the bladder and the urethra

voiding ____/___/___/___/____
WR CV WR CV S

11. x-ray imaging the bladder

_____/___/____
WR   CV   S

12. x-ray image of the kidney

_____/___/____
WR   CV   S

13. instrument used to measure (the specific gravity of) urine

_____/___/____
WR   CV   S

14. (graphic) record of the kidney (produced by radioactivity after injecting a radiopharmaceutical material into the blood)

_____/___/____
WR   CV   S

15. x-ray imaging of the kidney

_____/___/____
WR   CV   S

16. x-ray image of the urinary tract (with contrast medium instilled through the urethral catheters in a direction opposite from normal)

retrograde ____/___/____
WR CV S

17. visual examination of the kidney

_____/___/____
WR   CV   S

EXERCISE 22

Spell each of the diagnostic terms. Have someone dictate the terms on pp. 179 and 181-182 to you. Think about the word parts before attempting to write the word. Study any words you have spelled incorrectly.

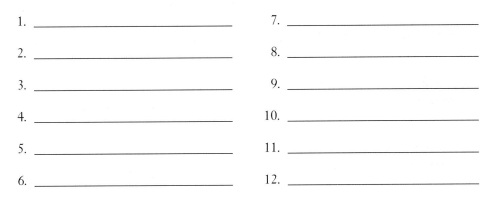

1. _____   7. _____

2. _____   8. _____

3. _____   9. _____

4. _____   10. _____

5. _____   11. _____

6. _____   12. _____

13. _____   16. _____

14. _____   17. _____

15. _____

Diagnostic Terms

Not Built from Word Parts

Term	Definition
Diagnostic Imaging	
KUB (kidney, ureter, and bladder)	a simple x-ray image of the abdomen. It is often used to view the kidneys, ureters, and bladder to determine size, shape, and location. Also used to identify calculi in the kidney ureters or bladder or to diagnose intestinal obstruction.
Laboratory	
blood urea nitrogen (BUN) .... (ū-RĒ-a) (NĪ-trō-jen)	a blood test that measures the amount of urea in the blood. Used to determine kidney function. An increased BUN indicates renal dysfunction.
creatinine .... (crē-AT-i-nen)	a blood test that measures the amount of creatinine in the blood. An elevated amount indicates impaired kidney function.
specific gravity (SG) .... (spe-SIF-ik) (GRAV-i-tē)	a test performed on a urine specimen to measure the concentrating or diluting ability of the kidneys
urinalysis (UA) .... (ū-rin-AL-is-is)	multiple routine tests performed on a urine specimen

Practice saying each of the words aloud. To hear the terms, access the **PRONOUNCE IT** activity for this chapter on the Student CD that accompanies this text. Or, to hear the terms and their definitions with a CD player or computer, obtain the Pronunciation CD designed for use with this text.

Learn the definitions and spellings of the diagnostic terms by completing exercises 23, 24, and 25.

EXERCISE 23

Fill in the blanks with the correct terms.

1. The x-ray image of the abdomen used to view the kidneys, ureters, and bladder to determine size, shape, and location is called _____.

2. A test performed on a urine specimen to measure concentrating and diluting ability of the kidneys is called _____ _____.

3. _____ _____ _____ measures the amount of urea in the blood.

4. Multiple routine tests performed on a urine specimen are referred to as a(n) _____ .

5. _____ is a blood test that measures the amount of creatinine in the blood.

EXERCISE 24

Match the terms in the first column with their correct definitions in the second column.

_____ 1. specific gravity

_____ 2. blood urea nitrogen

_____ 3. urinalysis

_____ 4. KUB

_____ 5. creatinine

a. an x-ray image of the kidneys, ureters, and bladder

b. a blood test used to determine kidney function

c. a urine test to measure concentrating or diluting abilities of the kidneys

d. multiple routine tests performed on a urine sample

e. an x-ray image of the kidneys, urethra, and bladder

f. a test on blood that if elevated indicates impaired kidney function

EXERCISE 25

Spell each of the diagnostic terms. Have someone dictate the terms on p. 186 to you. Study any words you have spelled incorrectly.

1. _____

2. _____

3. _____

4. _____

5. _____

Complementary Terms

Built from Word Parts

Term	Definition
albuminuria .... (*al*-bū-min-Ū-rē-a)	albumin in the urine (albumin is an important protein in the blood, but when found in the urine, it indicates a kidney problem)
anuria .... (an-Ū-rē-a)	absence of urine (failure of the kidney to produce urine)
azotemia .... (āz-ō-TĒ-mē-a)	(excessive) urea and nitrogenous substances in the blood

diuresis .... (dī-ū-RĒ-sis) (NOTE: the *a* is dropped from dia- because uresis begins with a vowel.)	condition of urine passing through (increased excretion of urine)
dysuria .... (dis-Ū-rē-a)	difficult or painful urination
glycosuria .... (glī-kō-SŪ-rē-a)	sugar (glucose) in the urine
hematuria .... (hem-a-TŪ-rē-a)	blood in the urine
meatal .... (mē-Ā-tal)	pertaining to the meatus
nephrologist .... (ne-FROL-ō-jist)	a physician who studies and treats diseases of the kidney
nephrology .... (ne-FROL-ō-jē)	study of the kidney (a branch of medicine dealing with disease of the kidney)
nocturia .... (nok-TŪ-rē-a)	night urination
oliguria .... (ol-ig-Ū-rē-a)	scanty urine (amount)
polyuria .... (pol-ē-Ū-rē-a)	much (excessive) urine
pyuria .... (pī-Ū-rē-a)	pus in the urine
urinary .... (Ū-rin-ā-rē)	pertaining to urine
urologist .... (ū-ROL-ō-jist)	a physician who studies and treats (diseases of) the urinary tract
urology .... (ū-ROL-ō-jē)	study of the urinary tract. (A branch of medicine dealing with diseases of the male and female urinary systems and the male reproductive system.)

Practice saying each of these terms aloud. To hear the terms, access the **PRONOUNCE IT** activity for this chapter on the Student CD that accompanies this text. Or, to hear the terms and their definitions with a CD player or computer, obtain the Pronunciation CD designed for use with this text.

Exercises 26, 27, and 28 will help you to learn the definitions and spellings of the complementary terms related to the urinary system.

EXERCISE 26

Analyze and define the following complementary terms.

1. nocturia _____

2. urologist _____

3. oliguria _____

4. azotemia _____

5. hematuria _____

6. urology _____

7. polyuria _____

8. albuminuria _____

9. anuria _____

10. diuresis _____

11. pyuria _____

12. urinary _____

13. glycosuria _____

14. meatal _____

15. dysuria _____

16. nephrology _____

17. nephrologist _____

EXERCISE 27

Build the complementary terms for the following definitions by using the word parts you have learned.

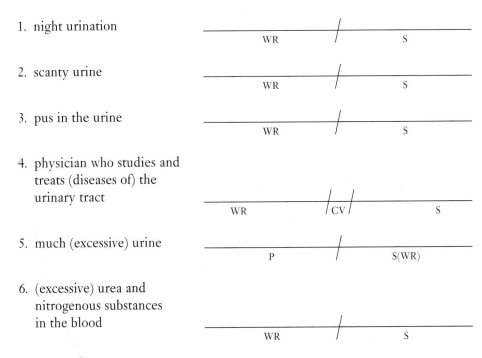

1. night urination
   _____ / _____
   WR   S

2. scanty urine
   _____ / _____
   WR   S

3. pus in the urine
   _____ / _____
   WR   S

4. physician who studies and treats (diseases of) the urinary tract
   _____ / _____ / _____
   WR   CV   S

5. much (excessive) urine
   _____ / _____
   P   S(WR)

6. (excessive) urea and nitrogenous substances in the blood
   _____ / _____
   WR   S

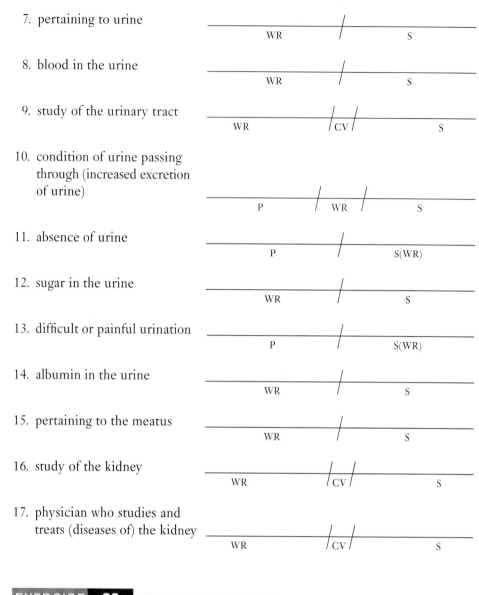

7. pertaining to urine

_____ / _____
WR   S

8. blood in the urine

_____ / _____
WR   S

9. study of the urinary tract

_____ / _____
WR   CV   S

10. condition of urine passing through (increased excretion of urine)

_____ / _____ / _____
P   WR   S

11. absence of urine

_____ / _____
P   S(WR)

12. sugar in the urine

_____ / _____
WR   S

13. difficult or painful urination

_____ / _____
P   S(WR)

14. albumin in the urine

_____ / _____
WR   S

15. pertaining to the meatus

_____ / _____
WR   S

16. study of the kidney

_____ / _____
WR   CV   S

17. physician who studies and treats (diseases of) the kidney

_____ / _____
WR   CV   S

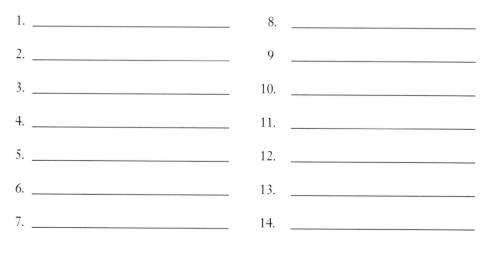

EXERCISE 28

Spell each of the complementary terms. Have someone dictate the terms on pp. 187-188 to you. Think about the word parts before attempting to write the word. Study any words you have spelled incorrectly.

1. _____

2. _____

3. _____

4. _____

5. _____

6. _____

7. _____

8. _____

9 _____

10. _____

11. _____

12. _____

13. _____

14. _____

15. _____   17. _____

16. _____

Complementary Terms

Not Built from Word Parts

Term	Definition
catheter (cath) (KATH-e-ter)	flexible, tubelike device, such as a urinary catheter, for withdrawing or instilling fluids
distended (dis-TEN-ded)	stretched out (a bladder is distended when filled with urine)
diuretic (dī-ū-RET-ik)	agent that increases the formation and excretion of urine
enuresis (en-ū-RĒ-sis)	involuntary urination (bed-wetting)
hemodialysis (HD) (hē-mō-dī-AL-i-sis)	procedure for removing impurities from the blood because of an inability of the kidneys to do so (Figure 6-12)
incontinence (in-KON-ti-nens)	inability to control bladder and/or bowels
micturate (MIK-tū-rāt)	to urinate or void
peritoneal dialysis (par-i-tō-NĒ-al) (dī-AL-i-sis)	procedure for removing toxic wastes when the kidney is unable to do so; the peritoneal cavity is used as the receptacle for the fluid used in the dialysis (Figure 6-13)

Catheter
is derived from the Greek **katheter**, meaning a **thing let down**. A catheter lets down the urine from the bladder.

Micturate
is derived from the Latin **mictus**, meaning **a making of water**. The noun form of micturate is **micturition**. Note the spelling of each. **Micturition** is often misspelled as **micturation**.

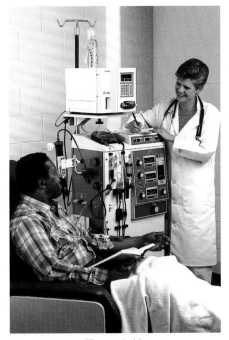

Figure 6-12
Hemodialysis.

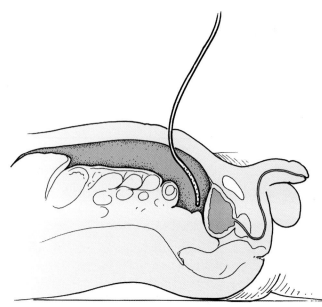

Figure 6-13

Peritoneal dialysis. A sterile dialyzing fluid is instilled into the peritoneal cavity by gravity and dwells there for the period ordered by the physician. The fluid, containing the nitrogenous wastes and excess water that a healthy kidney normally removes, is drained from the cavity.

stricture (STRIK-chŭr)	abnormal narrowing, such as a urethral stricture
urinal (Ū-rin-al)	receptacle for urine
urinary catheterization (*kath*-e-ter-i-ZĀ-shun)	passage of a catheter into the urinary bladder to withdraw urine (Exercise Figure K)
urodynamics (ū-rō-dī-NAM-iks)	pertaining to the force and flow of urine within the urinary tract
void (voyd)	to empty or evacuate waste material, especially urine

Practice saying each of these terms aloud. To hear the terms, access the **PRONOUNCE IT** activity for this chapter on the Student CD that accompanies this text. Or, to hear the terms and their definitions with a CD player or computer, obtain the Pronunciation CD designed for use with this text.

Learn the definitions and spellings of the complementary terms by completing exercises 29 through 32.

EXERCISE 29

Fill in the blanks with the correct terms.

1. A receptacle for urine is a(n) _____.

2. The procedure for removing impurities from the blood because of the inability of the kidneys to do so is called _____.

3. A _____ bladder is stretched out.

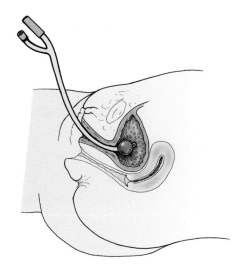

Exercise Figure K
Fill in the blanks to complete labeling of the diagram.
_____ / _____ catheterization. The catheter has been inserted through the urethra, and
urine / **pertaining to**
urine has been drained. The balloon on the end of the catheter has been inflated to hold the catheter
in the bladder for a period. This type of catheter is called a *retention catheter.*

4. A flexible, tubelike device for withdrawing or instilling fluids is a(n) _____.

5. The inability to control the bladder and/or bowels is called _____.

6. The passage of a catheter into the urinary bladder to withdraw urine is a(n) _____ _____.

7. To remove toxic wastes caused by kidney insufficiency by placing dialyzing fluid in the peritoneal cavity is called _____ _____.

8. To void is to _____ _____ _____.

9. An abnormal narrowing is a(n) _____.

10. An agent that increases the formation and excretion of urine is called a(n) _____.

11. Involuntary urination is called _____.

12. _____ is another word for void, or urinate.

13. _____ is the name given to the force and flow of urine.

EXERCISE 30

Match the terms in the first column with their correct definitions in the second column.

_____ 1. catheter

_____ 2. urinary catheterization

_____ 3. distended

a. increases the formation and excretion of urine

b. overdevelopment of the kidney

_____ 4. diuretic

_____ 5. hemodialysis

_____ 6. incontinence

_____ 7. void

c. inability to control the bladder and/or bowels

d. process for removing impurities from the blood when the kidneys are unable to do so

e. flexible, tubelike device for withdrawing or instilling fluids

f. stretched out

g. passage of a tubelike device into the urinary bladder to remove urine

h. to evacuate or empty waste material, especially urine

EXERCISE 31

Match the terms in the first column with their correct definitions in the second column.

_____ 1. micturate, or urinate

_____ 2. peritoneal dialysis

_____ 3. stricture

_____ 4. urinal

_____ 5. enuresis

_____ 6. urodynamics

a. to void liquid waste

b. receptacle for urine

c. force and flow of urine within the urinary tract

d. absence of urine

e. use of peritoneal cavity to hold dialyzing fluid in the removal of toxic wastes

f. involuntary urination

g. narrowing

EXERCISE 32

Spell each of the complementary terms. Have someone dictate the terms on pp. 191-192 to you. Study any words you have spelled incorrectly.

1. _____

2. _____

3. _____

4. _____

5. _____

6. _____

7. _____

8. _____

9. _____

10. _____

11. _____

12. _____

13. _____

Abbreviations

BUN	blood urea nitrogen
cath	catheterization, catheter
ESWL......................................	extracorporeal shock wave lithotripsy
HD	hemodialysis
IVU..	intravenous urogram
SG...	specific gravity
UA...	urinalysis
UTI..	urinary tract infection
VCUG	voiding cystourethrogram

EXERCISE 33

1. When imaging is used to diagnose obstructive uropathy, a KUB is usually performed first. An **IVU** _____ _____ is usually best for confirming or excluding obstruction and determining its level and cause. For further examination a **VCUG** _____ _____ may be performed to evaluate the posterior urethra and check for vesicoureteral reflux.

2. **SG** _____ _____ is one of many tests performed on the urine specimen during a **UA** _____. It measures the concentration of particles, including water and electrolytes in the urine.

3. **BUN** _____ _____ _____ is a laboratory test done on a blood sample to determine kidney function.

4. The number, size, and type of stones are important in determining if **ESWL** _____ _____ _____ _____ is the best method for treating renal calculi.

5. Bladder **cath** _____ carries the risk of **UTI** _____ _____ _____ ; therefore it is sometimes preferable to use other methods for obtaining urine specimens and managing incontinence.

6. Peritoneal dialysis, **HD** _____, and renal transplant are known as renal replacement therapies.

CHAPTER REVIEW

EXERCISE 34 *Interact with Medical Records*

Complete the discharge summary report by writing the medical terms in the blanks. Use the list of definitions with the corresponding numbers.

University Hospital and Medical Center
4700 North Main Street • Wellness, Arizona 54321 • (987) 555-3210

PATIENT NAME: Bruno Oliver   **CASE NUMBER:** 83658-URI
DATE OF BIRTH: 07/30/xx   **DATE OF ADMISSION:** 09/20/xx
                                                DATE OF DISCHARGE: 09/27/xx

DISCHARGE SUMMARY

Bruno Oliver is a 32-year-old white man, appearing his stated age, who was admitted to the hospital after presenting himself to the emergency department on 09/20/xx in acute distress. He complained of intermittent pain in the right posterior lumbar area, radiating to the right flank. He has a family history of 1. _____ and has been treated for this condition two other times in the past 10 years.

This patient was admitted to the 2. _____ Unit and was administered intravenous morphine sulfate for pain control. VITAL SIGNS: Low-grade temperature of 99.4. Initial blood pressure was 146/92.

The white blood count, hemoglobin, and hematocrit were normal. The urinalysis showed microscopic 3. _____ .

A 4. _____ revealed 5. _____ in the region of the right renal pelvis. A 6. _____ with a right retrograde 7. _____ confirmed the presence of the three stones in the right kidney. Minimal ureteral obstruction was present.

A percutaneous 8. _____ was completed with no complications. A ureteral stent was inserted as was an indwelling Foley 9. _____ . Drainage from the right kidney was pale yellow in 48 hours. The Foley catheter was removed 3 days postoperatively.

At discharge, the patient is 10. _____ without difficulty. The stones were sent to the laboratory for analysis. The report indicated that they were calcium oxalate.

The patient is to follow up with his urologist in a week to have his ureteral stent removed.

_____
Betsy Begay, MD

BB/mcm

---

1. condition of stones in the kidney
2. study of the urinary tract
3. blood in the urine
4. x-ray image of the abdomen
5. stones
6. visual examination of the bladder

7. x-ray image of the urinary tract
8. incision through the kidney into the renal pelvis to remove a stone
9. flexible, tubelike device
10. evacuating urine

EXERCISE 35 *Interpret Medical Terms*

To test your understanding of the terms introduced in this chapter, circle the words that correctly complete the sentences. The italicized words refer to the correct answer.

1. The patient was admitted with a *drooping kidney,* or (nephromegaly, nephrohypertrophy, nephroptosis).
2. The patient's x-ray image showed a *stone in the ureter,* or a condition known as (ureterocele, ureterolithiasis, ureterostenosis).
3. Because of Mrs. McLean's admission to the intensive care unit with pneumonia and her compromised immune system, her physicians were alert to signs of *pathogenic organisms entering the bloodstream,* or (fulguration, urodynamics, sepsis).
4. The physician first suspected diabetes when told of the *excessive amounts of urine* voided, or (oliguria, polyuria, dysuria).
5. The physician told the patient with the drooping kidney that it was necessary to *secure the kidney in place* by performing a (nephropexy, nephrolysis, nephrotripsy).
6. The patient had a *sudden stoppage of urine formation,* or (urinary suppression, urinary retention, azoturia).
7. The patient was scheduled for an *x-ray image of the urinary bladder,* or a (cystoscopy, cystogram, cystography).
8. The patient's mother informed the doctor of her son's *involuntary urination,* or (diuresis, dysuria, enuresis).
9. The patient was admitted to the hospital for *kidney and ureteral infection,* or (polycystic kidney disease, urinary retention, urinary tract infection).
10. *UA* is the abbreviation for (urine, urinary, urinalysis).

EXERCISE 36 *Read Medical Terms in Use*

Practice pronunciation of the terms by reading the following medical document. Use the pronunciation key following the medical terms to assist you in saying the word.

A 76-year-old woman consulted with her primary care physician because of **hematuria** (hēm-a-TŪ-rē-a) and **dysuria** (dis-Ū-rē-a). She was referred to a **urologist** (ū-ROL-ō-jist). **Urinalysis** (ū-rin-AL-is-is) disclosed 1+ albumin and mild **pyuria** (pī-Ū-rē-a) in addition to the hematuria. A spiral CT scan was obtained. Mild **nephrolithiasis** (*nef*-rō-lith-Ī-a-sis) was observed but no **hydronephrosis** (hī-drō-ne-FRŌ-sis). Finally a **cystoscopy** (sis-TOS-kō-pē) was performed, which showed mild **cystitis** (sis-TĪ-tis). A **urinary tract infection** was diagnosed and the patient responded favorably to antibiotics. The urologist did not advise **lithotripsy** (LITH-ō-trip-sē) for the **renal calculi** (RĒ-nal) (KAL-kū-lī).

EXERCISE 37 *Comprehend Medical Terms in Use*

Test your comprehension of terms in the previous medical document by circling the correct answer.

1. Symptoms that prompted the patient to seek treatment from the urologist were:
   a. scanty urine and painful urination
   b. painful urination and bloody urine
   c. pus and blood in the urine
   d. sugar and blood in the urine

2. Which of the following was rejected as treatment for kidney stones?
   a. urinalysis
   b. intravenous urogram
   c. cystoscopy
   d. lithotripsy

3. The CT image revealed which of the following was not present in the kidney?
   a. water
   b. blood
   c. stones
   d. tumor

For further practice or to evaluate what you have learned use the Student CD that accompanies this text.

COMBINING FORMS CROSSWORD PUZZLE

Across Clues

1. urine, urinary tract
5. glomerulus
6. sound
8. albumin
10. scanty
13. bladder
14. bladder
17. ureter
21. kidney
22. opening
23. sugar

Down Clues

2. cut, section
3. blood
4. night
5. sugar
7. urine, urinary tract
9. urethra
11. stone
12. water
15. urea, nitrogen
16. kidney
18. renal pelvis
20. blood

REVIEW OF WORD PARTS

Can you define and spell the following word parts?

Combining Forms

albumin/o	olig/o
azot/o	pyel/o
blast/o	ren/o
cyst/o	son/o
glomerul/o	tom/o
glyc/o	ureter/o
glycos/o	urethr/o
hydr/o	ur/o
lith/o	urin/o
meat/o	vesic/o
nephr/o	
noct/i	

Suffixes

-esis
-iasis
-lysis
-megaly
-ptosis
-rrhaphy
-tripsy
-trophy
-uria

REVIEW OF TERMS

Can you build, analyze, define, pronounce, and spell the following terms *built from word parts?*

Diseases and Disorders

cystitis
cystocele
cystolith
glomerulonephritis
hydronephrosis
nephritis
nephroblastoma
nephrohypertrophy
nephrolithiasis
nephroma
nephromegaly
nephroptosis
pyelitis
pyelonephritis
uremia
ureteritis
ureterocele
ureterolithiasis
ureterostenosis
urethrocystitis

Surgical

cystectomy
cystolithotomy
cystorrhaphy
cystostomy
cystotomy
lithotripsy
meatotomy
nephrectomy
nephrolysis
nephropexy
nephropyelolithotomy
nephrostomy
pyelolithotomy
pyeloplasty
ureterectomy
urethroplasty
vesicourethral suspension
vesicotomy

Diagnostic

cystogram
cystography
cystoscope
cystoscopy
intravenous urogram (IVU)
meatoscope
meatoscopy
nephrogram
nephrography
nephroscopy
nephrosonography
renogram
retrograde urogram
urethroscope
urinometer
voiding cystourethrography

Complementary

albuminuria
anuria
azotemia
diuresis
dysuria
glycosuria
hematuria
meatal
nephrologist
nephrology
nephrotomogram
nocturia
oliguria
polyuria
pyuria
urinary
urologist
urology

Can you define, pronounce, and spell the following terms *not built from word parts?*

Diseases and Disorders

epispadias
hypospadias
polycystic kidney disease
renal calculi
renal hypertension
sepsis
urinary retention
urinary suppression
urinary tract infection (UTI)

Surgical

extracorporeal shock
   wave lithotripsy
fulguration
renal transplant

Diagnostic

blood urea nitrogen (BUN)
creatinine
KUB
specific gravity (SG)
urinalysis (UA)

Complementary

catheter (cath)
distended
diuretic
enuresis
hemodialysis (HD)
incontinence
micturate
peritoneal dialysis
stricture
urinal
urinary catheterization
urodynamics
void

Male Reproductive System

OUTLINE

OBJECTIVES

On completion of this chapter you will be able to:

1. Identify the organs and other structures of the male reproductive system.
2. Define and spell the word parts presented in this chapter.
3. Build and analyze medical terms with word parts presented in this and previous chapters.
4. Define, pronounce, and spell the disease and disorder, diagnostic, surgical, and complementary terms for the male reproductive system.
5. Interpret the meaning of the abbreviations presented in this chapter.
6. Read medical documents and interpret medical terminology contained in them.

ANATOMY

Function

The function of the male reproductive system is to produce, sustain, and transport sperm, the male reproductive cell, and to secrete the hormone testosterone.

Organs of the Male Reproductive System

testis, or testicle (*pl.* testes, or testicles)	primary male sex organs, paired, oval-shaped, and enclosed in a sac called the *scrotum*. The testes produce spermatozoa (sperm cells) and the hormone testosterone (Figure 7-1).
sperm (spermatozoon, *pl.* spermatozoa)	the microscopic male germ cell, which, when united with the ovum, produces a zygote (fertilized egg) that with subsequent development becomes an *embryo*.
testosterone	the principle male sex hormone. Its chief function is to stimulate the development of the male reproductive organs and secondary sex characteristics such as facial hair.
seminiferous tubules	up to 900 coiled tubes within the testes in which spermatogenesis occurs
epididymis	a coiled 20-foot (6-m) tube atop each of the testes that carries the mature sperm up to the *vas deferens* (see Figure 7-1)
vas deferens, ductus deferens, or seminal duct	duct carrying the sperm from the epididymis to the urethra. (The urethra also connects with the urinary bladder and carries urine outside the body. A circular muscle constricts during intercourse to prevent urination.)
seminal vesicles	two main glands located at the base of the bladder that open into the vas deferens. The glands secrete a thick fluid, which forms part of the semen (see Figure 7-1).
prostate gland	encircles the upper end of the urethra. The prostate gland secretes a fluid that aids in the movement of the sperm and ejaculation (see Figure 7-1).
scrotum	sac suspended on both sides of and just behind the penis. The testes are enclosed in the scrotum (see Figure 7-1).
penis	male organ of urination and copulation (sexual intercourse) (see Figure 7-1)
glans penis	enlarged tip on the end of the penis

Prostate
is derived from the Greek **pro**, meaning **before**, and **statis**, meaning **standing** or **sitting**. Anatomically it is the gland standing before the bladder.

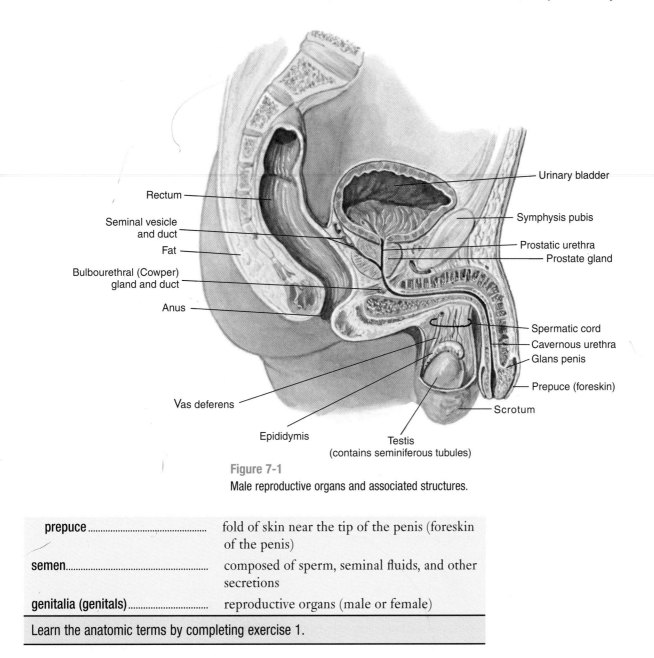

Figure 7-1
Male reproductive organs and associated structures.

prepuce	fold of skin near the tip of the penis (foreskin of the penis)
semen	composed of sperm, seminal fluids, and other secretions
genitalia (genitals)	reproductive organs (male or female)

Learn the anatomic terms by completing exercise 1.

EXERCISE 1

Match the anatomic terms in the first column with the correct definitions in the second column.

_____ 1. epididymis

_____ 2. glans penis

_____ 3. penis

_____ 4. prepuce, or foreskin

_____ 5. prostate gland

_____ 6. scrotum

_____ 7. semen

a. sac in which the testes are enclosed

b. structures in testes where the sperm originate

c. tube atop the testis that carries sperm to the vas deferens

d. reproductive organs (male or female)

e. male organ of copulation

_____ 8. seminal vesicles

_____ 9. seminiferous tubule

_____ 10. spermatic cord

_____ 11. testes

_____ 12. vas deferens

_____ 13. genitalia

_____ 14. sperm

_____ 15. testosterone

f. encircles upper end of urethra

g. glands that open into the vas deferens

h. primary male sex organs

i. large tip at end of male organ of copulation

j. the male germ cell

k. fold of skin at tip of penis

l. comprises sperm and secretions

m. male sex hormone

n. suspends testis in scrotum

o. engorgement of blood

p. duct that carries sperm to the urethra

WORD PARTS

Combining Forms of the Male Reproductive System

Study the word parts and their definitions listed below. Completing the exercises that follow will help you learn the terms.

Combining Form	Definition
balan/o	glans penis
epididym/o	epididymis
orchid/o, orchi/o, orch/o, test/o	testis, testicle
prostat/o	prostate gland
vas/o	vessel, duct
vesicul/o	seminal vesicle

Learn the anatomic locations and meanings of the combining forms by completing exercises 2 and 3 and Exercise Figure A.

EXERCISE 2

Write the definitions of the following combining forms.

1. test/o _____

2. vas/o _____

3. balan/o _____

4. prostat/o _____

5. orch/o _____

6. vesicul/o _____

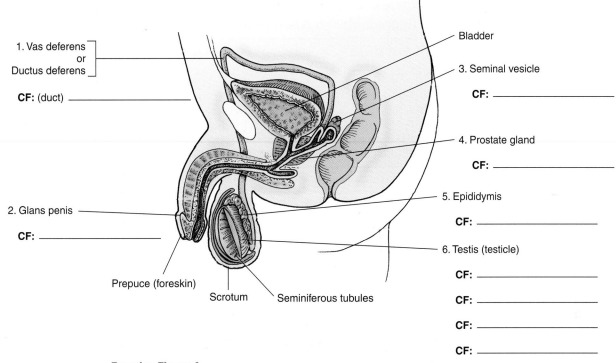

1. Vas deferens
   or
   Ductus deferens

   CF: (duct) _____

2. Glans penis _____

   CF: _____

Prepuce (foreskin)

Scrotum   Seminiferous tubules

Bladder

3. Seminal vesicle

   CF: _____

4. Prostate gland

   CF: _____

5. Epididymis

   CF: _____

6. Testis (testicle)

   CF: _____

   CF: _____

   CF: _____

   CF: _____

Exercise Figure A
Fill in the blanks with combining forms for the diagram of the male reproductive system.

7. orchi/o _____

8. epididym/o _____

9. orchid/o _____

EXERCISE   3

Write the combining form for each of the following terms.

1. vessel, duct   _____

2. prostate gland   _____

3. glans penis   _____

4. seminal vesicle   _____

5. epididymis   _____

6. testicle, or testis   a. _____

                            b. _____

                            c. _____

                            d. _____

Combining Forms Commonly Used with Male Reproductive System Terms

Combining Form	Definition
andr/o	male
sperm/o, spermat/o	spermatozoon (*pl.* spermatozoa), sperm (Figure 7-2)

Learn the combining forms by completing exercises 4 and 5.

EXERCISE 4

Write the definition of the following combining forms.

1. sperm/o _____

2. andr/o _____

3. spermat/o _____

EXERCISE 5

Write the combining form for each of the following.

1. sperm   a. _____

                  b. _____

2. male _____

Prefix and Suffix

Prefix	Definition
trans-	through, across, beyond

Suffix	Definition
-ism	state of

Refer to Appendix A and Appendix B for alphabetized word parts and their meanings. Learn the prefix and suffix by completing exercise 6.

Figure 7-2

Spermatozoon, or sperm. In normal ejaculation there may be as many as 300 million to 500 million sperm.

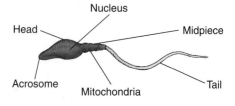

EXERCISE 6

Write the definitions for the prefix and the suffix.

1. -ism _____

2. trans- _____

MEDICAL TERMS

The terms you need to learn to complete this chapter are listed below. The exercises following each list will help you learn the definition and the spelling of each word.

Disease and Disorder Terms

Built from Word Parts

Term	Definition
anorchism (an-OR-kizm)	state of absence of testis (unilateral or bilateral)
balanitis (*bal*-a-NĪ-tis)	inflammation of the glans penis (Exercise Figure B)
balanorrhea (*bal*-a-nō-RĒ-a)	excessive discharge from the glans penis
benign prostatic hyperplasia (BPH) (bē-NĪN) (pros-TAT-ik) (*hī*-per-PLĀ-zhē-a)	excessive development pertaining to the prostate gland (nonmalignant enlargement of the prostate gland) (Figure 7-3)
cryptorchidism (kript-OR-kid-izm)	state of hidden testes. (During fetal development, testes are located in the abdominal area near the kidneys. Before birth they move down into the scrotal sac. Failure of the testes to descend from the abdominal cavity into the scrotum before birth results in cryptorchidism, or undescended testicles.) (Exercise Figure C)

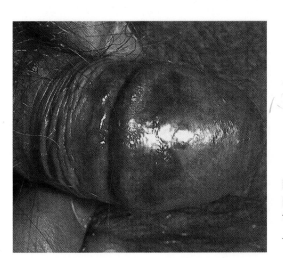

Exercise Figure B

Fill in the blanks with word parts to label the diagram.

_____ / _____
glans penis / inflammation

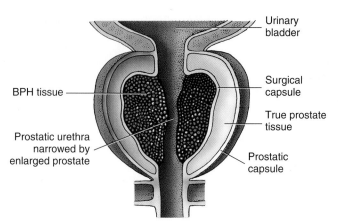
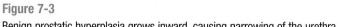
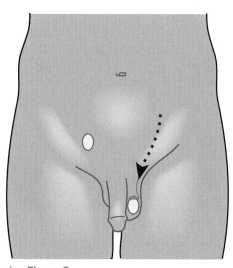

Figure 7-3
Benign prostatic hyperplasia grows inward, causing narrowing of the urethra.

Exercise Figure C
Fill in the blanks to complete labeling of the diagram.

_____ / _____ / _____ . The *arrow* shows the path
   hidden / **testis** / **state of**

the testis takes in its descent to the scrotal sac before birth.

Benign Prostatic Hypertrophy and Benign Prostatic Hyperplasia

As the male ages the prostate gland may undergo tissue changes called **prostatic hyperplasia,** which is the abnormal increase in the number of cells. The result is an enlarged prostate gland, referred to as **prostatic hypertrophy.** Benign prostatic hyperplasia is the correct term for the pathologic process, but **benign prostatic hypertrophy** is also currently used to describe this condition. As the gland enlarges it causes narrowing of the urethra, which interferes with the passage of urine. Symptoms include frequency of urination, nocturia, urinary retention, and incomplete emptying of the bladder.

---

epididymitis .... inflammation of an epididymis
(*ep*-i-*did*-i-MĪ-tis)

orchiepididymitis .... inflammation of the testis and epididymis
(*or*-kē-ep-i-did-i-MĪ-tis)

orchitis, orchiditis, or testitis .... inflammation of the testis or testicle
(or-KĪ-tis) (or-ki-DĪ-tis)
(tes-TĪ-tis)

prostatitis............................ (pros-ta-TĪ-tis)	inflammation of the prostate gland
prostatocystitis.............................. (pros-*ta*-tō-sis-TĪ-tis)	inflammation of the prostate gland and the bladder
prostatolith................................... (*pros*-TAT-ō-lith)	stone in the prostate gland
prostatorrhea............................. (pros-*tat*-ō-RĒ-a)	excessive discharge from the prostate gland
prostatovesiculitis.......................... (*pros*-ta-tō-ves-*ik*-ū-LĪ-tis)	inflammation of the prostate gland and seminal vesicles

Practice saying each of these terms aloud. To hear the terms, access the **PRONOUNCE IT** activity for this chapter on the Student CD that accompanies this text. Or, to hear the terms and their definitions with a CD player or computer, obtain the Pronunciation CD designed for use with this text.

Learn the definitions and spellings of the disease and disorder terms by completing exercises 7, 8, and 9.

EXERCISE   7

Analyze and define the following terms.

1. prostatolith _____

2. balanitis _____

3. (a) orchitis, (b) orchiditis, or (c) testitis _____

_____

4. prostatovesiculitis _____

5. prostatocystitis _____

6. orchiepididymitis _____

7. prostatorrhea _____

8. epididymitis _____

9. (benign) prostatic hyperplasia _____

10. cryptorchidism _____

11. balanorrhea _____

12. prostatitis _____

13. anorchism _____

EXERCISE **8**

Build disease and disorder terms for the following definitions with the word parts you have learned.

1. inflammation of the prostate gland and urinary bladder

  _____ / ____ / _____ / ____
  WR   CV   WR   S

2. stone in the prostate gland

  _____ / ____ / _____
  WR   CV   WR

3. inflammation of the testis   a. _____ / ____
                                     WR   S

   b. _____ / ____
      WR   S

   c. _____ / ____
      WR   S

4. (a nonmalignant) excessive development pertaining to the prostate gland

            benign
  _____ / ____   _____ / ____
  WR   S   P   S(WR)

5. state of hidden testes

  _____ / _____ / ____
  WR   WR   S

6. inflammation of the prostate gland and seminal vesicles

  _____ / ____ / _____ / ____
  WR   CV   WR   S

7. state of absence of testis

  _____ / _____ / ____
  P   WR   S

8. inflammation of the prostate gland

  _____ / ____
  WR   S

9. inflammation of the testis and the epididymis

  _____ / _____ / ____
  WR   WR   S

10. excessive discharge from the glans penis

  _____ / ____ / ____
  WR   CV   S

11. inflammation of an epididymis

  _____ / ____
  WR   S

12. inflammation of the glans penis

  _____ / ____
  WR   S

13. excessive discharge from the prostate gland

  _____ / ____ / ____
  WR   CV   S

EXERCISE 9

Spell each of the disease and disorder terms. Have someone dictate the terms on pp. 207-209 to you. Think about the word parts before attempting to write the word. Study any words you have spelled incorrectly.

1. _____   8. _____

2. _____   9. _____

3. _____   10. _____

4. _____   11. _____

5. _____   12. _____

6. _____   13. _____

7. _____

Disease and Disorder Terms

Not Built from Word Parts

Term	Definition
erectile dysfunction (ē-REK-tīl) (dis-FUNK-shun)	the inability of the male to attain or maintain an erection sufficient to perform sexual intercourse (formerly called *impotence*)
hydrocele (HĪ-drō-sēl)	scrotal swelling caused by a collection of fluid (Figure 7-4)
phimosis (fi-MŌ-sis)	a tightness of the prepuce (foreskin of the penis) that prevents its retraction over the glans. May be congenital or a result of balanitis. Circumcision is the usual treatment (Figure 7-5).
priapism (PRĪ-a-pizm)	persistent abnormal erection of the penis accompanied by pain and tenderness
prostate cancer (PROS-tāt)	cancer of the prostate gland (Figure 7-6)
testicular carcinoma (tes-TIK-ū-ler) (*kar*-sin-Ō-ma)	cancer of the testicle
testicular torsion (tes-TIK-ū-ler) (TOR-shun)	twisting of the spermatic cord causing decreased blood flow to the testis. Occurs most often during puberty. Because of lack of blood flow to the testis, it is often considered a surgical emergency.
varicocele (VAR-i-kō-sēl)	enlarged veins of the spermatic cord (Figure 7-7)

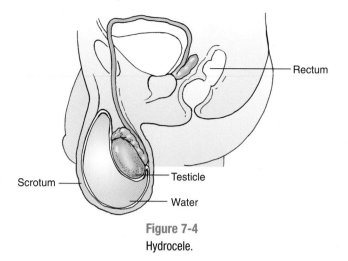

Figure 7-4
Hydrocele.

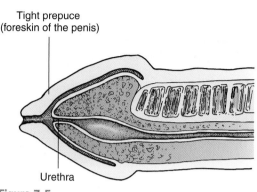

Figure 7-5
Phimosis. Cross section of the penis showing foreskin covering the opening.

Prostate cancer is the second most common cause of cancer deaths among American men and typically occurs after the age of 40 years. In the United States there are approximately 37,000 deaths and 180,000 new cases annually. Approximately 95% of all cancers of the prostate are adenocarcinomas arising from epithelial cells. Procedures used for detecting prostatic cancer are as follows:
1. digital rectal examination
2. prostate-specific antigen (PSA)
3. transrectal ultrasound
4. transrectal ultrasonically guided biopsy
5. magnetic resonance imaging with endorectal surface coil

Treatment includes prostatectomy, radiation therapy, hormonal therapy, bilateral orchidectomy, and chemotherapy. Hormonal therapy and bilateral orchidectomy are used to reduce production of testosterone, which fuels the prostate cancer. Treatment depends on the stage of prostate cancer, the age of the patient, and choices of treatment by the patient and his physician.

Practice saying each of these terms aloud. To hear the terms, access the **PRONOUNCE IT** activity for this chapter on the Student CD that accompanies this text. Or, to hear the terms and their definitions with a CD player or computer, obtain the Pronunciation CD designed for use with this text.

Learn the definitions and spellings of the disease and disorder terms by completing exercises 10, 11, and 12.

EXERCISE 10

Fill in the blanks with the correct terms.

1. Another way of referring to cancer of the testicle is _____ _____.

2. A tightness of the prepuce is called _____.

3. The condition of having enlarged veins of the spermatic cord is known medically as a(n) _____.

4. A scrotal swelling caused by a collection of fluid is called a(n) _____.

5. Cancer of the prostate gland is called _____ _____.

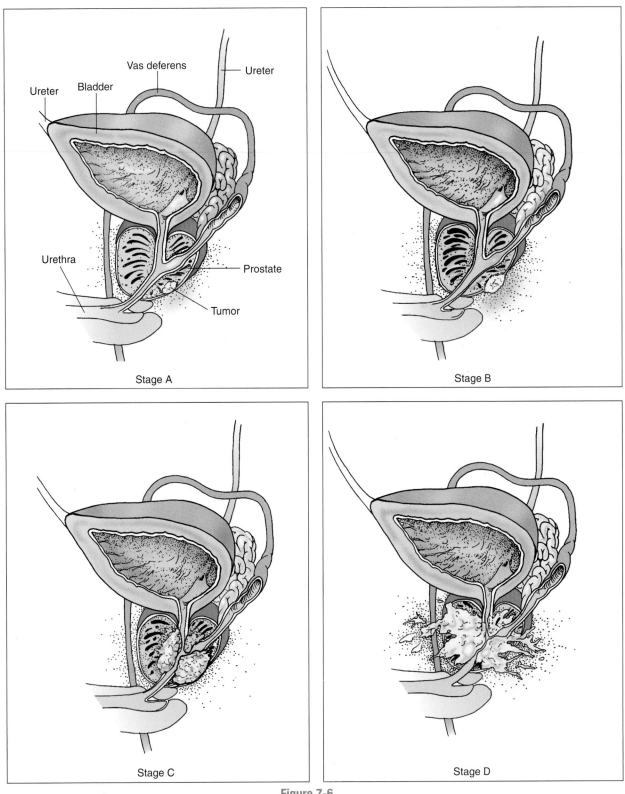

Figure 7-6
Prostate cancer.

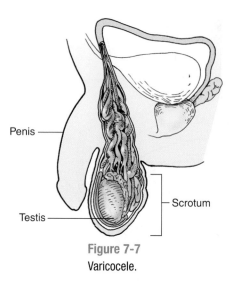

Figure 7-7
Varicocele.

6. Inability of the man to attain or maintain an erection is called

   _____ _____.

7. Persistent abnormal erection is called _____.

8. _____ _____ is the twisting of the spermatic cord.

EXERCISE 11

Match the terms in the first column with the correct definitions in the second column.

_____ 1. varicocele

_____ 2. phimosis

_____ 3. testicular carcinoma

_____ 4. erectile dysfunction

_____ 5. hydrocele

_____ 6. prostate cancer

_____ 7. testicular torsion

_____ 8. priapism

a. scrotal swelling caused by a collection of fluid

b. inability to attain or maintain an erection

c. a condition that prevents the retraction of the prepuce

d. enlarged veins of the spermatic cord

e. cancer of the testicle

f. cancer of the prostate gland

g. stone in the prostate gland

h. persistent abnormal erection

i. twisting of the spermatic cord

EXERCISE 12

Spell the disease and disorder terms. Have someone dictate the terms on p. 211 to you. Study any words you have spelled incorrectly.

1. _____

2. _____

3. _____

4. _____

5. _____   7. _____

6. _____   8. _____

Surgical Terms

Built from Word Parts

Term	Definition
balanoplasty .... (BAL-a-nō-plas-tē)	surgical repair of the glans penis
epididymectomy .... (ep-i-*did*-i-MEK-tō-mē)	excision of an epididymis
orchidectomy, orchiectomy .... (or-kid-EK-tō-mē) (or-kē-EK-tō-mē)	excision of the testis. (Bilateral orchidectomy also is called *castration*.)
orchidopexy, orchiopexy .... (OR-kid-ō-pek-sē) (OR-kē-ō-pek-sē)	surgical fixation of a testicle (performed to bring undescended testicle[s] into the scrotum)
orchidotomy, orchiotomy .... (or-kid-OT-ō-mē), (or-kē-OT-ō-mē)	incision into a testis
orchioplasty .... (OR-kē-ō-plas-tē)	surgical repair of a testis
prostatectomy .... (*pros*-ta-TEK-tō-mē)	excision of the prostate gland
prostatocystotomy .... (pros-*tat*-ō-sis-TOT-ō-mē)	incision into the prostate gland and bladder
prostatolithotomy .... (pros-*tat*-ō-li-THOT-ō-mē)	incision into the prostate gland to remove a stone
prostatovesiculectomy .... (*pros*-tat-ō-ves-*ik*-ū-LEK-tō-mē)	excision of the prostate gland and seminal vesicles
vasectomy .... (va-SEK-tō-mē)	excision of a duct (partial excision of the vas deferens bilaterally, resulting in male sterilization) (Exercise Figure D)
vasovasostomy .... (vas-ō-va-SOS-tō-mē)	creation of artificial openings between ducts (the severed ends of the vas deferens are reconnected in an attempt to restore fertility in men who have had a vasectomy)
vesiculectomy .... (ve-*sik*-ū-LEK-tō-mē)	excision of the seminal vesicle(s)

Practice saying each of these terms aloud. To hear the terms, access the **PRONOUNCE IT** activity for this chapter on the Student CD that accompanies this text. Or, to hear the terms and their definitions with a CD player or computer, obtain the Pronunciation CD designed for use with this text.

Learn the definitions and spellings of the surgical terms by completing exercises 13, 14, and 15.

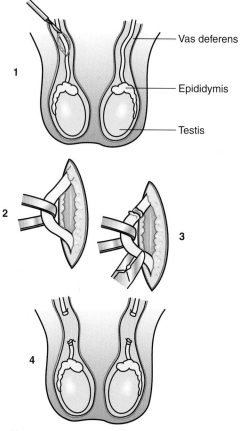

Vas deferens

Epididymis

Testis

Exercise Figure D

Fill in the blanks to complete labeling of the diagram.

_____ / _____ **1,** Incision is made into the covering of the vas.
    duct   **excision**

2, Vas is exposed. **3,** Segment of vas is excised. **4,** Vas is replaced and skin is sutured.

EXERCISE 13

Analyze and define the following surgical terms.

1. vasectomy _____

2. prostatocystotomy _____

3. orchidotomy, orchiotomy _____

4. epididymectomy _____

5. orchidopexy, orchiopexy _____

6. prostatovesiculectomy _____

7. orchioplasty _____

8. vesiculectomy _____

9. prostatectomy _____

10. balanoplasty _____

11. vasovasostomy _____

12. orchidectomy, orchiectomy _____

13. prostatolithotomy _____

EXERCISE 14

Build surgical terms for the following definitions by using the word parts you have learned.

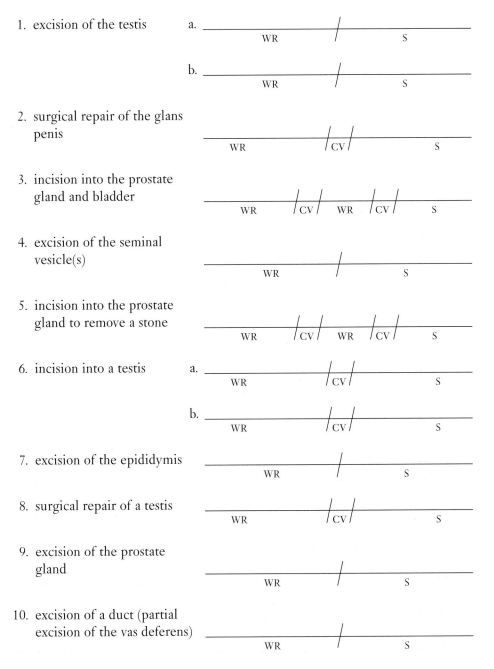

1. excision of the testis   a. _____
                                 WR   S

                    b. _____
                                 WR   S

2. surgical repair of the glans penis
    WR   /CV/   S

3. incision into the prostate gland and bladder
    WR /CV/ WR /CV/ S

4. excision of the seminal vesicle(s)
    WR   S

5. incision into the prostate gland to remove a stone
    WR /CV/ WR /CV/ S

6. incision into a testis   a. _____
                                   WR   /CV/   S

                    b. _____
                                 WR   /CV/   S

7. excision of the epididymis
    WR   S

8. surgical repair of a testis
    WR /CV/ S

9. excision of the prostate gland
    WR   S

10. excision of a duct (partial excision of the vas deferens)
    WR   S

11. excision of the prostate
gland and seminal vesicles

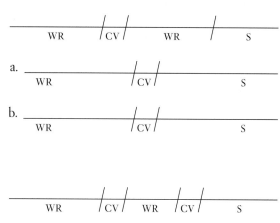

_____	/ ___ /	_____	/ ___	
WR	CV	WR		S

12. surgical fixation of a testicle   a.

_____	/ ___ /	_____	
WR	CV		S

     b.

_____	/ ___ /	_____	
WR	CV		S

13. creation of artificial open-
ings between the severed
ends of the vas deferens

_____	/ ___ /	___	/ ___ /	
WR	CV	WR	CV	S

EXERCISE 15

Spell each of the surgical terms. Have someone dictate the terms on p. 215 to you. Think about the word parts before attempting to write the word. Study any words you have spelled incorrectly.

1. _____   8. _____

2. _____   9. _____

3. _____   10. _____

4. _____   11. _____

5. _____   12. _____

6. _____   13. _____

7. _____

Surgical Terms

Not Built from Word Parts

Term	Definition
circumcision .... (*ser*-kum-SI-zhun)	surgical removal of the prepuce (foreskin) (Figure 7-8)
hydrocelectomy .... (*hī*-drō-sē-LEK-tō-mē)	surgical removal of a hydrocele
penile implant.. (PĒ-nīl) (im-PLANT)	surgical implantation of a penile prosthesis to correct erectile dysfunction (Figure 7-9)

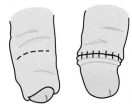

Figure 7-8
Circumcision.

In 1998 the first **oral therapy, Viagra** (sildenafil), became available for treatment of erectile dysfunction. Since 2002 more drugs, such as **Cialis** and **Levitra,** have become available for use. Oral therapies are currently the first-line treatment for erectile dysfunction and work by relaxing smooth muscle cells and, as such, increasing the flow of blood in the genital area.

suprapubic prostatectomy ....
  (su-pra-PŪ-bic)
  (*pros*-ta-TEK-tō-mē)

excision of the prostate gland through an abdominal incision made above the pubic bone. Used to treat benign prostatic hyperplasia and prostate cancer (Figure 7-10).

transurethral incision of the prostate gland (TUIP) ....
  (trans-ū-RĒ-thral)

a surgical procedure that widens the urethra by making a few small incisions in the bladder neck and the prostate gland. No prostate tissue is removed. TUIP may be used instead of TURP when the prostate gland is less enlarged.

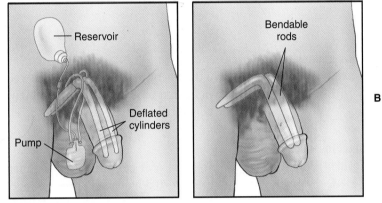

Figure 7-9
Penile implants. **A,** Surgical inflatable implant; **B,** surgical semirigid implants.

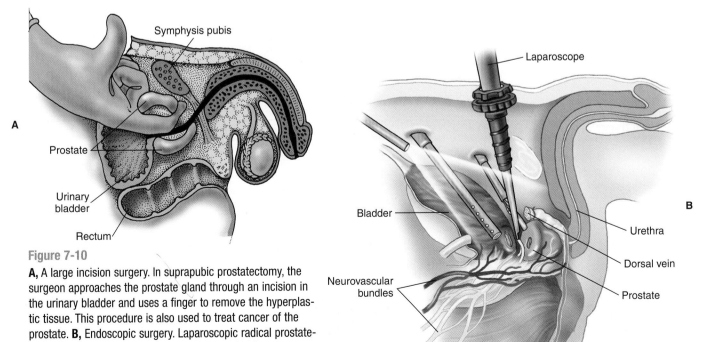

Figure 7-10
A, A large incision surgery. In suprapubic prostatectomy, the surgeon approaches the prostate gland through an incision in the urinary bladder and uses a finger to remove the hyperplastic tissue. This procedure is also used to treat cancer of the prostate. **B,** Endoscopic surgery. Laparoscopic radical prostatectomy is a new procedure used to treat early stages of prostate cancer and for men younger than 70 years.

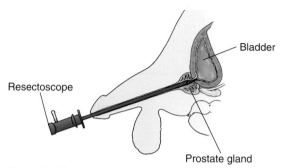

Figure 7-11
Transurethral resection of the prostate gland is used to treat benign prostatic hyperplasia. A resectoscope is inserted through the urethra to the prostate gland. The end of the instrument is equipped to remove small pieces of the enlarged prostate gland.

transurethral microwave thermotherapy (TUMT)................ (trans-ū-RE-thral) (mī-crō-WAVE) (ther-mō-THER-a-pē)	a treatment that eliminates excess cells present in benign prostatic hyperplasia by using heat generated by microwave (Figure 7-12)
transurethral resection of the prostate gland (TURP)................ (trans-ū-RE-thral) (rē-SEK-shun)	successive pieces of the prostate gland tissue are resected by using a resectoscope inserted through the urethra. The capsule is left intact. Usually performed when the enlarged prostate gland interferes with urination (Figure 7-11).

Surgical Treatments for Benign Prostatic Hyperplasia
Incisional
Transurethral resection of the prostate gland (TURP)
Prostatectomy
Transurethral incision of the prostate gland (TUIP)

Thermotherapy
Transurethral microwave thermotherapy (TUMT)
Cooled ThermoTherapy

Laser
Transurethral laser incision of the prostate gland (TULIP)
Visual laser incision of the prostate gland (VLIP)
Photoselective vaporization of the prostate gland (PVP)

Cooled ThermoTherapy
delivers precise microwavable energy to heat and destroy prostate tissue while a cooling mechanism protects surrounding tissue.

Practice saying each of these terms aloud. To hear the terms, access the **PRONOUNCE IT** activity for this chapter on the Student CD that accompanies this text. Or, to hear the terms and their definitions with a CD player or computer, obtain the Pronunciation CD designed for use with this text.

Learn the definitions and spellings of the surgical terms by completing exercises 16 and 17.

EXERCISE 16

Fill in the blanks with the correct term.

1. The surgery performed to remove the prostate gland is _____ _____.

2. The surgical procedure performed to remove the prepuce is called a(n) _____.

3. The surgery performed to correct erectile dysfunction is _____ _____.

4. Surgical removal of a hydrocele is _____.

5. _____ _____ _____ is a treatment for benign prostatic hyperplasia that uses heat generated by microwave.

6. A surgical procedure for benign prostatic hyperplasia that widens the urethra by making small incisions is called _____ _____ of the _____ _____.

7. Pieces of prostate gland tissue are removed with a resectoscope during the surgical procedure called _____ _____ of the _____ _____.

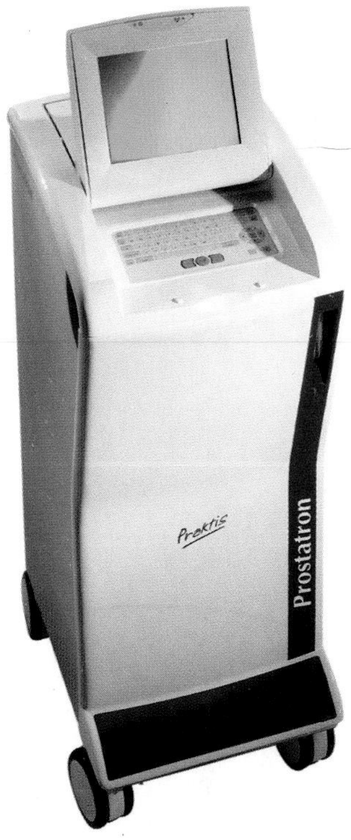

EXERCISE 17

Spell each of the surgical terms. Have someone dictate the terms on pp. 218-220 to you. Study any words you have spelled incorrectly.

1. _____   5. _____

2. _____   6. _____

3. _____   7. _____

4. _____

Figure 7-12
Cooled ThermoTherapy device used to treat benign prostatic hyperplasia.

Diagnostic Terms

Not Built from Word Parts

Term	Definition
Diagnostic Imaging	
transrectal ultrasound.................... (trans-REK-tal) (UL-tra-sownd)	an ultrasound procedure used to diagnose prostate cancer. Sound waves are obtained by placing a probe into the rectum. The sound waves are transformed into an image of the prostate gland.
Laboratory	
prostate-specific antigen (PSA)...... (PROS-tāt) (spe-SIF-ic) (AN-ti-jen)	a blood test that measures the level of prostate-specific antigen in the blood. Elevated test results may indicate the presence of prostate cancer.

Other

digital rectal examination (DRE) ....
    (DIJ-it-al) (REC-tal)
    (eg-*zam*-i-NĀ-shun)
	a physical examination in which the physician inserts a finger into the rectum and feels for the size and shape of the prostate gland through the rectal wall. Used to screen for BPH and cancer of the prostate. BPH usually presents as a uniform, nontender enlargement, whereas cancer usually presents as a stony hard nodule.

Practice saying each of the words aloud. To hear the terms, access the **PRONOUNCE IT** activity for this chapter on the Student CD that accompanies this text. Or, to hear the terms and their definitions with a CD player or computer, obtain the Pronunciation CD designed for use with this text.

Learn the definitions and spellings of the diagnostic terms by completing exercises 18, 19, and 20.

EXERCISE 18

Fill in the blanks with the correct terms.

1. A procedure in which the physician feels for the size and shape of the prostate gland through the rectal wall is called _____ _____ _____.

2. A blood test that, when elevated, may indicate the presence of prostate cancer is called _____ _____.

3. A diagnostic ultrasound procedure used to obtain images of the prostate gland is called _____ _____.

EXERCISE 19

Spell each of the diagnostic terms. Have someone dictate the terms on pp. 221-222 to you. Study any words you have spelled incorrectly.

1. _____   3. _____

2. _____

Complementary Terms

Built from Word Parts

Term	Definition
andropathy .... (an-DROP-a-thē)	diseases of the male (that is, peculiar to the male, such as a testitis)

oligospermia..............................	condition of scanty sperm (in the semen)
(ol-i-gō-SPER-mē-a)	
spermatolysis	dissolution (destruction) of sperm
(sper-ma-TOL-i-sis)	

Practice saying each of these terms aloud. To hear the terms, access the **PRONOUNCE IT** activity for this chapter on the Student CD that accompanies this text. Or, to hear the terms and their definitions with a CD player or computer, obtain the Pronunciation CD designed for use with this text.

Exercises 20, 21, and 22 will help you learn the definitions and spellings of the complementary terms related to the male reproductive system.

EXERCISE 20

Analyze and define the following complementary terms.

1. oligospermia _____

2. andropathy _____

3. spermatolysis _____

EXERCISE 21

Build the complementary terms for the following definitions by using the word parts you have learned.

1. dissolution (destruction) of
   sperm

   _____ / _____ / _____
   WR   CV   S

2. diseases of the male

   _____ / _____ / _____
   WR   CV   S

3. condition of scanty sperm
   (in the semen)

   _____ / ____ / _____ / ____
   WR   CV   WR   S

EXERCISE 22

Spell each of the complementary terms. Have someone dictate the terms on pp. 222-223 to you. Think about the word parts before attempting to write the word. Study any words you have spelled incorrectly.

1. _____   3. _____

2. _____

Complementary Terms

Not Built from Word Parts

Term	Definition
acquired immunodeficiency syndrome (AIDS).................... (*im*-ū-nō-de-FISH-en-sē) (SIN-drōm)	a disease that affects the body's immune system, transmitted by exchange of body fluid during the sexual act, reuse of contaminated needles, or receiving contaminated blood transfusions (also called *acquired immune deficiency syndrome*)
artificial insemination .... (ar-ti-FISH-al) (in-sem-i-NA-shun)	introduction of semen into the vagina by artificial means
chlamydia.................................... (klah-MID-ē-a)	a sexually transmitted disease, sometimes referred to as a *silent STD* because many people are not aware they have the disease. Symptoms that occur when the disease becomes serious are painful urination and discharge from the penis in men and genital itching, vaginal discharge, and bleeding between menstrual periods in women. The causative agent is *C. trachomatis.*
coitus.. (KŌ-i-tus)	sexual intercourse between male and female (also called *copulation*)
condom.. (KON-dum)	cover for the penis worn during coitus
ejaculation.................................. (ē-jak-ū-LA-shun)	ejection of semen from the male urethra
genital herpes............................ (JEN-i-tal) (HER-pēz)	sexually transmitted disease caused by *Herpesvirus hominis* type 2 (also called *herpes simplex virus*)
gonads.. (GŌ-nads)	male and female sex glands
gonorrhea.................................... (gon-or-RĒ-a)	contagious, inflammatory sexually transmitted disease caused by a bacterial organism that affects the mucous membranes of the genitourinary system
heterosexual.............................. (*het*-er-ō-SEKS-shū-al)	person who is attracted to a member of the opposite sex
homosexual .... (*hō*-mō-SEKS-shū-al)	person who is attracted to a member of the same sex
human immunodeficiency virus (HIV) .... (*im*-ū-nō-de-FISH-en-sē)	a type of retrovirus that causes AIDS. HIV infects T-helper cells of the immune system, allowing for opportunistic infections such as candidiasis, *P. carinii* pneumonia, tuberculosis, and Kaposi sarcoma.

human papilloma virus (HPV)..........................
 (HŪ-man) (pap-i-LŌ-ma)
 (VĪ-rus)

a prevalent sexually transmitted disease causing benign or cancerous growths in male and female genitals (also called *venereal warts*)

orgasm..........................
 (OR-gazm)

climax of sexual stimulation

prosthesis..........................
 (pros-THĒ-sis)

an artificial replacement of an absent body part

puberty..........................
 (PŪ-ber-tē)

period when secondary sex characteristics develop and the ability to reproduce sexually begins

sexually transmitted disease (STD)..........................
 (SEKS-ū-al-ē)
 (TRANS-mi-ted) (di-ZĒZ)

diseases, such as syphilis, gonorrhea, and genital herpes, transmitted during sexual contact (also called *venereal disease*)

sterilization..........................
 (star-il-i-ZĀ-shun)

process that renders an individual unable to produce offspring

syphilis..........................
 (SIF-i-lis)

infectious sexually transmitted disease having lesions that can affect any organ or tissue; a syphilitic mother may transmit the disease to her unborn infant because the causative organism is able to pass through the placenta

trichomoniasis..........................
 (trik-ō-mō-NĪ-a-sis)

a sexually transmitted disease caused by a one-cell organism, *Trichomonas.* It infects the genitourinary tract. Men may be asymptomatic or may develop urethritis, an enlarged prostate gland, or epididymitis. Women have vaginal itching, dysuria, and vaginal or urethral discharge.

Venereal
is derived from **Venus,** the goddess of love. In ancient times it was noted that the disease was part of the misfortunes of love.

List of Male and Female Sexually Transmitted Diseases
acquired immunodeficiency syndrome
human immunodeficiency virus infections
syphilis
genital herpes
venereal warts (human papilloma virus)
gonorrhea
chlamydia
trichomoniasis
cytomegalovirus infections

Practice saying each of these terms aloud. To hear the terms, access the **PRONOUNCE IT** activity for this chapter on the Student CD that accompanies this text. Or, to hear the terms and their definitions with a CD player or computer, obtain the Pronunciation CD designed for use with this text.

Learn the definitions and spellings of the complementary terms by completing exercises 23 through 26.

EXERCISE   23

Write the definitions of the following terms.

1. puberty _____

2. orgasm _____

3. gonorrhea _____

4. homosexual _____

5. coitus _____

6. genital herpes _____

7. heterosexual _____

8. syphilis _____

9. ejaculation _____

10. gonads _____

11. sexually transmitted disease _____

12. sterilization _____

13. human papilloma virus _____

14. acquired immunodeficiency syndrome _____

15. trichomoniasis _____

16. artificial insemination _____

17. chlamydia _____

18. condom _____

19. prosthesis _____

20. human immunodeficiency virus _____

EXERCISE   24

Match the terms in the first column with their correct definitions in the second column.

_____ 1. coitus   a. male and female sex glands

_____ 2. ejaculation   b. climax of sexual stimulation

_____ 3. human papilloma virus   c. one who is attracted to a member of the
                                              opposite sex
_____ 4. gonads

_____ 5. genital herpes   d. STD caused by *Herpesvirus hominis* type 2

_____ 6. gonorrhea

_____ 7. heterosexual

_____ 8. orgasm

_____ 9. condom

_____ 10. prosthesis

e. ejection of semen

f. an artificial replacement for an absent body part

g. sexual intercourse between man and woman

h. venereal warts

i. contagious and inflammatory STD

j. cover for the penis worn during coitus

k. one who is attracted to a member of the same sex

EXERCISE 25

Match the terms in the first column with their correct definitions in the second column.

_____ 1. homosexual

_____ 2. STD

_____ 3. sterilization

_____ 4. syphilis

_____ 5. puberty

_____ 6. AIDS

_____ 7. trichomoniasis

_____ 8. artificial insemination

_____ 9. chlamydia

_____ 10. HIV

a. abbreviation for diseases such as syphilis, gonorrhea, and genital herpes

b. a disease that affects the body's immune system

c. a type of retrovirus that causes AIDS

d. sexually transmitted disease that can affect any organ and that can be transmitted to an unborn infant

e. introduction of semen into the vagina by means other than intercourse

f. one who is attracted to members of the same sex

g. a prevalent STD caused by a bacterium, _C. trachomatis_ (silent STD)

h. process rendering an individual unable to produce offspring

i. an STD caused by a one-cell organism, _Trichomonas_

j. period when the ability to sexually reproduce begins

EXERCISE 26

Spell each of the complementary terms. Have someone dictate the terms on pp. 224-225 to you. Study any words you have spelled incorrectly.

1. _____   3. _____

2. _____   4. _____

5. _____   13. _____

6. _____   14. _____

7. _____   15. _____

8. _____   16. _____

9. _____   17. _____

10. _____   18. _____

11. _____   19. _____

12. _____   20. _____

Abbreviations

AIDS	acquired immunodeficiency syndrome
BPH	benign prostatic hyperplasia
DRE	digital rectal examination
HIV	human immunodeficiency virus
HPV	human papilloma virus
PSA	prostate-specific antigen
STD	sexually transmitted disease
TUIP	transurethral incision of the prostate
TUMT	transurethral microwave thermotherapy
TURP	transurethral resection of the prostate

Refer to Appendix D for a complete list of abbreviations.

EXERCISE   27

Write the meaning of the abbreviations in the following sentences.

1. The physician performed a **DRE** _____ _____ _____ on the patient to assist in diagnosing **BPH** _____ _____ _____. Surgical treatments for BPH include prostatectomy, **TURP** _____ _____ of the _____ gland, **TUMT** _____ _____ _____, and **TUIP** _____ _____ of the _____ gland.

2. **AIDS** _____ _____ _____ is an **STD** _____ _____ _____. **HIV** _____ _____ _____ is a type of retrovirus that causes AIDS. **HPV** _____ _____ _____ is an STD that causes female and male venereal warts.

3. **PSA** _____ _____ _____ is a laboratory test used to diagnose cancer of the prostate.

CHAPTER REVIEW

EXERCISE 28   *Interact with Medical Records*

Complete the emergency department report by writing the medical terms in the blanks. Use the list of definitions with the corresponding numbers.

University Hospital and Medical Center
4700 North Main Street • Wellness, Arizona 54321 • (987) 555-3210

PATIENT NAME: Andrew Nguyen   **CASE NUMBER:**   19504-MRS
DATE OF BIRTH: 07/27/xx   **DATE:**   08/23/xx

Emergency Department Report

CHIEF COMPLAINT: Severe lower abdominal pain and the inability to void for the past 12 hours.

PRESENT ILLNESS: Andrew Nguyen is a 75-year-old Asian American man who came into the emergency department at 3 AM stating that he was in great pain and could not urinate. He had not been seen by a physician for several years but claimed to be in good health except for "a little high blood pressure." The patient reports urinary frequency, 1. _____ × 2, hesitancy, intermittency, and diminished force and caliber of the urinary stream. He also has postvoid dribbling and the sensation of not having completely emptied the bladder. Earlier today, he had 2. _____ at the end of urination.

MEDICATION ALLERGIES: None

CURRENT MEDICATIONS: Benadryl 25 mg at bedtime.

PHYSICAL EXAM: Temperature, 98.6. Blood pressure, 140/90. Pulse, 98. Respirations, 24. Palpation of the abdomen shows a suprapubic mass approximately three fingerbreadths below the umbilicus, dull to percussion and slightly tender.

IMPRESSION: 3. _____ bladder distention caused by urinary outlet obstruction, probably from
4. _____ _____ _____.

PLAN:
Indwelling Foley catheter for relief of urinary obstruction.
5. _____ consult.

Eleanor Adams, MD

EA/mcm

---

1. night urination
2. blood in the urine
3. pertaining to urine

4. nonmalignant excessive development pertaining to the prostate gland (enlargement of the prostate gland)
5. study of the urinary tract

EXERCISE 29 *Interpret Medical Terms*

To test your understanding of the terms introduced in this chapter, circle the words that correctly complete the sentences. The italicized words refer to the correct answer.

1. A *discharge from the glans penis* is referred to medically as (balanorrhagia, balanorrhea, balanorrhaphy).
2. The surgical procedure circumcision is the removal of the *foreskin,* or (glans penis, testes, prepuce).
3. *A person who is attracted to a member of the opposite sex* is (heterosexual, homosexual).
4. The patient had a diagnosis of (oligospermia, phimosis, impotence), or *a narrowing of the opening of the prepuce.*
5. The *operation for the surgical fixation of the testicle* is (orchidopexy, orchidotomy, orchioplasty).
6. An *artificial replacement* or (condom, prosthesis, artificial insemination) is used to correct erectile dysfunction of the penis.
7. The following is a treatment for benign prostatic hyperplasia using heat (transurethral prostatectomy, suprapubic prostatectomy, transurethral microwave thermotherapy).

EXERCISE 30 *Read Medical Terms in Use*

Practice pronunciation of the terms by reading the following medical document. Use the pronunciation key following the medical term to assist you in saying the word.

A 62-year-old man was found to have an elevated **prostate-specific antigen test** (PROS-tāt) (spe-SIF-ic) (AN-ti-jen) during a routine physical examination. At the age of 42 years he underwent a **vasectomy** (va-SEK-tō-mē). The patient denies having nocturia or any significant change in his urinary stream. **Digital rectal** (DIJ-it-al) (REC-tal) **examination** revealed a mildly enlarged **prostate** (PROS-tāt) gland with a 1.0 cm nodule of the right lobe. The urologist performed a **transrectal** (trans-REK-tal) **ultrasound** and biopsy. A diagnosis of adenocarcinoma of the prostate was made. The patient elected to undergo a **suprapubic prostatectomy** (sū-pra-PŪ-bik) (*pros*-ta-TEK-tō-mē). Urinary incontinence complicated his postoperative course but this lasted for only 3 months. No **erectile dysfunction** (ē-REK-tīl) (dis-FUNK-shun) was reported. His prognosis for full recovery should be excellent.

EXERCISE 31 *Comprehend Medical Terms in Use*

Test your comprehension of the terms in the above medical document by circling the correct answer.

1. Before being diagnosed with cancer of the prostate the patient had surgery for:
   a. sterilization
   b. excision of the seminal vesicle
   c. removal of the prepuce
   d. repair of the glans penis
2. The patient chose which of the following types of treatment for prostate cancer?
   a. radiation
   b. chemotherapy
   c. surgery
   d. hormonal therapy
3. After surgery the patient:
   a. had absence of sperm
   b. had persistent abnormal erection
   c. had a narrowing of the opening of the prepuce of the glans penis
   d. was able to have an erection

For further practice or to evaluate what you have learned, use the Student CD that accompanies this text.

SUFFIXES CHAPTERS 2-4 CROSSWORD PUZZLE

Across Clues

2. instrument to measure
4. substance or agent that produces or causes
6. flow, excessive discharge
8. measurement
9. disease
10. surgical repair
11. sudden involuntary muscle contraction
13. pertaining to sound or voice
14. instrument to cut
15. instrument for visual examination
17. pertaining to
18. cell
19. pertaining to carbon dioxide
22. producing, originating, causing
24. chest
25. incision
28. abnormal condition
30. rapid flow of blood
32. inflammation
34. creation of an artificial opening
36. one who studies and treats
37. control, stop
38. process of imaging

Down Clues

1. softening
3. a stretching out, dilation
5. diseased state, abnormal state
7. excision
10. eating, swallowing
11. visual examination
12. breathing
13. surgical fixation, suspension
16. hernia or protrusion
17. blood condition
19. surgical puncture to aspirate fluid
20. pain
21. constriction, narrowing
23. tumor, swelling
26. resembling
27. record, x-ray imaging
29. pertaining to
31. pertaining to
33. study of
35. to view

REVIEW OF WORD PARTS

Can you define and spell the following word parts?

Combining Form		Prefix	Suffix
andr/o	prostat/o	trans-	-ism
balan/o	spermat/o		
epididym/o	sperm/o		
orch/o	test/o		
orchi/o	vas/o		
orchid/o	vesicul/o		

REVIEW OF TERMS

Can you build, analyze, define, pronounce, and spell the following terms *built from word parts?*

Diseases and Disorders

anorchism
balanitis
benign prostatic hyperplasia (BPH)
cryptorchidism
epididymitis
orchiepididymitis
orchitis, orchiditis, or testitis
prostatitis
prostatocystitis
prostatolith
prostatorrhea
prostatovesiculitis

Surgical

balanoplasty
epididymectomy
orchidectomy, or orchiectomy
orchidopexy, or orchiopexy
orchidotomy, or orchiotomy
orchioplasty
prostatectomy
prostatocystotomy
prostatolithotomy
prostatovesiculectomy
vasectomy
vasovasostomy
vesiculectomy

Complementary

andropathy
oligospermia
spermatolysis

Can you define, pronounce, and spell the following terms *not built from word parts?*

Diseases and Disorders

erectile dysfunction
hydrocele
phimosis
priapism
prostate cancer
testicular carcinoma
testicular torsion
varicocele

Surgical

circumcision
hydrocelectomy
penile implant
suprapubic
   prostatectomy
transurethral incision
   of the prostate
   gland (TUIP)
transurethral
   microwave
   thermotherapy
   (TUMT)
transurethral resection
   of the prostate
   gland (TURP)

Diagnostic

digital rectal
   examination (DRE)
prostate-specific anti-
   gen (PSA)
transrectal ultrasound

Complementary

acquired immunodeficiency syndrome
   (AIDS)
artificial insemination
chlamydia
coitus
condom
ejaculation
genital herpes
gonads
gonorrhea
heterosexual
homosexual
human immunodeficiency virus (HIV)
human papilloma virus (HPV)
orgasm
prosthesis
puberty
sexually transmitted disease (STD)
sterilization
syphilis
trichomoniasis

8

Female Reproductive System

OUTLINE

OBJECTIVES

On completion of this chapter you will be able to:

1. Identify the organs and other structures of the female reproductive system.
2. Define and spell the word parts presented in this chapter.
3. Build and analyze medical terms with word parts presented in this and previous chapters.
4. Define, pronounce, and spell the disease and disorder, diagnostic, surgical, and complementary terms for the female reproductive system.
5. Interpret the meaning of the abbreviations presented in this chapter.
6. Read medical documents and interpret medical terminology contained in them.

ANATOMY

Function

The female reproductive system produces the female egg cells and hormones and also provides for conception and pregnancy (Figures 8-1 and 8-2).

Internal Organs of the Female Reproductive System

ovaries	pair of almond-shaped organs located in the pelvic cavity. Egg cells are stored in the ovaries.
ovum (*pl.* ova)	female egg cell
graafian follicles	100,000 microscopic sacs that make up a large portion of the ovaries. Each follicle contains an immature ovum. Normally one graafian follicle develops to maturity monthly between puberty and menopause. It moves to the surface of the ovary and releases the ovum, which passes into the fallopian tube.
fallopian, or uterine, tubes	pair of 5-inch (12-cm) tubes, attached to the uterus, that provide a passageway for the ovum to move from the ovary to the uterus
fimbria (*pl.* fimbriae)	finger-like projection at the free end of the fallopian tube
uterus	pear-sized and pear-shaped muscular organ that lies in the pelvic cavity, except during pregnancy when it enlarges and extends up into the abdominal cavity. Its functions are menstruation, pregnancy, and labor.
endometrium	inner lining of the uterus
myometrium	muscular middle layer of the uterus
perimetrium	outer thin layer that covers the surface of the uterus
corpus, or body	large central portion of the uterus
fundus	rounded upper portion of the uterus
cervix (Cx)	narrow lower portion of the uterus
vagina	a 3-inch (7-8 cm) tube that connects the uterus to the outside of the body
hymen	fold of membrane found near the opening of the vagina
rectouterine pouch	pouch between the posterior wall of the uterus and the anterior wall of the rectum (also called *Douglas cul-de-sac*) (see Figure 8-1)

The Graafian Follicle is named for Dutch anatomist Reinier de **Graaf,** who discovered the sac in 1672.

The Fallopian Tube was named in honor of Gabriele Fallopius because he described it in his works. Fallopius also gave the **vagina** and the **placenta** their names.

Ever since I told a crowded room I had a Bavarian [Bartholin] cyst and not only did no one laugh, but two others had the same thing, I've been convinced that doctor and patient do not speak the same language. They speak Latin. We speak Reader's Digest.

Erma Bombeck, 1981

Glands of the Female Reproductive System

Bartholin glands..................................	pair of mucus-producing glands located on each side of the vagina and just above the vaginal opening

Bartholin Glands
were described by Thomas Bartholinus, a Danish anatomist, in 1675.

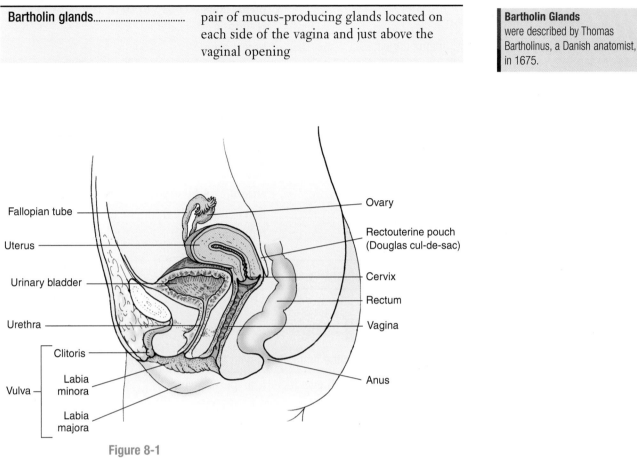

Figure 8-1
Female reproductive organs and associated structures.

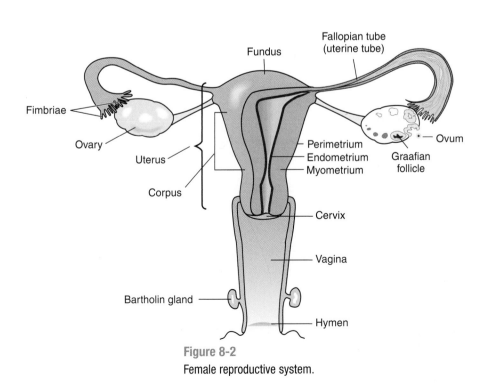

Figure 8-2
Female reproductive system.

mammary glands, or breasts...........	milk-producing glands of the female. Each breast consists of 15 to 20 divisions, or lobes (Figure 8-3).
mammary papilla...........................	breast nipple
areola..	pigmented area around the breast nipple

External Female Reproductive Structures

vulva, or external genitals...............	two pairs of lips (labia major and labia minora) that surround the vagina
clitoris..	highly erogenous erectile body located anterior to the urethra
perineum...	pelvic floor in both the male and female. In females it usually refers to the area between the vaginal opening and the anus.

Learn the anatomic terms by completing exercises 1 and 2.

EXERCISE   1

Match the definitions in the first column with the anatomic terms in the second column.

_____ 1. organs in which egg cells are formed

_____ 2. lower portion of the uterus

_____ 3. lining of the uterus

a. perimetrium

b. fundus

c. ovaries

d. perineum

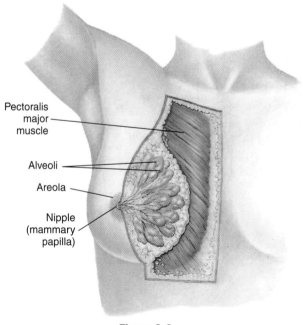

Pectoralis major muscle

Alveoli

Areola

Nipple (mammary papilla)

Figure 8-3
Female breast.

_____ 4. upper portion of the uterus

_____ 5. pelvic floor

_____ 6. ends of fallopian tubes

_____ 7. large central portion of the uterus

_____ 8. layer that covers the uterus

_____ 9. muscle layer of the uterus

e. fimbriae

f. cervix

g. endometrium

h. corpus

i. myometrium

j. ovum

EXERCISE 2

Match the definitions in the first column with the anatomic terms in the second column.

_____ 1. connects the uterus to the outside of the body

_____ 2. mucus-producing gland located on each side of the vagina

_____ 3. breast

_____ 4. female egg cells

_____ 5. external genitals

_____ 6. passageway for ovum

_____ 7. pigmented area around the nipple

_____ 8. microscopic sacs in the ovaries

_____ 9. muscular organ

_____ 10. nipples

_____ 11. rectouterine pouch

a. ovary

b. vagina

c. Bartholin glands

d. mammary gland

e. vulva

f. fallopian tube

g. areola

h. Douglas cul-de-sac

i. uterus

j. mammary papillae

k. ova

l. graafian follicles

WORD PARTS

Combining Forms of the Female Reproductive System

Study the word parts and their definitions listed below. Completing the exercises that follow and Exercise Figures A and B will help you learn the terms.

Combining Form	Definition
arche/o	first, beginning
cervic/o, trachel/o	cervix
(NOTE: _trachel/o_ also means _neck, necklike._)	

colp/o, vagin/o	vagina
culd/o	cul-de-sac
episi/o, vulv/o	vulva
gynec/o, gyn/o	woman

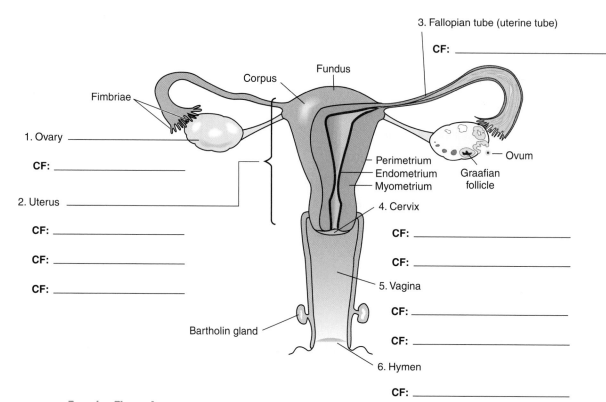

3. Fallopian tube (uterine tube)

CF: _____

Fundus

Corpus

Fimbriae

1. Ovary _____

CF: _____

2. Uterus _____

CF: _____

CF: _____

CF: _____

Perimetrium
Endometrium
Myometrium

Ovum

Graafian follicle

4. Cervix

CF: _____

CF: _____

5. Vagina

CF: _____

CF: _____

Bartholin gland

6. Hymen

CF: _____

Exercise Figure A

Fill in the blanks with combining forms in this diagram of the frontal view of the female reproductive system.

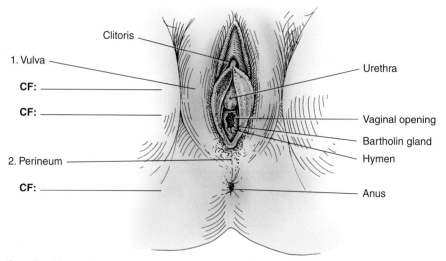

Clitoris

1. Vulva _____

CF: _____

CF: _____

Urethra

Vaginal opening

Bartholin gland

Hymen

2. Perineum _____

CF: _____

Anus

Exercise Figure B

Fill in the blanks with combining forms in this diagram showing the external reproductive organs.

| hymen/o | hymen |
| hyster/o,
metr/o,
metr/i,
uter/o | uterus |

(NOTE: the combining vowel
i or *o* may be used with metr/.)

mamm/o, mast/o	breast
men/o	menstruation
oophor/o	ovary
perine/o	perineum
salping/o	fallopian tube (uterine tube) (Figure 8-4)

Learn the anatomic locations and definitions of the combining forms by completing exercises 3 and 4 and Exercise Figures A and B.

EXERCISE 3

Write the definitions of the following combining forms.

1. vagin/o _____

2. oophor/o _____

3. metr/o, metr/i _____

4. uter/o _____

5. hymen/o _____

6. hyster/o _____

7. men/o _____

8. episi/o _____

9. cervic/o _____

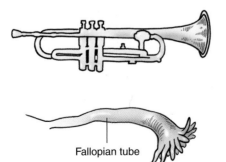

Fallopian tube

Figure 8-4

Salpinx is derived from *salpinx,* the Greek term for *trumpet.* The term was used for the fallopian tubes because of their trumpetlike shape.

10. colp/o _____

11. gynec/o _____

12. mamm/o _____

13. perine/o _____

14. salping/o _____

15. vulv/o _____

16. mast/o _____

17. arche/o _____

18. culd/o _____

19. gyn/o _____

20. trachel/o _____

EXERCISE 4

Write the combining form for each of the following terms.

1. vulva

   a. _____

   b. _____

2. breast

   a. _____

   b. _____

3. menstruation _____

4. ovary _____

5. fallopian tube _____

6. perineum _____

7. vagina

   a. _____

   b. _____

8. uterus

   a. _____

   b. _____

   c. _____

9. woman

   a. _____

   b. _____

10. hymen _____

11. cul-de-sac _____

12. cervix   a. _____

b. _____

13. beginning _____

Prefix and Suffixes

Prefix	Definition
peri-...	surrounding (outer)

Suffixes	Definition
-atresia.....................................	absence of a normal body opening; occlusion; closure
-ial..	pertaining to
-salpinx....................................	fallopian tube (see Figure 8-4)
(NOTE: for learning purposes *salpinx* and *atresia* are presented as suffixes.)	

Atresia
literally means **no perforation or hole.** It is composed of the Greek words **a,** meaning **without,** and **tresis,** meaning **perforation.** The term may be used alone, as in "atresia of vagina," or combined with other word parts, as in "gynatresia," meaning closure of a part of the female genital tract, usually the vagina.

Learn the prefix and suffixes by completing exercises 5 and 6.

EXERCISE 5

Write the prefix or suffix for each of the following.

1. fallopian tube _____

2. pertaining to _____

3. surrounding _____

4. absence of a normal body
   opening _____

EXERCISE 6

Write the definitions of the following prefix and suffixes.

1. -salpinx _____

2. peri- _____

3. -ial _____

4. -atresia _____

Refer to Appendix A and Appendix B for alphabetized word parts and their meanings.

MEDICAL TERMS

The terms you need to learn to complete this chapter are listed below. The exercises following each list will help you learn the definition and spelling of each word.

Disease and Disorder Terms

Built from Word Parts

Term	Definition
amenorrhea (ā-*men*-ō-RĒ-a)	absence of menstrual discharge (menostasis)
Bartholin adenitis (BAR-tō-lin) (*ad*-e-NĪ-tis)	inflammation of a Bartholin gland
cervicitis (*ser*-vi-SĪ-tis)	inflammation of the cervix
colpitis, vaginitis (kol-PĪ-tis), (vaj-i-NĪ-tis)	inflammation of the vagina
dysmenorrhea (*dis*-men-ō-RĒ-a)	painful menstrual discharge
endocervicitis (*en*-dō-*ser*-vi-SĪ-tis)	inflammation of the inner (lining) of the cervix
endometritis (*en*-dō-mē-TRĪ-tis)	inflammation of the inner (lining) of the uterus (endometrium)
hematosalpinx (*hem*-a-tō-SAL-pinks)	blood in the fallopian tube
hydrosalpinx (hī-drō-SAL-pinks)	water in the fallopian tube
hysteratresia (his-ter-a-TRĒ-zē-a)	closure of the uterus (uterine cavity)
mastitis (*mas*-TĪ-tis)	inflammation of the breast
menometrorrhagia (*men*-ō-*met*-rō-RĀ-jē-a)	rapid flow of blood from the uterus at menstruation (and between menstrual cycles)
metrorrhea (me-trō-RĒ-a)	excessive discharge from the uterus
myometritis (mī-o-mē-TRĪ-tis)	inflammation of the uterine muscle (myometrium)
oophoritis (ō-of-ō-RĪ-tis)	inflammation of the ovary
perimetritis (*per*-i-mē-TRĪ-tis)	inflammation surrounding the uterus (perimetrium)
pyosalpinx (pī-o-SAL-pinks)	pus in the fallopian tube
salpingitis (*sal*-pin-JĪ-tis)	inflammation of the fallopian tube (Exercise Figure C)

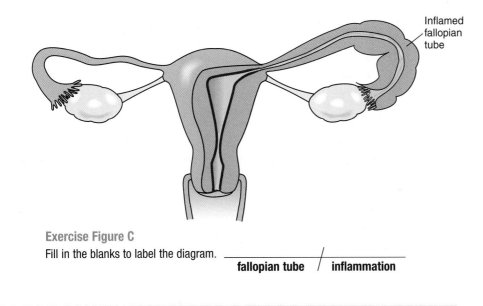

Inflamed
fallopian
tube

Exercise Figure C
Fill in the blanks to label the diagram. ————————/————————
fallopian tube / inflammation

salpingocele	hernia of the fallopian tube
(sal-PING-gō-sēl)	
vulvovaginitis	inflammation of the vulva and vagina
(*vul*-vō-vaj-i-NĪ-tis)	

Practice saying each of these terms aloud. To hear the terms, access the **PRONOUNCE IT** activity for this chapter on the Student CD that accompanies this text. Or, to hear the terms and their definitions with a CD player or computer, obtain the Pronunciation CD designed for use with this text.

Learn the definitions and spellings of the disease and disorder terms by completing exercises 7, 8, and 9.

EXERCISE 7

Analyze and define the following terms.

1. colpitis _____

2. cervicitis _____

3. hydrosalpinx _____

4. hematosalpinx _____

5. metrorrhea _____

6. oophoritis _____

7. (Bartholin) adenitis _____

8. vulvovaginitis _____

9. salpingocele _____

10. menometrorrhagia _____

11. amenorrhea _____

12. dysmenorrhea _____

13. mastitis _____

14. perimetritis _____

15. myometritis _____

16. endometritis _____

17. endocervicitis _____

18. pyosalpinx _____

19. hysteratresia _____

20. salpingitis _____

21. vaginitis _____

EXERCISE 8

Build disease and disorder terms for the following definitions with the word parts you have learned.

1. inflammation of the breast

   _____ / _____
   WR   S

2. excessive discharge from the uterus

   _____ / _____ / _____
   WR   CV   S

3. inflammation of the fallopian tube

   _____ / _____
   WR   S

4. inflammation of the vulva and vagina

   _____ / ___ / _____ / _____
   WR   CV   WR   S

5. absence of menstrual discharge

   _____ / _____ / ___ / _____
   P   WR   CV   S

6. inflammation of the cervix

   _____ / _____
   WR   S

7. inflammation of (Bartholin) gland

   _____ / _____
   (Bartholin)   WR   S

8. water in the fallopian tube

   _____ / _____ / _____
   WR   CV   S

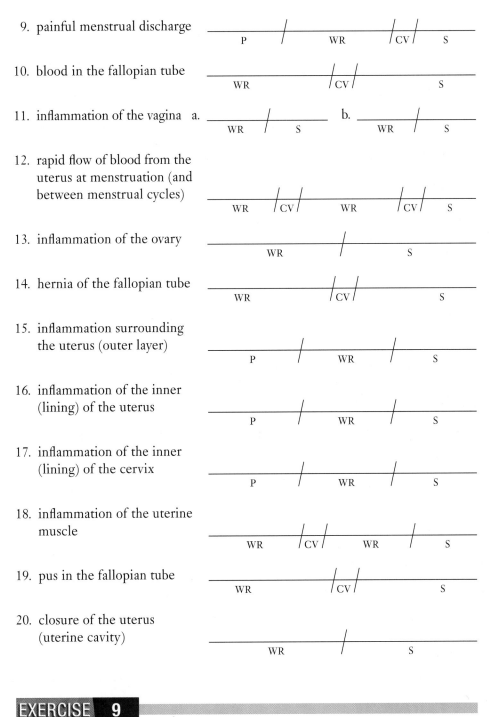

9. painful menstrual discharge ___P___ / ___WR___ /CV/ ___S___

10. blood in the fallopian tube ___WR___ /CV/ ___S___

11. inflammation of the vagina a. ___WR___ / ___S___ b. ___WR___ / ___S___

12. rapid flow of blood from the uterus at menstruation (and between menstrual cycles) ___WR___ /CV/ ___WR___ /CV/ ___S___

13. inflammation of the ovary ___WR___ / ___S___

14. hernia of the fallopian tube ___WR___ /CV/ ___S___

15. inflammation surrounding the uterus (outer layer) ___P___ / ___WR___ / ___S___

16. inflammation of the inner (lining) of the uterus ___P___ / ___WR___ / ___S___

17. inflammation of the inner (lining) of the cervix ___P___ / ___WR___ / ___S___

18. inflammation of the uterine muscle ___WR___ /CV/ ___WR___ / ___S___

19. pus in the fallopian tube ___WR___ /CV/ ___S___

20. closure of the uterus (uterine cavity) ___WR___ / ___S___

EXERCISE 9

Spell each of the disease and disorder terms. Have someone dictate the terms on pp. 242-243 to you. Think about the word parts before attempting to write the word. Study any words you have spelled incorrectly.

1. _____   5. _____

2. _____   6. _____

3. _____   7. _____

4. _____   8. _____

9. _____   16. _____

10. _____   17. _____

11. _____   18. _____

12. _____   19. _____

13. _____   20. _____

14. _____   21. _____

15. _____

Disease and Disorder Terms

Not Built from Word Parts

Term	Definition
adenomyosis (ad-e-nō-mī-O-sis)	growth of endometrium into the muscular portion of the uterus
breast cancer (brest) (KAN-cer)	malignant tumor of the breast
cervical cancer (SER-vi-k'l) (KAN-cer)	malignant tumor of the cervix
endometrial cancer (en-dō-ME-trē-al) (KAN-cer)	malignant tumor of the endometrium. Also called *uterine cancer*.
endometriosis (*en*-dō-*mē*-trē-O-sis)	abnormal condition in which endometrial tissue grows in various areas in the pelvic cavity, including ovaries, fallopian tubes, intestines, and uterus (Figure 8-5)
fibrocystic breast disease (fī-brō-SIS-tik) (di-ZEZ)	a disorder characterized by one or more benign cysts in the breast
fibroid tumor (FI-broyd) (TU-mor)	benign fibroid tumor of the uterine muscle (also called *myoma of the uterus* or *leiomyoma*) (Figure 8-6)

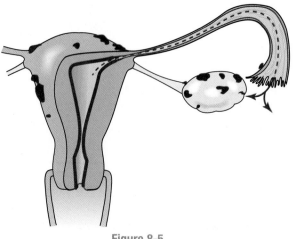

Figure 8-5
Endometriosis.

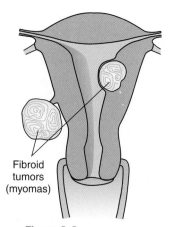

Fibroid
tumors
(myomas)

Figure 8-6
Fibroid tumors (myomas).

ovarian cancer........................... malignant tumor of the ovary
   (ō-VAR-ē-an) (KAN-cer)

pelvic inflammatory disease
(PID)... inflammation of the female pelvic organs
   (PEL-vik) (in-FLAM-a-tor-ē) (Figure 8-7)
   (di-ZĒZ)

prolapsed uterus .... downward displacement of the uterus in the va-
   (PRŌ-lapsd) (Ū-ter-us) gina (also called *hysteroptosis*) (Exercise Figure D)

toxic shock syndrome (TSS)............ a severe illness characterized by high fever,
   (TOX-ic) (shok) (SIN-drōm) rash, vomiting, diarrhea, and myalgia, followed by hypotension and, in severe cases,
   shock and death. Usually affects menstruating
   women using tampons. Caused by *Staphylococcus
   aureus* and *Streptococcus pyogenes.*

vesicovaginal fistula .... abnormal opening between the bladder and
   (*ves*-i-kō-VAJ-i-nal) (FIS-tū-la) the vagina (Exercise Figure E)

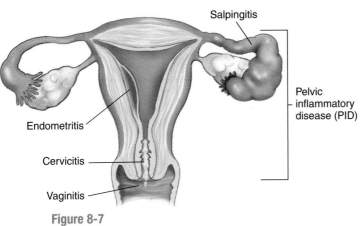

Figure 8-7
Ascending infection of the female reproductive system.

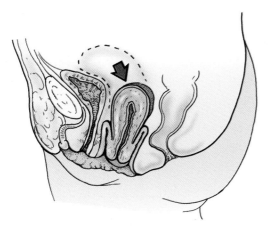

Exercise Figure D
Fill in the blanks to complete labeling of the diagram. Prolapsed
uterus, or

_____/___/_____
uterus /**cv** / **prolapsed**

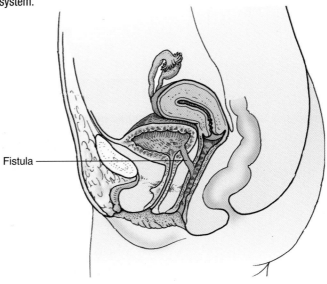

Exercise Figure E
Fill in the blanks to complete labeling of the diagram.
A _____/___/_____/_____ fistula.
bladder / **cv** / **vagina** / **pertaining to**

Practice saying each of these terms aloud. To hear the terms, access the **PRONOUNCE IT** activity for this chapter on the Student CD that accompanies this text. Or, to hear the terms and their definitions with a CD player or computer, obtain the Pronunciation CD designed for use with this text.

Learn the definitions and spellings of the disease and disorder terms by completing exercises 10, 11, and 12.

EXERCISE 10

Fill in the blanks with the correct definitions.

1. prolapsed uterus _____

2. pelvic inflammatory disease _____

3. vesicovaginal fistula _____

4. fibroid tumor _____

5. endometriosis _____

6. adenomyosis _____

7. toxic shock syndrome _____

8. fibrocystic breast disease _____

9. ovarian cancer _____

10. breast cancer _____

11. cervical cancer _____

12. endometrial cancer _____

EXERCISE 11

Write the term for each of the following.

1. abnormal opening between the bladder and the vagina _____
_____

2. benign tumor of the uterine muscle _____ _____

3. inflammation of the female pelvic organs _____
_____ _____

4. downward displacement of the uterus in the vagina _____
_____

5. endometrial tissue in the pelvic cavity _____

6. growth of endometrium into the muscular portion of the uterus
_____

7. affects menstruating women using tampons _____

_____ _____

8. one or more benign cysts in the breast _____

_____ _____

9. a malignant tumor of the breast _____ _____

10. also called uterine cancer _____ _____

11. malignant tumor of the ovaries _____ _____

12. malignant tumor of the cervix _____ _____

EXERCISE 12

Spell the disease and disorder terms. Have someone dictate the terms on pp. 246-247 to you. Study any words you have spelled incorrectly.

1. _____	7. _____
2. _____	8. _____
3. _____	9. _____
4. _____	10. _____
5. _____	11. _____
6. _____	12. _____

Surgical Terms

Built from Word Parts

Term	Definition
cervicectomy................................ (*ser*-vi-SEK-tō-mē)	excision of the cervix
colpoperineorrhaphy..................... (*kōl*-pō-*păr*-i-nē-OR-a-fē)	suture of the vagina and perineum (performed to mend perineal vaginal tears)
colpoplasty.................................... (KOL-pō-*plas*-tē)	surgical repair of the vagina
colporrhaphy................................. (*kōl*-POR-a-fē)	suture of the vagina (wall of the vagina)
episioperineoplasty....................... (e-*piz*-ē-ō-*păr*-i-nē-o-PLAST-ē)	surgical repair of the vulva and perineum
episiorrhaphy................................ (e-*piz*-ē-OR-a-fē)	suture of (a tear in) the vulva
hymenectomy................................ (*hī*-men-EK-tō-mē)	excision of the hymen
hymenotomy.................................. (*hī*-men-OT-ō-mē)	incision of the hymen

hysterectomy .... (*his*-te-REK-tō-mē)	excision of the uterus (see Exercise Figure F)
hysteropexy .... (HIS-ter-ō-*pek*-sē)	surgical fixation of the uterus
hysterosalpingo-oophorectomy ...... (*his*-ter-ō-sal-*ping*-gō-ō-*of*-ō-REK-tō-mē)	excision of the uterus, fallopian tubes, and ovaries (Exercise Figure F)
mammoplasty .... (MAM-ō-*plas*-tē)	surgical repair of the breast (performed to enlarge or reduce in size, to lift, or to reconstruct after removal of a tumor)
mammotome .... (MAM-ō-tōm)	instrument used to cut breast (tissue)
mastectomy .... (mas-TEK-tō-mē)	surgical removal of a breast
oophorectomy .... (ō-of-ō-REK-tō-mē)	excision of an ovary
perineorrhaphy .... (*păr*-i-nē-OR-a-fē)	suture of (a tear in) the perineum
salpingectomy .... (*sal*-pin-JEK-tō-mē)	excision of a fallopian tube
salpingostomy .... (*sal*-ping-GOS-tō-mē)	creation of an artificial opening in a fallopian tube (performed to restore patency)
salpingo-oophorectomy .... (sal-ping-gō-o-*of*-ō-REK-tō-mē)	excision of the fallopian tube and ovary (see Exercise Figure F)
trachelectomy .... (*trā*-ke-LEK-tō-mē)	excision of the cervix
trachelorrhaphy .... (trā-ke-LOR-a-fē)	suture of the cervix
vulvectomy .... (vul-VEK-tō-mē)	excision of the vulva

---

Types of Hysterectomies

Subtotal hysterectomy—excision of the uterus, excluding cervix; rarely performed

Total hysterectomy—excision of the uterus (abdominal, vaginal, or laparoscopic)

Panhysterectomy—excision of the uterus, ovaries, and fallopian tubes (abdominal)

Radical hysterectomy—excision of the uterus, ovaries, fallopian tubes, lymph nodes, upper portion of the vagina, and the surrounding tissues (abdominal)

Laparoscopic-assisted vaginal hysterectomy—vaginal excision of the uterus and the use of the laparoscope to view the abdominalpelvic cavity to perform the procedure and to use the laparoscopic instruments to sever the ligaments that hold the uterus in place to determine the presence of disease

---

CAM TERM

Massage therapy is the manual manipulation of soft tissue incorporating stroking, kneading, and percussion motions. Massage therapy may benefit the patient by reducing lymphedema resulting from breast cancer treatments.

Types of Surgery Performed to Treat Malignant Breast Tumors

Radical mastectomy—removal of breast tissue, nipple, underlying muscle, and lymph nodes; also called *Halsted mastectomy* (seldom used)

Modified radical mastectomy—removal of breast tissue, nipple, and lymph nodes

Simple mastectomy—removal of breast tissue and usually the nipple; referred to as a *total mastectomy*

Subcutaneous mastectomy—removal of breast tissue, preserving the overlying skin, nipple, and areola, so that the breast may be reconstructed

Lumpectomy—removal of the cancerous lesion only; also called *tylectomy*

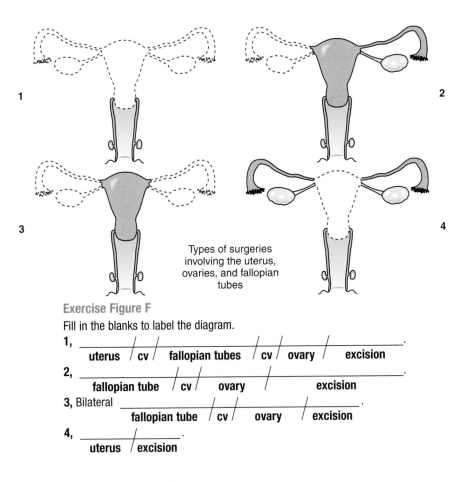

Types of surgeries
involving the uterus,
ovaries, and fallopian
tubes

Exercise Figure F

Fill in the blanks to label the diagram.

1, _____ / _____ / _____ / _____ .
   uterus / cv / fallopian tubes / cv / ovary / excision

2, _____ / _____ / _____ .
   fallopian tube / cv / ovary / excision

3, Bilateral _____ / _____ / _____ .
   fallopian tube / cv / ovary / excision

4, _____ / _____ .
   uterus / excision

Practice saying each of these terms aloud. To hear the terms, access the **PRONOUNCE IT** activity for this chapter on the Student CD that accompanies this text. Or, to hear the terms and their definitions with a CD player or computer, obtain the Pronunciation CD designed for use with this text.

Learn the definitions and spellings of the surgical terms by completing exercises 13, 14, and 15.

EXERCISE 13

Analyze and define the following surgical terms.

1. colporrhaphy _____

2. colpoplasty _____

3. episiorrhaphy _____

4. hymenotomy _____

5. hysteropexy _____

6. vulvectomy _____

7. perineorrhaphy _____

8. salpingostomy _____

9. salpingo-oophorectomy _____

10. oophorectomy _____

11. mastectomy _____

12. salpingectomy _____

13. cervicectomy _____

14. colpoperineorrhaphy _____

15. episioperineoplasty _____

16. hymenectomy _____

17. hysterosalpingo-oophorectomy _____

18. hysterectomy _____

19. mammoplasty _____

20. mammotome _____

21. trachelorrhaphy _____

22. trachelectomy _____

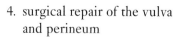 **EXERCISE 14**

Build surgical terms for the following definitions by using the word parts you have learned.

1. suture of the vagina

2. excision of the cervix

3. suture of the vulva

4. surgical repair of the vulva and perineum

5. surgical repair of the vagina

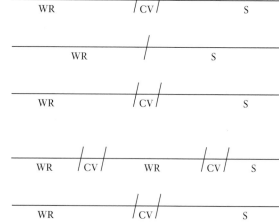

6. suture of the vagina and
   perineum

   ___/ /___/ /_____/ /___/ /_____
   WR   CV   WR   CV   S

7. excision of the uterus,
   ovaries, and fallopian tubes

   ___/ /___/ /___WR___/ /___/ /___WR___/ /___
   WR   CV   WR   CV   WR   S

8. surgical fixation of the
   uterus

   _____/ /___/ /_____
   WR   CV   S

9. excision of the hymen

   _____/ /_____
        WR   /   S

10. incision of the hymen

    _____/ /___/ /_____
         WR   CV   S

11. excision of the uterus

    _____/ /_____
         WR   /   S

12. excision of the ovary

    _____/ /_____
         WR   /   S

13. surgical removal of a breast

    _____/ /_____
         WR   /   S

14. excision of a fallopian tube

    _____/ /_____
         WR   /   S

15. suture of the perineum

    _____/ /___/ /_____
         WR   CV   S

16. excision of the fallopian
    tube and ovary

    _____/ /___/ /___WR___/ /_____
        WR   CV   WR   S

17. creation of an artificial
    opening in the fallopian tube

    _____/ /___/ /_____
         WR   CV   S

18. excision of the vulva

    _____/ /_____
         WR   /   S

19. surgical repair of the breast

    _____/ /___/ /_____
         WR   CV   S

20. instrument used to cut
    breast (tissue)

    _____/ /___/ /_____
         WR   CV   S

21. suture of the cervix

    _____/ /___/ /_____
         WR   CV   S

22. excision of the cervix

    _____/ /_____
         WR   /   S

EXERCISE **15**

Spell each of the surgical terms. Have someone dictate the terms on pp. 249-250 to you. Think about the word parts before attempting to write the word. Study any words you have spelled incorrectly.

1. _____   12. _____

2. _____   13. _____

3. _____   14. _____

4. _____   15. _____

5. _____   16. _____

6. _____   17. _____

7. _____   18. _____

8. _____   19. _____

9. _____   20. _____

10. _____   21. _____

11. _____   22. _____

Surgical Terms

Not Built from Word Parts

Term	Definition
anterior and posterior colporrhaphy (A&P repair) (kōl-POR-a-fē)	when a weakened vaginal wall results in a cystocele (protrusion of the bladder against the anterior wall of the vagina) and a rectocele (protrusion of the rectum against the posterior wall of the vagina), an A&P repair corrects the condition (Exercise Figure G)
conization (kō-ni-ZA-shun)	the surgical removal of a cone-shaped area of the cervix. Used in the treatment for noninvasive cervical cancer.
cryosurgery (krī-ō-SER-jer-ē)	the destruction of tissue by using extreme cold. Used in the treatment of early stages of cervical cancer.
dilation and curettage (D&C) (dī-LA-shun) (kū-re-TAHZH)	dilation (widening) of the cervix and scraping of the endometrium with an instrument called a *curette*. It is performed to diagnose disease, to correct bleeding, and to empty uterine contents (Figure 8-8).

Dilation or Dilatation
are both used in the presentation of dilation and curettage. Dilation is the more common usage and is used in this text.

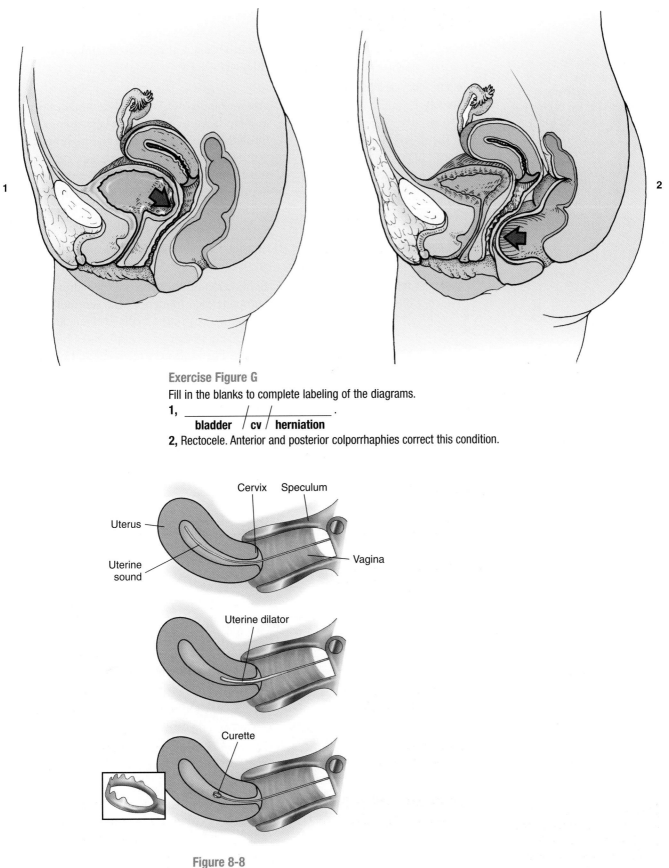

Exercise Figure G

Fill in the blanks to complete labeling of the diagrams.

1, _____ .
　　　bladder / cv / herniation

2, Rectocele. Anterior and posterior colporrhaphies correct this condition.

Uterus

Cervix   Speculum

Uterine sound

Vagina

Uterine dilator

Curette

Figure 8-8
Dilation and curettage.

Ablation

is from the Latin **ablatum**, meaning **to carry away**. In surgery **ablation** means **removal** or **excision**, especially by cutting with laser or electrical energy.

endometrial ablation ....
(en-dō-MĒ-trē-al)
(ab-LA-shun)

a procedure to destroy or remove the endometrium by use of laser or thermal energy. Used to treat abnormal uterine bleeding (Figure 8-9).

laparoscopy or laparoscopic surgery ....
(*lap*-a-ROS-kō-pē)
(lap-a-RŌ-skop-ic)

visual examination of the abdominal cavity, accomplished by inserting a laparoscope through a tiny incision near the umbilicus. It is used for surgical procedures such as tubal sterilization (blocking of the fallopian tubes), hysterectomy, oophorectomy, or biopsy of the ovaries. It may also be used to diagnose endometriosis (Figure 8-10).

myomectomy ....
(mī-ō-MEK-tō-mē)

excision of a fibroid tumor (myoma) from the uterus

sentinel lymph node biopsy ....
(sen-TIN-el) (nōd) (bī-op-sē)

an injection of blue dye and/or radioactive isotope is used to identify the sentinel lymph nodes, the first in the axillary chain, and most likely to contain metastasis of breast cancer. The nodes are removed and microscopically examined. If negative no more nodes are removed. (Figure 8-11).

stereotactic breast biopsy ....
(ster-ē-ō-TAC-tic)

a technique that combines mammography and computer-assisted biopsy to obtain tissue from a breast lesion (Figure 8-12)

tubal ligation ....
(lī-GĀ-shun)

closure of the fallopian tubes for sterilization

Sentinel lymph node biopsy was first developed for patients with melanoma. It is now used to determine metastasis of breast cancer to the lymph nodes. Previously, surgeons would remove 10 to 20 lymph nodes to determine the spread of cancer, often causing lymphedema, which can lead to painful and permanent swelling of the arm. With sentinel lymph node biopsy, if negative, no more lymph nodes are removed.

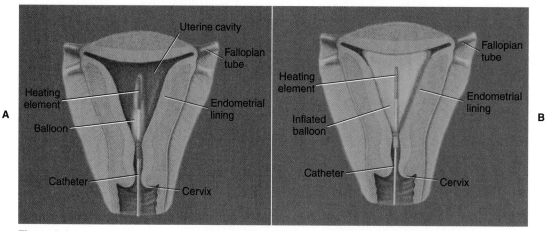

Figure 8-9
Thermal endometrial ablation. **A,** The balloon catheter (deflated) is inserted through the cervix into the uterine cavity. **B,** The balloon is inflated with a solution of 5% dextrose and water and heated to 87° C for 8 minutes, ablating the endometrial lining.

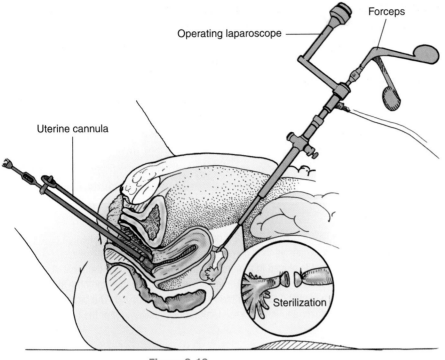

Figure 8-10
Laparoscopic tubal sterilization.

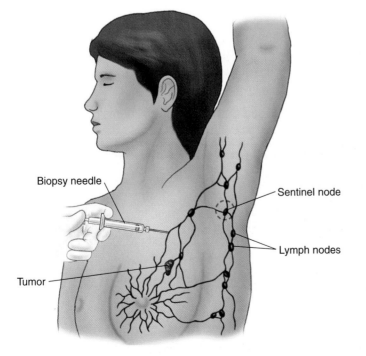

Figure 8-11
Sentinel lymph node biopsy.

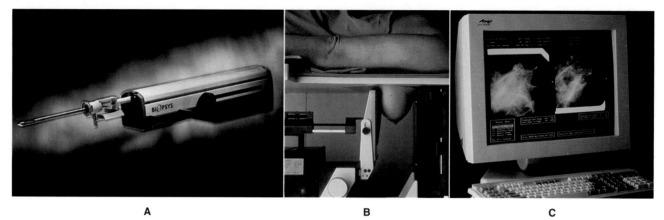

A   **B**   **C**

Figure 8-12
Stereotactic breast biopsy is the least invasive method of obtaining tissue to determine if a nonpalpable breast lesion is benign or malignant. Less pain and scarring and shorter recovery time occur, and it is less expensive than conventional surgery. The patient is placed prone on a special table with the breast suspended through an opening. The breast is placed in a mammography machine under the table. A digital mammogram is produced on a computer monitor to identify the exact location of the lesion. The machine guides the mammotome in obtaining tissue from the lesion to be used for examination. **A,** The mammotome is used to obtain the specimen for biopsy. **B,** The patient is positioned for stereotactic breast biopsy. **C,** The mammogram is placed on a digitizer and is then used to determine placement of the biopsy needle.

Uterine Artery Embolization (UAE) Procedure
Uterine artery embolization, also known as **uterine fibroid embolization,** is a relatively new, minimally invasive procedure used to treat fibroids of the uterus by blocking arteries that supply blood to the fibroids. First an arteriogram is used to identify the vessels. Once identified, tiny gelatin beads, about the size of grains of sand, are inserted into the vessels to create a blockage. The blockage stops the blood supply to the fibroids, causing them to shrink in size.
UAE provides an alternative to hysterectomy as a treatment for fibroid tumors. A hysterectomy is a major surgery involving general anesthesia and has considerably more recovery time. UAE is performed with local anesthesia and is often done on an outpatient basis.

Practice saying each of these terms aloud. To hear the terms, access the **PRONOUNCE IT** activity for this chapter on the Student CD that accompanies this text. Or, to hear the terms and their definitions with a CD player or computer, obtain the Pronunciation CD designed for use with this text.

Learn the definitions and spellings of the surgical terms by completing exercises 16, 17, and 18.

EXERCISE 16

Fill in the blanks with the correct term.

1. Two procedures used for sterilization of the woman are _____ and
   _____ _____ .

2. The surgery used to repair a cystocele and rectocele is a(n) _____
   and _____ _____.

3. D&C is the abbreviation for _____ and _____.

4. _____ _____ _____ is a technique used to
   obtain tissue from a breast lesion.

5. Excision of a fibroid tumor from the uterus is called _____.

6. A procedure to destroy endometrium by laser or thermal energy is called
   _____ _____.

7. The use of extreme cold to destroy tissue is called _____.

8. Surgical removal of a cone-shaped area of the cervix is called
   _____.

9. A procedure to identify metastasis of breast cancer in the axillary lymph nodes
   for biopsy is called _____ _____ _____
   _____.

EXERCISE 17

Match the surgical procedures in the first column with the corresponding organs in the second column. You may use the answers in the second column more than once.

_____ 1. dilation and curettage

_____ 2. laparoscopic surgery
         for sterilization

_____ 3. tubal ligation

_____ 4. anterior and posterior
         colporrhaphy repair

_____ 5. myomectomy

_____ 6. stereotactic breast biopsy

_____ 7. conization

_____ 8. endometrial ablation

_____ 9. sentinel lymph node
         biopsy

_____ 10. cryosurgery

a. fallopian tubes

b. vagina

c. uterus

d. ovaries

e. vulva

f. mammary glands

g. lymph nodes

EXERCISE 18

Spell each of the surgical terms. Have someone dictate the terms on pp. 254 and 256 to you. Study any words you have spelled incorrectly.

1. _____

2. _____

3. _____

4. _____

5. _____

6. _____

7. _____

8. _____

9. _____

10. _____

Diagnostic Terms

Built from Word Parts

Term	Definition
Diagnostic Imaging	
hysterosalpingogram (*his*-ter-ō-*sal*-PING-gō-gram)	x-ray image of the uterus and fallopian tubes (after an injection of a contrast agent) (Exercise Figure H)
mammogram (MAM-ō-gram)	x-ray image of the breast (Figure 8-13)
mammography (ma-MOG-ra-fē)	x-ray imaging of the breast (see Figure 8-10)
sonohysterography (son-ō-hyst-er-OG-ra-fē)	process of recording the uterus by use of sound (an ultrasound procedure)

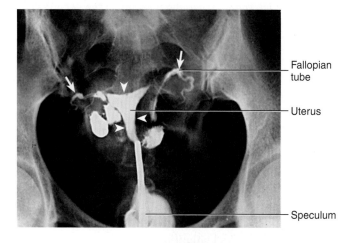

Fallopian tube

Uterus

Speculum

Exercise Figure H

Fill in the blanks to complete labeling of the diagram.

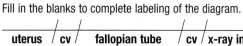

_____ / ___ / _____ / ___ / _____ reveals
uterus / cv / fallopian tube / cv / x-ray image

hydrosalpinx of the fallopian tubes. Liquid contrast material is injected through the vagina and used to outline the uterus and fallopian tubes before the x-ray image is made. This procedure is usually performed to determine whether an obstruction exists in the fallopian tubes that may cause sterility.

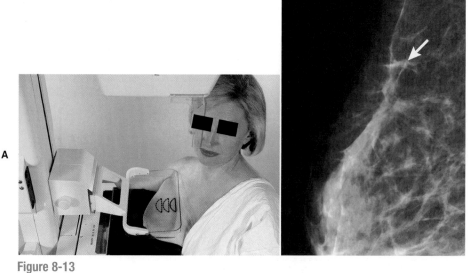

A

B

Figure 8-13

A, Mammography. **B,** Mammogram. *Arrow* points to a lesion confirmed by biopsy to be infiltrating ductal carcinoma.

Endoscopy

colposcope .... instrument used for visual examination of
(KOL-pō-skōp)   the vagina (and cervix)

colposcopy .... visual examination (with a magnified view)
(kol-POS-kō-pē)   of the vagina (and cervix)

culdoscope .... instrument used for visual examination of
(KUL-dō-skōp)   Douglas cul-de-sac (rectouterine pouch)

culdoscopy .... visual examination of Douglas cul-de-sac
(kul-DOS-kō-pē)   (Exercise Figure I)

hysteroscope .... instrument used for visual examination of
(HIS-ter-ō-skōp)   the uterus (uterine cavity)

hysteroscopy .... visual examination of the uterus (uterine
(*his*-ter-OS-kō-pē)   cavity)

Other

culdocentesis .... surgical puncture to remove fluid from
(*kul*-dō-sen-TĒ-sis)   Douglas cul-de-sac (see Exercise Figure I)

> **Endoscopy**
> dates back to the time of
> Hippocrates (460-375 BC), who
> mentions using a speculum to
> look into a rectum to see where it
> was affected. By the end of the
> nineteenth century, **cystoscopy,
> proctoscopy, laryngoscopy,** and
> **esophagoscopy** were well estab-
> lished. Use of the **endoscope** for
> surgery was not widely practiced
> in the United States until the
> 1970s when gynecologists started
> performing **laparoscopic tubal
> sterilization.** The first ectopic
> pregnancy was removed by
> laparoscopic surgery in 1973,
> the first **laparoscopic appendec-
> tomy** occurred in 1983, and the
> first laparoscopic **cholecystec-
> tomy** in 1989.

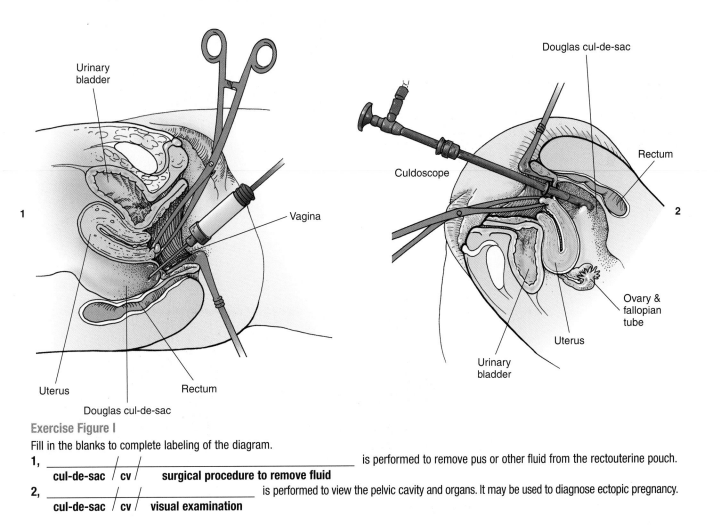

Exercise Figure I

Fill in the blanks to complete labeling of the diagram.

1, _____ / ___ / _____ is performed to remove pus or other fluid from the rectouterine pouch.
   cul-de-sac / cv / surgical procedure to remove fluid

2, _____ / ___ / _____ is performed to view the pelvic cavity and organs. It may be used to diagnose ectopic pregnancy.
   cul-de-sac / cv / visual examination

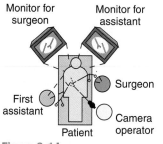

Monitor for surgeon

Monitor for assistant

First assistant

Surgeon

Camera operator

Patient

Figure 8-14

Operative setup for laparoscopic hysterectomy.

Sonohysterography is a technique for evaluating the uterine cavity. Saline solution is injected into the uterine cavity, followed by transvaginal sonography. It is used preoperatively to assess polyps, myomas, and adhesions.

Practice saying each of these words aloud. To hear the terms, access the **PRONOUNCE IT** activity for this chapter on the Student CD that accompanies this text. Or, to hear the terms and their definitions with a CD player or computer, obtain the Pronunciation CD designed for use with this text.

Learn the definitions and spellings of the procedural terms by completing exercises 19, 20, and 21.

Endoscopic Surgery

Endoscopic surgery includes the use of a slender, flexible fiberoptic endoscope that is inserted into a natural body cavity, such as the mouth, or other body areas through a small incision. Three or four other tiny incisions may be made to accommodate visualization equipment that projects the patient's internal organs and structures onto a television screen and to accommodate other instruments and devices needed to complete the surgery (Figure 8-14).

Because the surgeon performs endoscopic surgery, sometimes referred to as *videoscopic surgery,* by viewing a television screen, the surgeon must master a new set of skills. Although it is thought that endoscopic surgery will not replace large-incision surgery, its use is in demand because of the reduced trauma and medical cost to the patient. Continued advances in technology will improve and expand its use.

Types of Endoscopic Surgery

Instrument	Procedure	Type of Surgery
arthroscope	arthroscopy or arthroscopic surgery	biopsy ligament repair meniscus repair synovectomy
colonoscope	colonoscopy	polypectomy
hysteroscope	hysteroscopy	myomectomy polypectomy
laparoscope	laparoscopy or laparoscopic surgery	adhesiolysis appendectomy cholecystectomy herniorrhaphy hysterectomy myomectomy oophorectomy ovarian biopsy ovarian cystectomy prostatectomy splenectomy tubal sterilization
thoracoscope	thoracoscopy	biopsy wedge resection of the lung

EXERCISE 19

Analyze and define the following diagnostic terms.

1. colposcopy _____

2. mammogram _____

3. colposcope _____

4. hysteroscopy _____

5. hysterosalpingogram _____

6. culdoscope _____

7. culdoscopy _____

8. culdocentesis _____

9. mammography _____

10. hysteroscope _____

11. sonohysterography _____

EXERCISE   20

Build diagnostic terms that correspond to the following definitions by using the word parts you have learned.

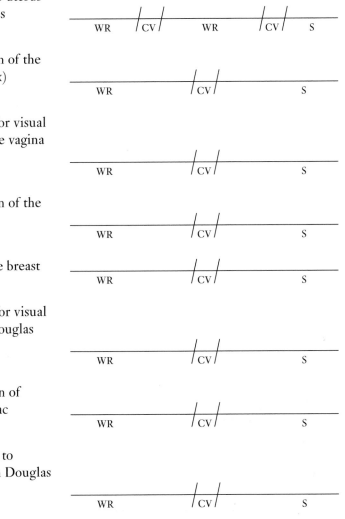

1. x-ray image of the uterus
   and fallopian tubes

   _____ / ___ / _____ / ___ / ___
   WR   CV   WR   CV   S

2. visual examination of the
   vagina (and cervix)

   _____ / ___ / ___
   WR   CV   S

3. instrument used for visual
   examination of the vagina
   (and cervix)

   _____ / ___ / ___
   WR   CV   S

4. visual examination of the
   uterus

   _____ / ___ / ___
   WR   CV   S

5. x-ray image of the breast

   _____ / ___ / ___
   WR   CV   S

6. instrument used for visual
   examination of Douglas
   cul-de-sac

   _____ / ___ / ___
   WR   CV   S

7. visual examination of
   Douglas cul-de-sac

   _____ / ___ / ___
   WR   CV   S

8. surgical puncture to
   remove fluid from Douglas
   cul-de-sac

   _____ / ___ / ___
   WR   CV   S

9. instrument used for visual
   examination of the uterus

   _____ /___/ _____
   WR   CV   S

10. x-ray imaging of the breast

   _____ /___/ _____
   WR   CV   S

11. process of recording the
    uterus with sound

   _____ /___/ _____ /___/ _____
   WR   CV   WR   CV   S

EXERCISE 21

Spell each of the diagnostic terms. Have someone dictate the terms on pp. 260-261 to you. Think about the word parts before attempting to write the word. Study any words you have spelled incorrectly.

1. _____   7. _____

2. _____   8. _____

3. _____   9. _____

4. _____   10. _____

5. _____   11. _____

6. _____

Diagnostic Terms

Not Built from Word Parts

Term	Definition
Laboratory	
CA-125 (cancer antigen-125 tumor marker)	a blood test used in the detection of ovarian cancer. It is also used to monitor treatment and to determine the extent of the disease.
Pap smear	a cytological study of cervical and vaginal secretions used to determine the presence of abnormal or cancerous cells. Most commonly used to detect cancers of the cervix (also called *Papanicolaou* [pap-a-nik-kō-LA-oo] *smear* and *Pap test)* (Figure 8-15).
transvaginal sonography (TVS) (trans-VAJ-i-nal) (so-NOG-ra-fē)	an ultrasound procedure that uses a transducer placed in the vagina to obtain images of the ovaries, uterus, cervix, fallopian tubes, and surrounding structures. Used to diagnose masses such as ovarian cysts or tumors, to monitor pregnancy, and to evaluate ovulation for the treatment of infertility (Figure 8-16).

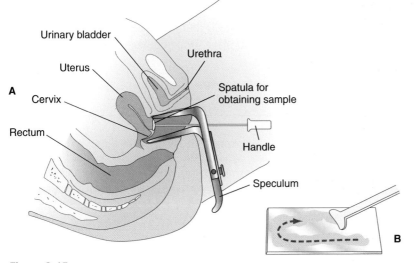

Figure 8-15

Pap smear. **A,** Obtaining the specimen. **B,** Transferring the specimen to a glass slide where it will be stained and studied under a microscope in the laboratory.

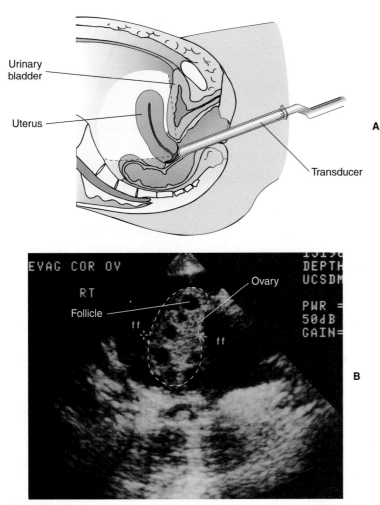

Figure 8-16

Transvaginal sonography. **A,** Transducer placed in the vagina. **B,** Transvaginal sagittal image of the right ovary with multiple follicles, showing free fluid surrounding the ovary.

Practice saying each of the words aloud. To hear the terms, access the **PRONOUNCE IT** activity for this chapter on the Student CD that accompanies this text. Or, to hear the terms and their definitions with a CD player or computer, obtain the Pronunciation CD designed for use with this text.

Learn the definitions and spelling to diagnostic terms by completing exercises 22, 23, and 24.

Pap smear is named after Dr George N. Papanicolaou (1883-1962), a Greek physician practicing in the United States, who developed the cell smear method for the diagnosis of cancer in 1943. The test may be used for tissue specimen from any organ but is most commonly used on cervical and vaginal secretions. The Pap smear is 95% accurate in detecting cervical carcinoma. In 1966 a liquid-based screening system was approved by the Food and Drug Administration as an alternative for the conventional Pap smear. This system improves detection of squamous intraepithelial lesions.

EXERCISE 22

Fill in the blanks with the correct definition.

1. Pap smear _____

2. transvaginal sonography _____

3. CA-125 _____

EXERCISE 23

Write the term for each of the following.

1. study of cervical and vaginal secretions _____   _____

2. blood test used to detect ovarian cancer _____

3. obtains images of the ovaries, uterus, cervix, uterine tubes, and surrounding structures _____   _____

EXERCISE 24

Spell each of the diagnostic terms. Have someone dictate the terms on p. 264 to you. Think about the word parts before attempting to write the word. Study any words you have spelled incorrectly.

1. _____   3. _____

2. _____

Complementary Terms
Built from Word Parts

Term	Definition
gynecologist......................... (gīn-e-KOL-ō-jist)	a physician who studies and treats diseases of women (female reproductive system)

gynecology (GYN)............ (gīn-e-KOL-ō-jē)	study of women (a branch of medicine dealing with diseases of the female reproductive system)
gynopathic.................... (gīn-ō-PATH-ik)	pertaining to disease of women
leukorrhea.................... (lū-kō-RĒ-a)	white discharge (from the vagina)
mastalgia.................... (mas-TAL-jē-a)	pain in the breast
mastoptosis.................... (mas-tō-TŌ-sis)	sagging breast
menarche.................... (me-NAR-kē)	beginning of menstruation (occurring between the ages of 11 and 16)
oligomenorrhea............ (ol-i-gō-men-ō-RĒ-a)	scanty menstrual flow
vaginal.................... (VAJ-i-nal)	pertaining to the vagina
vulvovaginal.................... (vul-vō-VAJ-i-nal)	pertaining to the vulva and vagina

Practice saying each of these terms aloud. To hear the terms, access the **PRONOUNCE IT** activity for this chapter on the Student CD that accompanies this text. Or, to hear the terms and their definitions with a CD player or computer, obtain the Pronunciation CD designed for use with this text.

Exercises 25, 26, and 27 will help you learn the definitions and spellings of the complementary terms related to the female reproductive system.

EXERCISE 25

Analyze and define the following complementary terms.

1. gynecologist _____

2. gynecology _____

3. vulvovaginal _____

4. mastalgia _____

5. menarche _____

6. leukorrhea _____

7. oligomenorrhea _____

8. gynopathic _____

9. mastoptosis _____

10. vaginal _____

EXERCISE **26**

Build complementary terms that correspond to the following definitions by using the word parts you have learned.

1. scanty menstrual flow

       WR   CV   WR   CV   S

2. white discharge (from the vagina)

       WR   CV   S

3. beginning of menstruation

       WR   WR

4. pain in the breast

       WR   S

5. pertaining to the vulva and vagina

       WR   CV   WR   S

6. a physician who studies and treats (diseases of) women

       WR   CV   S

7. study of women (branch of medicine dealing with diseases of the female reproductive system)

       WR   CV   S

8. sagging breast

       WR   CV   S

9. pertaining to disease of women

       WR   CV   WR   S

10. pertaining to the vagina

       WR   S

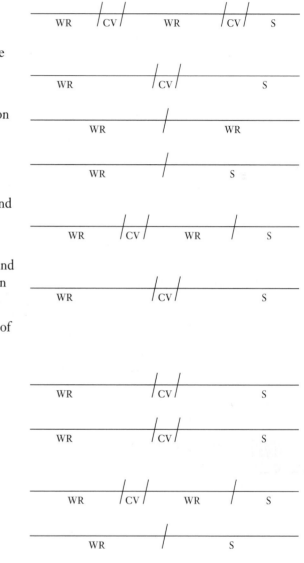

EXERCISE **27**

Spell each of the complementary terms. Have someone dictate the terms on pp. 266-267 to you. Think about the word parts before attempting to write the word. Study any words you have spelled incorrectly.

1. _____   6. _____

2. _____   7. _____

3. _____   8. _____

4. _____   9. _____

5. _____   10. _____

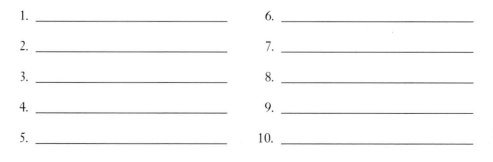

Complementary Terms

Not Built from Word Parts

Term	Definition
dyspareunia .... (*dis*-pa-RŪ-nē-a)	difficult or painful intercourse
estrogen replacement therapy (ERT) .... (ES-trō-jen)	replacement of hormones to treat menopause (also called *hormone replacement therapy* [HRT])
fistula .... (FIS-tū-la)	abnormal passageway between two organs or between an internal organ and the body surface
menopause .... (MEN-o-pawz)	cessation of menstruation, usually around the ages of 48 to 53 years
premenstrual syndrome (PMS) .... (prē-MEN-stroo-al) (SIN-drŏm)	a syndrome involving physical and emotional symptoms occurring in the 10 days before menstruation. Symptoms include nervous tension, irritability, mastalgia, edema, and headache. Its cause is not fully understood.
speculum .... (SPEK-ū-lum)	instrument for opening a body cavity to allow visual inspection (Figure 8-17)

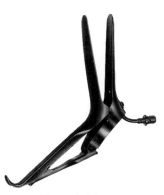

Figure 8-17
Vaginal speculum.

Practice saying each of these terms aloud. To hear the terms, access the **PRONOUNCE IT** activity for this chapter on the Student CD that accompanies this text. Or, to hear the terms and their definitions with a CD player or computer, obtain the Pronunciation CD designed for use with this text.

Learn the definitions and spellings of the complementary terms by completing exercises 28, 29, and 30.

EXERCISE   28

Write the definitions of the following terms.

1. menopause _____

2. dyspareunia _____

3. fistula _____

4. premenstrual syndrome _____

5. speculum _____

6. estrogen replacement therapy_____

EXERCISE   29

Write the term for each of the following.

1. abnormal passageway   _____

2. painful intercourse   _____

3. cessation of menstruation   _____

4. syndrome involving physical and emotional symptoms   _____ _____

5. instrument for opening a body cavity   _____

6. hormone replacement   _____ _____ _____

EXERCISE 30

Spell each of the complementary terms. Have someone dictate the terms on p. 269 to you. Study any words you have spelled incorrectly.

1. _____   4. _____

2. _____   5. _____

3. _____   6. _____

Abbreviations

A&P repair	anterior and posterior colporrhaphy
Cx	cervix
D&C	dilation and curettage
ERT	estrogen replacement therapy
FBD	fibrocystic breast disease
GYN	gynecology
PID	pelvic inflammatory disease
PMS	premenstrual syndrome
SHG	sonohysterogram
TAH/BSO	total abdominal hysterectomy/bilateral salpingo-oophorectomy
TSS	toxic shock syndrome
TVH	total vaginal hysterectomy
TVS	transvaginal sonography

EXERCISE 31

Write the meaning for each of the abbreviations in the following sentences.

1. To repair a cystocele and rectocele the patient is scheduled in surgery for an
   A&P repair _____ & _____ _____.

2. Following a **TAH/BSO** _____ _____
   _____ and _____ _____
   the gynecologist ordered **ERT** _____ _____
   _____ for the patient.

3. **SHG** _____ and **TVS** _____ _____
   are diagnostic ultrasound procedures used to assist in diagnosing diseases and
   disorders of the female reproductive organs.

4. When performing a **TVH** _____ _____
   _____ the surgeon removes the uterus through the vagina without a
   surgical incision into the abdomen.

5. **D&C** _____ & _____ is the dilation of the
   Cx _____ and scraping of the endometrium.

6. **FBD** _____ _____ _____ is the most common breast problem of women in their 20s.

7. A female patient with probable **PID** _____ _____
   _____ was referred to the **GYN** _____ clinic for evaluation and care.

8. The medical management of **PMS** _____ _____ em-
   phasizes the relief of symptoms.

CHAPTER REVIEW

EXERCISE 32 *Interact with Medical Records*

Complete the progress note by writing the medical terms in the blanks. Use the list of definitions with the corresponding numbers. See the next page for a list of medical terms to be used with this exercise.

University Hospital and Medical Center
4700 North Main Street • Wellness, Arizona 54321 • (987) 555-3210

PATIENT NAME: Sandra Garcia   **CASE NUMBER:** 05632-FRS
DATE OF BIRTH: 11/01/xx   **DATE:** 11/14/xx

PROGRESS NOTE

Sandra Garcia is a 48-year-old Puerto Rican woman is here for follow-up after a suspicious mass in the left breast was discovered during routine 1. _____ .

Family history is positive for 2. _____ in a maternal aunt.

Past medical history includes 3. _____ for 4. _____ and 5. _____ . She has been on 6. _____ since age 46 years.

The patient consented to a 7. _____ _____ _____ .

Pathology report is as follows:

GROSS DESCRIPTION: Received labeled "breast biopsy" is an ovoid mass of predominantly adipose breast tissue measuring 4.5 × 3.0 × 1.3 cm. Sectioning reveals a focal area of suspicious 8. _____ . Frozen section reveals fat 9. _____ and evidence of malignancy in an area measuring 0.25 cm in the center of the specimen. The surgeon is so informed.

MICROSCOPIC DESCRIPTION: Microscopic examination of the frozen section specimen confirms the presence of fat necrosis. There is focal duct epithelial 10. _____ exhibiting a papillomatous pattern. A well-differentiated adenocarcinoma was found in this area. Occasional breast parenchymal fragments are also identified and show fibrocystic changes. These are predominantly nonproliferative, although in slide D, a small radial scar containing ducts showing proliferative fibrocystic changes with significant atypia and adjacent sclerosis adenosis is identified.

DIAGNOSIS: Left breast biopsy:
1. Radial scar.
2. Nonproliferative and proliferative fibrocystic changes with significant atypia.
3. Papillary ductal carcinoma, well differentiated.
4. Focal sclerosing adenosis.

Marcus Weldon, MD

MW/mcm

1. x-ray imaging of the breast
2. cancerous tumor
3. excision of the uterus
4. growth of endometrium into the muscular portion of the uterus
5. abdominal condition in which endometrial tissue occurs in various areas of the pelvic cavity
6. abbreviation for replacement of hormones to treat menopause
7. combines mammography and computer-assisted biopsy to obtain tissue from a breast lesion
8. abnormal hard spot
9. abnormal condition of death (dead tissue because of disease)
10. excessive development (of cells)

EXERCISE 33 *Interpret Medical Terms*

To test your understanding of the terms introduced in this chapter, circle the words that correctly complete the sentences. The italicized words refer to the correct answer.

1. The patient was diagnosed as having *painful menstruation*, or (oligomenorrhea, dysmenorrhea, amenorrhea).
2. *Inflammation of the inner lining of the uterus* is (endocervicitis, endometritis, endometriosis).
3. The patient is scheduled in surgery for a *salpingectomy,* which is the *excision* of the (fallopian tube, ovary, uterus).
4. An *episiorrhaphy* is a (suture of the vulva, discharge from the vulva, rapid discharge from the vulva).
5. A surgical procedure to *reduce breast size* is called reduction (mammogram, mammography, mammoplasty).
6. A *hysterosalpingo-oophorectomy* is the excision of the (uterus, fallopian tubes, and ovaries; uterus, ovaries, and cervix; uterus, fallopian tubes, and vagina).
7. *Blood in the fallopian tube* is called (hematosalpinx, hydrosalpinx, pyosalpinx).
8. *Endometrial tissue occurring in various areas of the pelvic cavity* is called (adenomyosis, endometriosis, hysteratresia).
9. The doctor requested a (hysteroscope, colposcope, speculum) *to open the vagina for visual examination.*
10. A severe illness *that may affect menstruating women after using tampons* is (TVS, TSS, TVH).

EXERCISE 34 *Read Medical Terms in Use*

Practice pronunciation of the terms by reading the following information on cancers of the female reproductive system. Use the pronunciation key following the medical terms to assist you in saying the words.

Cancers of the Female Reproductive System
Breast Cancer
The breast is the second most common site of cancer in women. More than 80% of **breast cancer** is infiltrating ductal cancer (IDC), which originates in the mammary ducts. The rate of growth depends on hormonal influences. As long as the cancer remains in the duct, it is considered noninvasive and is called *ductal carcinoma in situ (DCIS)*.

    Mammography (ma-MOG-ra-fē) is the most common method used for diagnosing cancer of the breast. Confirmation is done with a biopsy obtained by conventional surgery or **stereotactic** (ster-ē-ō-TAC-tic) **breast biopsy.** Treatment may include lumpectomy, **mastectomy** (mas-TEK-tō-mē), chemotherapy, and radiation therapy.

Continued

Cancers of the Female Reproductive System—cont'd

Cervical Cancer

In many regions of the world **cervical** (SER-vi-k'l) **cancer** is the leading cause of death in women. Cervical cancer resembles a sexually transmitted disease, a feature that distinguishes it from other cancers. Abnormal **vaginal** (VAJ-i-nal) bleeding is the most common symptom. **Pap smear** followed by **colposcopy** (kōl-POS-kō-pē) biopsy is used to diagnose this disease. Surgical treatment options are **conization** (kō-ni-ZA-shun), **cryosurgery** (krī-ō-SER-jer-ē), laser **ablation** (ab-LA-shun), and **hysterectomy** (his-te-REC-tō-mē). Chemotherapy and radiation therapy may also be used. **Trachelectomy** (trā-kē-LEK-tō-mē) may be performed in patients with small primary tumors who may wish to bear children in the future.

Endometrial Cancer

Currently 75% of women diagnosed with **endometrial** (en-dō-ME-trē-al) **cancer** are postmenopausal. Inappropriate bleeding is the only warning sign; hence early diagnosis is common. Pelvic examination, Pap smear, and endometrial sampling are used to diagnose this disease. Treatment is **hysterosalpingo-oophorectomy** (his-ter-ō-sal-ping-gō-ō-of-ō-REK-tō-mē), which may be followed by chemotherapy and radiation therapy. Laparoscopic-assisted vaginal hysterectomy may also be used.

Ovarian Cancer

Ovarian (ō-VAR-ē-an) **cancer** is the sixth most common form of cancer in women. Early symptoms are often absent or associated with other problems; thus early diagnosis is uncommon. Early symptoms include abdominal discomfort and bloating; later stages include abdominal or pelvic pain and urinary or menstrual irregularities. **CA-125** and **transvaginal** (trans-VAJ-i-nal) **sonography** (so-NOG-ra-fē) are used in diagnosing this disease. Treatment is total abdominal **hysterectomy** and **bilateral salpingo-oophorectomy** (sal-ping-gō-ō-of-ō-REK-tō-mē) and removal of as much additional involved tissue as possible.

Chemotherapy is usually prescribed, followed a year later by a second-look **laparoscopy** (lap-a-ROS-kō-pē) to determine the presence or absence of the tumor.

EXERCISE 35 *Comprehend Medical Terms in Use*

Test your comprehension of the terms in the box above by circling the correct answer.

1. Which of the following diagnostic tests would the physician use to diagnose ovarian cancer?
   a. colposcopy biopsy
   b. transvaginal sonography
   c. Pap smear
   d. mammography
2. T F   Surgery is a treatment option for breast, cervical, endometrial, and ovarian cancer.
3. T F   Excision of the uterus, fallopian tubes, and ovaries is an accepted surgical treatment for both endometrial and ovarian cancer.
4. An instrument for visualization of the vagina is used to obtain a biopsy to confirm the diagnosis of cancer of the:
   a. ovary
   b. breast
   c. uterus
   d. cervix

For further practice or to evaluate what you have learned, use the Student CD that accompanies this text.

COMBINING FORMS CROSSWORD PUZZLE (CHAPTERS 7 AND 8)

Across Clues

1. vagina
2. prostate
5. vulva
8. cervix
9. fallopian tube
11. male
14. epididymis
17. uterus
18. ovary
22. sperm
24. vulva
25. glans penis
26. breast

Down Clues

3. sperm
4. cul-de-sac
6. vessel, duct
7. menstruation
10. perineum
12. woman
13. seminal vesicles
15. testis
16. first, beginning
19. testis, testicle
20. uterus
21. testis

REVIEW OF WORD PARTS

Can you define and spell the following word parts?

Combining Forms

arche/o	men/o
cervic/o	metr/i
colp/o	metr/o
culd/o	oophor/o
episi/o	perine/o
gyn/o	salping/o
gynec/o	trachel/o
hymen/o	uter/o
hyster/o	vagin/o
mamm/o	vulv/o
mast/o	

Prefix

peri-

Suffixes

-atresia
-ial
-salpinx

REVIEW OF TERMS

Can you build, analyze, define, pronounce, and spell the following terms *built from word parts?*

Diseases and Disorders	Surgical	Diagnostic	Complementary
amenorrhea	cervicectomy	colposcope	gynecologist
Bartholin adenitis	colpoperineorrhaphy	colposcopy	gynecology (GYN)
cervicitis	colpoplasty	culdocentesis	gynopathic
colpitis	colporrhaphy	culdoscope	leukorrhea
dysmenorrhea	episioperineoplasty	culdoscopy	mastalgia
endocervicitis	episiorrhaphy	hysterosalpingogram	mastoptosis
endometritis	hymenectomy	hysteroscope	menarche
hematosalpinx	hymenotomy	hysteroscopy	oligomenorrhea
hydrosalpinx	hysterectomy	mammogram	vaginal
hysteratresia	hysteropexy	mammography	vulvovaginal
mastitis	hysterosalpingo-	sonohysterography	
menometrorrhagia	oophorectomy		
metrorrhea	mammoplasty		
myometritis	mammotome		
oophoritis	mastectomy		
perimetritis	oophorectomy		
pyosalpinx	perineorrhaphy		
salpingitis	salpingectomy		
salpingocele	salpingo-oophorectomy		
vaginitis	salpingostomy		
vulvovaginitis	trachelectomy		
	trachelorrhaphy		
	vulvectomy		

Can you define, pronounce, and spell the following terms *not built from word parts?*

Diseases and Disorders	Surgical	Diagnostic	Complementary
adenomyosis	anterior and posterior	CA-125	dyspareunia
breast cancer	colporrhaphy (A&P	Pap smear	estrogen replacement therapy
cervical cancer	repair)	transvaginal sonography	(ERT)
endometrial cancer	conization		fistula
endometriosis	cryosurgery		menopause
fibrocystic breast disease (FBD)	dilation and curettage		premenstrual syndrome (PMS)
fibroid tumor	(D&C)		speculum
ovarian cancer	endometrial ablation		
pelvic inflammatory disease (PID)	laparoscopy		
prolapsed uterus	myomectomy		
toxic shock syndrome (TSS)	sentinel lymph node		
vesicovaginal fistula	biopsy		
	stereotactic breast biopsy		
	tubal ligation		

9

Obstetrics and Neonatology

OUTLINE

OBJECTIVES

On completion of this chapter you will be able to:

1. Identify the organs and other structures relating to pregnancy.
2. Define and spell the word parts presented in this chapter.
3. Build and analyze medical terms with word parts presented in this and previous chapters.
4. Define, pronounce, and spell the disease and disorder, diagnostic, surgical, and complementary terms related to obstetrics and neonatology.
5. Interpret the meanings of the abbreviations presented in this chapter.
6. Read medical documents and interpret medical terminology contained in them.

ANATOMY

Obstetrics is the branch of medicine that deals with childbirth and the care of the mother before, during, and after birth. **Neonatology** is the branch of medicine that deals with the diagnosis and treatment of disorders of the newborn.

Terms Relating to Pregnancy

gamete	mature germ cell, either sperm (male) or ovum (female)
ovulation	expulsion of a mature ovum from an ovary (Figure 9-1)
conception, or fertilization	beginning of pregnancy, when the sperm enters the ovum. Fertilization normally occurs in the fallopian tubes (see Figure 9-1).
zygote	cell formed by the union of the sperm and the ovum
embryo	unborn offspring in the stage of development from implantation of the zygote to the end of the second month of pregnancy. This period is characterized by rapid growth of the embryo.
fetus	unborn offspring from the beginning of the third month of pregnancy until birth (Figure 9-2)
gestation, pregnancy	development of a new individual from conception to birth
gestation period	duration of pregnancy
implantation, nidation	embedding of the zygote in the uterine lining. The process normally begins about 7 days after fertilization and continues for several days (see Figure 9-1).
placenta, or afterbirth	a structure that grows on the wall of the uterus during pregnancy and allows for nourishment of the unborn child (see Figure 9-1)
amniotic, or amnionic, sac (also known as *bag of water*)	membranous bag that surrounds the fetus before delivery (see Figure 9-1)
chorion	outermost layer of the fetal membrane
amnion	innermost layer of the fetal membrane
amniotic fluid	fluid within the amniotic sac, which surrounds the fetus

Learn the anatomic terms by completing exercise 1.

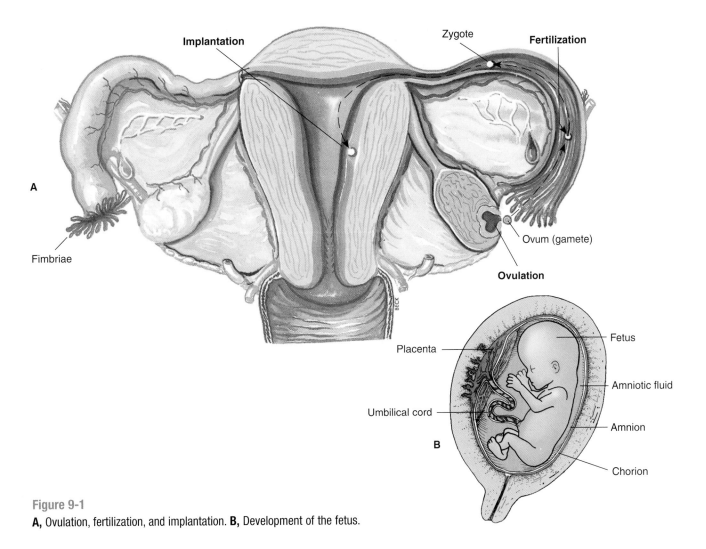

Figure 9-1
A, Ovulation, fertilization, and implantation. **B,** Development of the fetus.

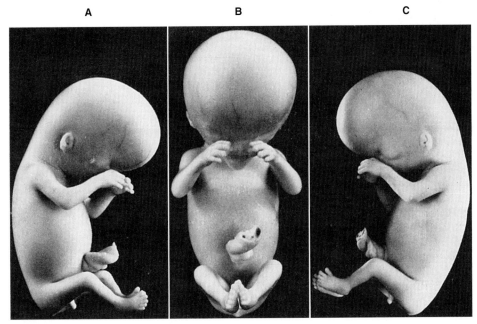

Figure 9-2
Human (male) fetus at 68 days (47 mm). **A,** Right; **B,** front; **C,** left.

EXERCISE   1

Fill in the blanks with the correct terms.

1. The expulsion of a mature ovum, or _____, from an ovary is called _____. When the male gamete enters the female gamete, _____ occurs, and a(n) _____ is formed. This marks the beginning of the _____ period.

2. Once the zygote is implanted, it becomes a(n) _____ until the end of the second month of gestation. The unborn offspring from the beginning of the third month until birth is called a(n) _____.

3. The fetus is surrounded by a(n) _____ sac, which has an outermost layer, called the _____, and an innermost layer, called the _____. This sac contains the _____ fluid that surrounds the fetus.

WORD PARTS

Combining Forms for Obstetrics and Neonatology

Study the word parts and their definitions listed below. Completing the exercises that follow and Exercise Figure A will help you to learn the terms.

Combining Form	Definition
amni/o, amnion/o	amnion, amniotic fluid
chori/o	chorion
embry/o	embryo, to be full (Figure 9-3)
fet/o, fet/i	fetus, unborn child
(NOTE: both *i* and *o* may be used as combining vowels with *fet.*)	

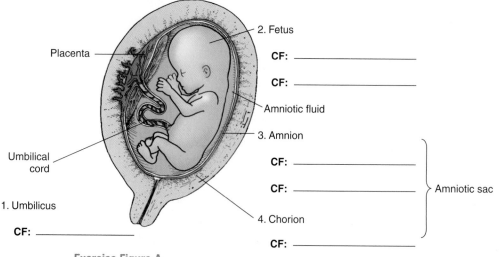

Placenta

Umbilical cord

1. Umbilicus

CF: _____

2. Fetus

CF: _____

CF: _____

Amniotic fluid

3. Amnion

CF: _____

CF: _____

4. Chorion

CF: _____

Amniotic sac

Exercise Figure A

Fill in the blanks with combining forms in this diagram of fetal development.

gravid/o	pregnancy
lact/o	milk
nat/o	birth
omphal/o	umbilicus, navel
par/o, part/o	bear, give birth to; labor, childbirth
puerper/o	childbirth

Learn the anatomic locations and definitions of the combining forms by completing exercises 2 and 3.

> **Puerper**
> is made up of two Latin word roots: **puer**, meaning **child**, and **per**, meaning **through.**

EXERCISE   2

Write the definitions of the following combining forms.

1. fet/o, fet/i _____

2. lact/o _____

3. par/o, part/o _____

4. omphal/o _____

5. amni/o, amnion/o _____

6. puerper/o _____

7. gravid/o _____

8. nat/o _____

9 chori/o _____

10. embry/o _____

EXERCISE   3

Write the combining form for each of the following terms.

1. milk _____

2. fetus _____   _____

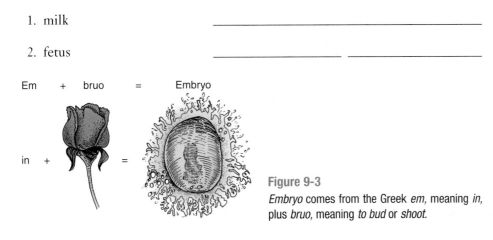

Em   +   bruo   =   Embryo

in   +   =

Figure 9-3
Embryo comes from the Greek *em,* meaning *in,* plus *bruo,* meaning *to bud* or *shoot.*

3. chorion _____

4. amnion, amniotic fluid   a. _____

   b. _____

5. childbirth _____

6. give birth to   a. _____

   b. _____

7. pregnancy _____

8. embryo _____

9. birth _____

10. umbilicus, or navel _____

Combining Forms Commonly Used in Obstetrics and Neonatology

Combining Form	Definition
cephal/o	head
esophag/o	esophagus (tube leading from the throat to the stomach) (see Figure 11-1)
pelv/i, pelv/o (NOTE: both i and o may be used as the combining vowel with pelv.)	pelvic bone, pelvis (see Chapter 14 Exercise Figure A and Exercise Figure B)
prim/i (NOTE: the combining vowel is *i*)	first
pseud/o	false
pylor/o	pylorus (pyloric sphincter) (see Figure 11-2)

Learn the combining forms by completing exercises 4 and 5.

EXERCISE 4

Write the definition of the following combining forms.

1. prim/i _____

2. pylor/o _____

3. cephal/o _____

4. esophag/o _____

5. pseud/o _____

6. pelv/o _____

EXERCISE 5

Write the combining form for each of the following.

1. head   _____

2. pylorus   _____

3. false   _____

4. esophagus   _____

5. first   _____

6. pelvic bone, pelvis   _____, _____

Prefixes

Prefix	Definition
ante-, pre-	before
micro-	small
multi-	many
nulli-	none
post-	after

Learn the prefixes by completing exercises 6 and 7.

EXERCISE 6

Write the definitions of the following prefixes.

1. post- _____

2. multi- _____

3. nulli- _____

4. micro- _____

5. ante- _____

6. pre- _____

EXERCISE 7

Write the prefix for each of the following definitions.

1. none   _____

2. small   _____

3. many _____

4. before a. _____

 b. _____

5. after _____

Suffixes

Suffix	Definition
-amnios	amnion, amniotic fluid
-cyesis	pregnancy
-e	noun suffix, no meaning
-is	noun suffix, no meaning
-partum	childbirth, labor
-rrhexis	rupture
-tocia	birth, labor
-um	noun suffix, no meaning
-us	noun suffix, no meaning

-rrhexis
is the last of the four **-rrh** suffixes to be learned. The other three introduced in earlier chapters are **-rrhea** (excessive flow or discharge), **-rrhagia** (raid flow [of blood]), and **-rrhaphy** (suturing, repair).

Refer to Appendix A and Appendix B for alphabetized word parts and their meanings. Learn the suffixes by completing exercises 8 and 9.

EXERCISE 8

Write the definitions of the following suffixes.

1. -rrhexis _____

2. -tocia _____

3. -cyesis _____

4. -partum _____

5. -amnios _____

EXERCISE 9

Write the suffix for each of the following definitions.

1. birth, labor _____

2. rupture _____

3. childbirth, labor _____

4. pregnancy _____

5. amnion, amniotic fluid _____

MEDICAL TERMS

The terms you need to learn to complete this chapter are listed next. The exercises following each list will help you learn the definition and the spelling of each word.

Obstetric Disease and Disorder Terms

Built from Word Parts

Term	Definition
amnionitis .... (*am*-nē-ō-NĪ-tis)	inflammation of the amnion
chorioamnionitis .... (kō-rē-ō-*am*-nē-ō-NĪ-tis)	inflammation of the chorion and amnion
choriocarcinoma .... (kō-rē-ō-*kar*-si-NŌ-ma)	cancerous tumor of the chorion
dystocia .... (dis-TŌ-sē-a)	difficult labor
embryotocia .... (*em*-brē-ō-TŌ-sē-a)	birth of an embryo (abortion)
hysterorrhexis .... (his-ter-ō-REK-sis)	rupture of the uterus
oligohydramnios .... (*ol-i*-gō-hī-DRAM-nē-os)	scanty amnion water (less than the normal amount of amniotic fluid; 500 ml or less)
polyhydramnios .... (*pol*-ē-hī-DRAM-nē-os)	much amnion water (more than the normal amount of amniotic fluid; 2000 ml or more) (also called *hydramnios*)
salpingocyesis .... (sal-PING-gō-sī-ē-sis)	pregnancy occurring in the fallopian tube (also called *ectopic pregnancy*) (Exercise Figure B)

Practice saying each of these terms aloud. To hear the terms, access the **PRONOUNCE IT** activity for this chapter on the Student CD that accompanies this text. Or, to hear the terms and their definitions with a CD player or computer, obtain the Pronunciation CD designed for use with this text.

Learn the definitions and spellings of the disease and disorder terms by completing exercises 10, 11, and 12.

EXERCISE   10

Analyze and define the following disease and disorder terms.

1. chorioamnionitis _____

2. choriocarcinoma _____

3. dystocia _____

4. amnionitis _____

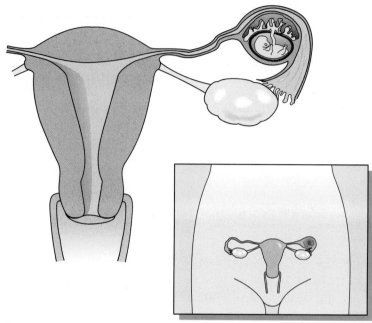

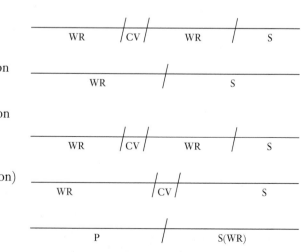

Exercise Figure B

Fill in the blanks to complete labeling of the diagram. Ectopic pregnancy in the fallopian tube or

_____ / _____ / _____
fallopian tube / **cv** / **pregnancy**

5. hysterorrhexis _____

6. embryotocia _____

7. salpingocyesis _____

8. oligohydramnios _____

9. polyhydramnios _____

EXERCISE 11

Build disease and disorder terms for the following definitions by using the word parts you have learned.

1. cancerous tumor of the
   chorion

   _____ / ___ / _____ / ___
   WR / CV / WR / S

2. inflammation of the amnion

   _____ / _____
   WR / S

3. inflammation of the chorion
   and amnion

   _____ / ___ / _____ / ___
   WR / CV / WR / S

4. birth of an embryo (abortion)

   _____ / ___ / _____
   WR / CV / S

5. difficult labor

   _____ / _____
   P / S(WR)

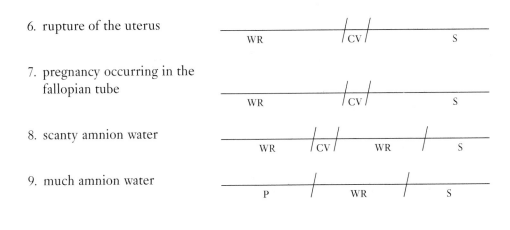

6. rupture of the uterus

_____ / CV / _____
WR   S

7. pregnancy occurring in the
   fallopian tube

_____ / CV / _____
WR   S

8. scanty amnion water

_____ / CV / _____ / _____
WR   WR   S

9. much amnion water

_____ / _____ / _____
P   WR   S

EXERCISE 12

Spell each of the disease and disorder terms. Have someone dictate the terms on
p. 285 to you. Think about the word parts before attempting to write the word. Study
any words you have spelled incorrectly.

1. _____   6. _____

2. _____   7. _____

3. _____   8. _____

4. _____   9. _____

5. _____

Obstetric Disease and Disorder Terms

Not Built from Word Parts

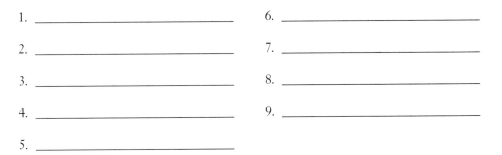

Term	Definition
abortion (ab-OR-shun)	termination of pregnancy by the expulsion from the uterus of an embryo before fetal viability, usually before 20 weeks of gestation.
abruptio placentae (ab-RUP-shē-ō) (pla-SEN-tē)	premature separation of the placenta from the uterine wall (Figure 9-4)
eclampsia (ē-KLAMP-sē-a)	severe complication and progression of preeclampsia characterized by convulsion and coma (see _preeclampsia_ on next page). Eclampsia is a potentially life-threatening disorder.

Types of Abortion
Spontaneous abortion is the termination of pregnancy that occurs naturally. It is commonly referred to as _miscarriage._
Induced abortion is the intentional termination of pregnancy by surgical or medical intervention.
Therapeutic abortion is an induced abortion performed because of health risks to the mother or for fetal disease.
Elective abortion is an induced abortion performed at the request of the woman.

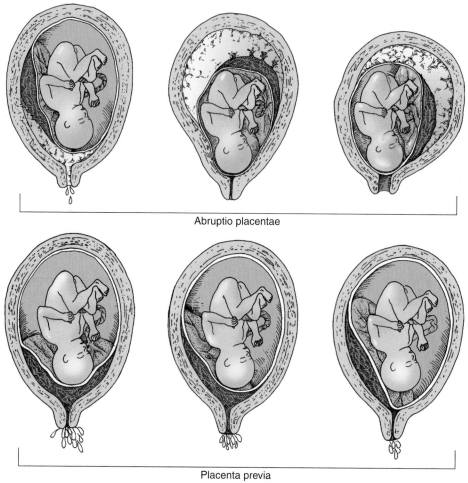

Abruptio placentae

Placenta previa

Figure 9-4

Various stages of abruptio placentae and placenta previa.

ectopic pregnancy (ek-TOP-ik) (PREG-nan-cē)	pregnancy occurring outside the uterus, commonly in the fallopian tubes (also called *salpingocyesis*) (see Exercise Figure B)
placenta previa (pla-SEN-ta) (PRĒV-ē-a)	abnormally low implantation of the placenta on the uterine wall. (Dilatation of the cervix can cause separation of the placenta from the uterine wall, resulting in bleeding. With severe hemorrhage, a cesarean section may be necessary to save the mother's life.) (Figure 9-4)
preeclampsia (prē-ē-KLAMP-sē-a)	abnormal condition encountered during pregnancy or shortly after delivery characterized by high blood pressure, edema, and proteinuria, but with no convulsions or coma. The cause is unknown; if not successfully treated the condition will progress to eclampsia. Eclampsia is the third most common cause of maternal death in the United States after hemorrhage and infection.

Practice saying each of these terms aloud. To hear the terms, access the **PRONOUNCE IT** activity for this chapter on the Student CD that accompanies this text. Or, to hear the terms and their definitions with a CD player or computer, obtain the Pronunciation CD designed for use with this text.

Learn the definitions and spellings of the disease and disorder terms by completing exercises 13, 14, and 15.

EXERCISE   13

Write the definitions of the following terms.

1. abruptio placentae _____

2. abortion _____

3. placenta previa _____

4. eclampsia _____

5. ectopic pregnancy _____

6. preeclampsia _____

EXERCISE   14

Write the term for each of the following definitions.

1. premature separation of the placenta from the uterine wall   _____

2. severe complication and progression of preeclampsia   _____

3. termination of pregnancy by the expulsion from the uterus of an embryo   _____

4. pregnancy occurring outside the uterus   _____

5. abnormally low implantation of the placenta on the uterine wall   _____

6. characterized by high blood pressure, edema, and proteinuria, but with no convulsions or coma   _____

EXERCISE 15

Spell the disease and disorder terms. Have someone dictate the terms on pp. 287-288 to you. Study any words you have spelled incorrectly.

1. _____   4. _____

2. _____   5. _____

3. _____   6. _____

Neonatology Disease and Disorder Terms

Built from Word Parts

Term	Definition
microcephalus .... (mī-krō-SEF-a-lus)	(fetus with a very) small head
omphalitis.................................... (om-fa-LĪ-tis)	inflammation of the umbilicus
omphalocele.............................. (om-FAL-ō-sēl)	herniation at the umbilicus (a part of the intestine protrudes through the abdominal wall at birth) (Exercise Figure C)
pyloric stenosis......................... (pī-LOR-ik) (ste-NŌ-sis)	narrowing pertaining to the pyloric sphincter. (Congenital pyloric stenosis occurs in 1 of every 200 newborns.)
tracheoesophageal fistula................ (TRĀ-kē-ō-ē-sof-a-jē-al) (FIS-tū-la)	abnormal passageway pertaining to the esophagus and the trachea (between the esophagus and trachea)

Practice saying each of these terms aloud. To hear the terms, access the **PRONOUNCE IT** activity for this chapter on the Student CD that accompanies this text. Or, to hear the terms and their definitions with a CD player or computer, obtain the Pronunciation CD designed for use with this text.

Learn the definitions and spellings of the neonatology disease and disorder terms by completing exercises 16, 17, and 18.

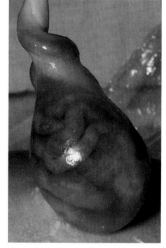

Exercise Figure C
Fill in the blanks to label the diagram.

_____ / __ / _____
umbilicus / **cv** / **herniation**

EXERCISE 16

Analyze and define the following disease and disorder terms.

1. pyloric stenosis _____

2. omphalocele _____

3. omphalitis _____

4. microcephalus_____

5. tracheoesophageal fistula _____

EXERCISE 17

Build disease and disorder terms for the following definitions by using the word parts you have learned.

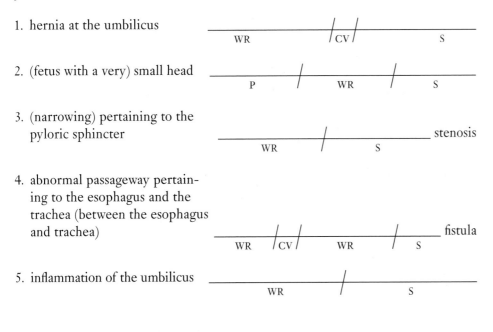

1. hernia at the umbilicus

    _____ /___/___/ _____
    WR   CV   S

2. (fetus with a very) small head

    _____ /_____/_____/ _____
    P   WR   S

3. (narrowing) pertaining to the
   pyloric sphincter

    _____ /_____/ _____ stenosis
    WR   S

4. abnormal passageway pertaining to the esophagus and the
   trachea (between the esophagus
   and trachea)

    _____ /___/___ /_____/ _____ fistula
    WR   CV   WR   S

5. inflammation of the umbilicus

    _____ /_____/ _____
    WR   S

EXERCISE 18

Spell each of the disease and disorder terms. Have someone dictate the terms on p. 290 to you. Think about the word parts before attempting to write the word. Study any words you have spelled incorrectly.

1. _____   4. _____

2. _____   5. _____

3. _____

Neonatology Disease and Disorder Terms

Not Built from Word Parts

Term	Definition
cleft lip and palate	congenital split of the lip and roof of the mouth (*cleft* indicates a fissure)
Down syndrome (down) (SIN-drōme)	congenital condition characterized by varying degrees of mental retardation and multiple defects (formerly called *mongolism*)
erythroblastosis fetalis (e-*rith*-rō-blas-TŌ-sis) (fē-TAL-is)	condition of the newborn characterized by hemolysis of the erythrocytes. The condition is usually caused by incompatibility of the infant's and mother's blood, occurring when the mother's blood is Rh negative and the infant's blood is Rh positive.

esophageal atresia.......................... congenital absence of part of the esophagus.
(ē-*sof*-a-JĒ-al) (a-TRĒ-zē-a)   Food cannot pass from the baby's mouth to the stomach (Figure 9-5).

gastroschisis.................................... a congenital fissure of the abdominal wall not
(gas-TROS-ki-sis)   at the umbilicus. Enterocele, protrusion of the intestine, is usually present (Figure 9-6).

respiratory distress syndrome (RDS)... a respiratory complication in the newborn,
(RES-pir-a-tōr-ē)   especially in premature infants. In premature
(di-STRESS) (SIN-drōm)   infants RDS is caused by normal immaturity of the respiratory system resulting in compromised respiration (formerly called *hyaline membrane disease*).

spina bifida (divided spine)............. congenital defect in the vertebral column
(SPĪ-na) (BIF-i-da)   caused by the failure of the vertebral arch to close. If the meninges protrude through the opening the condition is called *meningocele*. Protrusion of both the meninges and spinal cord is called *meningomyelocele*. Both terms are covered in Chapter 15 (Figure 9-7).

Practice saying each of these terms aloud. To hear the terms, access the **PRONOUNCE IT** activity for this chapter on the Student CD that accompanies this text. Or, to hear the terms and their definitions with a CD player or computer, obtain the Pronunciation CD designed for use with this text.

Learn the definitions and spellings of the disease and disorder terms by completing exercises 19 and 20.

EXERCISE 19

Match the terms in the first column with their correct definitions in the second column.

_____ 1. Down syndrome   a. defect of the vertebral column

_____ 2. cleft lip and palate   b. respiratory complication

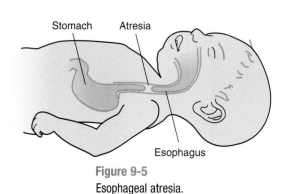

Figure 9-5
Esophageal atresia.

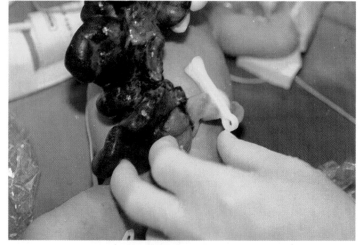

Figure 9-6
Gastroschisis.

_____ 3. spina bifida

_____ 4. erythroblastosis fetalis

_____ 5. respiratory distress syndrome

_____ 6. esophageal atresia

_____ 7. gastroschisis

c. split of the lip and roof of the mouth

d. caused by incompatibility of the infant's and the mother's blood

e. congenital fissure of the abdominal wall

f. congenital condition characterized by mental retardation

g. congenital absence of part of the esophagus

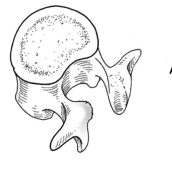

A

EXERCISE 20

Spell the disease and disorder terms. Have someone dictate the terms on pp. 291-292 to you. Study any words you have spelled incorrectly.

1. _____

2. _____

3. _____

4. _____

5. _____

6. _____

7. _____

Obstetric Surgical Terms

Built from Word Parts

Term	Definition
amniotomy............................... (*am*-nē-OT-ō-mē)	incision into the amnion (rupture of the fetal membrane to induce labor)
episiotomy............................... (e-*piz*-ē-OT-ō-mē)	incision of the vulva (perineum), usually performed during delivery to prevent tearing of the perineum (also called *perineotomy*) (Figure 9-8)

Obstetric Diagnostic Terms

Built from Word Parts

Term	Definition
Diagnostic Imaging	
pelvic sonography............................... (PEL-vik) (so-NOG-ra-fē)	pertaining to the pelvis, process of recording sound (pelvic ultrasound is used to evaluate the fetus and pregnancy) (Figure 9-9)

> **Pelvic sonography,** also called **ultrasonography, ultrasound,** or **obstetric ultrasonography,** is used extensively to evaluate the fetus and the pregnancy. It is noninvasive, harmless, and especially suited for this evaluation because the presence of amniotic fluid enhances sound. Some specific uses for pelvic sonography are:
> 1. to diagnose an abnormal pregnancy early
> 2. to determine the age of the fetus
> 3. to measure fetal growth and rate
> 4. to determine fetal position

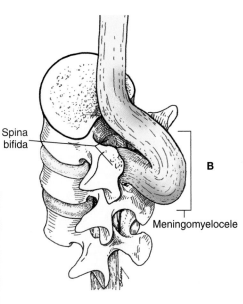

Spina bifida

Meningomyelocele

B

Figure 9-7
A, Spina bifida;
B, meningomyelocele.

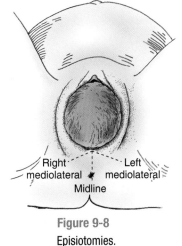

Right mediolateral

Left mediolateral

Midline

Figure 9-8
Episiotomies.

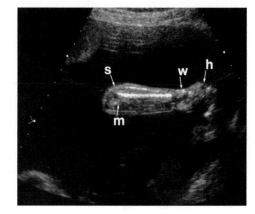

Figure 9-9
An ultrasound image showing the forearm of a fetus. The skinline (*s*), muscle (*m*), wrist (*w*), and hand (*h*) are in view. The first ultrasound examination was used in obstetrics in 1958.

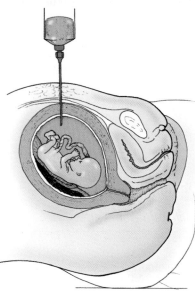

Exercise Figure D
Fill in the blanks to label the diagram.

| amniotic fluid | / cv / | surgical puncture to aspirate fluid |

Other

amniocentesis .... surgical puncture to aspirate amniotic fluid
(*am*-nē-ō-sen-TĒ-sis) (the needle is inserted through the abdominal and uterine walls, using ultrasound to guide the needle). The fluid is used for the assessment of fetal health and maturity to aid in diagnosing fetal abnormalities (Exercise Figure D).

amnioscope .... instrument used for visual examination of
(AM-nē-ō-skōp) the amniotic fluid (and the fetus)

amnioscopy .... visual examination of amniotic fluid (and the
(*am*-nē-OS-kō-pē) fetus)

Practice saying each of these terms aloud. To hear the terms, access the **PRONOUNCE IT** activity for this chapter on the Student CD that accompanies this text. Or, to hear the terms and their definitions with a CD player or computer, obtain the Pronunciation CD designed for use with this text.

Learn the definitions and spellings of the surgical and procedural terms by completing exercises 21, 22, and 23.

EXERCISE 21

Analyze and define the following diagnostic and surgical terms.

1. episiotomy _____

2. amniotomy _____

3. amnioscope _____

4. pelvic sonography _____

5. amniocentesis _____

6. amnioscopy _____

EXERCISE 22

Build surgical and diagnostic terms for the following definitions by using the word parts you have learned.

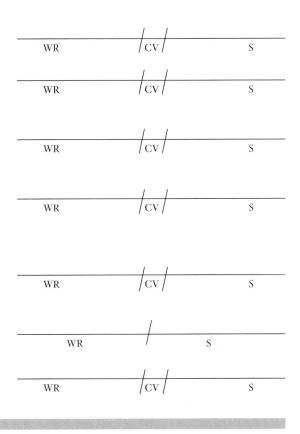

1. incision into the fetal
   membrane

   WR ____ / CV / ____ S

2. incision of the vulva

   WR ____ / CV / ____ S

3. visual examination of the
   amniotic fluid (and fetus)

   WR ____ / CV / ____ S

4. surgical puncture to
   aspirate amniotic fluid

   WR ____ / CV / ____ S

5. instrument used for visual
   examination of the amniotic
   fluid (and fetus)

   WR ____ / CV / ____ S

6. pertaining to the pelvis,
   process of recording sound

   WR ____ / ____ S

   WR ____ / CV / ____ S

EXERCISE 23

Spell each of the surgical and diagnostic terms. Have someone dictate the terms on pp. 293-294 to you. Think about the word parts before attempting to spell the word. Study any words you have spelled incorrectly.

1. _____   4. _____

2. _____   5. _____

3. _____   6. _____

Complementary Terms

Built from Word Parts

Term	Definition
amniochorial (*am*-nē-ō-KŌ-rē-al)	pertaining to the amnion and chorion
amniorrhea (*am*-nē-ō-RĒ-a)	discharge (escape) of amniotic fluid
amniorrhexis (*am*-nē-ō-REK-sis)	rupture of the amnion
antepartum (*an*-tē-PAR-tum)	before childbirth (reference to the mother)
embryogenic (*em*-brē-ō-JEN-ik)	producing an embryo
embryoid (EM-brē-oyd)	resembling an embryo
fetal (FĒ-tal)	pertaining to the fetus
gravida (GRAV-i-da)	pregnant (woman)
gravidopuerperal (*grav*-i-dō-pū-ER-per-al)	pertaining to pregnancy and the childbirth (from delivery until reproductive organs return to normal)
intrapartum (*in*-tra-PAR-tum)	within (during) labor and childbirth
lactic (LAK-tik)	pertaining to milk
lactogenic (*lak*-tō-JEN-ik)	producing milk (by stimulation)
lactorrhea (*lak*-tō-RĒ-a)	(spontaneous) discharge of milk
multigravida (*mul*-ti-GRAV-i-da)	many pregnancies (a woman who has been pregnant two or more times)
multipara (multip) (mul-TIP-a-ra)	many births (a woman who has given birth to two or more viable offspring)
natal (NĀ-tal)	pertaining to birth
neonate (NĒ-ō-nāt)	new birth (an infant from birth to 4 weeks of age) (synonymous with *newborn* [NB])
neonatologist (nē-ō-nā-TOL-ō-jist)	physician who studies and treats disorders of the newborn
neonatology (*nē*-ō-nā-TOL-ō-jē)	study of the newborn (branch of medicine that deals with diagnosis and treatment of disorders in newborns)
nulligravida (*nul*-li-GRAV-i-da)	no pregnancies (a woman who has never been pregnant)

nullipara (nu-LIP-a-ra)	no births (a woman who has not given birth to a viable offspring)
para (PAR-a)	birth (a woman who has given birth to a viable offspring)
postnatal (pōst-NĀ-tal)	pertaining to after birth (reference to the newborn)
postpartum (pōst-PAR-tum)	after childbirth (reference to the mother)
prenatal (prē-NĀ-tal)	pertaining to before birth (reference to the newborn)
primigravida (prī-mi-GRAV-i-da)	first pregnancy (a woman in her first pregnancy)
primipara (prī-MIP-a-ra)	first birth (a woman who has given birth to one viable offspring)
pseudocyesis (sū-dō-sī-Ē-sis)	false pregnancy
puerpera (pū-ER-per-a)	childbirth (a woman who has just given birth)
puerperal (pū-ER-per-al)	pertaining to (immediately after) childbirth

Practice saying each of these terms aloud. To hear the terms, access the **PRONOUNCE IT** activity for this chapter on the Student CD that accompanies this text. Or, to hear the terms and their definitions with a CD player or computer, obtain the Pronunciation CD designed for use with this text.

Learn the definitions and spellings of the complementary terms by completing exercises 24, 25, and 26.

EXERCISE 24

Analyze and define the following complementary terms.

1. puerpera _____

2. amniorrhexis _____

3. antepartum _____

4. pseudocyesis _____

5. prenatal _____

6. lactic _____

7. lactorrhea _____

8. amniorrhea _____

9. multipara _____

10. embryogenic _____

11. embryoid _____

12. fetal _____

13. gravida _____

14. amniochorial _____

15. multigravida _____

16. lactogenic _____

17. natal _____

18. gravidopuerperal _____

19. neonatology _____

20. nullipara _____

21. para _____

22. primigravida _____

23. postpartum _____

24. neonate _____

25. primipara _____

26. puerperal _____

27. nulligravida _____

28. intrapartum _____

29. postnatal _____

30. neonatologist _____

EXERCISE 25

Build the complementary terms for the following definitions by using the word parts you have learned.

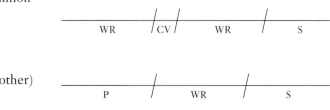

1. pertaining to the amnion
   and chorion
   _____ / ___ / _____ / ___
   WR   CV   WR   S

2. before childbirth
   (reference to the mother)
   _____ / _____ / ___
   P   WR   S

3. producing an embryo

_____ / _____
WR   /CV/   S

4. pertaining to the fetus

_____ / _____
WR   /   S

5. pertaining to before birth
(reference to the newborn)

_____ / _____ / _____
P   /   WR   /   S

6. pertaining to milk

_____ / _____
WR   /   S

7. (spontaneous) discharge
of milk

_____ / _____
WR   /CV/   S

8. discharge (escape) of
amniotic fluid

_____ / _____
WR   /CV/   S

9. false pregnancy

_____ / _____
WR   /CV/   S

10. (stimulating) the
production of milk

_____ / _____
WR   /CV/   S

11. rupture of the amnion

_____ / _____
WR   /CV/   S

12. resembling an embryo

_____ / _____
WR   /   S

13. pregnant (woman)

_____ / _____
WR   /   S

14. pertaining to pregnancy
and the childbirth

_____ / __ / _____ / _____
WR   /CV/   WR   /   S

15. many births

_____ / _____ / _____
P   /   WR   /   S

16. pertaining to birth

_____ / _____
WR   /   S

17. new birth (an infant from
birth to 4 weeks of age)

_____ / _____ / _____
P   /   WR   /   S

18. study of the newborn

_____ / _____ / __ / _____
P   /   WR   /CV/   S

19. no births

_____ / _____ / _____
P   /   WR   /   S

20. birth

|_____/_____|
     WR   /   S

21. first pregnancy

|_____/____/_____/_____|
    WR   /CV/   WR   /   S

22. after childbirth
    (reference to the mother)

|_____/_____/_____|
    P   /   WR   /   S

23. first birth

|_____/___/_____/_____|
    WR /CV/   WR   /   S

24. many pregnancies

|_____/_____/_____|
    P   /   WR   /   S

25. pertaining to (immediately
    after) childbirth

|_____/_____|
      WR   /   S

26. no pregnancies

|_____/_____/_____|
    P   /   WR   /   S

27. childbirth

|_____/_____|
      WR   /   S

28. within (during) labor and
    childbirth

|_____/_____/_____|
    P   /   WR   /   S

29. physician who studies
    and treats disorders of
    the newborn

|_____/_____/___/_____|
    P   /   WR   /CV/   S

30. pertaining to after birth
    (reference to the newborn)

|_____/_____/_____|
    P   /   WR   /   S

EXERCISE 26

Spell each of the complementary terms. Have someone dictate the terms on pp. 296-297 to you. Think about the word parts before attempting to write the word. Study any words you have spelled incorrectly.

1. _____   7. _____

2. _____   8. _____

3. _____   9. _____

4. _____   10. _____

5. _____   11. _____

6. _____   12. _____

13. _____ 22. _____

14. _____ 23. _____

15. _____ 24. _____

16. _____ 25. _____

17. _____ 26. _____

18. _____ 27. _____

19. _____ 28. _____

20. _____ 29. _____

21. _____ 30. _____

Complementary Terms
Not Built from Word Parts

Term	Definition
breech presentation (brēch)	parturition (act of giving birth) in which the buttocks, feet, or knees emerge first (Figure 9-10)
cesarean section **(CS, C-section)** (se-ZAR-ē-an)	the birth of a baby through an incision in the mother's abdomen and uterus (may also be spelled *caesarean*)
congenital anomaly (kon-JEN-i-tal) (a-NOM-a-lē)	abnormality present at birth
lochia (LŌ-kē-a)	vaginal discharge after childbirth
meconium (me-KŌ-nē-um)	first stool of the newborn (greenish black)
obstetrician (*ob*-ste-TRISH-an)	physician who specializes in obstetrics
obstetrics (OB) (ob-STET-riks)	medical specialty dealing with pregnancy, childbirth, and puerperium
parturition (*par*-tū-RISH-un)	act of giving birth
premature infant	infant born before completing 37 weeks of gestation
puerperium (pū-er-PĒ-rē-um)	period from delivery until the reproductive organs return to normal (approximately 6 weeks)

> **Cesarean Section (C-Section)**
> The origin of this term has no relation to the birth of Julius Caesar, as is commonly believed. One suggested etymology is that from 715 to 672 BC it was Roman law that the operation be performed on dying women in the last few months of pregnancy in the hope of saving the child. At that time the operation was called a **caeso matris utero**, which means **the cutting of the mother's uterus.**

Practice saying each of these terms aloud. To hear the terms, access the **PRONOUNCE IT** activity for this chapter on the Student CD that accompanies this text. Or, to hear the terms and their definitions with a CD player or computer, obtain the Pronunciation CD designed for use with this text.

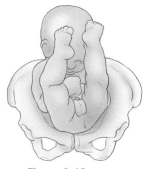

Figure 9-10
Breech presentation.

Learn the definitions and spellings of the complementary terms by completing exercises 27, 28, and 29.

EXERCISE 27

Match the definitions in the first column with the correct terms in the second column.

_____ 1. vaginal discharge

_____ 2. medical specialty

_____ 3. abnormality present at birth

_____ 4. period after delivery

_____ 5. giving birth

_____ 6. physician specializing in obstetrics

_____ 7. buttocks, feet, or knees first

_____ 8. first stool

_____ 9. born before completing 37 weeks of gestation

_____ 10. birth through an abdominal incision

a. lochia

b. obstetrician

c. premature infant

d. meconium

e. obstetrics

f. parturition

g. puerperium

h. cesarean section

i. congenital anomaly

j. breech presentation

EXERCISE 28

Write the definitions of the following terms.

1. meconium _____

2. obstetrics _____

3. premature infant _____

4. lochia _____

5. puerperium _____

6. parturition _____

7. obstetrician _____

8. congenital anomaly _____

9. breech presentation _____

10. cesarean section _____

EXERCISE 29

Spell each of the complementary terms. Have someone dictate the terms on p. 301 to you. Study any words you have spelled incorrectly.

1. _____   6. _____

2. _____   7. _____

3. _____   8. _____

4. _____   9. _____

5. _____   10. _____

Abbreviations

C/S, C-section	cesarean section
DOB	date of birth
EDD	expected (estimated) date of delivery
LMP	last menstrual period
LNMP	last normal menstrual period
multip	multipara
NB	newborn
OB	obstetrics
RDS	respiratory distress syndrome

Refer to Appendix D for a complete list of abbreviations.

EXERCISE 30

Write the definition of the following abbreviations.

1. OB _____

2. EDD _____ _____ of _____

3. LMP _____ _____ _____

4. DOB _____ _____ _____

5. NB _____

6. multip _____

7. C/S, C-section _____ _____

8. LNMP _____ _____ _____ _____

9. RDS _____ _____ _____

CHAPTER REVIEW

EXERCISE 31 *Interact with Medical Records*

Complete the progress note by writing the medical terms in the blanks. Use the list of definitions with the corresponding numbers.

University Hospital and Medical Center
4700 North Main Street • Wellness, Arizona 54321 • (987) 555-3210

PATIENT NAME: Gloria Cisneros   **CASE NUMBER:**   17432-OBN
DATE OF BIRTH: 08/26/xx   **VISIT/EVENT DATE:**   09/23/xx

PROGRESS NOTE

HISTORY: Gloria Cisneros is a 24-year-old married Latina 1. _____ 3 2. _____ 2 who is here today with her husband. Her 3. _____ is 1 week from today. She has received 4. _____ care here at the Medical Center Obstetrics Clinic since her second month of pregnancy. This 5. _____ has been uncomplicated with no spotting, albuminuria, hypertension, edema, or glycosuria. Patient has attended Lamaze classes with her husband.

PHYSICAL EXAM: Her breasts are large. She has gained 2 pounds since her last visit and she has gained 25 pounds throughout her pregnancy. Her current weight is 164 pounds. Her cervix is 1 cm dilated. Routine 6. _____ _____ reveals a single 7. _____ and indicates adequate pelvis for normal size delivery. 8. _____ presentation is cephalic.

PLAN: Patient will return to clinic once a week until delivery.

_____

Heather Strom, MD

HS/mcm

---

1. pregnant (woman)
2. birth
3. abbreviation for expected delivery date
4. pertaining to before birth (reference to the newborn)
5. development of a new individual from conception to birth
6. pertaining to the pelvis, process of recording sound
7. unborn offspring from second month of pregnancy
8. pertaining to the fetus

EXERCISE 32   *Interpret Medical Terms*

To test your understanding of the terms introduced in this chapter, circle the words that correctly complete the sentences. The italicized words refer to the correct answer.

1. The premature infant was diagnosed as having *respiratory distress syndrome,* a disease of the (umbilicus, erythrocytes, lungs).
2. Because of inadequate uterine contractions, the patient was experiencing *difficult labor,* or (dysphasia, dystocia, dysuria).
3. Down syndrome was diagnosed prenatally by laboratory analysis of *amniotic fluid removed by surgical puncture,* or (amniocentesis, amnioscopy, amnioscope).
4. The word that means *before childbirth* (reference to the mother) is (intrapartum, antepartum, antipartum).
5. *Nulligravida* is a woman who (has never been pregnant, has not given birth).
6. *Multipara* is a woman who has (given birth to two or more viable offspring, been pregnant two or more times).
7. *Primigravida* is a woman (in her first pregnancy, who has given birth to one child).
8. The word that means the *act of giving birth* is (parturition, puerperium, gravidopuerperal).
9. *Rupture of the uterus* is called (hysterorrhaphy, hysterorrhexis, hysteroptosis).

EXERCISE 33   *Read Medical Terms in Use*

Practice pronunciation of the terms by reading the following medical document. Use the pronunciation key following the medical term to assist you in saying the words.

> Jane Anne is a 34-year-old **gravida** (GRAV-i-da) 2 **para** (PAR-a) 1 woman. Her LMP was April 20, 20xx. The EDD is January 2, 20xx. The **obstetrician** (*ob*-ste-TRISH-an) prescribed folic acid to prevent **spina bifida** (SPĪ-na) (BIF-i-da). The patient's first pregnancy was complicated by **preeclampsia** (prē-ē-KLAMP-sē-a) and a **breech** (brēch) presentation, which required a **cesarean section** (se-ZĀR-ē-an) (SEK-shun). **Pelvic sonography** (PEL-vik) (so-NOG-ra-fē) showed a single female fetus with normal development. She went on to deliver a healthy baby 3 days before her expected delivery date.

EXERCISE 34   *Comprehend Medical Terms in Use*

Test your comprehension of terms in the above medical document by circling the correct answer.

1. T   F   Jane Anne has been pregnant twice and has given birth once.
2. The obstetrician prescribed folic acid to prevent congenital:
    a. split of the lip and roof of the mouth
    b. mental retardation
    c. absence of part of the esophagus
    d. defect of the vertebral column
3. During her first pregnancy the patient had:
    a. abnormally low implantation of the placenta on the uterine wall
    b. high blood pressure, edema, and proteinuria
    c. premature separation of the placenta from the uterine wall
    d. convulsions and coma
4. T   F   The fetal presentation of the patient's first pregnancy was cephalic.

COMBINING FORMS CROSSWORD PUZZLE

Across Clues

1. pregnancy
4. childbirth
6. first
8. amnion
11. umbilicus
12. bear, give birth
13. head

Down Clues

2. amnion
3. fetus, unborn child
4. pelvis
5. chorion
6. false
7. milk
9. embryo
10. birth

REVIEW OF WORD PARTS

Can you define and spell the following word parts?

Combining Forms

amni/o	lact/o
amnion/o	nat/o
cephal/o	omphal/o
chori/o	par/o
embry/o	part/o
esophag/o	pelv/o, pelv/i
fet/i	prim/i
fet/o	pseud/o
gravid/o	puerper/o
	pylor/o

Prefixes

ante-
micro-
multi-
nulli-
post-
pre-

Suffixes

-amnios
-cyesis
-partum
-rrhexis
-tocia

REVIEW OF TERMS

Can you build, analyze, define, pronounce, and spell the following terms *built from word parts?*

Diseases and Disorders (Obstetrics)	Diseases and Disorders (Neonatology)	Surgical (Obstetrics)	Diagnostic (Obstetrics)	Complementary (Obstetrics and Neonatology)	
amnionitis	microcephalus	amniotomy	amniocentesis	amniochorial	multigravida
chorioamnionitis	omphalitis	episiotomy	amnioscope	amniorrhea	multipara (multip)
choriocarcinoma	omphalocele		amnioscopy	amniorrhexis	natal
dystocia	pyloric stenosis		pelvic	antepartum	neonate
embryotocia	tracheoesophageal		sonography	embryogenic	neonatologist
hysterorrhexis	fistula			embryoid	neonatology
oligohydramnios				fetal	nulligravida
polyhydramnios				gravida	nullipara
salpingocyesis				gravidopuerperal	para
				intrapartum	postnatal
				lactic	postpartum
				lactogenic	prenatal
				lactorrhea	primigravida
					primipara
					pseudocyesis
					puerpera
					puerperal

Can you define, pronounce, and spell the following terms *not built from word parts?*

Diseases and Disorders (Obstetrics)	Diseases and Disorders (Neonatology)	Complementary
abortion	cleft lip and palate	breech presentation
abruptio placentae	Down syndrome	cesarean section (CS), C-section
eclampsia	erythroblastosis fetalis	congenital anomaly
ectopic pregnancy	esophageal atresia	lochia
placenta previa	gastroschisis	meconium
preeclampsia	respiratory distress syndrome (RDS)	obstetrician
	spina bifida	obstetrics (OB)
		parturition
		premature infant
		puerperium

10 Cardiovascular and Lymphatic Systems

OBJECTIVES

On completion of this chapter you will be able to:

1. Identify the organs and other structures of the cardiovascular and lymphatic systems.
2. Define and spell the word parts presented in this chapter.
3. Build and analyze medical terms with word parts presented in this and previous chapters.
4. Define, pronounce, and spell the disease and disorder, diagnostic, surgical, and complementary terms for the cardiovascular and lymphatic systems.
5. Interpret the meaning of the abbreviations presented in this chapter.
6. Read medical documents and interpret medical terminology contained in them.

ANATOMY

Cardiovascular System

Function

The cardiovascular system is composed of the heart, blood vessels, and blood. The function of the system is to nourish the body by transporting nutrients and oxygen to the cells and removing carbon dioxide and other waste products (Figure 10-1).

Structures of the Cardiovascular System

heart..	muscular organ the size of a fist, located behind the sternum (breast bone) and between the lungs. The pumping action of the heart circulates blood throughout the body. The heart consists of two upper chambers, the

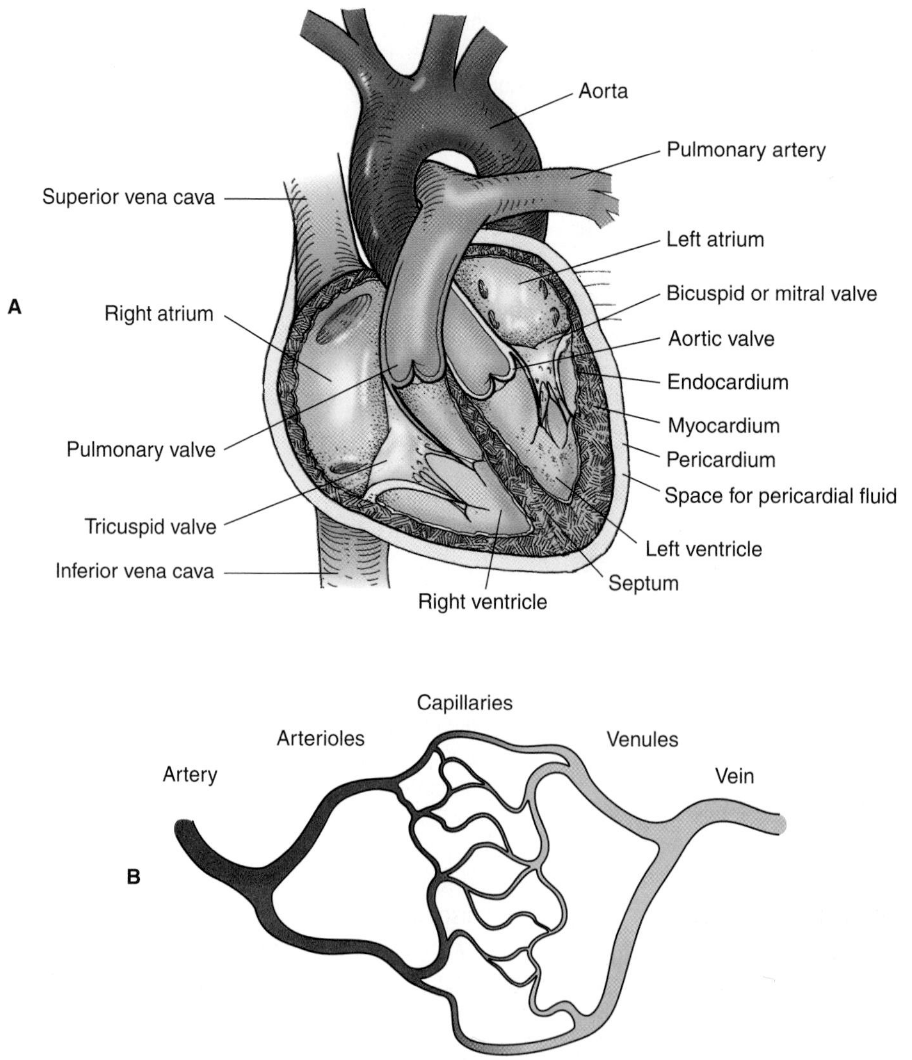

Figure 10-1
A, Interior of the heart. **B,** Microcirculation.

heart (cont'd)	*right atrium* (*pl.* atria) and the *left atrium,* and two lower chambers, the *right ventricle* and the *left ventricle.* Valves of the heart keep the blood flowing in one direction. The *cardiac septum* separates the right and left sides of the heart.
tricuspid valve	located between the right atrium and right ventricle
bicuspid valve	located between the left atrium and left ventricle (also called *mitral valve*)
semilunar valves	located between the right ventricle and the pulmonary artery and between the left ventricle and the aorta

three layers of the heart

pericardium	two-layer sac *(pericardial sac)* covering the heart *(pericardial fluid* allows the layers to move without friction)
visceral pericardium	lies closest to the myocardium
epicardium (parietal pericardium)	lines the pericardial sac
myocardium	middle, thick, muscular layer
endocardium	inner lining of the heart
blood vessels	tubelike structures that carry blood throughout the body
arteries	blood vessels that carry blood away from the heart. All arteries, with the exception of the pulmonary artery, carry oxygen and other nutrients from the heart to the body cells. The pulmonary artery, in contrast, carries carbon dioxide and other waste products from the heart to the lungs.
arterioles	smallest arteries
aorta	largest artery in the body, originating at the left ventricle and descending through the thorax and abdomen
veins	blood vessels that carry blood back to the heart. All veins, with the exception of the pulmonary veins, carry blood containing carbon dioxide and other waste products. The pulmonary veins carry oxygenated blood from the lungs to the heart.
venules	smallest veins
venae cavae	largest veins in the body. The *inferior vena cava* carries blood to the heart from body parts below the diaphragm, and the *superior vena cava* returns the blood to the heart from the upper part of the body.

capillaries	microscopic blood vessels that connect arterioles with venules. Materials are passed between the blood and tissue through the capillary walls.
blood	composed of *plasma* and *formed elements,* such as erythrocytes, leukocytes, and thrombocytes (platelets)
plasma	liquid portion of blood in which cells are suspended
cells (formed elements)	
erythrocytes	red blood cells that carry oxygen
leukocytes	white blood cells that fight infection
platelets (thrombocytes)	one of the formed elements in the blood that is responsible for aiding in the clotting process

Lymphatic System

Function

The major function of the lymphatic system is removal of excessive tissue fluid, which develops from increased metabolic activity. Lymphatics, or lymph vessels, are found throughout most of the body (Figure 10-2).

Structures of the Lymphatic System

lymph	transparent, usually colorless, tissue fluid
lymph nodes	small, spherical bodies made up of lymphoid tissue. They are found singularly or may be grouped together. The nodes act as filters in keeping substances such as bacteria from the blood.
spleen	located in the left side of the abdominal cavity between the stomach and the diaphragm. In adulthood, the spleen is the largest lymphatic organ in the body.
thymus gland	one of the primary lymphatic organs, it is located anterior to the ascending aorta and posterior to the sternum between the lungs. It plays an important role in the development of the body's immune system, particularly from infancy to puberty. Around puberty the thymus gland atrophies into connective tissue and does not function.

Learn the anatomic terms by completing exercises 1 and 2.

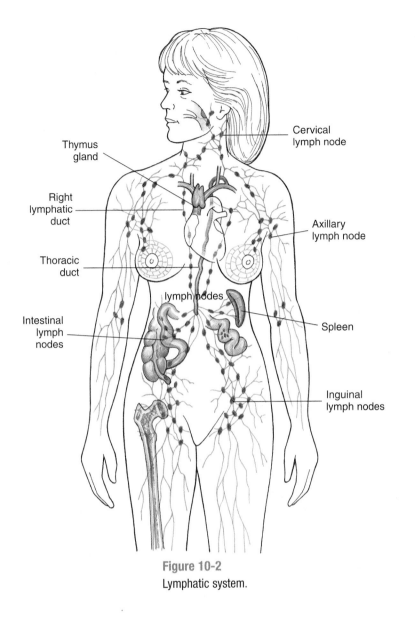

Figure 10-2
Lymphatic system.

EXERCISE   1

Match the anatomic terms in the first column with the correct definitions in the second column.

_____ 1. aorta

_____ 2. arteries

_____ 3. arterioles

_____ 4. atria

_____ 5. bicuspid valve

_____ 6. blood

_____ 7. capillaries

_____ 8. endocardium

a. white blood cells

b. lies between the left atrium and left ventricle

c. outer layer of the pericardial sac

d. pumps blood throughout the body

e. smallest arteries

f. inner lining of the heart

g. largest artery in the body

_____ 9. visceral pericardium

_____ 10. erythrocytes

_____ 11. heart

_____ 12. leukocytes

_____ 13. lymph

h. red blood cells

i. connect arterioles with venules

j. blood vessels that carry blood away from the heart

k. composed of plasma and formed elements

l. layer of the pericardial sac that lies closest to the myocardium

m. upper chambers of the heart

n. colorless tissue fluid

EXERCISE 2

Match the anatomic terms in the first column with the correct definitions in the second column.

_____ 1. lymph nodes

_____ 2. myocardium

_____ 3. parietal pericardium

_____ 4. pericardium

_____ 5. plasma

_____ 6. platelet

_____ 7. semilunar valves

_____ 8. cardiac septum

_____ 9. spleen

_____ 10. tricuspid valve

_____ 11. veins

_____ 12. ventricles

_____ 13. venules

_____ 14. vena cava

_____ 15. thymus gland

a. carries blood back to the heart

b. two-layer sac covering the heart

c. thrombocyte

d. largest lymphatic organ in the body

e. smallest veins

f. act as filters to keep substances such as bacteria from the blood

g. plays an important role in the development of the body's immune system

h. lines the pericardial sac

i. lower chambers of the heart

j. largest vein in the body

k. allows the double layer of the covering of the heart to move without friction

l. located between the right ventricle and the pulmonary artery and between the left ventricle and the aorta

m. liquid portion of the blood

n. carries oxygenated blood away from the heart

o. located between the right atrium and the right ventricle

p. muscular layer of the heart

q. separates heart into right and left sides

WORD PARTS

Combining Forms of the Cardiovascular and Lymphatic Systems

Study the word parts and their definitions listed below. Completing the exercises that follow will help you learn the terms.

Combining Form	Definition
angi/o	vessel (usually refers to blood vessel)
aort/o	aorta
arteri/o	artery
atri/o	atrium
cardi/o	heart
lymph/o	lymph, lymph gland
phleb/o, ven/o	vein
plasm/o	plasma
splen/o	spleen
(NOTE: only one *e* in the word root for spleen.)	
thym/o	thymus gland
valv/o, valvul/o	valve
ventricul/o	ventricle

Learn the anatomic locations and meanings of the combining forms by completing exercises 3 and 4 and Exercise Figure A.

Vital Air
It was believed in ancient times that arteries carried air. Vital air, or **pneuma**, did not allow blood in the arteries. A cut in an artery allowed vital air to escape and blood to replace it. The Greek **arteria**, meaning **windpipe**, was given for this reason.

Ventricle
is derived from the Latin **venter**, meaning **little belly.** It was first applied to the belly and then to the stomach. Later it was extended to mean any small cavity in an organ or body.

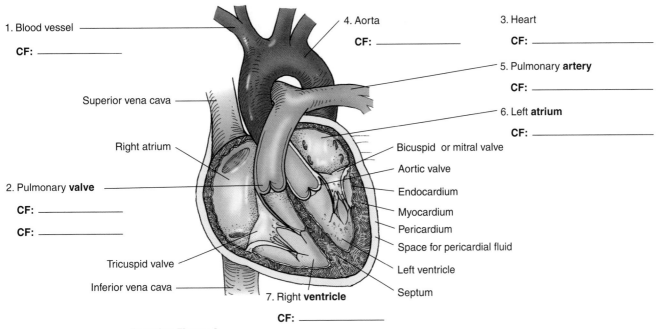

1. Blood vessel
   CF: _____

4. Aorta
   CF: _____

3. Heart
   CF: _____

5. Pulmonary **artery**
   CF: _____

6. Left **atrium**
   CF: _____

Superior vena cava

Right atrium

2. Pulmonary **valve**
   CF: _____
   CF: _____

Tricuspid valve

Inferior vena cava

7. Right **ventricle**
   CF: _____

Bicuspid or mitral valve
Aortic valve
Endocardium
Myocardium
Pericardium
Space for pericardial fluid
Left ventricle
Septum

Exercise Figure A
Fill in the blanks with combining forms in this diagram of a cutaway section of the heart.

EXERCISE 3

Write the definitions of the following combining forms.

1. cardi/o _____

2. atri/o _____

3. plasm/o _____

4. angi/o _____

5. ven/o _____

6. aort/o _____

7. valv/o _____

8. splen/o _____

9. thym/o _____

10. phleb/o _____

11. ventricul/o _____

12. arteri/o _____

13. valvul/o _____

14. lymph/o _____

EXERCISE 4

Write the combining form for each of the following terms.

1. artery _____

2. vein a. _____

    b. _____

3. heart _____

4. atrium _____

5. ventricle _____

6. lymph, lymph gland _____

7. aorta _____

8. vessel (usually blood vessel) _____

9. valve   a. _____

                            b. _____

10. spleen   _____

11. plasma   _____

12. thymus gland   _____

Combining Forms Commonly Used with the Cardiovascular and Lymphatic Systems

Combining Form	Definition
ather/o	yellowish, fatty plaque
ech/o	sound
electr/o	electricity, electrical activity
isch/o	deficiency, blockage
therm/o	heat
thromb/o	clot

Learn the combining forms by completing exercises 5 and 6.

EXERCISE 5

Write the definition of the following combining forms.

1. ech/o _____

2. thromb/o _____

3. isch/o _____

4. therm/o _____

5. ather/o _____

6. electr/o _____

EXERCISE 6

Write the combining form for each of the following.

1. clot   _____

2. sound   _____

3. deficiency, blockage   _____

4. yellowish, fatty plaque _____

5. heat _____

6. electricity, electrical activity _____

Prefixes

Prefix	Definition
brady-..	slow
tachy-..	fast, rapid

Learn the prefixes by completing exercises 7 and 8.

EXERCISE 7

Write the definitions of the following prefixes.

1. tachy- _____

2. brady- _____

EXERCISE 8

Write the prefix for each of the following.

1. fast, rapid _____

2. slow _____

Suffixes

Suffix	Definition
-ac..	pertaining to
-apheresis..	removal
-crit..	to separate
-graph..	instrument used to record (see Chapter 5 and the box on the next page for suffixes *-gram* and *-graphy*)
-odynia..	pain
-penia..	abnormal reduction in number
-poiesis..	formation
-sclerosis..	hardening

Refer to Appendix A and Appendix B for alphabetical lists of word parts and their meanings.

Comparing -graph, -graphy, and -gram
   -graph is the instrument used to record, i.e., the machine, as in **telegraph** or **electrocardiograph**.
   -graphy is the process of recording, the act of setting down or registering a record, as in **photography** or **electroencephalography**.
   -gram is the recording (picture, x-ray image, or tracing), as in **telegram** or **electrocardiogram**.

Learn the suffixes by completing exercises 9 and 10.

EXERCISE 9

Write the definitions of the following suffixes.

1. -crit _____

2. -graph _____

3. -penia _____

4. -sclerosis _____

5. -odynia _____

6. -apheresis _____

7. -poiesis _____

8. -ac _____

EXERCISE 10

Write the suffix for each of the following.

1. formation   _____

2. pertaining to   _____

3. hardening   _____

4. instrument used to record   _____

5. abnormal reduction in
   number   _____

6. pain   _____

7. separate   _____

8. removal   _____

MEDICAL TERMS

The terms you need to learn to complete this chapter are listed below. The exercises following each list will help you learn the definition and the spelling of each word.

Disease and Disorder Terms

Built from Word Parts

Term	Definition
Heart and Blood Vessels	
angiocarditis.................. (*an*-jē-ō-kar-DĪ-tis) (NOTE: the *i* in cardi/o is dropped because the suffix begins with an *i.*)	inflammation of the blood vessels and heart
angioma.......................... (an-jē-Ō-ma)	tumor composed of blood vessels
angiospasm..................... (AN-jē-ō-spazm)	spasm (contraction) of the blood vessels
angiostenosis.................. (an-jē-ō-ste-NŌ-sis)	narrowing of a blood vessel
aortic stenosis................ (ā-OR-tik) (ste-NŌ-sis)	narrowing pertaining to aorta (narrowing of the aortic valve) (Figure 10-3)
arteriorrhexis.................. (ar-*te*-rē-ō-REK-sis)	rupture of an artery
arteriosclerosis .... (ar-*te*-rē-ō-skle-*RŌ*-sis)	hardening of the arteries
atherosclerosis................ (*ath*-er-ō-skle-RŌ-sis)	hardening of fatty plaque (deposited on the arterial wall) (Exercise Figure B)
bradycardia..................... (brād-ē-KAR-dē-a) (NOTE: the *i* in cardi/o has been dropped.)	condition of a slow heart (rate less than 60 beats per minute)
cardiodynia .... (*kar*-dē-ō-DIN-ē-a)	pain in the heart
cardiomegaly................... (*kar*-dē-ō-MEG-a-lē)	enlargement of the heart
cardiomyopathy .... (kar-dē-ō-mī-OP-a-thē)	disease of the heart muscle
cardiovalvulitis............... (kar-dē-ō-val-vū-LĪ-tis)	inflammation of the valves of the heart
endocarditis.................... (en-dō-kar-DĪ-tis)	inflammation of the inner (lining) of the heart (particularly heart valves)
ischemia.......................... (is-KĒ-mē-a)	deficiency of blood (flow)
myocarditis .... (mī-ō-kar-DĪ-tis)	inflammation of the muscle of the heart

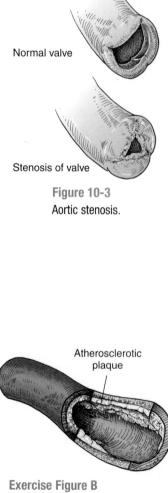

Normal valve

Stenosis of valve

Figure 10-3
Aortic stenosis.

Atherosclerotic plaque

Exercise Figure B
Fill in the blanks to label the diagram.

___**fatty** / **cv** / **hardening**___
plaque

pericarditis................................. inflammation of the outer sac of the heart
   (par-i-kar-DĪ-tis) (see Figure 10-8)

phlebitis..................................... inflammation of a vein
   (fle-BĪ-tis)

polyarteritis.............................. inflammation of many (sites in the) arteries
   (pol-ē-ar-te-RĪ-tis)
   (NOTE: the *i* in arteri/o has
   been dropped.)

tachycardia............................... abnormal state of rapid heart (rate of more
   (*tak*-i-KAR-dē-a) than 100 beats/min)
   (NOTE: the *i* in cardi/o has
   been dropped.)

thrombophlebitis .... inflammation of a vein associated with a clot
   (*throm*-bō-fle-BĪ-tis)

Blood and Lymphatic Systems

hematocytopenia...................... abnormal reduction in the number of blood
   (*hēm*-a-tō-sī-tō-PĒ-nē-a) cells

hematoma .... tumor of blood (mass of blood resulting from
   (*hēm*-a-TŌ-ma) a broken blood vessel)

lymphadenitis .... inflammation of the lymph glands
   (*limf*-ad-en-Ī-tis)

lymphadenopathy...................... disease of the lymph glands. Lymphade-
   (lim-*fad*-e-NOP-a-thē) nopathy syndrome (LAS) is a persistent,
    generalized swelling of the lymph nodes
    often preceding the development of
    AIDS.

lymphoma.................................. tumor of lymphatic tissue (malignant)
   (limf-Ō-ma)

pancytopenia............................. abnormal reduction of all (blood) cells
   (pan-sī-tō-PĒ-nē-a)

splenomegaly............................. enlargement of the spleen
   (*sple*-nō-MEG-a-lē)

thrombosis................................. abnormal condition of a (blood) clot
   (throm-BŌ-sis)

thrombus.................................... (blood) clot (attached to the interior wall of
   (THROM-bus) an artery or vein)
   (NOTE: -*us* is a noun suffix
   and has no meaning.)

thymoma.................................... tumor of the thymus gland
   (thī-MŌ-ma)

Practice saying each of these terms aloud. To hear the terms, access the **PRONOUNCE IT** activity for this chapter on the Student CD that accompanies this text. Or, to hear the terms and their definitions with a CD player or computer, obtain the Pronunciation CD designed for use with this text.

Learn the definitions and spellings of the disease and disorder terms by completing exercises 11, 12, and 13.

CAM TERM

Music therapy is the use of music within a therapeutic relationship to address physical, emotional, cognitive, and social needs of individuals. Music therapy may be used by patients with heart disease to affect heart rate, stress levels, and anxiety.

Embolus, Thrombus
An **embolus** circulates in the bloodstream until it becomes lodged in a vessel, whereas a **thrombus** is attached to the interior wall of a vessel. When a **thrombus** breaks away and circulates in the bloodstream, it becomes known as an **embolus**.

EXERCISE 11

Analyze and define the following terms.

1. endocarditis _____

2. bradycardia _____

3. cardiomegaly _____

4. arteriosclerosis _____

5. cardiovalvulitis _____

6. angiocarditis _____

7. arteriorrhexis _____

8. tachycardia _____

9. angiostenosis _____

10. thrombus _____

11. ischemia _____

12. pericarditis _____

13. cardiodynia _____

14. aortic stenosis _____

15. thrombosis _____

16. atherosclerosis _____

17. myocarditis _____

18. angioma _____

19. thymoma _____

20. hematocytopenia _____

21. lymphoma _____

22. lymphadenitis _____

23. splenomegaly _____

24. hematoma _____

25. polyarteritis _____

26. cardiomyopathy_____

27. angiospasm _____

28. lymphadenopathy _____

29. thrombophlebitis _____

30. phlebitis _____

31. pancytopenia _____

EXERCISE 12

Build disease and disorder terms for the following definitions by using the word parts you have learned.

1. rupture of an artery

   _____ / _____ / _____
   WR   CV   S

2. enlargement of the heart

   _____ / _____ / _____
   WR   CV   S

3. deficiency of blood (flow)

   _____ / _____
   WR   S

4. inflammation of the blood
   vessels and the heart

   _____ / CV / _____ / _____
   WR   WR   S

5. inflammation of the inner
   (layer) of the heart

   _____ / _____ / _____
   P   WR   S

6. condition of slow heart rate

   _____ / _____ / _____
   P   WR   S

7. hardening of the arteries

   _____ / _____ / _____
   WR   CV   S

8. abnormal condition of a
   (blood) clot

   _____ / _____
   WR   S

9. pain in the heart

   _____ / _____
   WR   S

10. inflammation of the muscle
    of the heart

    _____ / CV / _____ / _____
    WR   WR   S

11. narrowing of blood vessels

    _____ / _____ / _____
    WR   CV   S

12. abnormal state of a rapid heart rate

_____ / _____ / _____
P   WR   S

13. hardening of fatty plaque (deposited on the arterial wall)

_____ / / _____
WR   CV /   S

14. tumor composed of blood vessels

_____ / _____
WR   S

15. inflammation of the valves of the heart

_____ / / _____ / _____
WR   CV /   WR   S

16. pertaining to the aorta, narrowing

_____ / _____   _____
WR   S

17. inflammation of the outer layer of the heart

_____ / _____ / _____
P   WR   S

18. abnormal reduction in number of blood cells

_____ / / _____ / / _____
WR   CV / WR   CV /   S

19. tumor of lymphatic tissue

_____ / _____
WR   S

20. tumor of the thymus gland

_____ / _____
WR   S

21. enlargement of the spleen

_____ / / _____
WR   CV /   S

22. tumor (mass) of blood

_____ / _____
WR   S

23. inflammation of lymph glands

_____ / _____ / _____
WR   WR   S

24. disease of the heart muscle

_____ / / _____ / / _____
WR   CV / WR   CV /   S

25. inflammation of many (sites in the) arteries

_____ / _____ / _____
P   WR   S

26. spasm of the blood vessels

_____ / / _____
WR   CV /   S

27. disease of the lymph glands

   _____/_____/___/_____
   WR   WR   CV   S

28. inflammation of a vein associated with a clot

   _____/___/_____/_____
   WR   CV   WR   S

29. inflammation of a vein

   _____/_____
   WR   S

30. (blood) clot

   _____/_____
   WR   S

31. abnormal reduction of all (blood) cells

   _____/_____/___/_____
   P   WR   CV   S

EXERCISE 13

Spell each of the disease and disorder terms. Have someone dictate the terms on pp. 320-321 to you. Think about the word parts before attempting to write the word. Study any words you have spelled incorrectly.

1. _____   17. _____

2. _____   18. _____

3. _____   19. _____

4. _____   20. _____

5. _____   21. _____

6. _____   22. _____

7. _____   23. _____

8. _____   24. _____

9. _____   25. _____

10. _____   26. _____

11. _____   27. _____

12. _____   28. _____

13. _____   29. _____

14. _____   30. _____

15. _____   31. _____

16. _____

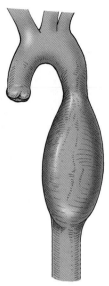

Figure 10-4
Aneurysm.

Acute Coronary Syndrome (ACS)
is an umbrella term used when a patient seeks care at an emergency care facility for symptoms of **acute angina** or **myocardial infarction not yet diagnosed.** Treatment includes rapid assessment to determine the diagnosis and treatment of symptoms to possibly minimize heart damage.

Angina Pectoris
was believed by the ancients to be a disorder of the breast. The Latin **angere,** meaning **to throttle,** was used to represent the sudden pain and was added to **pectus,** meaning **breast.**

Coronary
is derived from the Latin **coronalis,** meaning **crown** or **wreath.** It describes the arteries encircling the heart.

Disease and Disorder Terms

Not Built from Word Parts

Term	Definition
acute coronary syndrome (ACS) (a-KŪT) (KOR-ō-na-rē) (SIN-drōme)	sudden symptoms of insufficient blood supply to the heart indicating unstable angina or myocardial infarction
anemia (a-NĒ-mē-a)	reduction in the amount of hemoglobin in the red blood cells
aneurysm (AN-ū-rizm)	ballooning of a weakened portion of an arterial wall (Figure 10-4)
angina pectoris (an-JĪ-na) (PEK-to-ris)	chest pain, which may radiate to the left arm and jaw, that occurs when there is an insufficient supply of blood to the heart muscle
cardiac arrest (KAR-dē-ak) (a-REST)	sudden cessation of cardiac output and effective circulation, which requires cardiopulmonary resuscitation (CPR)
cardiac tamponade (KAR-dē-ak) (tam-pō-NĀD)	acute compression of the heart caused by fluid accumulation in the pericardial cavity
coarctation of the aorta (kō-ark-TA-shun)	congenital cardiac condition characterized by a narrowing of the aorta (Figure 10-5)
congenital heart disease (kon-JEN-i-tal)	heart abnormality present at birth
congestive heart failure (CHF) (kon-JES-tiv)	inability of the heart to pump enough blood through the body to supply the tissues and organs
coronary occlusion (KOR-ō-na-rē) (o-KLŪ-zhun)	obstruction of an artery of the heart, usually from atherosclerosis (can lead to *heart attack*)
deep vein thrombosis (DVT) (throm-BŌ-sis)	condition of thrombus in a deep vein of the body. Most often occurs in the lower extremities.
dysrhythmia (dis-RITH-mē-a)	any disturbance or abnormality in the heart's normal rhythmic pattern (arrhythmia)
embolus, *pl.* **emboli** (EM-bō-lus), (EM-bō-lī)	blood clot or foreign material, such as air or fat, that enters the bloodstream and moves until it lodges at another point in the circulation
fibrillation (fi-bril-Ā-shun)	rapid, quivering, noncoordinated contractions of the atria or ventricles
hemochromatosis (hē-mō-krō-ma-TŌ-sis)	an iron metabolism disorder that occurs when too much iron is absorbed from food, resulting in excessive deposits of iron in the tissue. Can cause congestive heart failure, diabetes, cirrhosis, or cancer of the liver.
hemophilia (hē-mō-FIL-ē-a)	inherited bleeding disease most commonly caused by a deficiency of the coagulation factor VIII

hemorrhoid......................................
(HEM-ō-royd)

varicose vein in the rectal area, which may be internal or external (Figure 10-6)

Hodgkin disease ....
(HOJ-kin)

malignant disorder of the lymphatic tissue characterized by progressive enlargement of the lymph nodes, usually beginning in the cervical nodes

hypertensive heart disease (HHD)..
(hī-per-TEN-siv)

disorder of the heart brought about by persistent high blood pressure

intermittent claudication ....
(klaw-di-KĀ-shun)

pain and discomfort in calf muscles while walking. A condition seen in occlusive artery disease.

leukemia...
(lū-KĒ-mē-a)

malignant disease characterized by excessive increase in abnormal white blood cells formed in the bone marrow

mitral valve stenosis..........................
(MĪ-tral) (ste-NŌ-sis)

a narrowing of the mitral (bicuspid) valve from scarring, usually caused by episodes of rheumatic fever

myocardial infarction (MI)................
(mī-ō-KAR-dē-al)
(in-FARK-shun)

death (necrosis) of a portion of the myocardium caused by lack of oxygen resulting from an interrupted blood supply (also called *heart attack*)

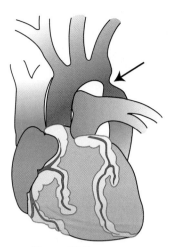

Figure 10-5
Coarctation of the aorta.

Hodgkin Disease
was first described in 1832 by Thomas Hodgkin, a pathologist at Guy's Hospital in London. In 1865 the name **Hodgkin disease** was given to the condition by another English physician, Sir Samuel Wilks.

Raynaud (rā-NŌ) Disease
is classified as a peripheral artery disease (PAD). The condition was first described by Maurice Raynaud, a French physician, in 1862. Symptoms include intermittent, symmetric attacks of cyanosis and pallor of the distal ends of the fingers and toes.

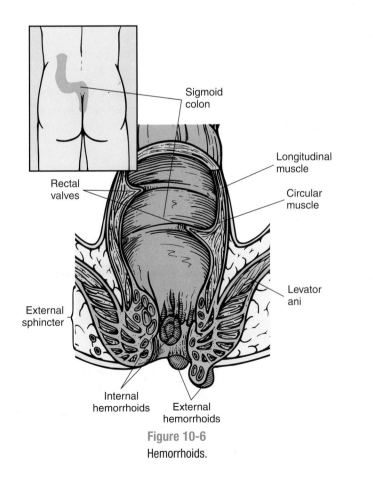

Sigmoid colon

Longitudinal muscle

Circular muscle

Rectal valves

Levator ani

External sphincter

Internal hemorrhoids

External hemorrhoids

Figure 10-6
Hemorrhoids.

peripheral arterial disease (PAD) (pe-RIF-er-al) (ar-TĒ-rē-al)	disease of the arteries, other than those of the heart and brain, that affects blood circulation, such as atherosclerosis and Raynaud disease. The most common symptom of peripheral atherosclerosis is intermittent claudication.
rheumatic fever (rū-MAT-ik)	an inflammatory disease, usually occurring in children and often after an upper respiratory tract streptococcal infection
rheumatic heart disease (rū-MAT-ik) (hart) (di-ZĒZ)	damage to the heart muscle or heart valves caused by one or more episodes of rheumatic fever
sickle cell anemia (SIK-el) (sel) (a-NĒ-mē-a)	a hereditary, chronic hemolytic disease characterized by crescent- or sickle-shaped red blood cells (incurable disease)
varicose veins (varicosities) (VAR-i-kōs) (vāns)	distended or tortuous veins usually found in the lower extremities (Figure 10-7)

Varicose Veins and Current Treatment

Varicose veins usually occur in the superficial veins of the legs, which return approximately 15% of the blood back to the heart. One-way valves in the veins help move the blood upward. When these valves fail, or the veins lose their elasticity, the blood flows backward, pools, and forms varicose veins. Approximately 80 million Americans, mostly women, have varicose veins or small, shallow spider veins. Causes are heredity, obesity, pregnancy, illness, or injury. Ligation and stripping was previously considered the primary surgical procedure for treatment.

Current Treatment

Ambulatory phlebectomy—Tiny punctures are made in the skin through which the varicose veins are pulled out. Local anesthetic is used, and the procedure is minimally invasive.

Sclerotherapy—Sclerotherapy takes less than an hour and requires no anesthesia. A solution is injected into the varicose vein and destroys it over several months. Sclerotherapy isn't effective on varicose veins that extend into the groin area.

Laser or intense pulsed light—This noninvasive technique is used to remove spider veins. The light causes the veins to shrink and collapse.

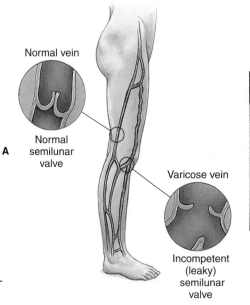

A

Normal vein

Normal semilunar valve

Varicose vein

Incompetent (leaky) semilunar valve

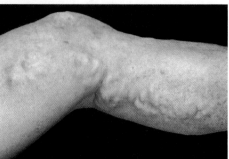

B

Figure 10-7

A, Normal and varicose veins. **B,** Appearance of varicose veins.

Practice saying each of these terms aloud. To hear the terms, access the **PRONOUNCE IT** activity for this chapter on the Student CD that accompanies this text. Or, to hear the terms and their definitions with a CD player or computer, obtain the Pronunciation CD designed for use with this text.

Learn the definitions and spellings of the disease and disorder terms by completing exercises 14 through 17.

EXERCISE 14

Fill in the blanks with the correct terms.

1. A congenital cardiac condition characterized by a narrowing of the aorta is called _____ of the aorta.

2. A blood clot or foreign material that enters the bloodstream and moves until it lodges at another point in the circulation is called a(n) _____.

3. Sudden cessation of cardiac output and effective circulation is referred to as a(n) _____ _____.

4. _____ heart disease is the name given to a heart abnormality present at birth.

5. Veins that are distended or tortuous are called _____ _____.

6. Obstruction of an artery of the heart, usually from atherosclerosis, is called a(n) _____ _____.

7. _____ is the name given to the ballooning of a weakened portion of an artery wall.

8. _____ disease is the name given to a malignant disorder of lymphatic tissue characterized by enlarged lymph nodes.

9. Varicose veins in the rectal area are called _____.

10. _____ _____ is a cardiac condition characterized by chest pain caused by an insufficient blood supply to the cardiac muscle.

11. Death of a portion of myocardial muscle caused by lack of oxygen resulting from an interrupted blood supply is called a(n) _____ _____.

12. The condition in which the atria or ventricles have rapid, quivering, noncoordinated contractions is called _____.

13. Any disturbance or abnormality in the heart's normal rhythmic pattern is called a(n) _____.

14. A disorder of the heart brought about by a persistently high blood pressure is called _____ heart disease.

15. _____ _____ _____ is the inability of the heart to pump enough blood through the body to supply tissues and organs.

16. _____ _____ _____ is a disease of the arteries that affects blood circulation.

17. _____ is an inherited bleeding disease most commonly caused by a deficiency of the coagulation factor VIII.

18. _____ is a disease in which the number of abnormal white blood cells formed in the bone marrow is excessively increased.

19. A reduction in the amount of hemoglobin in the red blood cells results in a condition known as _____.

20. A hereditary, chronic hemolytic disease in which the red blood cells are crescent shaped is called _____ _____ _____.

21. _____ _____ is a condition in which a patient has pain and discomfort in calf muscles while walking.

22. Acute compression of the heart caused by fluid accumulation in the pericardial cavity is known as _____ _____.

23. Episodes of rheumatic fever can cause _____ _____ _____ and _____ _____ _____.

24. _____ _____ _____ usually occurs in the deep veins of the lower extremities.

25. An inflammatory disease usually occurring in children is _____ _____.

26. _____ is an iron metabolism disorder.

27. _____ _____ _____ is insufficient blood supply to the heart, indicating unstable angina or myocardial infarction.

EXERCISE 15

Match the terms in the first column with the correct definitions in the second column.

_____ 1. anemia

_____ 2. aneurysm

_____ 3. angina pectoris

_____ 4. dysrhythmia

_____ 5. cardiac arrest

_____ 6. cardiac tamponade

_____ 7. coarctation of the aorta

_____ 8. congenital heart disease

_____ 9. congestive heart failure

_____ 10. coronary occlusion

_____ 11. intermittent claudication

_____ 12. deep vein thrombosis

a. sudden cessation of cardiac output and effective circulation

b. obstruction of an artery of the heart, usually from atherosclerosis

c. ballooning of a weak portion of an arterial wall

d. reduction of the amount of hemoglobin in the blood

e. any disturbance or abnormality in the heart's normal rhythmic pattern

f. chest pain occurring because of insufficient blood supply to the heart muscle

g. inability of the heart to pump enough blood through the body to supply tissues or organs

h. pain in calf muscles while walking

_____ 13. hemochromatosis

_____ 14. peripheral arterial disease

i. congenital cardiac condition with narrowing of the aorta

j. acute compression of the heart caused by fluid in the pericardial cavity

k. heart abnormality present at birth

l. clot in a deep vein

m. disease of the arteries, such as atherosclerosis, that affects blood circulation

n. may cause congestive heart failure, diabetes, or cirrhosis of the liver

EXERCISE 16

Match the terms in the first column with the correct definitions in the second column.

_____ 1. embolus

_____ 2. fibrillation

_____ 3. hemophilia

_____ 4. hemorrhoids

_____ 5. Hodgkin disease

_____ 6. hypertensive heart disease

_____ 7. leukemia

_____ 8. myocardial infarction

_____ 9. sickle cell anemia

_____ 10. acute coronary syndrome

_____ 11. varicose veins

_____ 12. mitral valve stenosis and rheumatic heart disease

_____ 13. rheumatic fever

a. inherited bleeding disease most commonly caused by a deficiency of the coagulation factor VIII

b. heart disorder brought on by persistent high blood pressure

c. distended or tortuous veins

d. excessive increase of abnormal white blood cells formed in the bone marrow

e. rapid, quivering, noncoordinated contractions of the atria or ventricles

f. caused by episodes of rheumatic fever

g. symptoms indicating unstable angina or myocardial infarction

h. varicose veins in the rectal area

i. blood clot or foreign material that enters the bloodstream and moves until it lodges at another point

j. malignant disorder of lymphatic tissue with enlargement of lymph nodes

k. death of a portion of myocardium caused by lack of oxygen resulting from an interrupted blood supply

l. chronic hemolytic disease having crescent-shaped blood cells

m. often follows an upper respiratory streptococcal infection

EXERCISE 17

Spell the disease and disorder terms. Have someone dictate the terms on pp. 326-328 to you. Study any words you have spelled incorrectly.

1. _____   15. _____

2. _____   16. _____

3. _____   17. _____

4. _____   18. _____

5. _____   19. _____

6. _____   20. _____

7. _____   21. _____

8. _____   22. _____

9. _____   23. _____

10. _____   24. _____

11. _____   25. _____

12. _____   26. _____

13. _____   27. _____

14. _____   28. _____

Surgical Terms
Built from Word Parts

Term	Definition
angioplasty .... (AN-jē-ō-plas-tē)	surgical repair of a blood vessel
angiorrhaphy .... (an-jē-OR-a-fē)	suturing of a blood vessel
atherectomy .... (ath-er-EK-tō-mē)	excision of fatty plaque (from a blocked artery using a specialized catheter and a rotary cutter)
endarterectomy .... (*end*-ar-ter-EK-tō-mē) (NOTE: the *o* from *endo-* is dropped for easier pronunciation.)	excision within the artery (excision of plaque from the arterial wall). This procedure is usually named for the artery to be cleaned out, such as carotid endarterectomy, which means removal of plaque from the wall of the carotid artery (Exercise Figure C).

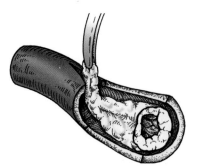

Exercise Figure C

Fill in the blanks to label the diagram.

_____ / _____ / _____
within / **artery** / **excision**

pericardiocentesis .... (par̄-i-kar-dē-ō-sen-TĒ-sis)	surgical puncture to aspirate fluid from (within) the outer sac of the heart (pericardium). (Used to treat cardiac tamponade.) (Figure 10-8)
phlebectomy................................. (fle-BEK-tō-mē)	excision of a vein
phlebotomy.................................. (fle-BOT-ō-mē)	incision into a vein (to remove blood or to give blood or intravenous fluids) (also called *venipuncture*)
splenectomy................................ (sple-NEK-tō-mē)	excision of the spleen
splenopexy.................................. (SPLE-nō-*peks-ē*)	surgical fixation of the spleen
thymectomy................................. (thī-MEK-tō-mē)	excision of the thymus gland

Practice saying each of these terms aloud. To hear the terms, access the **PRONOUNCE IT** activity for this chapter on the Student CD that accompanies this text. Or, to hear the terms and their definitions with a CD player or computer, obtain the Pronunciation CD designed for use with this text.

Learn the definitions and spellings of the surgical terms by completing exercises 18, 19, and 20.

EXERCISE   18

Analyze and define the following surgical terms.

1. pericardiocentesis _____

2. thymectomy _____

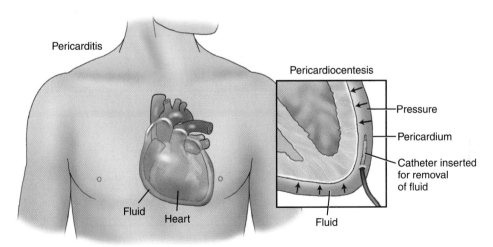

Figure 10-8

Pericarditis may produce excess fluid in the pericardium. If the fluid seriously affects the heart's ability to pump blood, pericardiocentesis may be performed to remove the fluid.

3. angioplasty _____

4. splenopexy _____

5. angiorrhaphy _____

6. endarterectomy _____

7. phlebotomy _____

8. splenectomy _____

9. phlebectomy _____

10. atherectomy _____

EXERCISE 19

Build surgical terms for the following definitions by using the word parts you have learned.

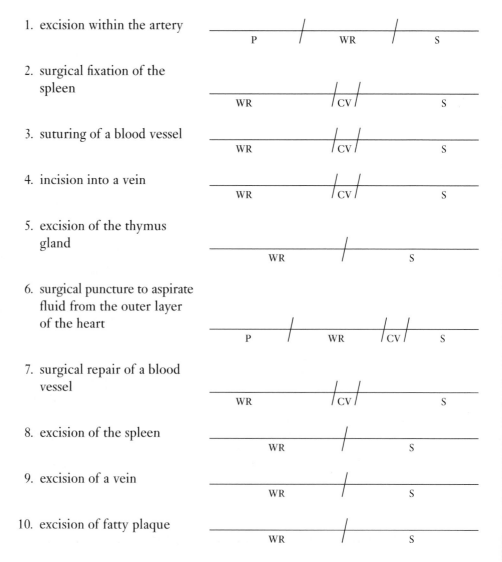

1. excision within the artery

    P   WR   S

2. surgical fixation of the spleen

    WR   CV   S

3. suturing of a blood vessel

    WR   CV   S

4. incision into a vein

    WR   CV   S

5. excision of the thymus gland

    WR   S

6. surgical puncture to aspirate fluid from the outer layer of the heart

    P   WR   CV   S

7. surgical repair of a blood vessel

    WR   CV   S

8. excision of the spleen

    WR   S

9. excision of a vein

    WR   S

10. excision of fatty plaque

    WR   S

EXERCISE 20

Spell each of the surgical terms. Have someone dictate the terms on pp. 332-333 to you. Think about the word parts before attempting to write the word. Study any words you have spelled incorrectly.

1. _____   6. _____

2. _____   7. _____

3. _____   8. _____

4. _____   9. _____

5. _____   10. _____

Surgical Terms

Not Built from Word Parts

Term	Definition
aneurysmectomy................................. (*an*-ū-riz-MEK-tō-mē)	surgical excision of an aneurysm
bone marrow transplant.................... (bōn) (MAR-ō) (TRANS-plant)	infusion of normal bone marrow cells from a donor with matching cells and tissue to a recipient with a certain type of leukemia or anemia
cardiac pacemaker............................ (KAR-dē-ak) (pās-MĀK-r)	battery-powered or nuclear-powered apparatus implanted under the skin to regulate the heart rate (Figure 10-9)

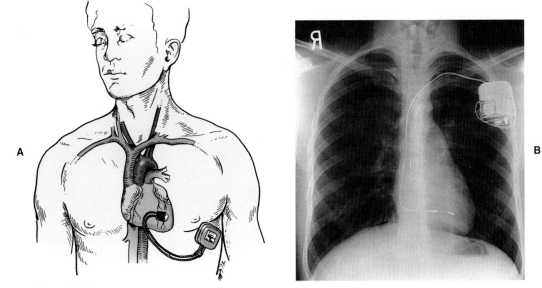

A, Cardiac pacemaker. **B,** Chest radiograph of a patient with a cardiac pacemaker.

Figure 10-9

coronary artery bypass graft (CABG) .... surgical technique to bring a new blood supply to heart muscle by detouring around blocked arteries (Figure 10-10)
(KOR-ō-na-rē)
(AR-ter-ē) (BĪ-pas) (graft)

coronary stent .... a supportive scaffold device implanted in the coronary artery. Used to prevent closure of the artery after angioplasty or atherectomy (Figure 10-11).
(KOR-ō-na-rē) (stent)

defibrillation .... application of an electric shock to the myocardium through the chest wall to restore normal cardiac rhythm (Figure 10-12)
(dē-fib-ri-LĀ-shun)

embolectomy .... excision of an embolus or clot
(em-bō-LEK-tō-mē)

femoropopliteal bypass .... surgery to establish an alternate route from femoral artery to popliteal artery to bypass an obstruction (Figure 10-13)
(FEM-or-ō-pop-li-TĒ-al)

hemorrhoidectomy .... excision of hemorrhoids, the varicosed veins in the rectal region
(hem-ō-royd-EK-tō-mē)

implantable cardiac defibrillator .... a device implanted in the body that continuously monitors the heart rhythm. If life-threatening dysrhythmias occur the device delivers an electric shock to convert the dysrhythmia back to a normal rhythm (Figure 10-14).
(im-PLANT-a-bl)
(KAR-dē-ak)
(de-FIB-ri-lā-tōr)

intracoronary thrombolytic therapy .... an injection of an intravenous medication to dissolve blood clots in coronary (blood) vessels
(in-tra-KOR-ō-na-rē)
(throm-BŌ-li-tik) (THER-a-pē)

laser angioplasty .... the use of *l*ight *a*mplification by *s*timulated *e*mission of *r*adiation (laser beam) to open blocked arteries, especially in lower extremities
(LĀ-zer) (AN-jē-ō-*plas*-tē)

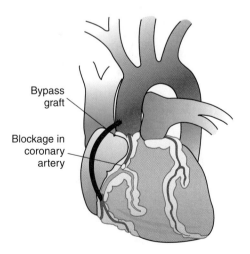

Figure 10-10
Coronary artery bypass graft.

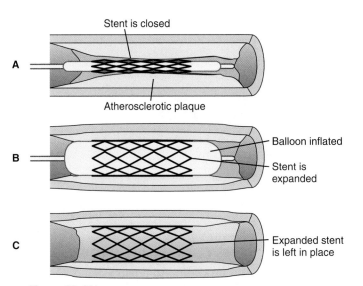

Figure 10-11
Coronary stent. **A,** Stent at the site of plaque formation. **B,** Inflated balloon and expanded stent. **C,** Implanted stent with balloon removed.

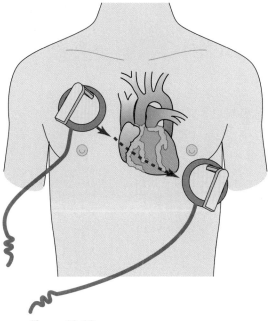

Figure 10-12
Placement of defibrillator paddles on the chest.

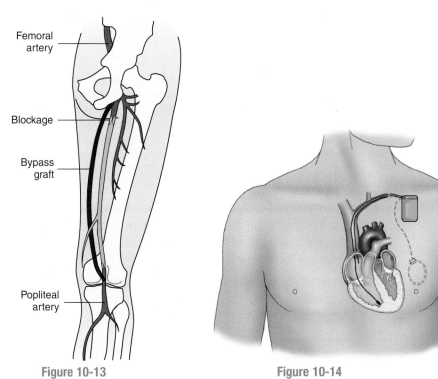

Figure 10-13
Femoropopliteal bypass.

Figure 10-14
An implantable cardiac defibrillator.

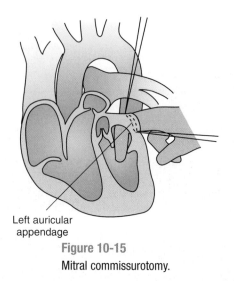

Left auricular
appendage

Figure 10-15
Mitral commissurotomy.

mitral commissurotomy.................... (MĪ-tral) (*kom*-i-shūr-OT-ō-mē)	surgical procedure to repair a stenosed mitral valve by breaking apart the leaves (commissures) of the valve (Figure 10-15)
percutaneous transluminal coronary angioplasty (PTCA)........... (*per*-kū-TA-nē-us) (trans-LUM-in-al) (KOR-ō-na-rē) (AN-jē-ō-*plas*-tē)	procedure in which a balloon is passed through a blood vessel into a coronary artery to the area where plaque is formed. Inflation of the balloon compresses the plaque against the vessel wall, expanding the inner diameter of the blood vessel, which allows the blood to circulate more freely (also called *balloon angioplasty*) (Figure 10-16).

Thrombolytic Therapy for Myocardial Infarction

Intracoronary thrombolytic therapy is the administration of a medication that breaks blood clots apart (thrombolysis) before they become hardened. It is used in the treatment of myocardial infarction in emergency departments and is administered immediately after the diagnosis is made. The drugs, such as streptokinase, t-PA (Activase), or recombinant tissue plasminogen activator (rTPA) (reteplase), are administered intravenously. The greatest benefit occurs when the drug is administered 3 to 6 hours after the myocardial infarction. Thrombolytic therapy restores blood flow and is known to reduce mortality rate, preserve the myocardium, and restore ventricular function.

Practice saying each of these terms aloud. To hear the terms, access the **PRONOUNCE IT** activity for this chapter on the Student CD that accompanies this text. Or, to hear the terms and their definitions with a CD player or computer, obtain the Pronunciation CD designed for use with this text.

Learn the definitions and spellings of these surgical terms by completing exercises 21, 22, and 23.

EXERCISE 21

1. Surgical excision of hemorrhoids is called a(n) _____.

2. The procedure in which a balloon is passed through a blood vessel into a coronary artery (where plaque is formed) to compress plaque against the

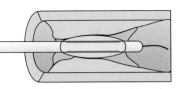

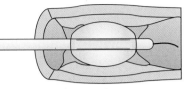

A

Balloon catheter positioned
in stenotic area

Inflated balloon presses
plaque against arterial wall
expanding the size of
vessel opening

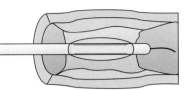

Balloon is deflated and
blood flow reestablished

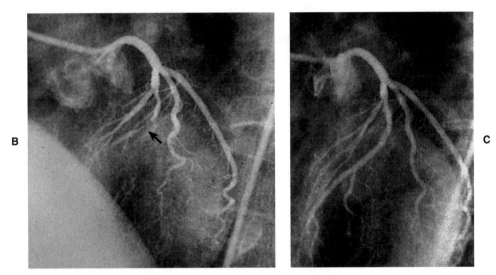

B

C

Figure 10-16

Percutaneous transluminal coronary angioplasty. **A,** Balloon dilation. **B,** Coronary arteriogram before PTCA. The *arrow* indicates the stenotic area, estimated at 95% minimum blood flow distal to the lesion. **C,** Coronary arteriogram after PTCA in the same patient. Blood flow is estimated to be 100%.

vessel wall when the balloon is inflated is called _____
_____ _____ _____.

3. To regulate the heart rate, the physician may insert a(n) _____
_____ under the patient's skin.

4. A mitral _____ is the name of the surgery performed to repair a stenosed mitral valve.

5. The surgery performed to detour blood around a blocked artery so that a new blood supply can be given to heart muscles is called _____
_____ _____ _____.

6. The surgical excision of an aneurysm is called a(n) _____.

7. A(n) _____ _____ is the name of the surgery performed to establish an alternate route from femoral artery to popliteal artery to bypass an obstruction.

8. _____ _____ is the name of the procedure to open blocked arteries with a laser beam.

9. An injection of a medication in a blocked coronary vessel to dissolve blood clots is called _____ _____ therapy.

10. _____ is the application of electric shock to the myocardium through the chest wall to restore cardiac rhythm.

11. _____ _____ _____ is a procedure to transfuse bone marrow cells to a recipient from a donor with matching tissue and cells.

12. _____ is the excision of an embolus, or clot.

13. A supportive scaffold device used to prevent closure of a coronary artery is called a _____ _____.

14. _____ _____ _____ is used to treat life-threatening dysrhythmias.

EXERCISE 22

Match the terms in the first column with their correct definitions in the second column.

_____ 1. aneurysmectomy

_____ 2. coronary artery bypass graft

_____ 3. femoropopliteal bypass

_____ 4. hemorrhoidectomy

_____ 5. cardiac pacemaker

_____ 6. mitral commissurotomy

_____ 7. percutaneous transluminal coronary angioplasty

_____ 8. defibrillation

_____ 9. laser angioplasty

_____ 10. bone marrow transplant

_____ 11. intracoronary thrombolytic therapy

_____ 12. embolectomy

_____ 13. coronary stent

_____ 14. implantable cardiac defibrillator

a. compressing plaque against a blood vessel wall by inflating a balloon passed through the blood vessel

b. use of medication to dissolve blood clots in a blocked coronary vessel

c. application of electric shock to the myocardium through the chest wall to restore cardiac rhythm

d. apparatus implanted under the skin to regulate the heartbeat

e. procedure performed to open blocked arteries with a laser beam

f. monitors and corrects heart rhythms

g. supportive scaffold device implanted in an artery

h. excision of a weakened, ballooning blood vessel wall

i. normal bone marrow cells infused from a donor with matching tissues and cells into a recipient with leukemia

j. excision of an embolus

k. surgical procedure to establish an alternate route from the femoral artery to the popliteal artery to bypass an obstruction

l. surgical excision of varicose veins in the rectal area

m. surgical procedure to break apart the leaves of the mitral valve

n. surgical removal of a thickened artery

o. diverts blood past a blocked artery in the heart

EXERCISE   23

Spell each of the surgical terms. Have someone dictate the terms on pp. 335-336 and 338 to you. Study any words you have spelled incorrectly.

1. _____   8. _____

2. _____   9. _____

3. _____   10. _____

4. _____   11. _____

5. _____   12. _____

6. _____   13. _____

7. _____   14. _____

Diagnostic Terms

Built from Word Parts

Term	Definition
Heart and Blood Vessels	
Diagnostic Imaging	
angiography................................ (an-jē-OG-ra-fē)	x-ray imaging of a blood vessel (after an injection of contrast medium; the procedure is named for the vessel to be studied, for example, *femoral angiography*)
angioscope................................ (AN-jē-ō-skōp)	instrument used for visual examination of a blood vessel
angioscopy................................ (an-jē-OS-kō-pē)	visual examination of a blood vessel
aortogram................................ (ā-OR-tō-gram)	x-ray image of the aorta (after an injection of contrast medium)
arteriogram................................ (ar-TE-rē-ō-gram)	x-ray image of an artery (after an injection of contrast medium) (Figure 10-17)
venogram................................ (VĒ-nō-gram)	x-ray image of a vein (after an injection of contrast medium) (Figure 10-18)
venography................................ (vē-NOG-ra-fē)	x-ray imaging of a vein (after an injection of contrast medium)
Cardiovascular Procedures	
echocardiogram (ECHO).................... (ek-ō-KAR-dē-ō-gram)	record of the heart (structure and motion) using sound. Used to detect valvular disease and evaluate the heart during stress testing.
electrocardiogram **(ECG, EKG)**................................ (e-*lek*-trō-KAR-dē-ō-gram)	record of the electrical activity of the heart (Exercise Figure D)

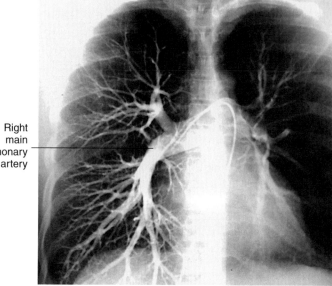

Right
main
pulmonary
artery

Figure 10-17

Arteriogram showing the right main pulmonary artery. This procedure (arteriography) involves injection of contrast material.

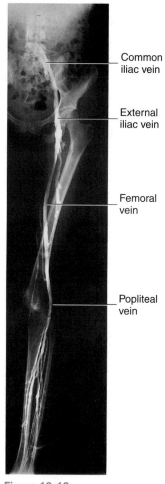

Common
iliac vein

External
iliac vein

Femoral
vein

Popliteal
vein

Figure 10-18

Normal venogram, lower left limb.

electrocardiograph .... instrument used to record the electrical activity of the heart
(e-*lek*-trō-KAR-dē-ō-graf)

electrocardiography .... process of recording the electrical activity of the heart
(e-*lek*-trō-*kar*-dē-OG-ra-fē)

Blood and Lymphatic Systems

Laboratory

erythrocyte count (RBC) .... red cell count (number of red blood cells per cubic millimeter of blood)
(e-RITH-rō-sīt)

hematocrit (HCT) .... separated blood (volume percentage of erythrocytes in whole blood after separation by centrifuge)
(hē-MAT-ō-krit)

leukocyte count (WBC) .... white cell count (number of white blood cells per cubic millimeter of blood)
(LŪ-kō-sīt)

Diagnostic Imaging

lymphangiography .... x-ray imaging of the lymphatic vessels (after an injection of contrast medium)
(lim-*fan*-jē-OG-ra-fē)

Lead II

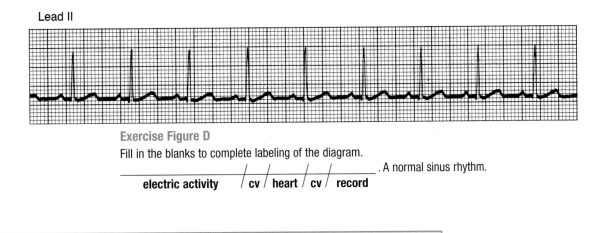

Exercise Figure D

Fill in the blanks to complete labeling of the diagram.

_____ / cv / heart / cv / record . A normal sinus rhythm.

electric activity

Lymphangiography is being replaced by CT scanning but is still used to determine the extent of lymphoma metastasis or to evaluate radiation therapy or chemotherapy.

Practice saying each of these words aloud. To hear the terms, access the **PRONOUNCE IT** activity for this chapter on the Student CD that accompanies this text. Or, to hear the terms and their definitions with a CD player or computer, obtain the Pronunciation CD designed for use with this text.

Learn the definitions and spellings of the diagnostic terms by completing exercises 24, 25, and 26.

EXERCISE 24

Analyze and define the following diagnostic terms.

1. electrocardiograph _____

2. venogram _____

3. angiography _____

4. echocardiogram _____

5. aortogram _____

6. electrocardiogram _____

7. arteriogram _____

8. electrocardiography _____

9. erythrocyte count _____

10. hematocrit _____

11. leukocyte count _____

12. lymphangiography _____

13. angioscopy_____

14. venography _____

15. angioscope_____

EXERCISE 25

Build diagnostic terms that correspond to the following definitions by using the word parts you have learned.

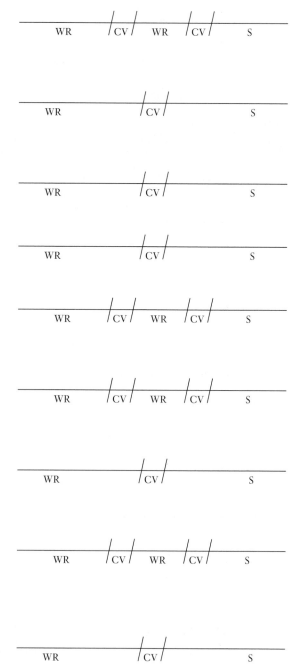

1. instrument used to record the electrical activity of the heart

    _____ / CV / WR / CV / _____
    WR   WR   S

2. x-ray image of an artery (after an injection of contrast medium)

    _____ / CV / _____
    WR   S

3. x-ray image of a vein (after an injection of contrast medium)

    _____ / CV / _____
    WR   S

4. x-ray imaging of a blood vessel

    _____ / CV / _____
    WR   S

5. record of the electrical activity of the heart

    _____ / CV / WR / CV / _____
    WR   WR   S

6. record of the heart (structure and motion) by using sound

    _____ / CV / WR / CV / _____
    WR   WR   S

7. x-ray image of the aorta (after an injection of contrast medium)

    _____ / CV / _____
    WR   S

8. process of recording the electrical activity of the heart

    _____ / CV / WR / CV / _____
    WR   WR   S

9. separated blood (volume percentage of erythrocytes in whole blood after separation by centrifuge)

    _____ / CV / _____
    WR   S

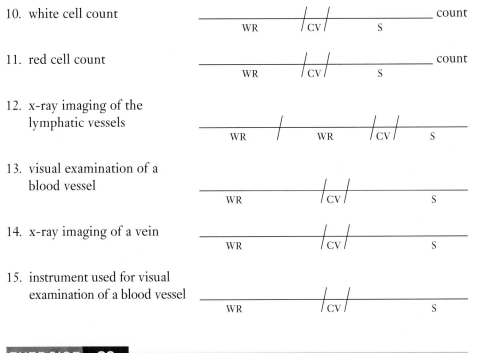

10. white cell count

    WR   CV   S   count

11. red cell count

    WR   CV   S   count

12. x-ray imaging of the lymphatic vessels

    WR   WR   CV   S

13. visual examination of a blood vessel

    WR   CV   S

14. x-ray imaging of a vein

    WR   CV   S

15. instrument used for visual examination of a blood vessel

    WR   CV   S

EXERCISE 26

Spell each of the diagnostic terms. Have someone dictate the terms on pp. 341-342 to you. Think about the word parts before attempting to write the word. Study any words you have spelled incorrectly.

1. _____   9. _____

2. _____   10. _____

3. _____   11. _____

4. _____   12. _____

5. _____   13. _____

6. _____   14. _____

7. _____   15. _____

8. _____

Diagnostic Terms

Not Built from Word Parts

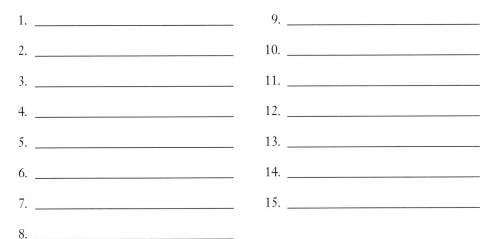

Term	Definition
Heart and Blood Vessels	
Diagnostic Imaging	
digital subtraction angiography (DSA)........................ (DIJ-it-l) (sub-TRAK-shun) (an-jē-OG-ra-fē)	a process of digital x-ray imaging of the blood vessels that "subtracts" or removes structures not being studied

> **Digital Subtraction Angiography**
> First an image is taken and stored in the computer, then contrast medium is injected into the artery or vein. A second image is taken and stored in the computer. The computer compares the two images and subtracts the first image from the second, removing structures not being studied. DSA enables better visualization of the arteries than regular angiography (Figure 10-19).

Chemical Stress Testing is the use of drugs to simulate the stress of physical exercise in the body. It is used to study patients who are unable to exercise.

Doppler ultrasound...............
(DOP-ler) (UL-tra-sound)

a study that uses sound for detection of blood flow within the vessels. Used to assess intermittent claudication, deep vein thrombosis, and other blood flow abnormalities (Figure 10-20).

exercise stress test...........
(EK-ser-sīz) (stres) (test)

a study that evaluates cardiac function during physical stress by riding a bike or walking on a treadmill. Electrocardiography, echocardiography, and nuclear medicine scanning are three types of tests performed to measure cardiac function while exercising. Echocardiography is fast becoming the preferred choice of testing over electrocardiography.

single-photon emission computed tomography (SPECT)..........
(SING-el-fō-ton) (Ē-mis-on)
(com-PŪ-td)
(tō-MOG-ra-fē)

a nuclear medicine scan that visualizes the heart from several different angles. A tracer substance such as sestamibi or thallium is injected intravenously. The SPECT scanner creates images from the tracer absorbed by the body tissues. It is used to assess damage to cardiac tissue (Figure 10-21).

thallium test...........
(THĀL-ē-um) (test)

a nuclear medicine test used to diagnose coronary artery disease and assess revascularization after coronary artery bypass surgery. Thallium, a radioactive isotope, is injected

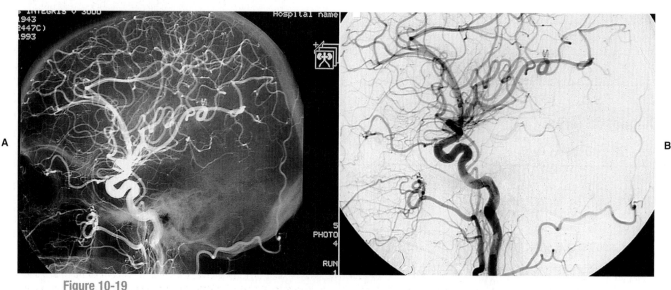

Figure 10-19

Digital subtraction angiography. **A,** Lateral digital *nonsubtracted* carotid artery. **B,** Lateral digital *subtracted* carotid artery.

thallium test—cont'd

into the body intravenously; a radiation detector is placed over the heart and images are recorded. Thallium is taken up by the normal myocardial cells, but not in ischemia or infarction. These areas are identified as "cold" spots on the images produced. Thallium testing can be performed when the patient is at rest or it can be part of a stress test.

transesophageal echocardiogram (TEE)..

(trans-e-sof-a-JĒ-al)
(ek-ō-KAR-dē-ō-gram)

an ultrasound test that examines cardiac function and structure by using an ultrasound probe placed in the esophagus, which provides views of the heart structures

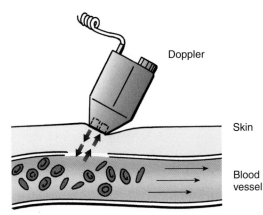

Doppler

Skin

Blood vessel

Figure 10-20

Doppler ultrasound showing the red blood cells reflecting sound.

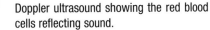

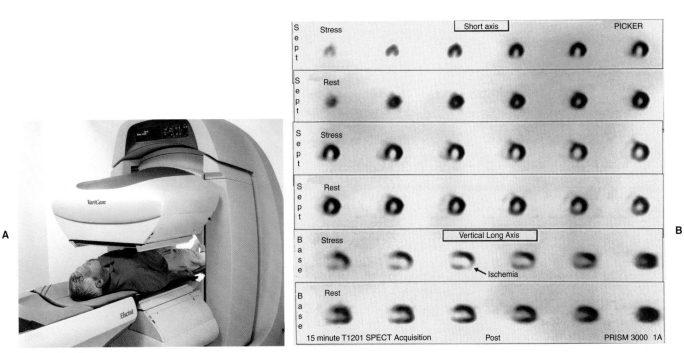

Figure 10-21

A, Single-photon emission computed tomography (SPECT) camera system. **B,** Thallium-201 myocardial perfusion scan comparing stress and redistribution (resting) images in various planes of the heart (short axis and long axis). A perfusion defect is identified in the stress images but not seen in the redistribution (rest) images. This finding is indicative of ischemia.

Stethoscope
is a term derived from the Greek **stethos,** meaning **chest,** and **scopeo,** meaning **to view** or **examine.** It means **to see** what is in the body by listening to the body sounds. The stethoscope was first called a **baton** or **cylinder.**

Cardiovascular Studies

cardiac catheterization.....................
(KAR-dē-ak)
(*kath*-e-ter-i-ZĀ-shun)

an examination to determine the condition of the heart and surrounding blood vessels. A catheter is passed into the heart through a blood vessel and is used to record pressures and inject a contrast medium, enabling the visualization of the great vessels and the heart chambers. Used most frequently to evaluate chest pain and coronary artery disease (Figure 10-24).

impedance plethysmography (IPG)...
(im-PĒD-ans)
(pleth-iz-MOG-rā-fē)

measures venous flow of the extremities with a plethysmograph to detect clots by measuring changes in blood volume and resistance (impedance) in the vein. Used to detect deep vein thrombosis.

Other

sphygmomanometer............................
(*sfig*-mō-ma-NOM-e-ter)

device used for measuring blood pressure (Figure 10-22)

stethoscope...
(STETH-ō-scope)

an instrument used to hear sounds produced by the heart, lungs, and bowels

Blood and Lymphatic Systems

Laboratory

coagulation time...................................
(kō-ag-ū-LĀ-shun)

blood test to determine the time it takes for blood to form a clot

complete blood count (CBC).............

basic blood screening that includes tests on hemoglobin, hematocrit, red blood cell morphology (size and shape), leukocyte count, and white blood cell differential (types of WBCs)

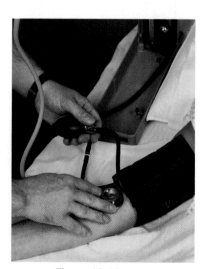

Figure 10-22
Sphygmomanometer.

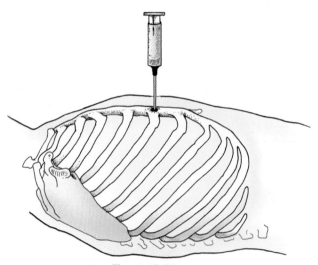

Figure 10-23
Bone marrow for biopsy.

hemoglobin (Hgb)..............................
(HĒ-mō-glō-bin)

blood test used to determine the concentration of oxygen-carrying components (hemoglobin) in red blood cells

prothrombin time (PT)..........................
(prō-THROM-bin)

blood test used to determine certain coagulation activity defects and to monitor anticoagulation therapy for patients taking Coumadin, an oral anticoagulant medication. (Activated partial thromboplastin time [PTT] is used to monitor anticoagulation therapy for patients taking heparin, an intravenous anticoagulant medication.)

Other

bone marrow biopsy...........................

needle puncture to remove bone marrow for study, usually from the sternum or ilium. Used to diagnose blood cell diseases, such as leukemia and anemia (Figure 10-23).

Practice saying each of these terms aloud. To hear the terms, access the **PRONOUNCE IT** activity for this chapter on the Student CD that accompanies this text. Or, to hear the terms and their definitions with a CD player or computer, obtain the Pronunciation CD designed for use with this text.

Learn the definitions and spellings of these procedural terms by completing exercises 27, 28, and 29.

EXERCISE 27

Fill in the blanks with the correct terms.

1. A device for measuring blood pressure is called a(n) _____.

2. _____ _____ is a blood test that determines the time it takes for blood to form a clot.

3. _____ _____ _____ is the name of a basic blood-screening test.

4. A study that uses sound for detection of blood flow within blood vessels is called _____ _____.

5. _____ is an instrument used to hear heart, lung, and bowel sounds.

6. _____ _____ _____ is used to diagnose blood diseases such as leukemia.

7. A blood test used to determine certain coagulation activity defects and to monitor oral anticoagulation therapy is called _____ _____.

8. _____ _____ is a procedure in which a catheter is introduced into the heart to record pressure and enable the visualization of the heart chambers.

9. A blood test used to determine the oxygen-carrying component in the red blood cells is called _____.

10. _____ _____ measures venous flow of the extremities.

11. A nuclear medicine test used to diagnose coronary artery disease is _____ _____.

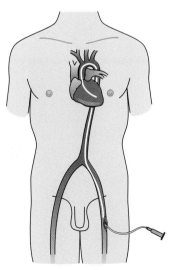

Figure 10-24
Cardiac catherization.

12. _____ _____ is a test in which an ultrasound probe provides views of the heart structures from the esophagus.

13. A nuclear medicine test that visualizes the heart from different angles is called a(n) _____ _____

    _____ _____.

14. _____ _____ _____ evaluates cardiac function during physical stress.

15. A process of x-ray imaging of blood vessels that removes structures not being studied is called _____ _____ _____.

EXERCISE 28

Match the terms in the first column with their correct definition in the second column.

_____ 1. cardiac catheterization

_____ 2. stethoscope

_____ 3. complete blood count

_____ 4. coagulation time

_____ 5. hemoglobin

_____ 6. Doppler ultrasound

_____ 7. prothrombin time

_____ 8. sphygmomanometer

_____ 9. bone marrow biopsy

_____ 10. digital subtraction angiography

_____ 11. thallium test

_____ 12. transesophageal echocardiogram

_____ 13. single-photon emission computed tomography

_____ 14. exercise stress test

_____ 15. impedance plethysmography

a. device used for measuring blood pressure

b. procedure using echocardiography, electrocardiography, or nuclear medicine scanning

c. test to determine certain coagulation activity defects

d. passage of a catheter into the heart to evaluate coronary artery disease

e. visualizes the heart from several different angles

f. used to assess revascularization after CABG

g. oxygen-carrying component of the red blood cell

h. basic blood-screening test

i. an ultrasound test that provides views of the heart from the esophagus

j. study in which sound is used to determine the flow of blood within the vessels

k. used to diagnose certain blood cell diseases, such as leukemia

l. test to determine the number of red blood cells

m. measures venous flow of the extremities

n. used to hear heart, lung, and bowel sounds

o. determines the time it takes for blood to form a clot

p. digital x-ray imaging of blood vessels

EXERCISE 29

Spell each of the diagnostic terms. Have someone dictate the terms on pp. 345-349 to you. Study any words you have spelled incorrectly.

1. _____   9. _____

2. _____   10. _____

3. _____   11. _____

4. _____   12. _____

5. _____   13. _____

6. _____   14. _____

7. _____   15. _____

8. _____

Complementary Terms

Built from Word Parts

Term	Definition
atrioventricular (AV) (ā-trē-ō-ven-TRIK-ū-ler)	pertaining to the atrium and ventricle
cardiac (KAR-dē-ak)	pertaining to the heart
cardiogenic (*kar*-dē-ō-JEN-ik)	originating in the heart
cardiologist (*kar*-dē-OL-ō-jist)	physician who studies and treats diseases of the heart
cardiology (*kar*-dē-OL-ō-jē)	study of the heart (a branch of medicine that deals with diseases of the heart and blood vessels)
hematologist (*hē*-ma-TOL-ō-jist)	physician who studies and treats diseases of the blood
hematology (*hē*-ma-TOL-ō-jē)	study of the blood (a branch of medicine that deals with diseases of the blood)
hematopoiesis (*hē*-ma-tō-poy-Ē-sis)	formation of blood (cells)
hemolysis (*hē*-MOL-i-sis)	dissolution of (red) blood (cells)
hemostasis (*hē*-mō-STĀ-sis)	stoppage of bleeding
hypothermia (*hī*-pō-THER-mē-a)	condition of (body) temperature that is below (normal sometimes induced for various surgical procedures, such as bypass surgery)

intravenous (IV).................................... (in-tra-VĒ-nus)	pertaining to within the vein
plasmapheresis.................................... (plaz-ma-fe-RĒ-sis)	removal of plasma (from withdrawn blood)
tachypnea.. (tak-IP-nē-a)	rapid breathing
thrombolysis.. (throm-BOL-i-sis)	dissolution of a clot

Practice saying each of these terms aloud. To hear the terms, access the **PRONOUNCE IT** activity for this chapter on the Student CD that accompanies this text. Or, to hear the terms and their definitions with a CD player or computer, obtain the Pronunciation CD designed for use with this text.

Learn the definitions and spellings of the complementary terms by completing exercises 30, 31, and 32.

EXERCISE   30

Analyze and define the following complementary terms.

1. hypothermia _____

2. hematopoiesis _____

3. cardiology _____

4. cardiologist _____

5. hemolysis _____

6. hematologist _____

7. cardiac _____

8. hematology _____

9. plasmapheresis _____

10. hemostasis _____

11. cardiogenic _____

12. tachypnea _____

13. thrombolysis _____

14. atrioventricular _____

15. intravenous _____

EXERCISE 31

Build the complementary terms for the following definitions by using the word parts you have learned.

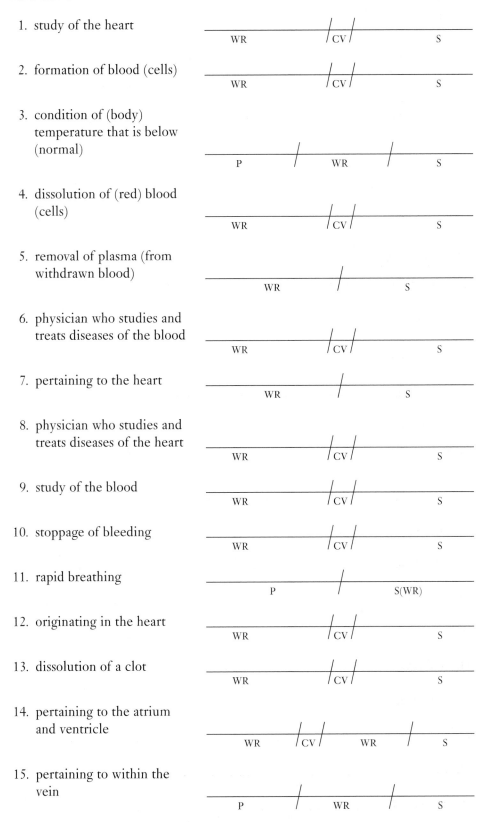

1. study of the heart
   WR / CV / S

2. formation of blood (cells)
   WR / CV / S

3. condition of (body) temperature that is below (normal)
   P / WR / S

4. dissolution of (red) blood (cells)
   WR / CV / S

5. removal of plasma (from withdrawn blood)
   WR / S

6. physician who studies and treats diseases of the blood
   WR / CV / S

7. pertaining to the heart
   WR / S

8. physician who studies and treats diseases of the heart
   WR / CV / S

9. study of the blood
   WR / CV / S

10. stoppage of bleeding
    WR / CV / S

11. rapid breathing
    P / S(WR)

12. originating in the heart
    WR / CV / S

13. dissolution of a clot
    WR / CV / S

14. pertaining to the atrium and ventricle
    WR / CV / WR / S

15. pertaining to within the vein
    P / WR / S

EXERCISE 32

Spell each of the complementary terms. Have someone dictate the terms on pp. 351-352 to you. Think about the word parts before attempting to write the word. Study any words you have spelled incorrectly.

1. _____   9. _____

2. _____   10. _____

3. _____   11. _____

4. _____   12. _____

5. _____   13. _____

6. _____   14. _____

7. _____   15. _____

8. _____

Complementary Terms

Not Built from Word Parts

Term	Definition
Heart and Blood Vessels	
auscultation	hearing sounds within the body through a stethoscope
(*aws*-kul-TĀ-shun)	
blood pressure (BP)	pressure exerted by the blood against the blood vessel walls. A blood pressure measurement written as systolic pressure (120)/diastolic pressure (80) is commonly recorded as 120/80 (see Figure 10-22).
cardiopulmonary resuscitation (CPR)	emergency procedure consisting of artificial ventilation and external cardiac massage
(*kar*-dē-ō-PUL-mō-nar-ē) (rē-*sus*-i-TĀ-shun)	

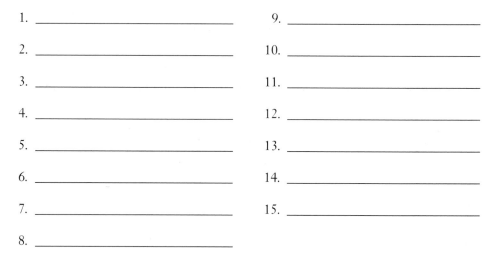

New Blood Pressure Guidelines
In 2003 the National Heart, Lung, and Blood Institute recommended new guidelines for measurements. They are:

$$\text{Normal: } \leq \frac{120}{80}$$

$$\text{Prehypertension: } \frac{120\text{-}139}{80\text{-}89}$$

$$\text{Stage 1 Hypertension: } \frac{140\text{-}159}{90\text{-}99}$$

$$\text{Stage 2 Hypertension: } \geq \frac{160}{100}$$

diastole (dī-AS-tō-lē)	phase in the cardiac cycle in which the ventricles relax between contractions (diastolic is the lower number of a blood pressure reading)
extracorporeal (*ek*-stra-kōr-PŌ-rē-al)	occurring outside the body. During open-heart surgery extracorporeal circulation occurs when blood is diverted outside the body to a heart-lung machine.
extravasation (eks-trav-a-SĀ-shun)	escape of blood from the blood vessel into the tissue
heart murmur (MER-mer)	a short-duration humming sound of cardiac or vascular origin
hypertension (*hī*-per-TEN-shun)	blood pressure that is above normal (greater than 140/90)
hypotension (*hī*-pō-TEN-shun)	blood pressure that is below normal (less than 90/60)
lumen (LŪ-men)	space within a tubular part or organ, such as the space within a blood vessel
occlude (o-KLŪD)	to close tightly, to block
percussion (per-KUSH-un)	tapping of a body surface with the fingers to determine the density of the part beneath (Figure 10-25)
systole (SIS-tō-lē)	phase in the cardiac cycle in which the ventricles contract (systolic is the upper number of a blood pressure reading)
vasoconstrictor (*vās*-ō-kon-STRIK-tor)	agent or nerve that narrows the blood vessels
vasodilator (*vās*-ō-DĪ-lā-tor)	agent or nerve that enlarges the blood vessels
venipuncture (VEN-i-*punk*-chūr)	puncture of a vein to remove blood, instill a medication, or start an intravenous infusion

Blood and Lymphatic Systems

anticoagulant (*an*-ti-kō-AG-ū-lant)	agent that slows the clotting process
dyscrasia (dis-KRĀ-zhē-a)	abnormal or pathologic condition of the blood
hemorrhage (HEM-or-ij)	rapid flow of blood
plasma (PLAZ-ma)	liquid portion of the blood in which elements or cells are suspended and that contains some of the clotting factors
serum (SER-um)	liquid portion of the blood without the clotting factors

Practice saying each of these terms aloud. To hear the terms, access the **PRONOUNCE IT** activity for this chapter on the Student CD that accompanies this text. Or, to hear the terms and their definitions with a CD player or computer, obtain the Pronunciation CD designed for use with this text.

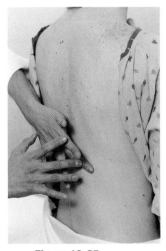

Figure 10-25
Percussion technique.

Learn the definitions and spellings of these complementary terms by completing exercises 33, 34, and 35.

EXERCISE 33

Write the term for each of the following definitions.

1. agent that narrows the blood vessels _____

2. space within a tubelike structure _____

3. emergency procedure consisting of artificial ventilation and external cardiac massage _____ _____

4. phase in the cardiac cycle in which the ventricles relax _____

5. pressure exerted by blood against blood vessel walls _____ _____

6. blood pressure that is below normal _____

7. escape of blood from the blood vessel into the tissue _____

8. puncture of a vein to remove blood _____

9. phase in the cardiac cycle in which the ventricles contract _____

10. agent that enlarges the blood vessels _____

11. blood pressure that is above normal _____

12. to close tightly _____

13. tapping of a body surface with the fingers to determine the density of the part beneath _____

14. listening to sounds within the body through a stethoscope _____

15. liquid portion of the blood
    that contains clotting factors   _____

16. rapid flow of blood   _____

17. agent that slows the
    clotting process   _____

18. liquid portion of the blood
    without the clotting factors   _____

19. pathologic condition of the
    blood   _____

20. a humming sound of
    cardiac or vascular origin   _____   _____

21. occurring outside the body   _____

EXERCISE 34

Write the definitions of the following terms.

1. lumen   _____

2. extravasation   _____

3. blood pressure   _____

4. venipuncture   _____

5. vasodilator   _____

6. hypertension   _____

7. cardiopulmonary resuscitation   _____

8. systole   _____

9. hypotension   _____

10. vasoconstrictor   _____

11. diastole   _____

12. auscultation   _____

13. occlude   _____

14. percussion   _____

15. serum   _____

16. dyscrasia   _____

17. plasma _____

18. hemorrhage _____

19. anticoagulant _____

20. extracorporeal _____

21. heart murmur _____

EXERCISE 35

Spell each of the complementary terms. Have someone dictate the terms on pp. 354-355 to you. Study any words you have spelled incorrectly.

1. _____   12. _____

2. _____   13. _____

3. _____   14. _____

4. _____   15. _____

5. _____   16. _____

6. _____   17. _____

7. _____   18. _____

8. _____   19. _____

9. _____   20. _____

10. _____   21. _____

11. _____

Abbreviations

ACS	acute coronary syndrome
AV	atrioventricular
BP	blood pressure
CABG	coronary artery bypass graft
CAD	coronary artery disease
CBC	complete blood count
CCU	coronary care unit
CHF	congestive heart failure
CPR	cardiopulmonary resuscitation
DSA	digital subtraction angiography
DVT	deep vein thrombosis

ECG, EKG	electrocardiogram
ECHO	echocardiogram
HCT	hematocrit
Hgb	hemoglobin
HHD	hypertensive heart disease
IPG	impedance plethysmography
IV	intravenous
MI	myocardial infarction
PAD	peripheral arterial disease
PT	prothrombin time
PTCA	percutaneous transluminal coronary angioplasty
RBC	red blood cell (erythrocyte)
SPECT	single-photon emission computed tomography
TEE	transesophageal echocardiogram
WBC	white blood cell (leukocyte)

Refer to Appendix D for a complete list of abbreviations.

EXERCISE 36

Write the meaning of the abbreviation in the blanks.

1. **CAD** _____ _____ _____ has received growing interest over the past 20 years. Diagnostic procedures for new patients usually begin with an exercise **ECG** _____. Patients whose stress tests are borderline usually proceed to noninvasive imaging such as **SPECT** _____ _____ _____ _____ _____ and stress **ECHO** _____.

2. **DVT** _____ _____ _____ is common in hospitalized patients. Early detection is important because **DVT** can result in death from a pulmonary embolism. Doppler ultrasound and **IPG** _____ _____ are two noninvasive diagnostic procedures used to diagnose DVT. MRI and venography may be used as well.

3. The **CBC** _____ _____ _____ and differential are a series of automated laboratory tests of the peripheral blood that provide a great deal of information about the blood and other body organs. Tests performed as part of the CBC are **RBC** _____ _____ _____ count, **WBC** _____ _____ _____ count and differential, **Hgb** _____, and **HCT** _____.

4. Standard surgical treatment for CAD includes **CABG** _____ _____ _____ _____. There is a growth in the use of minimally invasive techniques to treat CAD, which include transmyocardial laser revascularization and **PTCA** _____ _____ _____ _____, atherectomy, and stent insertion.

5. Hospitalized patients diagnosed with **MI** _____ _____ are cared for in the **CCU** _____ _____ _____.

6. A sphygmomanometer is used to measure **BP** _____ _____.

7. Diagnosis used to indicate that a patient's heart is unable to pump enough blood through the body to supply tissues is **CHF** _____ _____ _____.

8. If the patient's heart and/or lungs have ceased to function, the medical team must begin **CPR** _____ _____.

9. A patient with persistently elevated blood pressure is likely to be diagnosed with **HHD** _____ _____ _____.

10. When scheduling blood tests for a patient on oral anticoagulant medication, the doctor is likely to include a **PT** _____ _____.

11. Any interruption of the conduction of electrical impulses from the atria to the ventricles is called **AV** _____ block.

12. The treatment of **ACS** _____ _____ _____ is aimed at preventing thrombus formation and restoring blood flow to the occluded coronary artery.

13. Stopping smoking, exercising, and proper diet are important in the medical management of **PAD** _____ _____ _____.

14. **DSA** _____ _____ _____ is especially valuable in cardiac applications.

15. The physician ordered a **TEE** _____ _____ to examine the patient's heart structure and function.

CHAPTER REVIEW

EXERCISE 37   *Interact with Medical Records*

Complete the inpatient progress note by writing the medical terms in the blanks. Use the list of definitions with the corresponding numbers. See the next page for a list of medical terms to be used with this exercise.

University Hospital and Medical Center
4700 North Main Street • Wellness, Arizona 54321 • (987) 555-3210

PATIENT NAME: Natalie Wells	**CASE NUMBER:** 20922-CVR
DATE OF BIRTH: 01/14/xx	**DATE:** 04/07/xx

INPATIENT PROGRESS NOTE

CHIEF COMPLAINT: Natalie Wells is a 76-year-old white woman who was admitted to the hospital for recurrent chest pain.

HISTORY OF PRESENT ILLNESS: The patient has a long history of stable 1. _____ _____. She had a positive treadmill stress test in 1988. A 2. _____ _____ in 1998 showed reversible 3. _____ . In May 1992 she underwent cataract surgery, and during her postoperative care she developed severe chest pain. An ECG at that time showed ischemic ST changes in the anterior leads. Subsequent coronary 4. _____ revealed a 90% focal 5. _____ left anterior descending coronary artery. The patient then underwent 6. _____ of this lesion. The 90% stenosis was dilated to a 20% stenosis. The patient had an uncomplicated course.

Over the last 10 days the patient has had at least five episodes of chest pain, all relieved by rest or a single nitroglycerin tablet. She had an episode yesterday while gardening, which lasted almost 5 minutes before subsiding after a second nitroglycerin tablet. She went to her 7. _____ office yesterday. 8. _____ was performed, which showed marked anterior T-wave inversion in the anterior leads, and she was immediately sent to this hospital for further evaluation. Atherogenic risk factors for her age include hypercholesterolemia and hypertension; she also smokes one pack of cigarettes per day. She is not a diabetic. Her family history reveals a brother who has had a coronary artery bypass graft.

PHYSICAL EXAM:
On exam today, blood pressure is 138/86. She has tachycardia with a pulse of 120. She is in no acute distress. Her lungs are clear and she has regular rhythm without a murmur. There is no edema or distention of neck veins.

CURRENT MEDICATIONS:
1. Lovastatin 20 mg with evening meal.
2. Enalapril 20 mg bid.
3. Nifedipine 10 mg tid.
4. nitroglycerin 0.4 mg sublingual prn.

PLAN:
9. _____ _____ with possible coronary stent if necessary.
Serial ECGs and enzymes will be obtained to rule out 10. _____ _____ .

_____
Emily Watson, MD

EW/mcm

1. chest pain, occurs when there is an insufficient supply of blood to the heart muscle
2. a nuclear medicine test used to determine blood flow to the myocardium
3. deficient supply of blood to the heart's blood vessels
4. x-ray imaging a blood vessel
5. narrowing
6. surgical repair of a blood vessel
7. physician who studies and treats diseases of the heart
8. process of recording electrical activity of the heart
9. introduction of a catheter into the heart by way of a blood vessel to determine coronary artery disease
10. death of a portion of the myocardial muscle caused by lack of oxygen resulting from an interrupted blood supply

EXERCISE 38 *Interpret Medical Terms in Use*

To test your understanding of the terms introduced in this chapter, circle the words that correctly complete the sentences. The italicized words refer to the correct answer.

1. *Yellowish, fatty plaque within the arteries* is (arteriosclerosis, atherosclerosis, aortosclerosis).
2. *Inflammation of a vein associated with a clot* is called a (thrombosis, phlebitis, thrombophlebitis).
3. *Inflammation of the middle muscular layer of the heart* is (endocarditis, myocarditis, pericarditis).
4. Another name for a *heart attack* is (myocardial infarction, coronary fibrillation, angina pectoris).
5. The *surgical excision of a thickened artery interior* is an (arteriorrhaphy, angioplasty, endarterectomy).
6. *Varicose veins in the rectal area* are (plasma, thrombi, hemorrhoids).
7. *Reduction of body temperature to a level below normal* results in a condition called (hypothermia, hypertension, hyperthermia).
8. (Impedance plethysmography, cardiac scan, aortogram) is used to *determine if a patient has a blood clot in the femoral vein.*
9. *A humming sound* or (hemorrhage, murmur, auscultation) originating *in the heart* is sometimes the result of many episodes of rheumatic fever, an inflammatory disease occurring in children.
10. The doctor uses an (echocardiograph, electrocardiogram, angioscope) to *visualize the blood vessel* and guide the laser beam to open blocked arteries; this procedure is called (echocardiography, angioscopy).
11. The following is *a nuclear medicine test used to diagnose coronary artery disease* (coronary stent, thallium test, transesophageal echocardiogram).

For further practice or to evaluate what you have learned, use the Student CD that accompanies this text.

EXERCISE 39 Read Medical Terms in Use

Practice pronunciation of terms by reading the following medical document. Use the pronunciation key following the medical terms to assist you in saying the word.

A 55-year-old man presented to his doctor with pain in the calf and swelling in the left foot and ankle. A total of 5 days before, the patient had traveled by air across the country, spending several hours in a sitting position. He has a history of **varicose** (VAR-i-kōs) **veins** (vāns). No previous history of **hypertension** (hī-per-TEN-shun) or **thrombophlebitis** (throm-bō-fle-BĪ-tis) existed. Physical examination revealed an edematous left lower extremity and a tender calf. The pedal pulse was intact. A **Doppler ultrasound** (DOP-ler) (UL-tra-sound) was obtained, which revealed **deep vein thrombosis** (throm-BŌ-sis). The patient was hospitalized and subcutaneous low molecular weight heparin was begun. Concurrently, Coumadin was started and will continue for 6 months. The oral **anticoagulant** (an-ti-cō-AG-ū-lant) therapy will be monitored monthly by **prothrombin** (prō-THROM-bin) **time.**

EXERCISE 40 Comprehend Medical Terms in Use

Test your comprehension of the terms in the previous medical document by circling the correct answer.

1. T   F   An x-ray image was used to diagnose deep vein thrombosis.
2. The patient was diagnosed with:
   a. inflammation of the vein
   b. vascular inflammatory disorder
   c. a clot in a vein in the lower extremity
   d. a clot in the blood vessels of the heart
3. A blood test will be used to determine:
   a. bleeding time
   b. the time it takes for blood to form a clot
   c. the oxygen-carrying capacity of the red blood cell
   d. certain coagulation activity defects
4. It was noted the patient has no previous history of:
   a. low blood pressure and inflammation of a vein with a clot
   b. high blood pressure and inflammation of a vein with a clot
   c. high blood pressure and distended veins in the rectal area
   d. low blood pressure and distended veins in the rectal area

For additional information on heart disease, visit the American Heart Association at www.americanheart.org.

COMBINING FORMS CROSSWORD PUZZLE

Across Clues

1. yellowish, fatty plaque
2. heart
6. ventricle
9. clot
13. blockage, deficiency
14. spleen
15. aorta

Down Clues

3. vessel
4. valve
5. artery
7. electricity, electrical activity
8. plasma
10. valve
11. atrium
12. sound

REVIEW OF WORD PARTS

Can you define and spell the following word parts?

Combining Forms

angi/o	lymph/o
aort/o	phleb/o
arteri/o	plasm/o
ather/o	splen/o
atri/o	therm/o
cardi/o	thromb/o
ech/o	thym/o
electr/o	valv/o
isch/o	valvul/o
	ven/o
	ventricul/o

Prefixes

brady-
tachy-

Suffixes

-ac
-apheresis
-crit
-graph
-odynia
-penia
-poiesis
-sclerosis

REVIEW OF TERMS

Can you build, analyze, define, pronounce, and spell the following terms *built from word parts?*

Diseases and Disorders

Heart and Blood Vessels

angiocarditis
angioma
angiospasm
angiostenosis
aortic stenosis
arteriorrhexis
arteriosclerosis
atherosclerosis
bradycardia
cardiodynia
cardiomegaly
cardiomyopathy
cardiovalvulitis
endocarditis
ischemia
myocarditis
pericarditis
phlebitis
polyarteritis
tachycardia
thrombophlebitis

Blood and Lymphatic Systems

hematocytopenia
hematoma
lymphadenitis
lymphadenopathy
lymphoma
pancytopenia
splenomegaly
thrombosis
thrombus
thymoma

Surgical

angioplasty
angiorrhaphy
atherectomy
endarterectomy
pericardiocentesis
phlebectomy
phlebotomy
splenectomy
splenopexy
thymectomy

Diagnostic

Heart and Blood Vessels

angiography
angioscope
angioscopy
aortogram
arteriogram
echocardiogram (ECHO)
electrocardiogram (ECG, EKG)
electrocardiograph
electrocardiography
venogram
venography

Blood and Lymphatic Systems

erythrocyte count (RBC)
hematocrit (HCT)
leukocyte count (WBC)
lymphangiography

Complementary

atrioventricular (AV)
cardiac
cardiogenic
cardiologist
cardiology
hematologist
hematology
hematopoiesis
hemolysis
hemostasis
hypothermia
intravenous (IV)
plasmapheresis
tachypnea
thrombolysis

Can you define, pronounce, and spell the following terms *not built from word parts?*

Diseases and Disorders

acute coronary syndrome (ACS)
anemia
aneurysm
angina pectoris
cardiac arrest
cardiac tamponade
coarctation of the aorta
congenital heart disease
congestive heart failure (CHF)
coronary occlusion
deep vein thrombosis (DVT)
dysrhythmia
embolus, *pl.* emboli
fibrillation
hemochromatosis
hemophilia
hemorrhoid
Hodgkin disease
hypertensive heart disease (HHD)
intermittent claudication
leukemia
mitral valve stenosis
myocardial infarction (MI)
peripheral arterial disease (PAD)
rheumatic fever
rheumatic heart disease
sickle cell anemia
varicose veins

Surgical

aneurysmectomy
bone marrow transplant
cardiac pacemaker
coronary artery bypass graft (CABG)
coronary stent
defibrillation
embolectomy
femoropopliteal bypass
hemorrhoidectomy
implantable cardiac defibrillator
intracoronary thrombolytic therapy
laser angioplasty
mitral commissurotomy
percutaneous transluminal coronary angioplasty (PTCA)

Diagnostic

Heart and Blood Vessels

cardiac catheterization
digital subtraction angiography (DSA)
Doppler ultrasound
exercise stress test
impedance plethysmography (IPG)
single-photon emission computed tomography (SPECT)
sphygmomanometer
stethoscope
thallium test
transesophageal echocardiogram (TEE)

Blood and Lymphatic Systems

bone marrow biopsy
coagulation time
complete blood count (CBC)
hemoglobin (Hgb)
prothrombin time (PT)

Complementary

Heart and Blood Vessels

auscultation
blood pressure (BP)
cardiopulmonary resuscitation (CPR)
diastole
extracorporeal
extravasation
heart murmur
hypertension
hypotension
lumen
occlude
percussion
systole
vasoconstrictor
vasodilator
venipuncture

Blood and Lymphatic Systems

anticoagulant
dyscrasia
hemorrhage
plasma
serum

Digestive System

OUTLINE

OBJECTIVES

On completion of this chapter you will be able to:

1. Identify the organs and other structures of the digestive system.
2. Define and spell the word parts presented in this chapter.
3. Build and analyze medical terms with word parts presented in this and previous chapters.
4. Define, pronounce, and spell the disease and disorder, diagnostic, surgical, and complementary terms for the digestive system.
5. Interpret the meaning of abbreviations presented in this chapter.
6. Read medical documents and interpret medical terminology contained in them.

ANATOMY

Function

The digestive tract, also known as the *alimentary canal* or the *gastrointestinal tract*, sometimes abbreviated as *GI tract*, is made up of several digestive organs. The organs connect to form a continuous passageway from the mouth to the anus (Figure 11-1). With the help of

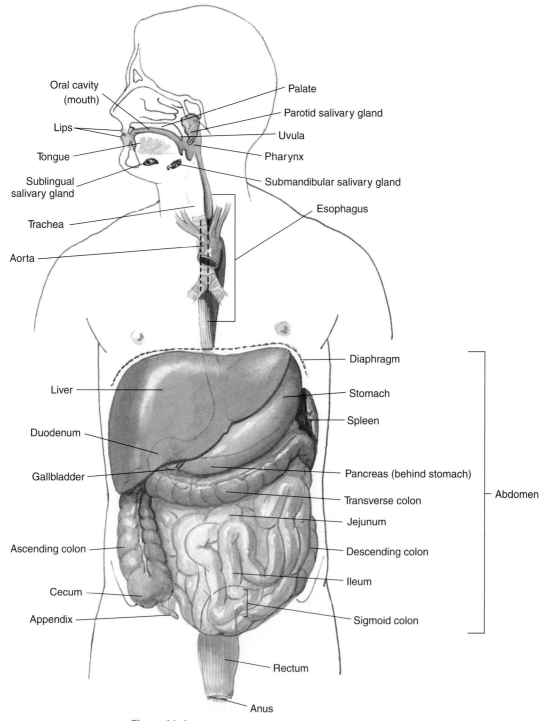

Figure 11-1

Organs of the digestive system and some associated structures.

accessory organs, the digestive tract prepares ingested food for use by the body cells through physical and chemical digestion and eliminates the solid waste products from the body.

Organs of the Digestive Tract

mouth	opening through which food passes into the body; breaks food into small particles by mastication (chewing) and mixing with saliva
tongue	consists mostly of skeletal muscle; attached in the posterior region of the mouth. It provides movement of food for mastication, directs food to the pharynx for swallowing, and is a major organ for taste and speech.
palate	separates the nasal cavity from the oral cavity
soft palate	posterior portion, not supported by bone
hard palate	anterior portion, supported by bone
uvula	soft V-shaped mass that extends from the soft palate. Directs food into the throat.
pharynx, throat	performs the swallowing action that passes food from the mouth into the esophagus
esophagus	10-inch (25-cm) tube that extends from the pharynx to the stomach
stomach	J-shaped sac that mixes and stores food. It secretes chemicals for digestion and hormones for local communication control (Figure 11-2).
cardia	area around the opening of the esophagus
fundus	uppermost domed portion of the stomach
body	central portion of the stomach
pylorus	lower part of the stomach that connects to the small intestine
antrum	portion of the pylorus that connects to the body of the stomach
pyloric sphincter	ring of muscle that guards the opening between the stomach and the duodenum
small intestine	20-foot (6-m) canal extending from the pyloric sphincter to the large intestine (see Figure 11-1)
duodenum	first 10 to 12 inches (25 cm) of the small intestine
jejunum	second portion of the small intestine, approximately 8 feet (2.4 m) long
ileum	third portion of the small intestine, approximately 11 feet (3.3 m) long, which connects with the large intestine
large intestine	canal that is approximately 5 feet (1.5 m) long and extends from the ileum to the anus (Figure 11-3)

Duodenum
is derived from the Latin **duodeni,** meaning **12 each,** a reference to its length. It was named in 240 BC by a Greek physician.

Jejunum is derived from the Latin **jejunus,** meaning **empty;** it was so named because the early anatomists always found it empty.

Ileum is derived from the Greek **eilein,** meaning **to roll,** a reference to the peristaltic waves that move food along the digestive tract. This term was first used in the early part of the seventeenth century.

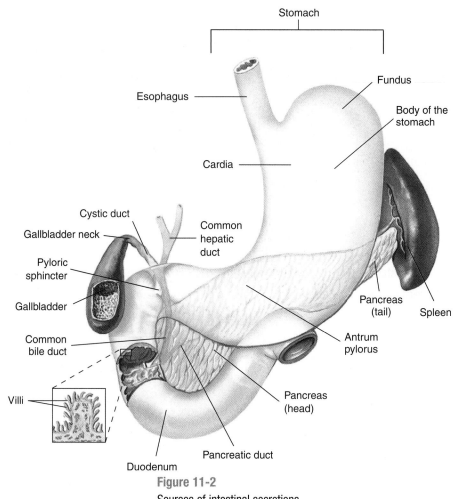

Figure 11-2
Sources of intestinal secretions.

cecum...	blind U-shaped pouch that is the first portion of the large intestine (see Figure 11-3)
colon...	next portion of the large intestine. The colon is divided into four parts: ascending colon, transverse colon, descending colon, and sigmoid colon (see Figure 11-3).
rectum...	remaining portion of the large intestine, approximately 8 to 10 inches (20 cm) long, extending from the sigmoid colon to the anus
anus...	sphincter muscle (ringlike band of muscle fiber that keeps an opening tight) at the end of the digestive tract

Accessory Organs

salivary glands....................................	produce saliva, which flows into the mouth (see Figure 11-1)

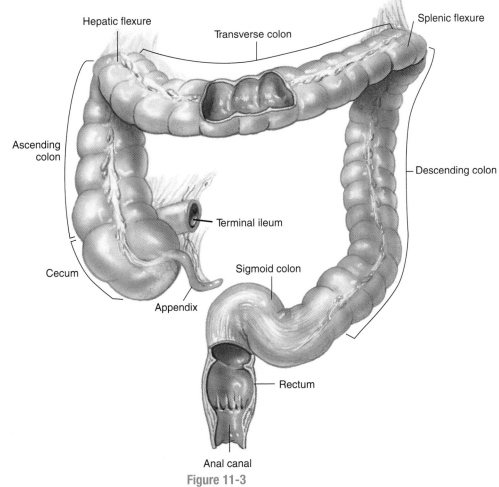

Hepatic flexure

Transverse colon

Splenic flexure

Ascending colon

Descending colon

Terminal ileum

Sigmoid colon

Cecum

Appendix

Rectum

Anal canal

Figure 11-3
Anatomy of the large intestine.

liver	produces bile, which is necessary for the digestion of fats. The liver performs many other functions concerned with digestion and metabolism (see Figure 11-1).
bile ducts	passageways that carry bile: the hepatic duct is a passageway for bile from the liver, and the cystic duct carries bile from the gallbladder. They join to form the common bile duct, which conveys bile to the duodenum (see Figure 11-2).
gallbladder	small, saclike structure that stores bile
pancreas	produces pancreatic juice, which helps digest all types of food and secretes insulin for carbohydrate metabolism

Other Structures

peritoneum	serous sac lining of the abdominal and pelvic cavities

Pancreas
is derived from the Greek **pan,** meaning **all,** and **krea,** meaning **flesh.** The pancreas was first described in 300 BC. It was so named because of its fleshy appearance.

| appendix | small pouch, which has no function in digestion, attached to the cecum (see Figures 11-1 and 11-3) |
| abdomen | portion of the body between the thorax and the pelvis |

Learn the anatomic terms by completing exercises 1 and 2.

EXERCISE 1

Fill in the blanks with the correct terms.

The digestive tract, also known as the (1) _____ _____, and (2) _____ _____, begins with the mouth, connects with the throat, or (3) _____, and continues on to a 10-inch tube called the (4) _____; this connects with the (5) _____, a **J**-shaped sac that mixes and stores food.

The small intestine, the next portion of the digestive tract, is made up of three portions. They are called the (6) _____, (7) _____, and (8) _____. The small intestine connects with the first portion of the large intestine, the (9) _____, and then connects with the colon, which is divided into four parts called (10) _____ _____, (11) _____ _____, (12) _____ _____, and (13) _____ _____. The (14) _____ extends from the sigmoid colon to the (15) _____.

EXERCISE 2

Match the definitions in the first column with the correct terms in the second column.

_____ 1. connects to the body of the stomach

_____ 2. hangs from the roof of the mouth

_____ 3. produce saliva

_____ 4. produces bile

_____ 5. separates the nasal cavity from the oral cavity

_____ 6. guards the opening between the stomach and the duodenum

_____ 7. secretes insulin for carbohydrate metabolism

a. salivary glands

b. pancreas

c. peritoneum

d. uvula

e. gallbladder

f. tongue

g. abdomen

h. liver

i. appendix

j. pyloric sphincter

k. fundus

l. antrum

m. palate

_____ 8. small pouch that has no
function in digestion

_____ 9. lining of the abdominal
and pelvic cavities

_____ 10. portion of the body
between the pelvis and
thorax

_____ 11. stores bile

_____ 12. uppermost domed
portion of the stomach

_____ 13. directs food to the
pharynx for swallowing

WORD PARTS

Combining Forms for the Digestive Tract

Study the word parts and their definitions listed below. Completing the exercises that
follow and Exercise Figure A will help you learn the terms.

Combining Form	Definition
an/o	anus
antr/o	antrum
cec/o	cecum
col/o, colon/o	colon (usually denoting the large intestine)
duoden/o	duodenum
enter/o	intestine (usually denoting the small intestine)
esophag/o (NOTE: *esophag/o* was covered in Chapter 9.)	esophagus
gastr/o	stomach
ile/o	ileum
jejun/o	jejunum
or/o, stomat/o	mouth
proct/o, rect/o	rectum
sigmoid/o	sigmoid colon

**Learn the anatomic locations and meanings of the combining forms by completing
exercises 3 and 4 and Exercise Figure A.**

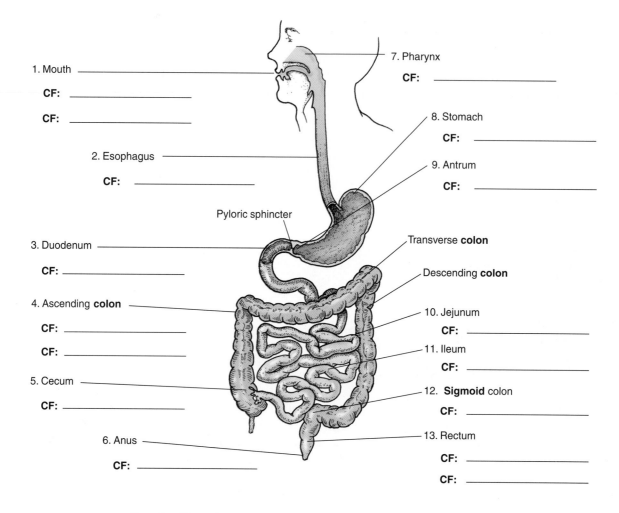

1. Mouth

   CF: _____

   CF: _____

2. Esophagus

   CF: _____

3. Duodenum

   CF: _____

4. Ascending **colon**

   CF: _____

   CF: _____

5. Cecum

   CF: _____

6. Anus

   CF: _____

7. Pharynx

   CF: _____

8. Stomach

   CF: _____

9. Antrum

   CF: _____

Pyloric sphincter

Transverse **colon**

Descending **colon**

10. Jejunum

    CF: _____

11. Ileum

    CF: _____

12. **Sigmoid** colon

    CF: _____

13. Rectum

    CF: _____

    CF: _____

Exercise Figure A
Fill in the blanks with combining forms in this diagram of the digestive system.

EXERCISE 3

Write the definitions of the following combining forms.

1. proct/o _____

2. gastr/o _____

3. an/o _____

4. cec/o _____

5. ile/o _____

6. stomat/o _____

7. duoden/o _____

8. col/o _____

9. or/o _____

10. enter/o _____

11. rect/o _____

12. antr/o _____

13. esophag/o _____

14. jejun/o _____

15. sigmoid/o _____

16. colon/o _____

EXERCISE 4

Write the combining form for each of the following terms.

1. cecum   _____

2. stomach   _____

3. ileum   _____

4. jejunum   _____

5. sigmoid colon _____

6. esophagus   _____

7. rectum   a. _____

             b. _____

8. intestines   _____

9. duodenum   _____

10. colon   a. _____

             b. _____

11. mouth   a. _____

             b. _____

12. anus   _____

13. antrum   _____

Combining Forms for the Accessory Organs/Combining Forms Commonly Used with Digestive System Terms

Combining Form	Definition
abdomin/o, celi/o, lapar/o	abdomen (abdominal cavity)
appendic/o	appendix
cheil/o	lip
cholangi/o	bile duct
chol/e (NOTE: the combining vowel is *e*.)	gall, bile
choledoch/o	common bile duct
diverticul/o	diverticulum, or blind pouch, extending from a hollow organ (*pl.* diverticula) (Figure 11-4)
gingiv/o	gum
gloss/o, lingu/o	tongue
hepat/o	liver
herni/o	hernia, or protrusion of an organ through a membrane or cavity wall (Figure 11-5)
palat/o	palate
pancreat/o	pancreas
peritone/o	peritoneum
polyp/o	polyp, small growth
pylor/o (NOTE: *pylor/o* was covered in Chapter 9.)	pylorus, pyloric sphincter

Hernia
The layman's term for hernia is **rupture.** Types include abdominal, hiatal, or diaphragmatic, inguinal, and umbilical hernia.

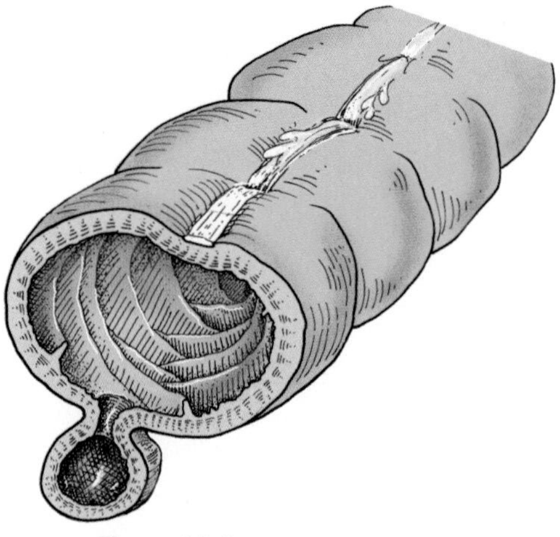

Figure 11-4
Diverticulum of the large intestine.

| sial/o .... | saliva, salivary gland |
| uvul/o .... | uvula |

Learn the anatomic locations and definitions of the combining forms by completing exercises 5 and 6 and Exercise Figure B.

EXERCISE   5

Write the definitions of the following combining forms.

1. herni/o _____

2. abdomin/o _____

3. sial/o _____

4. chol/e _____

5. diverticul/o _____

6. gingiv/o _____

7. appendic/o _____

8. gloss/o _____

9. hepat/o _____

10. cheil/o _____

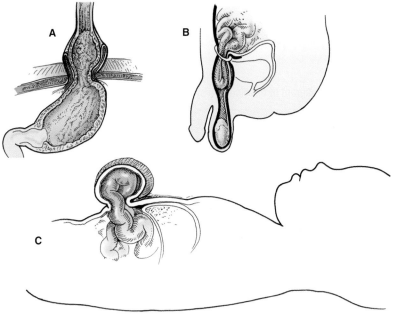

Figure 11-5
Types of hernias. **A,** Hiatal; **B,** inguinal; **C,** umbilical.

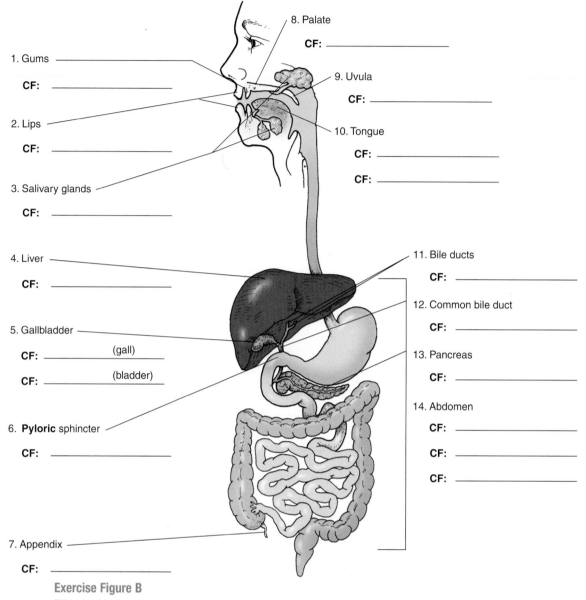

1. Gums ─────────

    CF: _____

2. Lips

    CF: _____

3. Salivary glands

    CF: _____

4. Liver

    CF: _____

5. Gallbladder

    CF: _____ (gall)

    CF: _____ (bladder)

6. **Pyloric** sphincter

    CF: _____

7. Appendix

    CF: _____

8. Palate

    CF: _____

9. Uvula

    CF: _____

10. Tongue

    CF: _____

    CF: _____

11. Bile ducts

    CF: _____

12. Common bile duct

    CF: _____

13. Pancreas

    CF: _____

14. Abdomen

    CF: _____

    CF: _____

    CF: _____

Exercise Figure B

Fill in the blanks with combining forms in this diagram of the digestive system and associated structures.

11. peritone/o _____

12. palat/o _____

13. pancreat/o _____

14. lapar/o _____

15. lingu/o _____

16. choledoch/o _____

17. pylor/o _____

18. uvul/o _____

19. cholangi/o _____

20. polyp/o _____

21. celi/o _____

EXERCISE 6

Write the combining form for each of the following.

1. palate   _____

2. saliva, salivary gland   _____

3. pancreas   _____

4. peritoneum   _____

5. tongue   a. _____

                             b. _____

6. gum   _____

7. pylorus, pyloric sphincter   _____

8. liver   _____

9. gall, bile   _____

10. abdomen   a. _____

                             b. _____

                             c. _____

11. hernia   _____

12. diverticulum   _____

13. lip   _____

14. appendix   _____

15. uvula   _____

16. bile duct   _____

17. common bile duct   _____

18. small growth   _____

Prefix

Prefix	Definition
hemi-	half

Suffix

Suffix	Definition
-pepsia	digestion

Learn the prefix and suffix by completing exercises 7 and 8. Refer to Appendix A and Appendix B for a complete listing of word parts.

EXERCISE 7

Write the definition of the following prefix and suffix.

1. -pepsia _____

2. hemi- _____

EXERCISE 8

Write the prefix and suffix for the following definition.

1. digestion _____

2. half _____

MEDICAL TERMS

The terms you need to learn to complete this chapter are listed below. The exercises following each list will help you learn the definition and the spelling of each word. Refer to Appendix J for terms relating to nutrition.

Disease and Disorder Terms

Built from Word Parts

Term	Definition
appendicitis (ap-*pen*-di-SĪ-tis)	inflammation of the appendix (Exercise Figure C)
cholangioma (kō-lan-jē-Ō-ma)	tumor of the bile duct
cholecystitis (kō-lē-sis-TĪ-tis)	inflammation of the gallbladder

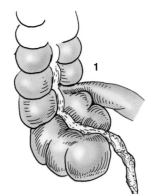

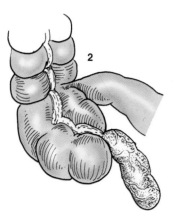

Exercise Figure C

Fill in the blanks to complete labeling of the diagram.

1, Normal appendix.

2, _____ .

appendix / **inflammation**

choledocholithiasis............................. (kō-led-ō-kō-lith-Ī-a-sis)	condition of stones in the common bile duct (Exercise Figure D)
cholelithiasis .... (kō-lē-lith-Ī-a-sis)	condition of gallstones (see Exercise Figure D)
diverticulitis..................................... (dī-ver-tik-ū-LĪ-tis)	inflammation of a diverticulum (see Figure 11-4)
diverticulosis.................................... (dī-ver-tik-ū-LŌ-sis)	abnormal condition of having diverticula (see Figures 11-4 and 11-13, B)
esophagitis.. (e-sof-a-JĪ-tis)	inflammation of the esophagus
gastritis... (gas-TRĪ-tis)	inflammation of the stomach
gastroenteritis .... (gas-trō-en-te-RĪ-tis)	inflammation of the stomach and intestines
gastroenterocolitis............................ (gas-trō-en-ter-ō-kō-LĪ-tis)	inflammation of the stomach, intestines, and colon
gingivitis.. (jin-ji-VĪ-tis)	inflammation of the gums
hepatitis... (hep-a-TĪ-tis)	inflammation of the liver
hepatoma.. (hep-a-TŌ-ma)	tumor of the liver
palatitis.. (pal-a-TĪ-tis)	inflammation of the palate
pancreatitis...................................... (pan-krē-a-TĪ-tis)	inflammation of the pancreas

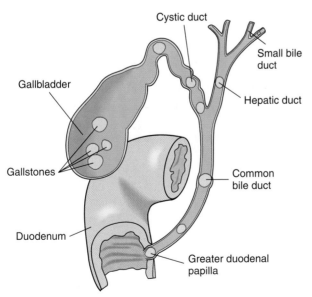

Exercise Figure D

Fill in the blanks to complete labeling of the diagram. Common sites of

_____ / ___ / _____ / _____ and _____ / ___ / _____ / _____ .
gall / cv / stone / condition   common bile duct / cv / stone / condition

peritonitis...................	inflammation of the peritoneum
(per-i-tō-NĪ-tis) (NOTE: the *e* is dropped from the combining form peritone/o.)	
polyposis....................	abnormal condition of (multiple) polyps (in the mucous membrane of the intestine, especially the colon; high potential for malignancy) (Figure 11-6)
(pol-ē-PŌ-sis)	
proctoptosis..............	prolapse of the rectum
(*prok*-top-TŌ-sis)	
rectocele....................	protrusion of the rectum
(REK-tō-sēl)	
sialolith.....................	stone in the salivary gland
(sī-AL-ō-lith)	
uvulitis.....................	inflammation of the uvula
(ū-vū-LĪ-tis)	

Practice saying each of these terms aloud. To hear the terms, access the **PRONOUNCE IT** activity for this chapter on the Student CD that accompanies this text. Or, to hear the terms and their definitions with a CD player or computer, obtain the Pronunciation CD designed for use with this text.

Learn the definitions and spellings of the disease and disorder terms by completing exercises 9, 10, and 11.

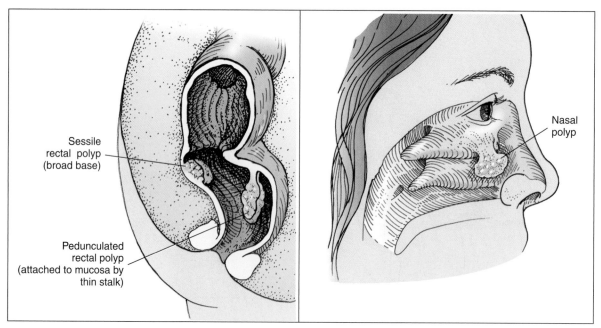

Sessile rectal polyp (broad base)

Pedunculated rectal polyp (attached to mucosa by thin stalk)

Nasal polyp

Figure 11-6
Polyp is a general term used to describe a protruding growth from a mucous membrane. Polyps are commonly found in the nose, uterus, intestines, and bladder.

EXERCISE   9

Analyze and define the following terms.

1. cholelithiasis _____

2. diverticulosis _____

3. sialolith _____

4. hepatoma _____

5. uvulitis _____

6. pancreatitis _____

7. proctoptosis _____

8. gingivitis _____

9. gastritis _____

10. rectocele _____

11. palatitis _____

12. hepatitis _____

13. appendicitis _____

14. cholecystitis _____

15. diverticulitis _____

16. gastroenteritis _____

17. gastroenterocolitis _____

18. choledocholithiasis _____

19. cholangioma _____

20. polyposis _____

21. esophagitis _____

22. peritonitis _____

EXERCISE 10

Build disease and disorder terms for the following definitions by using the word parts you have learned.

1. tumor of the liver

_____ / _____
      WR   S

2. inflammation of the stomach

_____ / _____
      WR   S

3. stone in the salivary gland

_____ /CV/ _____
      WR   WR

4. inflammation of the appendix

_____ / _____
      WR   S

5. inflammation of a diverticulum

_____ / _____
      WR   S

6. inflammation of the gallbladder

_____ /CV/ _____ / _____
      WR   WR   S

7. abnormal condition of having diverticula

_____ / _____
      WR   S

8. inflammation of the stomach and intestines

_____ /CV/ _____ / _____
      WR   WR   S

9. prolapse of the rectum

_____ /CV/ _____
      WR   S

10. protrusion of the rectum

_____ /CV/ _____
      WR   S

11. inflammation of the uvula

_____ / _____
      WR   S

12. inflammation of the gums

_____ / _____
      WR   S

13. inflammation of the liver

_____ / _____
      WR   S

14. inflammation of the palate

_____ / _____
      WR   S

15. condition of gallstones

_____ /CV/ _____ / _____
      WR   WR   S

16. inflammation of the stomach, intestines, and colon

_____ / _ / _____ / _ / _____ / _
WR /CV/ WR /CV/ WR / S

17. inflammation of the pancreas

_____ / _____
WR / S

18. tumor of the bile duct

_____ / _____
WR / S

19. inflammation of the esophagus

_____ / _____
WR / S

20. condition of stones in the common bile duct

_____ / _ / _____ / _____
WR /CV/ WR / S

21. abnormal condition of (multiple) polyps

_____ / _____
WR / S

22. inflammation of the peritoneum

_____ / _____
WR / S

EXERCISE 11

Spell each of the disease and disorder terms. Have someone dictate the terms on pp. 380-382 to you. Think about the word parts before attempting to write the word. Study any words you have spelled incorrectly.

1. _____   12. _____

2. _____   13. _____

3. _____   14. _____

4. _____   15. _____

5. _____   16. _____

6. _____   17. _____

7. _____   18. _____

8. _____   19. _____

9. _____   20. _____

10. _____   21. _____

11. _____   22. _____

Disease and Disorder Terms

Not Built from Word Parts

Term	Definition
adhesion (ad-HĒ-zhun)	abnormal growing together of two surfaces that normally are separated. This may occur after abdominal surgery; surgical treatment is called *adhesiolysis* or *adhesiotomy* (Figure 11-7, *A*).
anorexia nervosa (*an*-ō-REK-sē-a) (ner-VŌ-sa)	psychoneurotic disorder characterized by a prolonged refusal to eat, resulting in emaciation, amenorrhea in females, and abnormal fear of becoming obese. It occurs primarily in adolescents.
bulimia nervosa (bū-LĒ-mē-a) (ner-VŌ-sa)	an eating disorder involving gorging with food, followed by induced vomiting or laxative abuse (bingeing and purging)
cirrhosis (ser-RŌ-sis)	chronic disease of the liver with gradual destruction of cells, most commonly caused by alcoholism
Crohn disease (krōn) (di-ZĒZ)	chronic inflammation usually affecting the ileum, although it can affect any part of the gastrointestinal tract. It is characterized by cobblestone ulcerations along the intestinal

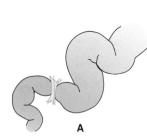
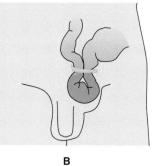
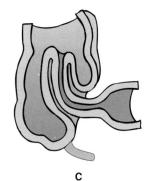

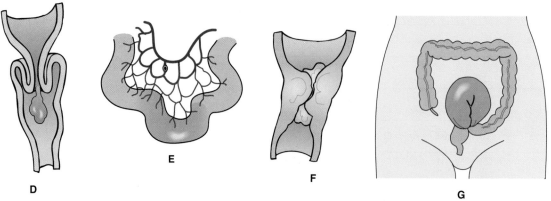

Figure 11-7

Causes of intestinal obstruction. **A,** Adhesions. **B,** Strangulated inguinal hernia. **C,** Ileocecal intussusception. **D,** Intussusception resulting from polyps. **E,** Mesenteric occlusion. **F,** Neoplasm. **G,** Volvulus of the sigmoid colon.

Gastroesophageal reflux disease (GERD) is estimated to be the most common gastrointestinal disorder. The acidity of the regurgitated stomach contents causes irritation and inflammation of the esophagus (reflux esophagitis).

Crohn disease (cont'd).....................	wall and the formation of scar tissue and may cause obstruction. It is also called *regional ileitis or regional enteritis.*
duodenal ulcer..................... (*dū*-o-DĒ-nal) (UL-ser)	ulcer in the duodenum (Figure 11-8)
gastric ulcer..................... (GAS-trik) (UL-ser)	ulcer in the stomach (see Figure 11-8)
gastroesophageal reflux disease (GERD)..................... (gas-trō-ē-sof-a-JĒ-al) (RĒ-fluks) (di-ZEZ)	the abnormal backward flow of the gastrointestinal contents into the esophagus, gradually breaking down the mucous barrier of the esophagus
ileus..................... (IL-ē-us)	obstruction of the intestine, often caused by failure of peristalsis
intussusception..................... (*in*-tus-sus-SEP-shun)	telescoping of a segment of the intestine (see Figure 11-7 *C* and *D*)
irritable bowel syndrome (IBS)..................... (ir-i-ta-BL) (BOW-el) (SIN-drōm)	periodic disturbances of bowel function, such as diarrhea and/or constipation, usually associated with abdominal pain
obesity..................... (ō-BĒ-si-tē)	excess of body fat (not body weight)

Obesity is when the BMI (body mass index) is greater than 30 kg/m². Overweight is defined as BMI between 25 and 29.9 kg/m². BMI is calculated by dividing weight in kilograms by the square of height in meters.

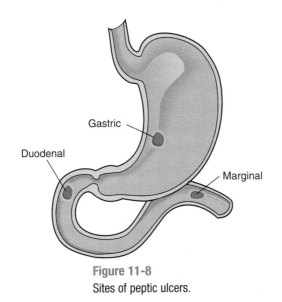

Gastric

Duodenal

Marginal

Figure 11-8
Sites of peptic ulcers.

peptic ulcer............................... (PEP-tik) (UL-ser)	another name for gastric or duodenal ulcer (see Figure 11-8)
polyp.. (POL-ip)	tumorlike growth extending outward from a mucous membrane. Usually benign; common sites are in the nose, throat, and intestines (see Figures 11-6 and 11-12).
ulcerative colitis...................... (UL-ser-a-tiv) (kōl-LĪ-tis)	inflammation of the colon with the formation of ulcers. The main symptom is diarrhea—as many as 15 to 29 stools per day. An ileostomy may be performed to treat this condition.
volvulus.................................. (VOL-vū-lus)	twisting or kinking of the intestine, causing intestinal obstruction (see Figure 11-7)

Practice saying each of these terms aloud. To hear the terms, access the **PRONOUNCE IT** activity for this chapter on the Student CD that accompanies this text. Or, to hear the terms and their definitions with a CD player or computer, obtain the Pronunciation CD designed for use with this text.

Learn the definitions and spellings of the disease and disorder terms by completing exercises 12, 13, and 14.

EXERCISE 12

Match the definitions in the first column with the correct terms in the second column.

_____ 1. prolonged refusal to eat

_____ 2. chronic disease of the liver

_____ 3. chronic inflammation that usually affects the ileum

_____ 4. abnormal growing together of two surfaces

_____ 5. twisted intestine

_____ 6. gastric or duodenal ulcer

_____ 7. telescoping of a segment of the intestine

_____ 8. tumorlike growth

_____ 9. formation of ulcers in the colon

_____ 10. eating disorder involving gorging food, followed by induced vomiting

a. intussusception

b. cirrhosis

c. gastroesophageal reflux disease

d. volvulus

e. Crohn disease

f. anorexia nervosa

g. peptic ulcer

h. ulcerative colitis

i. irritable bowel syndrome

j. bulimia nervosa

k. polyp

l. obesity

m. ileus

n. adhesion

o. duodenal ulcer

p. gastric ulcer

_____ 11. obstruction of the intestine

_____ 12. periodic disturbance of bowel function

_____ 13. abnormal backward flow of the gastrointestinal contents into the esophagus

_____ 14. excess of body fat

_____ 15. ulcer in the duodenum

_____ 16. ulcer in the stomach

EXERCISE 13

Write the definitions of the following terms.

1. peptic ulcer _____

2. anorexia nervosa _____

3. Crohn disease _____

4. volvulus _____

5. adhesion _____

6. cirrhosis _____

7. intussusception _____

8. gastric ulcer _____

9. duodenal ulcer _____

10. ulcerative colitis _____

11. bulimia nervosa _____

12. polyp _____

13. irritable bowel syndrome _____

14. ileus _____

15. gastroesophageal reflux disease _____

16. obesity _____

EXERCISE   14

Spell the disease and disorder terms. Have someone dictate the terms on pp. 386-388 to you. Study any words you have spelled incorrectly.

1. _____   9. _____

2. _____   10. _____

3. _____   11. _____

4. _____   12. _____

5. _____   13. _____

6. _____   14. _____

7. _____   15. _____

8. _____   16. _____

Surgical Terms

Built from Word Parts

Term	Definition
abdominoplasty..................................... (ab-DOM-i-nō-plas-tē)	surgical repair of the abdomen
anoplasty .... (A-nō-*plas*-tē)	surgical repair of the anus
antrectomy.. (an-TREK-tō-mē)	excision of the antrum
appendectomy....................................... (*ap*-en-DEK-tō-mē)	excision of the appendix
celiotomy .... (sē-lē-OT-ō-mē)	incision into the abdominal cavity
cheilorrhaphy.. (kī-LOR-a-fē)	suture of the lip
cholecystectomy.................................... (kō-lē-sis-TEK-tō-mē)	excision of the gallbladder (Figure 11-9)
choledocholithotomy .... (kō-led-ō-kō-li-THOT-ō-mē)	incision into the common bile duct to remove a stone
colectomy.. (kō-LEK-tō-mē)	excision of the colon

Cholecystectomy
was first performed in 1882 by a German surgeon. **Laparoscopic cholecystectomy** was first performed in 1987 in France.

Cholecystectomy is the most common abdominal surgery performed. Approximately 500,000 are performed in the United States each year.

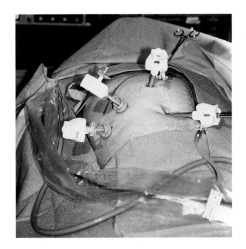

Figure 11-9
Laparoscopic cholecystectomy. Carbon dioxide is used to insufflate the surgical area for better visualization. A small incision is made in the folds of the umbilicus for the insertion of the laparoscope. Three additional small incisions are made for the insertion of operative sheaths to accommodate accessory instrumentation.

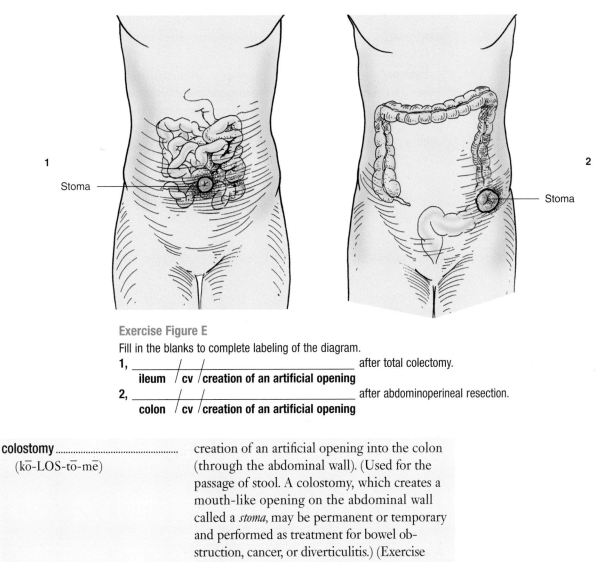

Exercise Figure E

Fill in the blanks to complete labeling of the diagram.

1, _____ / ___ / _____ after total colectomy.
      ileum / cv /creation of an artificial opening

2, _____ / ___ / _____ after abdominoperineal resection.
      colon / cv /creation of an artificial opening

colostomy................................. (kō-LOS-tō-mē)	creation of an artificial opening into the colon (through the abdominal wall). (Used for the passage of stool. A colostomy, which creates a mouth-like opening on the abdominal wall called a *stoma*, may be permanent or temporary and performed as treatment for bowel obstruction, cancer, or diverticulitis.) (Exercise Figure E)

Bariatric
contains the word roots **bar**, meaning **weight**, and **iatr**, meaning **treatment**.

Bariatric surgery is used to treat obesity, a condition in which a person has a BMI greater than 40 and other existing factors. Three types of surgeries performed in the United States are:
1. vertical banded **gastroplasty** (Figure 11-10)
2. gastric banding (lapband)
3. Roux-en-Y gastric bypass
During surgery, a small stomach pouch is created for the purpose of restricting the amount of food the individual can eat.

diverticulectomy .... (dī-ver-tik-ū-LEK-tō-mē)	excision of a diverticulum
enterorrhaphy .... (en-ter-OR-a-fē)	suture of the intestine
esophagogastroplasty .... (e-*sof*-a-gō-GAS-trō-plas-tē)	surgical repair of the esophagus and the stomach
gastrectomy .... (gas-TREK-tō-mē)	excision of the stomach (or part of the stomach) (Exercise Figure F)
gastrojejunostomy .... (*gas*-trō-je-jū-NOS-tō-mē)	creation of an artificial opening between the stomach and jejunum
gastroplasty .... (GAS-trō-*plas*-tē)	surgical repair of the stomach (Figure 11-10)
gastrostomy .... (gas-TROS-tō-mē)	creation of an artificial opening into the stomach (through the abdominal wall). (A tube is inserted through the opening for administration of food when swallowing is impossible.) (Figure 11-11)

Percutaneous Endoscopic Gastrostomy (PEG)
was first described in 1980. It is an alternative to **traditional gastrostomy**. An **endoscope** is used to place a tube in the stomach. Cost and discomfort to the patient are reduced when **PEG** is used instead of traditional gastrostomy.

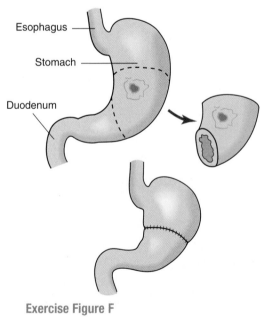

Exercise Figure F
Fill in the blanks to label the diagram.

_____ / _____
stomach   **surgical removal**

Esophagus

Stomach

Duodenum

gingivectomy...................................... surgical removal of gum (tissue)
  (*jin*-ji-VEK-tō-mē)

glossorrhaphy...................................... suture of the tongue
  (glo-SOR-a-fē)

hemicolectomy...................................... excision of half of the colon
  (*hem*-i-kō-LEK-tō-mē)

herniorrhaphy...................................... suturing of a hernia (for repair)
  (*her*-nē-OR-a-fē)

ileostomy...................................... creation of an artificial opening into the ileum
  (il-ē-OS-tō-mē)   (through the abdominal wall creating a stoma,
                            a mouthlike opening on the abdominal wall).
                            (Used for the passage of stool. It is performed
                            for ulcerative colitis, Crohn disease, or cancer.)
                            (see Exercise Figure E)

laparotomy...................................... incision into the abdomen
  (*lap*-a-ROT-ō-mē)

palatoplasty...................................... surgical repair of the palate
  (PAL-a-tō-*plas*-tē)

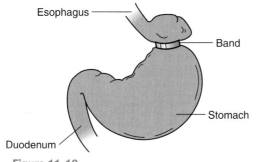

Figure 11-10
Vertical banded gastroplasty; used to treat obesity.

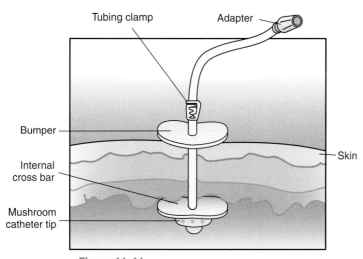

Figure 11-11
Percutaneous endoscopic gastrostomy (PEG).

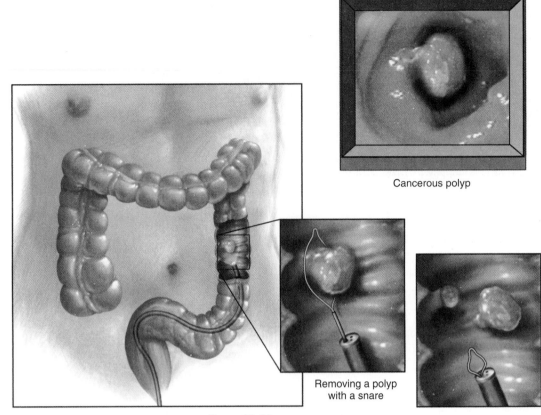

Cancerous polyp

Removing a polyp
with a snare

Figure 11-12
Colonoscopy and polypectomy.

polypectomy............................... (pol-ē-PEK-tō-mē)	excision of a polyp (Figure 11-12)
pyloromyotomy.................................... (pī-*lor*-ō-mī-OT-ō-mē)	incision into the pyloric muscle
pyloroplasty............................. (pī-LOR-ō-plas-tē)	surgical repair of the pylorus
uvulectomy............................. (ū-vū-LEK-tō-mē)	excision of the uvula
uvulopalatopharyngoplasty (UPPP)............................ (ū-vū-lō-*pal*-a-tō-*phar*-in-GO-plas-tē)	surgical repair of the uvula, palate, and pharynx (performed to correct obstructive sleep apnea) (see Figure 5-6)

Practice saying each of these terms aloud. To hear the terms, access the **PRONOUNCE IT** activity for this chapter on the Student CD that accompanies this text. Or, to hear the terms and their definitions with a CD player or computer, obtain the Pronunciation CD designed for use with this text.

Learn the definitions and spellings of the surgical terms by completing exercises 15, 16, and 17.

EXERCISE 15

Analyze and define the following surgical terms.

1. gastrectomy _____

2. esophagogastroplasty _____

3. diverticulectomy _____

4. antrectomy _____

5. palatoplasty _____

6. uvulectomy _____

7. gastrojejunostomy _____

8. cholecystectomy _____

9. colectomy _____

10. colostomy _____

11. pyloroplasty _____

12. anoplasty _____

13. appendectomy _____

14. cheilorrhaphy _____

15. gingivectomy _____

16. laparotomy _____

17. ileostomy _____

18. gastrostomy _____

19. herniorrhaphy _____

20. glossorrhaphy _____

21. choledocholithotomy _____

22. hemicolectomy _____

23. polypectomy _____

24. enterorrhaphy _____

25. abdominoplasty _____

26. pyloromyotomy _____

27. uvulopalatopharyngoplasty _____

28. celiotomy _____

29. gastroplasty _____

EXERCISE 16

Build surgical terms for the following definitions by using the word parts you have learned.

1. excision of the appendix _____ / _____
   WR   S

2. suture of the tongue _____ / CV / _____
   WR   S

3. surgical repair of the esophagus and stomach _____ / CV / WR / CV / _____
   WR   WR   S

4. excision of a diverticulum _____ / _____
   WR   S

5. artificial opening into the ileum _____ / CV / _____
   WR   S

6. surgical removal of gum tissue _____ / _____
   WR   S

7. incision into the abdomen _____ / CV / _____
   WR   S

8. surgical repair of the anus _____ / CV / _____
   WR   S

9. excision of the antrum _____ / _____
   WR   S

10. excision of the gallbladder _____ / CV / WR / _____
    WR   WR   S

11. excision of the colon _____ / _____
    WR   S

12. creation of an artificial opening into the colon _____ / CV / _____
    WR   S

13. excision of the stomach _____ / _____
    WR   S

14. creation of an artificial
    opening into the stomach

    _____/__/_____
    WR   CV   S

15. creation of an artificial
    opening between the
    stomach and jejunum

    _____/__/____/__/_____
    WR   CV   WR   CV   S

16. excision of the uvula

    _____/_____
         WR   S

17. surgical repair of the palate

    _____/__/_____
    WR   CV   S

18. surgical repair of the
    pylorus

    _____/__/_____
    WR   CV   S

19. suture of a hernia

    _____/__/_____
    WR   CV   S

20. suture of the lip

    _____/__/_____
    WR   CV   S

21. excision of half of the colon

    _____/____/_____
    P   WR   S

22. incision into the common
    bile duct to remove a stone

    _____/__/____/__/_____
    WR   CV   WR   CV   S

23. excision of a polyp

    _____/_____
         WR   S

24. suture of the intestine

    _____/__/_____
    WR   CV   S

25. surgical repair of the
    abdomen

    _____/__/_____
    WR   CV   S

26. incision into the abdominal
    cavity

    _____/__/_____
    WR   CV   S

27. incision into the pylorus
    muscle

    _____/__/____/__/_____
    WR   CV   WR   CV   S

28. surgical repair of the uvula,
    palate, and pharynx

    ____/__/____/__/_____/__/____
    WR CV WR CV   WR CV S

29. surgical repair of the
    stomach

    _____/__/_____
    WR   CV   S

EXERCISE 17

Spell each of the surgical terms. Have someone dictate the terms on pp. 390-394 to you. Think about the word parts before attempting to write the word. Study any words you have spelled incorrectly.

1. _____	16. _____
2. _____	17. _____
3. _____	18. _____
4. _____	19. _____
5. _____	20. _____
6. _____	21. _____
7. _____	22. _____
8. _____	23. _____
9. _____	24. _____
10. _____	25. _____
11. _____	26. _____
12. _____	27. _____
13. _____	28. _____
14. _____	29. _____
15. _____	

Surgical Terms

Not Built from Word Parts

Term	Definition
abdominoperineal resection (A&P resection) .... (ab-*dom*-in-ō-par-i-NĒ-el) (rē-SEK-shun)	removal of the colon and rectum through both abdominal and perineal approaches. Performed to treat colorectal cancer and inflammatory diseases of the lower large intestine. The patient will have a colostomy (see Exercise Figure F).
anastomosis .... (a-*nas*-tō-MŌ-sis)	surgical connection between two normally distinct structures
vagotomy .... (vā-GOT-ō-mē)	cutting of certain branches of the vagus nerve, performed with gastric surgery to reduce the amount of gastric acid produced and thus reduce the recurrence of ulcers

Practice saying each of the words aloud. To hear the terms, access the **PRONOUNCE IT** activity for this chapter on the Student CD that accompanies this text. Or, to hear the terms and their definitions with a CD player or computer, obtain the Pronunciation CD designed for use with this text.

Learn the definitions and spellings of the surgical terms by completing exercises 18 and 19.

EXERCISE   18

Write the term for each of the following definitions.

1. cutting certain branches of
   the vagus nerve   _____

2. surgical connection between
   two structures   _____

3. removal of the colon and
   rectum   _____

EXERCISE   19

Spell each of the surgical terms. Have someone dictate the terms on p. 398 to you. Study any words you have spelled incorrectly.

1. _____   3. _____

2. _____

Diagnostic Terms

Built from Word Parts

Term	Definition
Diagnostic Imaging	
cholangiogram.................................... (kō-LAN-jē-ō-gram)	x-ray image of bile ducts. (An injection of radiopaque material is used to outline the ducts.)
cholecystogram.................................... (kō-lē-SIS-tō-gram)	x-ray image of the gallbladder. (Oral cholecystogram is still used to diagnose cholelithiasis, but ultrasound is now the method of choice.) (Exercise Figure G)

Operative cholangiography is performed during surgery to check for residual stones after the removal of the gallbladder. Postoperative **cholangiography,** also called T-tube cholangiography, is performed in the radiology department after a cholecystectomy, also to check for residual stones. Both use the injection of contrast medium into the common bile duct.

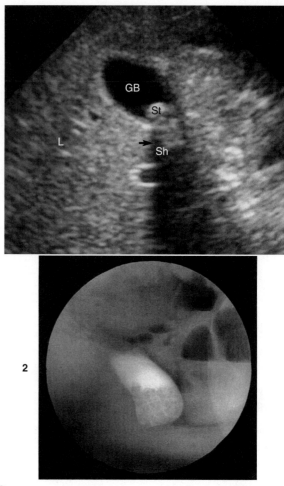

Exercise Figure G

Fill in the blanks to complete labeling of the diagram. **1,** Abdominal ultrasound showing cholelithiasis.
2, Oral _____ / ___ / _____ / ___ / _____ showing multiple small stones settled at the
        gall / **cv** / **bladder** / **cv** / **x-ray image**
bottom of the gallbladder.

Computerized tomography (CT) colonography, also called **virtual colonoscopy,** is a new method to
test for colon cancer. It involves using a CT scanner and computer software that allows the physician
to see the colon in multiple dimensions. It is less invasive than the conventional method of colonoscopy to
screen for colon cancer.

CT colonography.................................... (kō-lon-OG-ra-fē)	x-ray imaging of the colon
Endoscopy	
colonoscope... (kō-LON-ō-skōp)	instrument used for visual examination of the colon
colonoscopy... (kō-lon-OS-kō-pē)	visual examination of the colon (see Figures 11-12 and 11-13)
endoscope.. (EN-dō-skōp)	instrument used for visual examination within a hollow organ

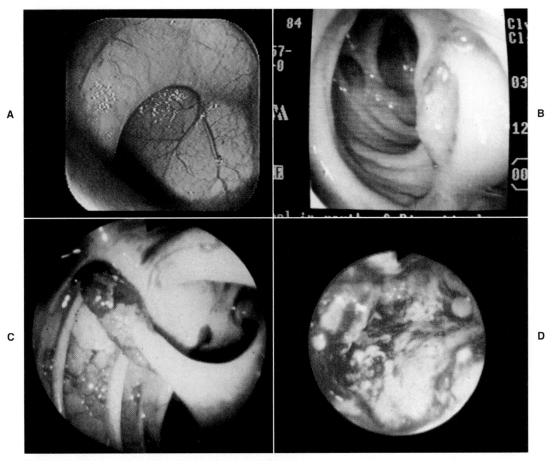

Figure 11-13
Endoscopic views obtained at colonoscopy reveal **A,** normal colon; **B,** diverticulosis; **C,** colon polyp; and **D,** colon cancer.

Capsule endoscopy, also known as **camera endoscopy,** was approved for use in 2001 by the Food and Drug Administration. Patients swallow a capsule containing a camera, about the size of a large vitamin pill. Pictures are taken by the camera every second as it moves naturally through the digestive tract. The images are recorded on a small device worn around the patient's waist. The recording device is returned to the physician's office after 8 hours. The images are transferred to a computer and examined. The video capsule is expelled in the bowel movement and not retrieved.

Capsule endoscopy replaces the standard endoscopy performed by pushing an endoscopic tube through the small intestine. It is especially helpful in identifying the cause of intestinal bleeding, revealing ulcers in Crohn disease, and diagnosing the causes of abdominal pain.

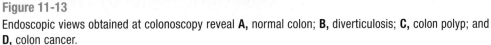

endoscopy .... (en-DOS-kō-pē)	visual examination within a hollow organ (see Figure 11-13)
esophagogastroduodenoscopy (EGD) .... (e-*sof*-a-gō-*gas*-trō-dū-od-e-NOS-kō-pē)	visual examination of the esophagus, stomach, and duodenum
esophagoscope .... (e-SOF-a-gō-skōp)	instrument for visual examination of the esophagus

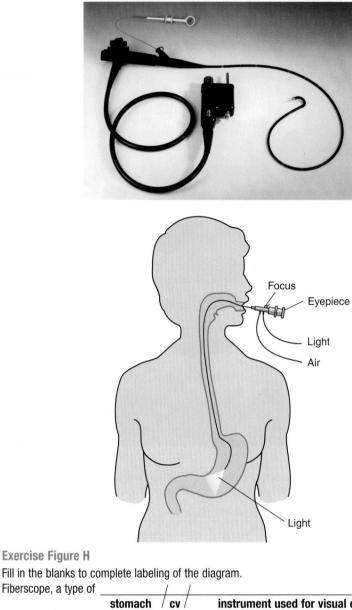

Exercise Figure H

Fill in the blanks to complete labeling of the diagram.

Fiberscope, a type of _____ that

<u>stomach</u> / **cv** / **instrument used for visual examination**

has glass fibers in a flexible tube, allows for light to be transmitted back to the examiner.

esophagoscopy.................................... (e-*sof*-a-GOS-kō-pē)	visual examination of the esophagus
gastroscope............................ (GAS-trō-skōp)	instrument used for visual examination of the stomach (Exercise Figure H)
gastroscopy............................ (gas-TROS-kō-pē)	visual examination of the stomach
laparoscope........................... (LAP-a-rō-skōp)	instrument used for visual examination of the abdominal cavity

The **laparoscope** is the instrument used to perform laparoscopic surgery, a modern method that sometimes replaces **laparotomy,** open abdominal incisional surgery (see Figures 8-10 and 11-9). Abdominal surgeries performed with a laparoscope include laparoscopic cholecystectomy, laparoscopic herniorrhaphy, laparoscopic appendectomy, and laparoscopic colectomy.

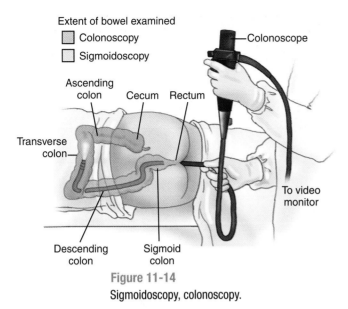

Extent of bowel examined
☐ Colonoscopy
☐ Sigmoidoscopy

Figure 11-14
Sigmoidoscopy, colonoscopy.

laparoscopy .... (lap-a-ROS-kō-pē)	visual examination of the abdominal cavity
proctoscope .... (PROK-tō-skōp)	instrument used for visual examination of the rectum
proctoscopy .... (prok-TOS-kō-pē)	visual examination of the rectum
sigmoidoscope .... (sig-MOY-dō-skōp)	instrument used for visual examination of the sigmoid colon
sigmoidoscopy .... (*sig*-moy-DOS-kō-pē)	visual examination of the sigmoid colon (Figure 11-14)

Practice saying each of these words aloud. To hear the terms, access the **PRONOUNCE IT** activity for this chapter on the Student CD that accompanies this text. Or, to hear the terms and their definitions with a CD player or computer, obtain the Pronunciation CD designed for use with this text.

Learn the definitions and spellings of the diagnostic terms by completing exercises 20, 21, and 22.

EXERCISE 20

Analyze and define the following diagnostic terms.

1. esophagoscope _____

2. esophagoscopy _____

3. gastroscope _____

4. gastroscopy _____

5. proctoscope _____

6. proctoscopy _____

7. endoscope _____

8. endoscopy _____

9. sigmoidoscope _____

10. sigmoidoscopy _____

11. cholecystogram _____

12. cholangiogram _____

13. esophagogastroduodenoscopy _____

14. colonoscope _____

15. laparoscope _____

16. colonoscopy _____

17. laparoscopy _____

18. CT colonography _____

EXERCISE 21

Build diagnostic terms that correspond to the following definitions by using the word parts you have learned.

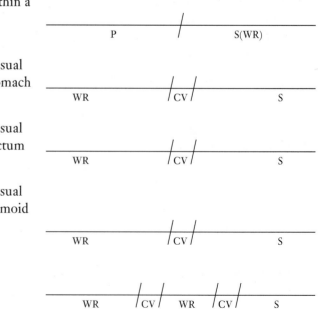

1. visual examination within a
   hollow organ

   _____ / _____
   P   S(WR)

2. instrument used for visual
   examination of the stomach

   _____ /_/ _____
   WR   CV   S

3. instrument used for visual
   examination of the rectum

   _____ /_/ _____
   WR   CV   S

4. instrument used for visual
   examination of the sigmoid
   colon

   _____ /_/ _____
   WR   CV   S

5. x-ray image of the
   gallbladder

   _____ /_/ _____ /_/ _____
   WR   CV   WR   CV   S

6. instrument used for visual examination within a hollow organ

_____ / _____
     P   S(WR)

7. instrument used for visual examination of the esophagus

_____ /CV/ _____
     WR   S

8. visual examination of the rectum

_____ /CV/ _____
     WR   S

9. visual examination of the esophagus

_____ /CV/ _____
     WR   S

10. visual examination of the sigmoid colon

_____ /CV/ _____
     WR   S

11. x-ray image of bile ducts

_____ /CV/ _____
     WR   S

12. visual examination of the stomach

_____ /CV/ _____
     WR   S

13. instrument used for visual examination of the abdominal cavity

_____ /CV/ _____
     WR   S

14. visual examination of the esophagus, stomach, and duodenum

___ /CV/ ___ /CV/ _____ /CV/ ___
WR   WR   WR   S

15. visual examination of the colon

_____ /CV/ _____
     WR   S

16. visual examination of the abdominal cavity

_____ /CV/ _____
     WR   S

17. instrument used for visual examination of the colon

_____ /CV/ _____
     WR   S

18. x-ray imaging of the colon

CT _____ /CV/ _____
        WR   S

EXERCISE **22**

Spell each of the diagnostic terms. Have someone dictate the terms on pp. 399-403 to you. Think about the word parts before attempting to write the word. Study any words you have spelled incorrectly.

1. _____   10. _____

2. _____   11. _____

3. _____   12. _____

4. _____   13. _____

5. _____   14. _____

6. _____   15. _____

7. _____   16. _____

8. _____   17. _____

9. _____   18. _____

Diagnostic Terms

Not Built from Word Parts

Term	Definition
Diagnostic Imaging	
barium enema (BE).............. (BAR-ē-um) (EN-e-ma)	series of x-ray images taken of the large in-testine after a barium enema has been admin-istered (Figure 11-15)
upper GI (gastrointestinal) series.......................................	series of x-ray images taken of the stomach and duodenum after barium has been swallowed
Endoscopy	
endoscopic retrograde cholangiopancreatography (ERCP).................................... (kō-lan-jē-ō-*pan*-krē-a-TOG-rah-fē)	radiographic (x-ray) examination of the bile and pancreatic ducts with contrast medium, fluoroscopy, and endoscopy (Figure 11-16)
endoscopic ultrasound (EUS)..........	a procedure using an endoscope fitted with an ultrasound probe that provides images of layers of the intestinal wall. Used to detect tumors and cystic growths and for staging of malignant tumors.

ERCP was first performed in 1968. ERCP is used to evaluate obstructions, pancreatic cancer, and unex-plained pancreatitis. It is used to diagnose stone diseases, strictures, and pancreatic neoplasms.

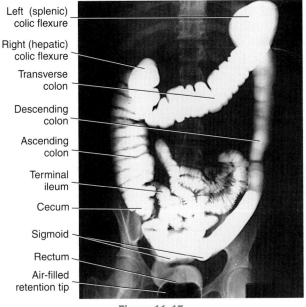

Left (splenic) colic flexure
Right (hepatic) colic flexure
Transverse colon
Descending colon
Ascending colon
Terminal ileum
Cecum
Sigmoid
Rectum
Air-filled retention tip

Figure 11-15
Barium enema.

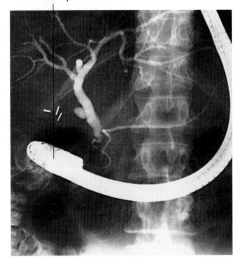

Endoscope

Figure 11-16
Endoscopic retrograde cholangiopancreatography (ERCP) is used to diagnose biliary and pancreatic pathologic conditions.

Abdominal ultrasound, which includes images of the **liver, gallbladder, biliary tract,** and **pancreas,** is a major diagnostic tool. It can detect liver cysts, abscesses, tumors, gallstones, an enlarged pancreas, and pancreatic tumors. High-frequency sound waves are used to visualize the size and structure of the internal organs. Abdominal ultrasound is replacing the use of the cholecystogram to diagnose the presence of cholelithiasis.

Laboratory

Helicobacter pylori (H. pylori)
antibodies test.................................
(hēl-i-kō-BAK-ter) (pī-LŌ-rē)
(AN-ti-bod-ēs)

a blood test to determine the presence of *H. pylori* bacteria. The bacteria can be found in the lining of the stomach and can cause peptic ulcers. Tests for *H. pylori* are also performed on biopsy specimens and by breath test.

fecal occult blood test
(also called *guaiac test*) ....
(FĒ-kl) (o-KULT)

a test to detect occult blood in feces. It is used to screen for colon cancer or polyps. Occult blood refers to blood that is present but can only be viewed microscopically. Trade names for commercial test kits include: *Hema-Check, Colo-Rect,* and *Hematest.*

Practice saying each of the words aloud. To hear the terms, access the **PRONOUNCE IT** activity for this chapter on the Student CD that accompanies this text. Or, to hear the terms and their definitions with a CD player or computer, obtain the Pronunciation CD designed for use with this text.

Learn the definitions and spellings of diagnostic terms by completing exercises 23 and 24.

EXERCISE 23

Write definitions for the following terms.

1. upper GI series _____

2. barium enema _____

3. endoscopic retrograde cholangiopancreatography _____

4. endoscopic ultrasound _____

5. *Helicobacter pylori* antibodies test _____

6. fecal occult blood test _____

EXERCISE 24

Match the procedures in the first column with their correct definitions in the second column.

_____ 1. fecal occult blood test   a. used to diagnose peptic ulcers

_____ 2. barium enema   b. x-ray image of the stomach and duodenum

_____ 3. *Helicobacter pylori* antibodies test   c. examination of bile and pancreatic ducts

    d. detects blood in feces

_____ 4. upper GI series   e. x-ray image of the esophagus

_____ 5. endoscopic retrograde cholangiopancreatography   f. x-ray image of the large intestine

EXERCISE 25

Spell each of the diagnostic terms. Have someone dictate the terms on pp. 406-407 to you. Study any words you have spelled incorrectly.

1. _____   4. _____

2. _____   5. _____

3. _____   6. _____

Complementary Terms

Built from Word Parts

Term	Definition
abdominal.. (ab-DOM-i-nal)	pertaining to the abdomen
abdominocentesis............................. (ab-*dom*-i-nō-sen-TĒ-sis)	surgical puncture to remove fluid from the abdominal cavity (also called *paracentesis*)
anal.. (A-nal)	pertaining to the anus

aphagia	without swallowing (the inability to)
(a-FĀ-jē-a)	
colorectal	pertaining to the colon and rectum
(kō-lō-REK-tal)	
dyspepsia	difficult digestion (often used to describe GI symptoms)
(dis-PEP-sē-a)	
dysphagia	difficult swallowing
(dis-FĀ-jē-a)	
gastrodynia	pain in the stomach
(*gas*-trō-DIN-ē-a)	
gastroenterologist	a physician who studies and treats diseases of the stomach and intestines (GI tract and accessory organs)
(*gas*-trō-en-ter-OL-ō-jist)	
gastroenterology	study of the stomach and intestines (a branch of medicine that deals with treating diseases of the GI tract and accessory organs)
(*gas*-trō-en-ter-OL-ō-jē)	
gastromalacia	softening of the stomach
(*gas*-trō-ma-LĀ-shē-a)	
glossopathy	disease of the tongue
(glo-SOP-a-thē)	
ileocecal	pertaining to the ileum and cecum
(*il*-ē-ō-SĒ-kal)	
nasogastric	pertaining to the nose and stomach
(*nā*-zō-GAS-trik)	
oral	pertaining to the mouth
(Ō-ral)	
pancreatic	pertaining to the pancreas
(*pan*-krē-AT-ik)	
peritoneal	pertaining to the peritoneum
(*par*-i-tō-NĒ-al)	
proctologist	physician who studies and treats diseases of the rectum
(prok-TOL-ō-jist)	
proctology	study of the rectum (a branch of medicine that deals with disorders of the rectum and anus)
(prok-TOL-ō-jē)	
rectal	pertaining to the rectum (a branch of medicine that deals with treating diseases of the rectum)
(REK-tal)	
stomatogastric	pertaining to the mouth and stomach
(*stō*-ma-tō-GAS-trik)	
sublingual	pertaining to under the tongue
(sub-LING-gwal)	

Practice saying each of these terms aloud. To hear the terms, access the **PRONOUNCE IT** activity for this chapter on the Student CD that accompanies this text. Or, to hear the terms and their definitions with a CD player or computer, obtain the Pronunciation CD designed for use with this text.

Exercises 26, 27, and 28 will help you learn the definitions and spellings of the complementary terms related to the digestive system.

EXERCISE 26

Analyze and define the following complementary terms.

1. aphagia _____

2. dyspepsia _____

3. anal _____

4. dysphagia _____

5. glossopathy _____

6. ileocecal _____

7. oral _____

8. stomatogastric _____

9. abdominocentesis _____

10. gastromalacia _____

11. pancreatic _____

12. gastrodynia _____

13. peritoneal _____

14. sublingual _____

15. proctology _____

16. nasogastric _____

17. abdominal _____

18. proctologist _____

19. gastroenterology _____

20. gastroenterologist _____

21. colorectal _____

22. rectal _____

EXERCISE 27

Build the complementary terms for the following definitions by using the word parts you have learned.

1. disease of the tongue _____ /CV/ _____
                          WR   S

2. without swallowing (the inability to)

_____ / _____
          P   S(WR)

3. pertaining to under the tongue

_____ / WR / _____
          P   S

4. pertaining to the nose and the stomach

_____ / CV / WR / _____
   WR   S

5. pertaining to the mouth and the stomach

_____ / CV / WR / _____
   WR   S

6. pertaining to the anus

_____ / _____
   WR   S

7. surgical puncture to remove fluid from the abdominal cavity

_____ / CV / _____
   WR   S

8. pertaining to the peritoneum

_____ / _____
   WR   S

9. pertaining to the abdomen

_____ / _____
   WR   S

10. difficult swallowing

_____ / _____
          P   S(WR)

11. pertaining to the ileum and cecum

_____ / CV / WR / _____
   WR   S

12. softening of the stomach

_____ / CV / _____
   WR   S

13. pain in the stomach

_____ / _____
   WR   S

14. physician who studies and treats diseases of the rectum

_____ / CV / _____
   WR   S

15. difficult digestion

_____ / _____
          P   S(WR)

16. pertaining to the pancreas

_____ / _____
   WR   S

17. study of the rectum

_____ / CV / _____
   WR   S

18. pertaining to the mouth

_____ / _____
　　　　　　　　　WR　　　　　　　S

19. physician who studies and
treats diseases of the
stomach and intestines

_____ /__/ _____ /__/ _____
　WR　　/CV/　WR　/CV/　　S

20. study of the stomach and
intestines

_____ /__/ _____ /__/ _____
　WR　　/CV/　WR　/CV/　　S

21. pertaining to the colon and
rectum

_____ /__/ _____ / _____
　WR　　/CV/　　WR　　　　S

22. pertaining to the rectum

_____ / _____
　　　　WR　　　　　　　S

EXERCISE 28

Spell each of the complementary terms. Have someone dictate the terms on pp. 408-409 to you. Think about the word parts before attempting to write the word. Study any words you have spelled incorrectly.

1. _____

2. _____

3. _____

4. _____

5. _____

6. _____

7. _____

8. _____

9. _____

10. _____

11. _____

12. _____

13. _____

14. _____

15. _____

16. _____

17. _____

18. _____

19. _____

20. _____

21. _____

22. _____

Complementary Terms

Not Built from Word Parts

Term	Definition
ascites... (a-SĪ-tēz)	abnormal collection of fluid in the peritoneal cavity

diarrhea .... (dī-a-RĒ-a) (NOTE: diarrhea is composed of *dia*, meaning through, and *rrhea*, meaning flow.)	frequent discharge of liquid stool
dysentery .... (DIS-en-ter-ē)	disorder that involves inflammation of the intestine associated with diarrhea and abdominal pain
feces .... (FĒ-sēz)	waste from the digestive tract expelled through the rectum (also called a *bowel movement, stool,* or *fecal matter*)
flatus .... (FLĀ-tus)	gas in the digestive tract or expelled through the anus
gastric lavage .... (la-VOZH)	washing out of the stomach
gavage .... (ga-VOZH)	process of feeding a person through a nasogastric tube
hematemesis .... (hēm-a-TEM-e-sis)	vomiting of blood
melena .... (me-LĒ-na)	black, tarry stool that contains digested blood. Usually a result of bleeding in the upper GI tract.
nausea .... (NAW-zē-a)	urge to vomit
peristalsis .... (per-i-STAL-sis)	involuntary wavelike contractions that propel food along the digestive tract
reflux .... (RĒ-fluks)	abnormal backward flow. In esophageal reflux, the stomach contents flow back into the esophagus.
vomit .... (VOM-it)	matter expelled from the stomach through the mouth (also called *vomitus* or *emesis*)

Practice saying each of these terms aloud. To hear the terms, access the **PRONOUNCE IT** activity for this chapter on the Student CD that accompanies this text. Or, to hear the terms and their definitions with a CD player or computer, obtain the Pronunciation CD designed for use with this text.

Learn the definitions and spellings of the complementary terms by completing exercises 29, 30, and 31.

EXERCISE 29

Match the definitions in the first column with the correct terms in the second column.

_____ 1. abnormal collection of fluid

_____ 2. matter expelled from the stomach

_____ 3. feeding a person through a tube

a. hematemesis

b. flatus

c. gastric lavage

d. reflux

e. vomit

_____ 4. washing out of the stomach

_____ 5. urge to vomit

_____ 6. frequent discharge of liquid stool

_____ 7. waste expelled from the rectum

_____ 8. vomiting of blood

_____ 9. abnormal backward flow

_____ 10. inflammation of the intestine associated with diarrhea and abdominal pain

_____ 11. gas expelled through the anus

_____ 12. involuntary wavelike contractions

_____ 13. black, tarry stools

f. gavage

g. melena

h. dysentery

i. diarrhea

j. peristalsis

k. feces

l. nausea

m. ascites

EXERCISE 30

Write definitions for each of the following terms.

1. ascites _____

2. gavage _____

3. gastric lavage_____

4. feces _____

5. nausea _____

6. vomit _____

7. dysentery _____

8. diarrhea _____

9. flatus _____

10. reflux _____

11. hematemesis _____

12. peristalsis _____

13. melena _____

EXERCISE   31

Spell each of the complementary terms. Have someone dictate the terms on pp. 412-413 to you. Study any words you have spelled incorrectly.

1. _____   8. _____

2. _____   9. _____

3. _____   10. _____

4. _____   11. _____

5. _____   12. _____

6. _____   13. _____

7. _____

Refer to Appendix J for a list of nutritional terms.

Abbreviations

A&P resection	abdominoperineal resection
BE	barium enema
EGD	esophagogastroduodenoscopy
ERCP	endoscopic retrograde cholangiopancreatography
EUS	endoscopic ultrasound
GERD	gastroesophageal reflux disease
GI	gastrointestinal
H. pylori	*Helicobacter pylori*
IBS	irritable bowel syndrome
N&V	nausea and vomiting
PEG	percutaneous endoscopic gastrostomy
UGI	upper gastrointestinal
UPPP	uvulopalatopharyngoplasty

Refer to Appendix D for a complete list of abbreviations.

EXERCISE   32

Write the meaning of the following abbreviations.

1. ERCP _____ _____ _____

2. EUS _____ _____

3. N&V _____ & _____

4. IBS _____ _____ _____

5. PEG _____ _____ _____

6. UGI _____ _____

7. UPPP _____

8. GERD _____ _____ _____

9. GI _____

10. *H. pylori* _____ _____

11. BE _____ _____

12. EGD _____

13. A&P resection _____ _____

CHAPTER REVIEW

EXERCISE   33   *Interact with Medical Records*

Complete the endoscopy report by writing the medical terms in the blanks. Use the list of definitions with the corresponding numbers.

University Hospital and Medical Center
4700 North Main Street • Wellness, Arizona 54321 • (987) 555-3210

PATIENT NAME: Ruth Clifton	**CASE NUMBER:** 77721-DIG
DATE OF BIRTH: 09/15/xx	**DATE:** 12/27/xx

ENDOSCOPY REPORT

CASE HISTORY: This is a 40-year-old African American woman who was referred to the 1. _____ clinic for evaluation. Patient reports 2. _____ and vomiting with upper abdominal pain. She has also had a problem with 3. _____ but denies any 4. _____ or 5. _____ . She has not used any alcohol or salicylates. She is currently taking several medications but they are not known for ulcerogenic side effects.

PROCEDURE: 6. _____ : The patient was given 2 mg of intravenous Versed along with lidocaine spray to the pharynx. After the patient was placed in the left lateral decubitus position, the Olympus 7. _____ was passed into the esophagus without difficulty. The esophagus in its entirety was essentially free of mucosal abnormalities. No evidence of 8. _____. The stomach was entered and some gastric juices were aspirated. The esophagus, the cardia, and the antrum body of the stomach were free of abnormalities. A biopsy of the gastric mucosa was taken for 9. _____ . In the distal antral area some mild erythematous changes were noted. The pylorus had normal peristaltic activity. The first part of the duodenum, however, revealed evidence of ulcerations, both anterosuperiorly as well as posteroinferiorly, with surrounding erythema. These 10. _____ were less than 1 cm in size. The second part of the duodenum was free of mucosal abnormalities. Withdrawing the scope confirmed the findings upon entry. The patient tolerated the procedure quite well and recovered uneventfully.

Vital signs will be taken every half hour for the next 2 hours.

POSTPROCEDURAL DIAGNOSIS:
11. _____
12. _____   _____

_____
Jesus Garcia, MD

JG/mcm

---

1. visual examination within a hollow organ
2. urge to vomit
3. difficult digestion
4. vomiting of blood
5. black, tarry stool that contains digested blood
6. visual examination of the esophagus, stomach, and duodenum
7. instrument used for visual examination of the stomach
8. abnormal backward flow
9. abbreviation for *Helicobacter pylori*
10. eroded sores
11. inflammation of the stomach
12. ulcer in the duodenum

EXERCISE 34 *Interpret Medical Terms*

To test your understanding of the terms introduced in this chapter, circle the words that correctly complete the sentences. The italicized words refer to the correct answer.

1. Mr. E. was admitted to the hospital with a diagnosis of *gallstones*, or (cholelithiasis, cholecystitis, sialolithiasis).
2. An abdominal ultrasound confirmed the admitting diagnosis, and Mr. E. is now scheduled for a laparoscopic *excision of the gallbladder*, or (cholecystostomy, cholecystectomy, colectomy).
3. The patient was diagnosed with a condition including the symptom of *inflammation of the colon and formation of ulcers*, called (cirrhosis, ulcerative colitis, peptic ulcer).
4. A *prolapse of the rectum* is (rectocele, intussusception, proctoptosis).
5. An *abnormal growing together of two surfaces* is (anastomosis, adhesion, amniocentesis).
6. Three surgical procedures that may be performed on a patient with peptic ulcers are (1) *excision of the stomach*, or (gastrotomy, gastrostomy, gastrectomy); (2) *surgical repair of the pylorus*, or (pyloroplasty, cheilorrhaphy, gastrojejunostomy); and (3) *cutting of certain branches of the vagus nerve*, or (colostomy, vagotomy, gingivectomy).
7. *Difficult digestion* is (dyspepsia, dysphagia, gastrodynia).
8. *Feeding* a person *through a gastric tube* is called (lavage, gavage, gastrostomy).
9. The *surgical procedure to remove the colon and rectum and create an artificial opening into the colon* is (colectomy and colostomy, abdominoperineal resection and colostomy, abdominoperineal resection and ileostomy).
10. To rule out cancer of the colon, the doctor performed a diagnostic procedure to *visually examine the colon* or (colonoscopy, colonoscope, colostomy).
11. The doctor diagnosed the patient as having *an obstruction of the intestine* or (polyp, irritable bowel syndrome, ileus).
12. The following test is used to screen for colon cancer (fecal occult blood, *Helicobacter pylori* antibodies test, upper GI series).

EXERCISE 35 *Read Medical Terms in Use*

Practice pronunciation of terms by reading the following discussion. Use the pronunciation key following the medical term to assist you in saying the word.

Colorectal Cancer

Colorectal (kō-lō-REK-tal) cancer begins in the colon or rectum and is the second leading cause of cancer deaths in the United States. Most are adenocarcinomas that originate as a benign, adenomatous **polyp** (POL-ip).

Many people have no symptoms until the tumor is quite advanced, and symptoms vary depending on the location of the tumor. Warning signs are altered bowel habits, **rectal** (REK-tal) bleeding, **abdominal** (ab-DOM-i-nal) cramps, **flatus** (FLĀ-tus) and bloating, iron deficiency anemia, and weight loss.

Screening and diagnostic tests for colorectal cancer include digital rectal examination, **fecal** (FĒ-kl) **occult** (o-KULT) blood test, **sigmoidoscopy** (sig-moy-DOS-kō-pē), **colonoscopy** (kō-lon-OS-kō-pē), and **barium** (BAR-ē-um) **enema** (EN-e-ma). As well as being an important diagnostic tool, colonoscopy may be used for biopsy and for the removal of **polyps** in the early stage of colon cancer. To perform a **polypectomy** (pol-e-PEK-tō-mē), a braided wire snare is inserted into the **colonoscope** (kō-LON-ō-skōp). A snare loop, like a noose, is placed around the stem of the polyp. With electrosurgical power attached to the snare, the polyp is detached. The polyp is removed from the colon for histologic examination.

For cancer beyond the early stage, conventional surgery is the main treatment. The type of surgery depends on the location and stage of the tumor. Types of surgeries performed are left- or right-sided **hemicolectomy** (hem-i-kō-LEK-tō-mē) with **anastomosis** (a-nas-tō-MŌ-sis), sigmoid **colectomy** (kō-LEK-tō-mē), and **abdominoperineal** (ab-dom-in-ō-par-i-NĒ-el) **resection** with **colostomy** (kō-LOS-tō-mē).

EXERCISE 36 *Comprehend Medical Terms in Use*

Test your comprehension of terms in the previous medical discussion by circling the correct answer.

1. Which of the following is used for diagnosing colorectal cancer?
   a. visual exam of the stomach
   b. series of x-rays of the small intestine
   c. visual exam of the colon
   d. x-ray image of the esophagus
2. T   F   A polypectomy may be performed during a colonoscopy.
3. T   F   Depending on the location of the tumor, a surgical treatment for colorectal cancer may be performed that creates an opening between the colon and abdominal wall for the passage of stool.
4. T   F   Vomiting blood is a warning sign for colorectal cancer.

> For further practice or to evaluate what you have learned, use the Student CD that accompanies this text.

COMBINING FORMS CROSSWORD PUZZLE

Across Clues

1. palate
3. abdomen
5. liver
9. peritoneum
11. intestine
13. ileum
14. cecum
16. diverticulum
19. pylorus
21. gum
24. jejunum
25. sigmoid
26. uvula

Down Clues

1. rectum
2. abdomen
4. tongue
5. hernia
6. stomach
7. antrum
8. appendix
9. pancreas
10. gall, bile
12. duodenum
15. lip
17. colon
18. mouth
20. rectum
21. tongue
22. saliva
23. anus

REVIEW OF WORD PARTS

Can you define and spell the following word parts?

Combining Forms

abdomin/o	duoden/o	or/o
an/o	enter/o	palat/o
antr/o	esophag/o	pancreat/o
appendic/o	gastr/o	peritone/o
cec/o	gingiv/o	polyp/o
celi/o	gloss/o	proct/o
cheil/o	hepat/o	pylor/o
cholangi/o	herni/o	rect/o
chol/e	ile/o	sial/o
choledoch/o	jejun/o	sigmoid/o
col/o	lapar/o	stomat/o
colon/o	lingu/o	uvul/o
diverticul/o		

Prefix

hemi-

Suffix

-pepsia

REVIEW OF TERMS

Can you build, analyze, define, pronounce, and spell the following terms *built from word parts?*

Diseases and Disorders	Surgical	Diagnostic	Complementary
appendicitis	abdominoplasty	cholangiogram	abdominal
cholangioma	anoplasty	cholecystogram	abdominocentesis
cholecystitis	antrectomy	colonoscope	anal
choledocholithiasis	appendectomy	colonoscopy	aphagia
cholelithiasis	celiotomy	CT colonography	colorectal
diverticulitis	cheilorrhaphy	endoscope	dyspepsia
diverticulosis	cholecystectomy	endoscopy	dysphagia
esophagitis	choledocholithotomy	esophagogastroduodenoscopy	gastrodynia
gastritis	colectomy	(EGD)	gastroenterologist
gastroenteritis	colostomy	esophagoscope	gastroenterology
gastroenterocolitis	diverticulectomy	esophagoscopy	gastromalacia
gingivitis	enterorrhaphy	gastroscope	glossopathy
hepatitis	esophagogastroplasty	gastroscopy	ileocecal
hepatoma	gastrectomy	laparoscope	nasogastric
palatitis	gastrojejunostomy	laparoscopy	oral
pancreatitis	gastroplasty	proctoscope	pancreatic
peritonitis	gastrostomy	proctoscopy	peritoneal
polyposis	gingivectomy	sigmoidoscope	proctologist
proctoptosis	glossorrhaphy	sigmoidoscopy	proctology
rectocele	hemicolectomy		rectal
sialolith	herniorrhaphy		stomatogastric
uvulitis	ileostomy		sublingual
	laparotomy		
	palatoplasty		
	polypectomy		
	pyloromyotomy		
	pyloroplasty		
	uvulectomy		
	uvulopalatopharyngoplasty (UPPP)		

Can you define, pronounce, and spell the following terms *not built from word parts?*

Diseases and Disorders

adhesion

anorexia nervosa

bulimia nervosa

cirrhosis

Crohn disease

duodenal ulcer

gastric ulcer

gastroesophageal reflux disease
  (GERD)

ileus

intussusception

irritable bowel syndrome (IBS)

obesity

peptic ulcer

polyp

ulcerative colitis

volvulus

Surgical

abdominoperineal resection
  (A&P resection)

anastomosis

vagotomy

Diagnostic

barium enema (BE)

endoscopic retrograde
  cholangiopancreatography
  (ERCP)

endoscopic ultrasound
  (EUS)

fecal occult blood test

Helicobacter pylori antibodies
  test *(H. pylori)*

upper GI (gastrointestinal)
  series

Complementary

ascites

diarrhea

dysentery

feces

flatus

gastric lavage

gavage

hematemesis

melena

nausea

peristalsis

reflux

vomit

12

Eye

OUTLINE

OBJECTIVES

On completion of this chapter you will be able to:

1. Identify the anatomy of the eye.
2. Define and spell the word parts presented in this chapter.
3. Build and analyze medical terms with word parts presented in this and previous chapters.
4. Define, pronounce, and spell the disease and disorder, diagnostic, surgical, and complementary terms for the eye.
5. Interpret the meaning of the abbreviations presented in this chapter.
6. Read medical documents and interpret medical terminology contained in them.

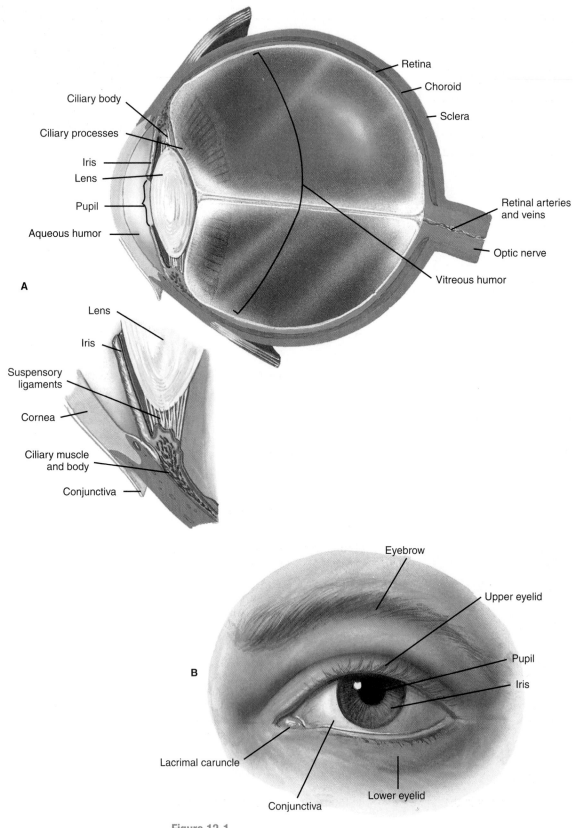

Figure 12-1
A, Anatomy of the eye; **B,** visible surface of the eye.

ANATOMY

Function

The eyes are organs of vision and are located in a bony protective cavity of the skull called the *orbit*. Only a small portion of the eye is visible from the exterior (Figure 12-1).

Structures of the Eye

sclera	outer protective layer of the eye; the portion seen on the anterior portion of the eyeball is referred to as the *white of the eye*
cornea	transparent anterior part of the sclera, which is in front of the aqueous humor and lies over the iris
choroid	middle layer of the eye, which is interlaced with many blood vessels
iris	the pigmented muscular structure that allows light to pass through
pupil	opening in the center of the iris
lens	lies directly behind the pupil. Its function is to focus and bend light.
retina	innermost layer of the eye, which contains the vision receptors (Figure 12-2)
aqueous humor	watery liquid found in the anterior cavity of the eye
vitreous humor	jellylike substance found behind the lens in the posterior cavity of the eye that maintains its shape
meibomian glands	oil glands found in the upper and lower edges of the eyelids that help lubricate the eye
lacrimal glands and ducts	produce and drain tears
optic nerve	carries visual impulses from the retina to the brain
conjunctiva	mucous membrane lining the eyelids and covering the anterior portion of the sclera

Learn the anatomic terms by completing exercises 1 and 2.

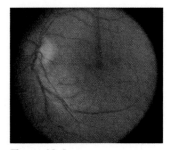

Figure 12-2
Ophthalmoscopic view of the retina.

Iris
was the special messenger of the Queen of Heaven according to Greek mythology. In this role she passed from heaven to earth over the rainbow while dressed in rainbow hues. Her name was applied to the **circular eye muscle** because of its varied colors.

EXERCISE   1

Match the anatomic terms in the first column with the correct definitions in the second column.

_____ 1. aqueous humor

_____ 2. choroid

_____ 3. conjunctiva

a. lies directly behind the pupil

b. the pigmented muscular structure

c. middle layer of the eye

_____ 4. cornea

_____ 5. iris

_____ 6. lacrimal glands

_____ 7. lens

d. watery liquid found in the anterior cavity of the eye

e. produce tears

f. mucous membrane lining the eyelids

g. jellylike substance behind the lens and in the posterior cavity

h. transparent anterior part of the sclera

EXERCISE 2

Match the anatomic terms in the first column with the correct definitions in the second column.

_____ 1. meibomian glands

_____ 2. optic nerve

_____ 3. orbit

_____ 4. pupil

_____ 5. retina

_____ 6. sclera

_____ 7. vitreous humor

a. outer protective layer of the eye

b. innermost layer of the eye

c. jellylike substance found behind the lens and in the posterior cavity of the eye

d. oil glands in eyelids that help lubricate the eye

e. opening in the center of the iris

f. carries visual impulses from the retina to the brain

g. middle layer of the eye

h. bony protective cavity of the skull in which the eye lies

WORD PARTS

Combining Forms for the Eye

Study the word parts and their definitions listed below. Completing the exercises that follow will help you learn the terms.

Combining Form	Definition
blephar/o.................................	eyelid
conjunctiv/o.................................	conjunctiva
cor/o, core/o, pupill/o................................. (NOTE: pupil has one *l*; the combining form has two *l*s.)	pupil
corne/o, kerat/o................................. (NOTE: *kerat/o* also means *hard* or *horny tissue*; see Chapter 4.)	cornea

dacry/o,	
lacrim/o	tear, tear duct
irid/o,	
iri/o	iris
ocul/o,	
ophthalm/o	eye
opt/o	vision
retin/o	retina
scler/o	sclera

Learn the anatomic locations and meanings of the combining forms by completing exercises 3 and 4 and Exercise Figure A.

Spelling Ophthalm
Look closely at the spelling of the word root **ophthalm.** Medical terms containing **ophthalm** are often misspelled by omitting the first h. **ph** Gives the **f** sound followed by the sound of **thal.**
Think pronunciation when spelling terms that contain **ophthalm,** as in ophthalmology (of(ph)-thal-MOL-ō-jē).

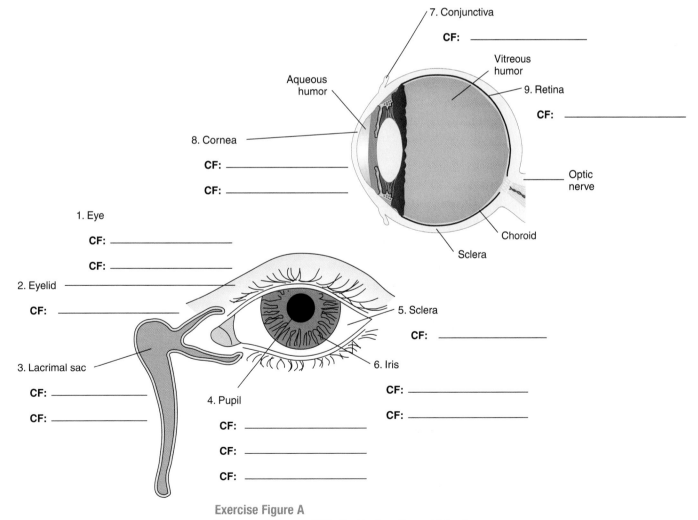

Exercise Figure A
Diagrams of the eye. Fill in the blanks with combining forms.

EXERCISE 3

Write the definitions of the following combining forms.

1. ocul/o _____

2. blephar/o _____

3. corne/o _____

4. lacrim/o _____

5. retin/o _____

6. pupill/o _____

7. scler/o _____

8. irid/o _____

9. conjunctiv/o _____

10. cor/o _____

11. ophthalm/o _____

12. kerat/o _____

13. iri/o _____

14. core/o _____

15. opt/o _____

16. dacry/o _____

EXERCISE 4

Write the combining form for each of the following terms.

1. eye
   a. _____

   b. _____

2. cornea
   a. _____

   b. _____

3. conjunctiva
   _____

4. tear duct, tear
   a. _____

   b. _____

5. eyelid   _____

6. pupil   a. _____

               b. _____

               c. _____

7. sclera   _____

8. retina   _____

9. iris   a. _____

               b. _____

10. vision   _____

Combining Forms Commonly Used With the Eye

Combining Form	Definition
cry/o	cold
dipl/o	two, double
phot/o	light
ton/o	tension, pressure

Learn the combining forms by completing exercises 5 and 6.

EXERCISE   5

Write the definitions of the following combining forms.

1. ton/o _____

2. phot/o _____

3. cry/o _____

4. dipl/o _____

EXERCISE   6

Write the combining form for each of the following.

1. cold   _____

2. tension, pressure _____

3. two, double   _____

4. light   _____

Prefixes and Suffixes

Prefixes	Definition
bi-, bin-	two

Suffixes	Definitions
-opia	vision (condition)
-phobia	abnormal fear of or aversion to specific things
-plegia	paralysis

Learn the prefixes and suffixes by completing exercises 7 and 8. Refer to Appendix A and Appendix B for a complete listing of word parts.

EXERCISE 7

Write the definition of the following prefixes and suffixes.

1. -opia _____

2. bi- _____

3. -plegia _____

4. -phobia _____

5. bin- _____

EXERCISE 8

Write the prefixes or suffixes for each of the following definitions.

1. paralysis _____

2. two a. _____

   b. _____

3. abnormal fear of or
   aversion to specific things _____

4. vision (condition) _____

MEDICAL TERMS

The terms you need to learn to complete this chapter are listed below. The exercises following each list will help you learn the definition and the spelling of each word.

Disease and Disorder Terms

Built from Word Parts

Term	Definition
blepharitis (*blef*-a-RĪ-tis)	inflammation of the eyelid (Exercise Figure B)
blepharoptosis (*blef*-ar-op-TŌ-sis)	drooping of the eyelid (Exercise Figure C) (commonly called *ptosis*)
conjunctivitis (kon-*junk*-ti-VĪ-tis)	inflammation of the conjunctiva (commonly called *pinkeye*)
dacryocystitis (*dak*-rē-ō-sis-TĪ-tis)	inflammation of the tear (lacrimal) sac (Exercise Figure D)
diplopia (di-PLŌ-pē-a)	double vision
endophthalmitis (en-dof-thal-MĪ-tis) (NOTE: the *o* in *endo* is dropped.)	inflammation within the eye
iridoplegia (īr-i-dō-PLĒ-jē-a)	paralysis of the iris
iritis (ī-RĪ-tis)	inflammation of the iris
keratitis (ker-a-TĪ-tis)	inflammation of the cornea
leukocoria (lū-kō-KŌ-rē-a)	condition of white pupil
oculomycosis (*ok*-ū-lō-mī-KŌ-sis)	abnormal condition of the eye caused by a fungus
ophthalmalgia (*of*-thal-MAL-jē-a)	pain in the eye
ophthalmoplegia (of-thal-mō-PLĒ-jē-a)	paralysis of the eye (muscle)

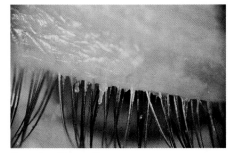

Exercise Figure B

Fill in the blanks to complete labeling of this diagram.

_____ / _____ with thickened
eyelid / inflammation

lids and crusts around the lashes.

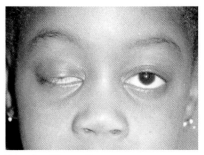

Exercise Figure C

Fill in the blanks to label the diagram.

_____ / __ / _____
eyelid / cv / drooping

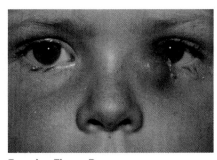

Exercise Figure D

Fill in the blanks to label the diagram.

_____ / __ / ___ / _____
tear / cv / sac / inflammation

photophobia................................... ($f\bar{o}$-t$\bar{o}$-F$\bar{O}$-b$\bar{e}$-a)	abnormal fear of (sensitivity to) light
retinoblastoma............................... (ret-i-n$\bar{o}$-blas-T$\bar{O}$-ma)	tumor arising from a developing retinal cell (a congenital, malignant tumor)
sclerokeratitis............................... (*skle*-r$\bar{o}$-kar-a-T$\bar{I}$-tis)	inflammation of the sclera and cornea
scleromalacia................................. (*skle*-r$\bar{o}$-ma-L$\bar{A}$-sh$\bar{e}$-a)	softening of the sclera

Practice saying each of these terms aloud. To hear the terms, access the **PRONOUNCE IT** activity for this chapter on the Student CD that accompanies this text. Or, to hear the terms and their definitions with a CD player or computer, obtain the Pronunciation CD designed for use with this text.

Learn the definitions and spellings of the disease and disorder terms by completing exercises 9, 10, and 11.

EXERCISE 9

Analyze and define the following terms.

1. sclerokeratitis _____

2. ophthalmalgia _____

3. blepharoptosis _____

4. diplopia _____

5. conjunctivitis _____

6. leukocoria _____

7. iridoplegia _____

8. scleromalacia _____

9. photophobia _____

10. blepharitis _____

11. oculomycosis _____

12. dacryocystitis _____

13. endophthalmitis _____

14. iritis _____

15. retinoblastoma _____

16. keratitis _____

17. ophthalmoplegia _____

EXERCISE 10

Build disease and disorder terms for the following definitions by using the word parts you have learned.

1. inflammation of the conjunctiva

   _____ / _____
   WR   S

2. abnormal eye condition caused by a fungus

   _____ / CV / _____ / _____
   WR   WR   S

3. pain in the eye

   _____ / _____
   WR   S

4. double vision

   _____ / _____
   WR   S

5. inflammation of the eyelid

   _____ / _____
   WR   S

6. condition of white pupil

   _____ / CV / _____ / _____
   WR   WR   S

7. paralysis of the iris

   _____ / CV / _____
   WR   S

8. drooping of the eyelid

   _____ / CV / _____
   WR   S

9. inflammation of the iris

   _____ / _____
   WR   S

10. tumor arising from a developing retinal cell

    _____ / CV / _____ / _____
    WR   WR   S

11. softening of the sclera

    _____ / CV / _____
    WR   S

12. inflammation of a tear (lacrimal) sac

    _____ / CV / _____ / _____
    WR   WR   S

13. inflammation of the sclera and cornea

    _____ / CV / _____ / _____
    WR   WR   S

14. abnormal fear of (sensitivity to) light

    _____ / CV / _____
    WR   S

15. inflammation of the cornea

    _____ / _____
    WR   S

16. inflammation within the eye _____ / _____ / _____
                                                               P   WR   S

17. paralysis of the eye (muscle) _____ / _____ / _____
                                                  WR   CV   S

EXERCISE 11

Spell each of the disease and disorder terms. Have someone dictate the terms on pp. 431-432 to you. Think about the word parts before attempting to write the word. Study any words you have spelled incorrectly.

1. _____   10. _____

2. _____   11. _____

3. _____   12. _____

4. _____   13. _____

5. _____   14. _____

6. _____   15. _____

7. _____   16. _____

8. _____   17. _____

9. _____

Disease and Disorder Terms

Not Built from Word Parts

Term	Definition
astigmatism (Ast) (a-STIG-ma-tizm)	defective curvature of the refractive surface of the eye
cataract (KAT-a-rakt)	clouding of the lens of the eye (Figure 12-3)

Cataract
is derived from the Greek **kato,** meaning **down,** and **raktos,** meaning **precipice.** Together, the words were interpreted as **waterfall.** The cataract sufferer sees things as through a watery veil of mist, or waterfall.

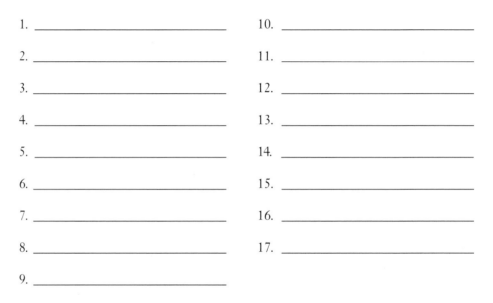

Figure 12-3
A, Snowflake cataract; **B,** senile cataract.

chalazion... (ka-LĀ-zē-on)	obstruction of an oil gland of the eyelid (also called *meibomian cyst*) (Figure 12-4)
detached retina.................................	separation of the retina from the choroid in back of the eye (Figure 12-5)
emmetropia (Em)............................... (em-e-TRŌ-pē-a)	normal refractive condition of the eye
glaucoma... (glaw-KŌ-ma)	eye disorder characterized by optic nerve damage usually caused by the abnormal increase of intraocular pressure. If not treated it will lead to blindness (Figure 12-6).
hyperopia... (*hī*-per-Ō-pē-a)	farsightedness (Figure 12-7)
macular degeneration....................... (MAC-ū-lar)	a progressive deterioration of the portion of the retina called the *macula lutea*, resulting in

Glaucoma
is composed of the Greek **glaukos**, meaning **blue-gray** or **sea green**, and **oma**, meaning a morbid condition. The term was given to any condition in which gray or green replaced the black in the pupil.

CAM TERM

Vitamin therapy is the use of nutrition, through diet and supplements, to decrease the incidence of disease and symptoms. Research sponsored by the National Institutes of Health found that people at high risk of developing advanced stages of age-related macular degeneration lowered their risk by 25% when treated with a high-dose combination of antioxidants and zinc.

Age-related macular degeneration (ARMD) is the leading cause of legal blindness in persons older than 65 years. Onset occurs between the ages of 50 and 60 (see Figure 12-8).

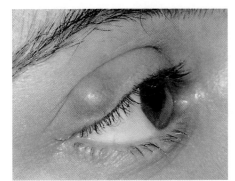

Figure 12-4
Chalazion (right upper eyelid).

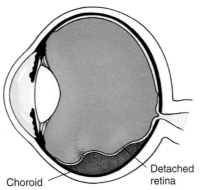

Choroid / Detached retina

Figure 12-5
Detached retina. Vitreous humor has seeped through a break in the retina, causing the retina to separate from the choroid coat.

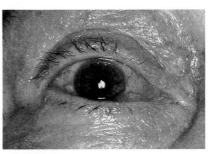

Figure 12-6
Appearance of the eye in acute glaucoma.

ERRORS OF REFRACTION

Cornea / Lens / Retina

Light waves / Image

Myopia (nearsightedness)
A

Hyperopia (farsightedness)
B

Astigmatism
C

Figure 12-7
Refraction errors. **A,** Myopia, nearsightedness; **B,** hyperopia, farsightedness; **C,** astigmatism.

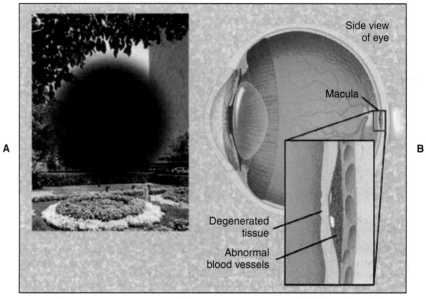

Figure 12-8
A, How a patient with age-related macular degeneration might see the world.
B, Macular degeneration.

	loss of central vision (Figure 12-8)
myopia .... (mī-Ō-pē-a)	nearsightedness (see Figure 12-7)
nyctalopia .... (nik-ta-LŌ-pē-a)	poor vision at night or in faint light
nystagmus .... (nis-TAG-mus)	involuntary, jerking movements of the eyes
presbyopia .... (*pres*-bē-Ō-pē-a)	impaired vision as a result of aging
pterygium .... (te-RIJ-ē-um)	thin tissue growing into the cornea from the conjunctiva, usually caused from sun exposure
retinitis pigmentosa .... (ret-i-NĪ-tis) (pig-men-TŌ-sa)	hereditary, progressive disease marked by night blindness with atrophy and retinal pigment changes
strabismus .... (stra-BIZ-mus)	abnormal condition of squint or crossed eyes caused by the visual axes not meeting at the same point
sty .... (stī)	infection of an oil gland of the eyelid (Figure 12-9) (also spelled *stye* and also called *hordeolum*)

Practice saying each of these terms aloud. To hear the terms, access the **PRONOUNCE IT** activity for this chapter on the Student CD that accompanies this text. Or, to hear the terms and their definitions with a CD player or computer, obtain the Pronunciation CD designed for use with this text.

Learn the definitions and spellings of the disease and disorder terms by completing exercises 12, 13, and 14.

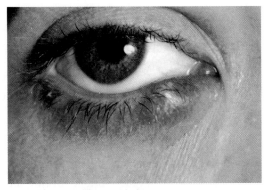

Figure 12-9
Hordoleum, sty, or stye.

EXERCISE 12

Fill in the blanks with the correct terms.

1. Another name for nearsightedness is _____.

2. Impaired vision as a result of aging is _____.

3. The abnormal condition of squinted or crossed eyes caused by visual axes not meeting at the same point is called _____.

4. An obstruction of an oil gland of the eyelid is called a(n) _____.

5. A defective curvature of the refractive surface of the eye causes a condition known as _____.

6. _____ is the name given to involuntary, jerking movements of the eye.

7. A clouding of the lens of the eye is called a(n) _____.

8. _____ is the name given to an infection of the oil gland of the eyelids.

9. A disorder usually caused by the abnormal increase of intraocular pressure is _____.

10. A(n) _____ _____ is a separation of the retina from the choroid in the back of the eye.

11. Another name for farsightedness is _____.

12. Normal refractive condition of the eye is called _____.

13. _____ _____ is a hereditary, progressive disease causing night blindness with retinal pigment changes and atrophy.

14. Poor vision at night or in faint light is called _____.

15. A thin tissue growing into the cornea from the conjunctiva is called a(n) _____.

16. _____ _____ is the progressive deterioration of the macula lutea.

EXERCISE 13

Match the terms in the first column with the correct definitions in the second column.

_____	1. astigmatism	a. infection of an oil gland of the eyelid
_____	2. cataract	b. deterioration of the macula lutea
_____	3. chalazion	c. crossed eyes or squinting caused by visual axes not meeting at the same point
_____	4. detached retina	
_____	5. glaucoma	
_____	6. myopia	d. involuntary, jerking movements of the eye
_____	7. nystagmus	e. impaired vision caused by aging
_____	8. hyperopia	f. defective curvature of the refractive surface of the eye
_____	9. presbyopia	
_____	10. strabismus	g. normal refractive condition of the eye
_____	11. sty, stye	h. clouding of a lens of the eye
_____	12. pterygium	i. hereditary progressive disease marked by night blindness
_____	13. retinitis pigmentosa	
_____	14. nyctalopia	j. nearsightedness
_____	15. emmetropia	k. obstruction of an oil gland of the eye
_____	16. macular degeneration	l. usually caused from sun exposure

m. eye disorder characterized by optic nerve damage

n. separation of the retina from the choroid in the back of the eye

o. poor vision at night or in faint light

p. farsightedness

q. double vision

EXERCISE 14

Spell the disease and disorder terms. Have someone dictate the terms on pp. 434-436 to you. Study any words you have spelled incorrectly.

1. _____	7. _____
2. _____	8. _____
3. _____	9. _____
4. _____	10. _____
5. _____	11. _____
6. _____	12. _____

13. _____   15. _____

14. _____   16. _____

Surgical Terms

Built from Word Parts

Term	Definition
blepharoplasty .... (BLEF-a-rō-plast-tē)	surgical repair of the eyelid
cryoretinopexy .... (*krī-ō*-re-tin-ō-PEK-sē)	surgical fixation of the retina by using extreme cold (carbon dioxide)
dacryocystorhinostomy .... (*dak*-rē-ō-*sis*-tō-rī-NOS-tō-mē)	creation of an artificial opening between the tear (lacrimal) sac and the nose (to restore drainage into the nose when the nasolacrimal duct is obstructed or obliterated)
dacryocystotomy .... (*dak*-rē-ō-sis-TOT-ō-mē)	incision into the tear sac
iridectomy .... (ir-i-DEK-tō-mē)	excision (of part) of the iris
keratoplasty .... (KER-a-tō-plas-tē)	surgical repair of the cornea (corneal transplant)
sclerotomy .... (skle-ROT-ō-mē)	incision into the sclera

Practice saying each of these terms aloud. To hear the terms, access the **PRONOUNCE IT** activity for this chapter on the Student CD that accompanies this text. Or, to hear the terms and their definitions with a CD player or computer, obtain the Pronunciation CD designed for use with this text.

Learn the definitions and spellings of the surgical terms by completing exercises 15, 16, and 17.

EXERCISE 15

Analyze and define the following surgical terms.

1. keratoplasty _____

2. sclerotomy _____

3. dacryocystotomy _____

4. cryoretinopexy _____

5. blepharoplasty _____

6. iridectomy _____

7. dacryocystorhinostomy _____

EXERCISE 16

Build surgical terms for the following definitions by using the word parts you have learned.

1. creation of an artificial opening between the tear (lacrimal) sac and the nose (to restore drainage when the nasolacrimal duct is obstructed)

   _____ / ___ / ___ / ___ / _____ / ___ / ___
   WR / CV / WR / CV /   WR / CV / S

2. excision of the iris

   _____ / _____
      WR /   S

3. surgical repair of the cornea

   _____ / ___ / _____
     WR / CV /   S

4. incision of the sclera

   _____ / ___ / _____
     WR / CV /   S

5. surgical repair of the eyelid

   _____ / ___ / _____
     WR / CV /   S

6. surgical fixation of the retina by a method using extreme cold

   _____ / ___ / ___ / ___ / _____
     WR / CV / WR / CV /   S

7. incision into the tear sac

   _____ / ___ / ___ / ___ / _____
     WR / CV / WR / CV /   S

EXERCISE 17

Spell each of the surgical terms. Have someone dictate the terms on p. 439 to you. Think about the word parts before attempting to write the word. Study any words you have spelled incorrectly.

1. _____   5. _____

2. _____   6. _____

3. _____   7. _____

4. _____

Surgical Terms

Not Built from Word Parts

Term	Definition
enucleation .... (e-*nū*-klē-Ā-shun)	surgical removal of the eyeball (also, the removal of any organ that comes out clean and whole)

LASIK (laser-assisted in situ keratomileusis)..................................
(LĀ-sik)

a laser procedure that reshapes the corneal tissue beneath the surface of the cornea to correct astigmatism, hyperopia, and myopia. LASIK is a combination of Excimer laser and lamellar keratoplasty. It differs from PRK in that it reshapes corneal tissue beneath the surface rather than on the surface (Figure 12-10).

phacoemulsification..........................
(fa-kō-ē-mul-si-fi-KĀ-shun)

method to remove cataracts in which an ultrasonic needle probe breaks up the lens, which is then aspirated

PRK (photorefractive keratectomy)...
(fō-tō-rē-FRAK-tiv)
(ker-a-TEK-tō-mē)

a procedure for the treatment of nearsightedness in which an Excimer laser is used to reshape (flatten) the corneal surface by removing a portion of the cornea (see Figure 12-10)

retinal photocoagulation...................
(RET-in-al)
(fo-tō-kō-ag-ū-LĀ-shun)

a procedure to repair tears in the retina by use of an intense, precisely focused light beam, which causes coagulation of the tissue protein

scleral buckling......................................
(SKLE-ral) (BUK-ling)

a procedure to repair a detached retina. A strip of sclera is resected, or a fold is made in the sclera. An exoplant is used to hold and buckle the sclera (Figure 12-11).

trabeculectomy.......................................
(tra-bek-ū-LEK-tō-mē)

surgical creation of a drain to reduce intraocular pressure (used to treat glaucoma)

vitrectomy...
(vi-TREK-tō-mē)

surgical removal of all or part of the vitreous humor (used to treat diabetic retinopathy)

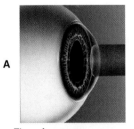

Flap of cornea

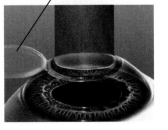

Figure 12-10
Surgical treatments for nearsightedness. **A,** LASIK shapes tissue below the surface of the cornea. **B,** PRK removes tissue from the surface of the cornea.

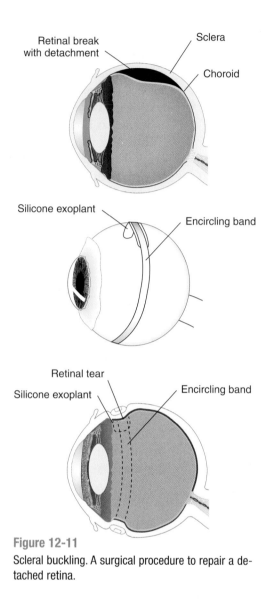

Figure 12-11
Scleral buckling. A surgical procedure to repair a detached retina.

Excimer Laser Treatments for Nearsightedness
PRK (photorefractive keratectomy): removes tissue from the surface of the cornea
LASIK (laser-assisted in situ keratomileusis): reshapes corneal tissue below the surface of the cornea
The Excimer laser was invented in the early 1980s. It is a computer-controlled ultraviolet beam of light that reshapes the cornea, allowing light to focus more directly on the retina. It has replaced **RK (radial keratotomy)**, a surgery in which spoke incisions are made to reshape the cornea. (See Figure 12-10.)

Practice saying each of these terms aloud. To hear the terms, access the **PRONOUNCE IT** activity for this chapter on the Student CD that accompanies this text. Or, to hear the terms and their definitions with a CD player or computer, obtain the Pronunciation CD designed for use with this text.

Learn the definitions and spellings of the surgical terms by completing exercises 18, 19, and 20.

EXERCISE 18

Fill in the blank with the correct terms.

1. The procedure performed to repair tears in the retina is called _____ _____.

2. Surgical removal of an eyeball is called a(n) _____.

3. _____ is the name given to the procedure that breaks up the lens with ultrasound and then aspirates it.

4. A procedure using the Excimer laser and lamellar keratoplasty to correct hyperopia, myopia, and astigmatism is called _____.

5. _____ is the surgical creation of a drain to reduce intraocular pressure.

6. An operation to repair a detached retina in which the sclera is folded or resected and an exoplant is used to buckle and hold the sclera is called _____ _____.

7. Surgery to remove vitreous humor from the eye is called _____.

8. _____ is a procedure for the treatment of nearsightedness in which an Excimer laser is used to reshape the corneal surface.

EXERCISE 19

Match the terms in the first column with their correct definitions in the second column.

_____ 1. LASIK
_____ 2. enucleation
_____ 3. trabeculectomy
_____ 4. retinal photocoagulation
_____ 5. phacoemulsification
_____ 6. scleral buckling
_____ 7. vitrectomy
_____ 8. PRK

a. procedure to repair tears in the retina

b. surgical creation of a permanent drain to reduce intraocular pressure

c. procedure for the treatment of nearsightedness in which an Excimer laser is used to reshape the cornea

d. procedure in which the lens is broken up by ultrasound and aspirated

e. procedure used to correct astigmatism, nearsightedness, and farsightedness

f. surgical removal of an eyeball

g. surgical removal of vitreous humor

h. operation in which a cataract is lifted from the eye with an extremely cold probe

i. detached retina surgery in which the sclera is folded and an exoplant is used to buckle and hold the sclera

j. surgical incision of the sclera

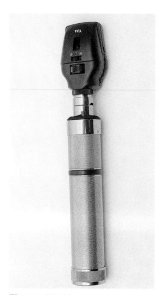

Figure 12-12
Ophthalmoscope used to view the retina.

Spell each of the surgical terms. Have someone dictate the terms on pp. 440-441 to you. Study any words you have spelled incorrectly.

1. _____   5. _____

2. _____   6. _____

3. _____   7. _____

4. _____   8. _____

Diagnostic Terms

Built from Word Parts

Term	Definition
Diagnostic Imaging	
fluorescein angiography .... (flō-RES-ē-in) (an-jē-OG-ra-fē)	process of recording (photographic) blood vessels (of the eye with fluorescing dye)
Ophthalmic Evaluation	
keratometer .... (*ker*-a-TOM-e-ter)	instrument used to measure (the curvature of) the cornea (used for fitting contact lenses)
ophthalmoscope .... (of-THAL-mō-skōp)	instrument used for visual examination (the interior) of the eye (Figure 12-12)
ophthalmoscopy .... (*of*-thal-MOS-kō-pē)	visual examination of the eye
optometry .... (op-TOM-e-trē)	measurement of vision (acuity and the prescribing of corrective lenses)
pupillometer .... (pū-pil-OM-e-ter)	instrument used to measure (the diameter of) the pupil
pupilloscope .... (pū-PIL-ō-skōp)	instrument used for visual examination of the pupil
tonometer .... (ton-OM-e-ter)	instrument used to measure pressure (within the eye, used to diagnose glaucoma) (Figure 12-13)
tonometry .... (ton-OM-e-trē)	measurement of pressure (within the eye)

Practice saying each of these words aloud. To hear the terms, access the **PRONOUNCE IT** activity for this chapter on the Student CD that accompanies this text. Or, to hear the terms and their definitions with a CD player or computer, obtain the Pronunciation CD designed for use with this text.

Learn the definitions and spellings of the diagnostic terms by completing exercises 21, 22, and 23.

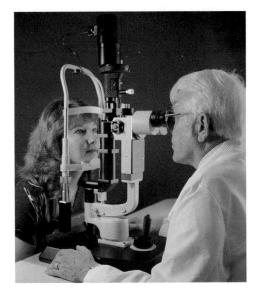

Figure 12-13
Tonometry.

EXERCISE 21

Analyze and define the following diagnostic terms.

1. pupilloscope _____

2. optometry _____

3. ophthalmoscope _____

4. tonometry _____

5. pupillometer _____

6. tonometer _____

7. keratometer _____

8. ophthalmoscopy _____

9. fluorescein angiography _____

EXERCISE 22

Build diagnostic terms that correspond to the following definitions by using the word parts you have learned.

1. measurement of pressure
   (within the eye)

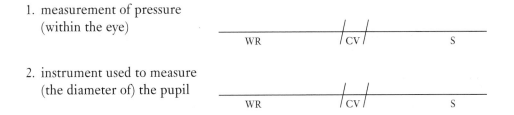

WR   CV   S

2. instrument used to measure
   (the diameter of) the pupil

WR   CV   S

3. instrument used to measure
   (the curvature of) the cornea

   _____ /___/ _____
   WR   CV   S

4. measurement of vision
   (acuity and the prescribing
   of corrective lenses)

   _____ /___/ _____
   WR   CV   S

5. instrument used for visual
   examination of the eye

   _____ /___/ _____
   WR   CV   S

6. instrument used to measure
   pressure (within the eye)

   _____ /___/ _____
   WR   CV   S

7. instrument used for visual
   examination of the pupil

   _____ /___/ _____
   WR   CV   S

8. visual examination of the eye

   _____ /___/ _____
   WR   CV   S

9. process of recording blood
   vessels (of the eye using
   fluorescing dye)

   fluorescein _____ /___/ _____
                    WR   CV   S

EXERCISE 23

Spell each of the diagnostic terms. Have someone dictate the terms on p. 444 to you. Think about the word parts before attempting to write the word. Study any words you have spelled incorrectly.

1. _____   6. _____

2. _____   7. _____

3. _____   8. _____

4. _____   9. _____

5. _____

Complementary Terms

Built from Word Parts

Term	Definition
binocular (bin-OK-ū-lar)	pertaining to two or both eyes
corneal (KOR-nē-al)	pertaining to the cornea

intraocular............................ (*in*-tra-OK-ū-lar)	pertaining to within the eye
lacrimal............................ (LAK-ri-mal)	pertaining to tears or tear ducts
nasolacrimal............................ (*nā*-zō-LAK-ri-mal)	pertaining to the nose and tear ducts
ophthalmic............................ (of-THAL-mik)	pertaining to the eye
ophthalmologist............................ (*of*-thal-MOL-ō-jist)	physician who studies and treats diseases of the eye
ophthalmology (Ophth)............................ (*of*-thal-MOL-ō-jē)	study of the eye (a branch of medicine that deals with treating diseases of the eye)
ophthalmopathy............................ (*of*-thal-MOP-a-thē)	(any) disease of the eye
optic............................ (OP-tik)	pertaining to vision
pupillary............................ (PŪ-pi-lar-ē)	pertaining to the pupil
retinal............................ (RET-i-nal)	pertaining to the retina
retinopathy............................ (*ret*-i-NOP-a-thē)	(any noninflammatory) disease of the retina (such as diabetic retinopathy)

Practice saying each of these terms aloud. To hear the terms, access the **PRONOUNCE IT** activity for this chapter on the Student CD that accompanies this text. Or, to hear the terms and their definitions with a CD player or computer, obtain the Pronunciation CD designed for use with this text.

Exercises 24, 25, and 26 will help you learn the definitions and spellings of the complementary terms related to the eye.

EXERCISE 24

Analyze and define the following complementary terms.

1. ophthalmology _____

2. binocular _____

3. lacrimal _____

4. pupillary _____

5. retinopathy _____

6. ophthalmologist _____

7. corneal _____

8. ophthalmic _____

9. nasolacrimal _____

10. optic _____

11. intraocular _____

12. retinal _____

13. ophthalmopathy _____

Build the complementary terms for the following definitions by using the word parts you have learned.

1. study of the eye

    _____ / ___ / _____
    WR   CV   S

2. pertaining to two or both eyes

    _____ / ___ / _____
    P   WR   S

3. pertaining to the retina

    _____ / _____
    WR   S

4. pertaining to within the eye

    _____ / ___ / _____
    P   WR   S

5. physician who studies and treats diseases of the eye

    _____ / ___ / _____
    WR   CV   S

6. pertaining to tears or tear ducts

    _____ / _____
    WR   S

7. pertaining to vision

    _____ / _____
    WR   S

8. (any noninflammatory) disease of the retina

    _____ / ___ / _____
    WR   CV   S

9. pertaining to the cornea

    _____ / _____
    WR   S

10. pertaining to the nose and tear ducts

    _____ / ___ / _____ / _____
    WR   CV   WR   S

11. any disease of the eye

    _____ / ___ / _____
    WR   CV   S

12. pertaining to the pupil

    _____ / _____
    WR   S

EXERCISE 26

Spell each of the complementary terms. Have someone dictate the terms on pp. 446-447 to you. Think about the word parts before attempting to write the word. Study any words you have spelled incorrectly.

1. _____   8. _____

2. _____   9. _____

3. _____   10. _____

4. _____   11. _____

5. _____   12. _____

6. _____   13. _____

7. _____

Complementary Terms

Not Built from Word Parts

Term	Definition
miotic .... (mī-OT-ik)	agent that constricts the pupil
mydriatic .... (*mid*-rē-AT-ik)	agent that dilates the pupil
oculus dexter (OD) .... (OK-ū-lus) (DEX-ter)	medical term for right eye
oculus sinister (OS) .... (OK-ū-lus) (sin-IS-ter)	medical term for left eye
oculus uterque (OU) .... (OK-ū-lus) (ū-TERK)	medical term for each eye
optician .... (op-TISH-in)	a specialist who fills prescriptions for lenses (cannot prescribe lenses)
optometrist .... (op-TOM-e-trist)	a health professional who prescribes corrective lenses and/or eye exercises
visual acuity (VA) .... (VIZH-ū-al) (a-KŪ-i-tē)	sharpness of vision for either distance or nearness

Optometrist
is derived from the Greek **optikos**, meaning **sight**, and **metron**, meaning **measure.** Literally, an optometrist is a person who measures sight.

Practice saying each of these terms aloud. To hear the terms, access the **PRONOUNCE IT** activity for this chapter on the Student CD that accompanies this text. Or, to hear the terms and their definitions with a CD player or computer, obtain the Pronunciation CD designed for use with this text.

Learn the definitions and spellings of the complementary terms by completing exercises 27, 28, and 29.

EXERCISE 27

Write the definitions for the following complementary terms.

1. oculus sinister _____

2. optometrist _____

3. mydriatic _____

4. oculus uterque _____

5. visual acuity _____

6. miotic _____

7. oculus dexter _____

8. optician _____

EXERCISE 28

Fill in the blanks with the correct terms.

1. The medical term for the left eye is _____ _____.

2. An agent that dilates a pupil is a(n) _____.

3. _____ _____ means each eye.

4. An agent that constricts a pupil is a(n) _____.

5. The medical term for the right eye is _____ _____.

6. A health professional who prescribes corrective lenses and/or eye exercises is a(n) _____.

7. Another term for sharpness of vision is _____ _____.

8. A specialist who fills prescriptions for lenses but who cannot prescribe lenses is a(n) _____.

EXERCISE 29

Spell each of the complementary terms. Have someone dictate the terms on p. 449 to you. Study any words you have spelled incorrectly.

1. _____   5. _____

2. _____   6. _____

3. _____   7. _____

4. _____   8. _____

Abbreviations

ARMD	age-related macular degeneration
Ast	astigmatism
Em	emmetropia
OD	right eye (oculus dexter)
Ophth	ophthalmology
OS	left eye (oculus sinister)
OU	each eye (oculus uterque)
VA	visual acuity

EXERCISE 30

Write the meaning of the following abbreviations in the spaces provided.

1. VA _____ _____

2. Ast _____

3. OD _____ _____

4. OS _____ _____

5. OU _____ _____

6. Em _____

7. Ophth _____

8. ARMD _____ _____ _____ _____

CHAPTER REVIEW

EXERCISE 31   *Interact with Medical Documents*

Complete the progress note by writing the medical terms in the blanks. Use the list of definitions with the corresponding numbers.

University Hospital and Medical Center
4700 North Main Street • Wellness, Arizona 54321 • (987) 555-3210

PATIENT NAME: William Graves   **CASE NUMBER:** 20066-OPH
DATE OF BIRTH: 06/27/xx   **DATE:** 04/05/xx

PROGRESS NOTE

SUBJECTIVE: Mr. Graves is a 66-year-old white male here today for his annual 1. _____ exam. He has no current complaints. He has a family history of 2. _____ in his brother. He has a history of hypertension and type 2 diabetes mellitus. A 3. _____ was removed from his right eye 5 years ago.

Current Medications: Glyburide 5 mg bid and Lopressor 50 mg bid. Allergies: None.

OBJECTIVE:
Visual Acuities: Aided: OD 2/25-2 OS 20/30-1 OU 20/25
                 Unaided: OD 20/100 OS 20/80-1 OU 20/80

Externals: 2 mm 4. _____ OD. PERLA (pupils equal and reactive to light and accommodation). EOMI (extraocular movements intact).

Ophthalmoscopic: Lens: OS showed early cortical spokes
                 Disk: margins normal
                 Cup-to-disk ratio: 0.2 OU
                 Fundus: Within normal limits, including DVM
                 Refraction: OD-1.00-0.50 $\times$ 90 20/20, OS-1.25-0.25 $\times$ 90 20/20
                 Tonometry: 14 mm Hg/OD, 13 mm Hg/OS

Visual Field: Full

ASSESSMENT: Patient has compound myopic 5. _____ and 6. _____ with diabetic 7. _____ and grade II hypertension. He also shows an early 8. _____ in the left eye.

PLAN: Provide prescription for corrective lenses. See patient for follow-up visit in 6 months to reevaluate diabetic retinopathy and cataract. Counseled patient to report any sudden changes in vision.

Milli Bentley, MD

MB/mcm

---

1. study of the eye
2. usually caused by abnormal increased intraocular pressure
3. thin tissue growing into the cornea from the conjunctiva
4. drooping of eyelid
5. defective curvature of the refractive surface of the eye
6. impaired vision as a result of aging
7. (any noninflammatory) disease of the retina
8. clouding of the lens of the eye

EXERCISE 32   *Interpret Medical Terms*

To test your understanding of the terms introduced in this chapter, circle the words that correctly complete the sentences. The italicized words refer to the correct answer.

1. The patient's *pupils* needed to be *dilated;* therefore the doctor requested that a (miotic, mydriatic, miopic) medication be placed in each eye.
2. A person with a *defective curvature of the refractive surface* of the eye has a(n) (astigmatism, glaucoma, strabismus).
3. The doctor diagnosed the patient with the *clouded lens* of the eye as having a(n) (nystagmus, astigmatism, cataract).
4. To *measure the pressure within the patient's eye,* the physician used a(n) (pupillometer, tonometer, keratometer).
5. A person who is *farsighted* has (hyperopia, myopia, diplopia).
6. An *obstruction of the oil gland of the eyelid* is called a(n) (sty, chalazion, conjunctivitis).
7. A patient with an *involuntary jerking movement of the eyes* has a condition known as (astigmatism, strabismus, nystagmus).
8. The name of the *surgery performed to create a permanent drain to reduce intraocular pressure* is (trabeculectomy, strabotomy, phacoemulsification).
9. The doctor ordered a *photographic imaging of the blood vessels of the eye* or a(n) (ophthalmoscopy, fluorescein angiography, optometer).

EXERCISE 33   *Read Medical Terms in Use*

Practice pronunciation of terms by reading the following medical document. Use the pronunciation key following the medical terms to help you say the word.

An elderly gentleman visited his **ophthalmologist** (*of*-thal-MOL-ō-jist) because of decreased vision. A **tonometry** (ton-OM-e-trē) examination showed borderline readings. **Visual acuity** (VIZH-ū-al) (a-KŪ-i-tē) measurement indicated a mild degree of **myopia** (mī-O-pē-a) and **presbyopia** (*pres*-bē-O-pē-a). A diagnosis of **glaucoma** (glaw-KŌ-ma) is suspect in this case and Timoptic eye drops were prescribed, one drop **oculus uterque** (OU) (OK-ū-lus) (ū-TERK) daily.

A **cataract** (KAT-a-rakt) of the **oculus dexter** (OD) (OK-ū-lus) (DEX-ter) was found. Lens implant surgery will be performed when the cataract matures sufficiently. Approximately 5 years ago the patient had a **detached retina** (RET-i-na) of the **oculus sinister** (OS) (OK-ū-lus) (sin-IS-ter). A **scleral buckling** (SKLE-ral) (BUK-ling) procedure was performed and was successful in halting the process of retinal detachment.

EXERCISE 34   *Comprehend Medical Terms in Use*

Test your comprehension of terms in the above medical document by circling the correct answer.

1. T   F   The ophthalmologist used an instrument to measure pressure within the patient's eyes to assist in the diagnosis of abnormally increased intraocular pressure.
2. Visual acuity measurement indicated:
   a. farsightedness and impaired vision as a result of aging
   b. nearsightedness and impaired vision as a result of aging
   c. poor night vision and farsightedness
   d. poor night vision and impaired vision because of aging

3. To treat glaucoma the patient would place Timoptic eye drops in:
   a. his left eye daily
   b. his right eye every other day
   c. each eye daily
   d. each eye every other day
4. T   F   A scleral buckling procedure was used to correct clouding of the lens in the right eye.

For further practice or to evaluate what you have learned use the Student CD that accompanies this text.

REVIEW OF WORD PARTS

Can you define and spell the following word parts?

Combining Forms		Prefixes	Suffixes
blephar/o	kerat/o	bi-	-opia
conjunctiv/o	lacrim/o	bin-	-phobia
core/o	ocul/o		-plegia
cor/o	ophthalm/o		
corne/o	opt/o		
cry/o	phot/o		
dacry/o	pupill/o		
dipl/o	retin/o		
iri/o	scler/o		
irid/o	ton/o		

REVIEW OF TERMS

Can you build, analyze, define, pronounce, and spell the following terms *built from word parts?*

Diseases and Disorders	Surgical	Diagnostic	Complementary
blepharitis	blepharoplasty	fluorescein angiography	binocular
blepharoptosis	cryoretinopexy	keratometer	corneal
conjunctivitis	dacryocystorhinostomy	ophthalmoscope	intraocular
dacryocystitis	dacryocystotomy	ophthalmoscopy	lacrimal
diplopia	iridectomy	optometry	nasolacrimal
endophthalmitis	keratoplasty	pupillometer	ophthalmic
iridoplegia	sclerotomy	pupilloscope	ophthalmologist
iritis		tonometer	ophthalmology (ophth)
keratitis		tonometry	ophthalmopathy
leukocoria			optic
oculomycosis			pupillary
ophthalmalgia			retinal
ophthalmoplegia			retinopathy
photophobia			
retinoblastoma			
sclerokeratitis			
scleromalacia			

Can you define, pronounce, and spell the following terms *not built from word parts?*

Diseases and Disorders

astigmatism (Ast)	myopia
cataract	nyctalopia
chalazion	nystagmus
detached retina	presbyopia
emmetropia (Em)	pterygium
glaucoma	retinitis pigmentosa
hyperopia	strabismus
macular degeneration	sty, stye (hordeolum)

Surgical

enucleation
LASIK
phacoemulsification
PRK
retinal photocoagulation
scleral buckling
trabeculectomy
vitrectomy

Complementary

miotic
mydriatic
oculus dexter (OD)
oculus sinister (OS)
oculus uterque (OU)
optician
optometrist
visual acuity (VA)

13

Ear

OUTLINE

OBJECTIVES

On completion of this chapter you will be able to:

1. Identify the anatomy of the ear.
2. Define and spell the word parts presented in this chapter.
3. Build and analyze medical terms with word parts presented in this and previous chapters.
4. Define, pronounce, and spell the disease and disorder, diagnostic, surgical, and complementary terms for the ear.
5. Interpret the meaning of abbreviations presented in this chapter.
6. Identify and use plural endings.
7. Read medical documents and interpret medical terminology in them.

ANATOMY

Function

The two functions of the ear are to hear and to provide the sense of balance. The ear is made up of three parts: the *external* ear, the *middle* ear, and the *inner* ear, also called the *labyrinth* (Figure 13-1). We hear because sound waves vibrate through the ear where they are transformed into nerve impulses that are then carried to the brain.

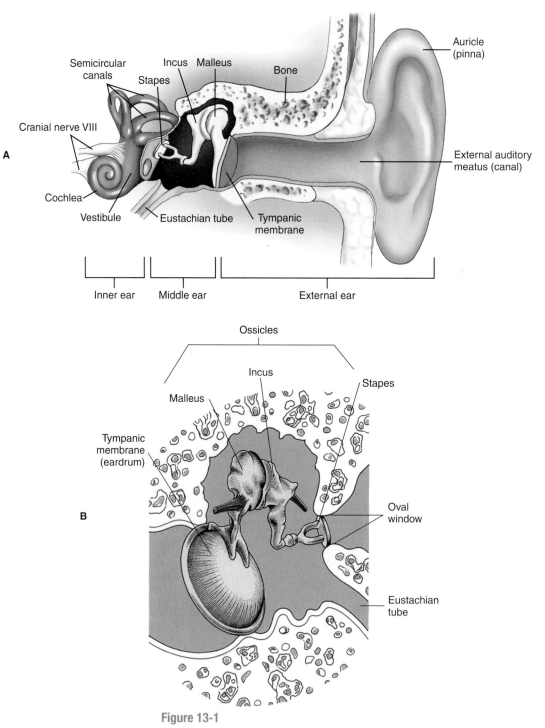

Figure 13-1
A, Gross anatomy of the ear; **B,** the middle ear.

Structures of the Ear

external ear

    auricle (pinna)..................... external structure located on both sides of the head. The auricle directs sound waves into the external auditory meatus.

    external auditory meatus
    (canal)................................... short tube that ends at the tympanic membrane. The inner part lies within the temporal bone of the skull and contains the glands that secrete earwax (cerumen).

middle ear

    tympanic membrane
    (eardrum)............................. semitransparent membrane that separates the external auditory meatus and the middle ear cavity (Figure 13-2)

    eustachian tube................... connects the middle ear and the pharynx. It equalizes air pressure on both sides of the eardrum.

    ossicles................................ bones of the middle ear that carry sound vibrations. The ossicles are composed of the malleus (hammer), incus (anvil), and stapes (stirrup). The stapes connects to the *oval window,* which transmits the sound vibrations to the inner ear.

labyrinth (inner ear)...................... bony spaces within the temporal bone of the skull. It contains the cochlea, semicircular canals, and vestibule.

    cochlea................................ is snail-shaped and contains the organ of hearing. The cochlea connects to the oval window in the middle ear

    semicircular canals and
    vestibule.............................. contains receptors and endolymph that help the body maintain its sense of balance (equilibrium)

mastoid bone and cells.................. located in the skull bone behind the external auditory meatus

Learn the anatomic terms by completing exercise 1.
Refer to Appendixes A and B for a complete list of word parts.

> **Tympanic Membrane**
> is derived from the Greek **tympanon,** meaning **drum,** because of its resemblance to a drum or tambourine.

> **Stapes**
> is Latin for **stirrup.** The anatomic stapes was so named for its stirruplike shape.

EXERCISE   1

Match the anatomic terms in the first column with the correct definitions in the second column.

_____ 1. auricle

_____ 2. cochlea

_____ 3. eustachian tube

_____ 4. external auditory meatus

a. contains receptors and endolymph, which help maintain equilibrium

b. equalizes air pressure on both sides of the eardrum

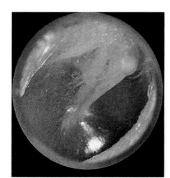

Figure 13-2
Normal tympanic membrane.

_____ 5. labyrinth

_____ 6. mastoid bone

_____ 7. ossicles

_____ 8. oval window

_____ 9. semicircular canals

_____ 10. tympanic membrane

c. separates the external auditory meatus and middle ear cavity

d. malleus, incus, and stapes

e. transmits sound vibration to the inner ear

f. contains glands that secrete earwax

g. external structure located on each side of the head

h. bony spaces within the temporal bone

i. relays messages to the brain

j. contains the organ of hearing

k. located in the skull behind the external auditory meatus

WORD PARTS

Combining Forms for the Ear

Study the word parts and their definitions listed below. Completing the exercises that follow will help you learn the terms.

Combining Form	Definition
acou/o, audi/o	hearing
aur/i, aur/o, ot/o	ear
labyrinth/o	labyrinth (inner ear)
mastoid/o	mastoid bone
myring/o	tympanic membrane (eardrum)
staped/o	stapes (middle ear bone)
tympan/o	tympanic membrane (eardrum), middle ear

Learn the anatomic locations and meanings of the combining forms by completing exercises 2 and 3 and Exercise Figure A.

EXERCISE 2

Write the definitions of the following combining forms.

1. staped/o _____

2. mastoid/o _____

3. audi/o _____

1. Ear
CF: _____
CF: _____
CF: _____

2. Labyrinth
CF: _____

3. Stapes
CF: _____

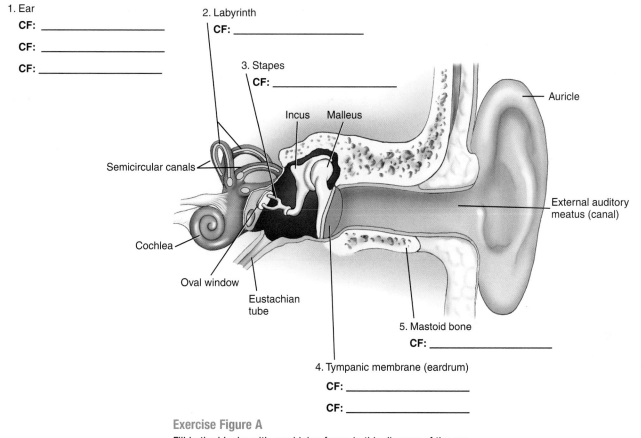

Semicircular canals

Incus   Malleus

Auricle

Cochlea

External auditory
meatus (canal)

Oval window

Eustachian
tube

5. Mastoid bone
CF: _____

4. Tympanic membrane (eardrum)
CF: _____
CF: _____

Exercise Figure A
Fill in the blanks with combining forms in this diagram of the ear.

4. aur/o, aur/i, ot/o _____

5. tympan/o _____

6. acou/o _____

7. labyrinth/o _____

8. myring/o _____

EXERCISE   3

Write the combining form for each of the following terms.

1. ear
    a. _____
    b. _____
    c. _____

2. mastoid bone
    _____

3. stapes
    _____

4. tympanic membrane
   (eardrum), middle ear   _____

5. labyrinth (inner ear)   _____

6. hearing   a. _____

   b. _____

7. tympanic membrane
   (eardrum)   _____

MEDICAL TERMS

The terms you need to learn to complete this chapter are listed below. The exercises following each list will help you learn the definition and spelling of each word.

Disease and Disorder Terms

Built from Word Parts

Term	Definition
labyrinthitis (*lab*-i-rin-THĪ-tis)	inflammation of the labyrinth (inner ear)
mastoiditis (*mas*-toyd-Ī-tis)	inflammation of the mastoid bone
myringitis (mir-in-JĪ-tis)	inflammation of the tympanic membrane (eardrum)
otalgia (ō-TAL-jē-a)	pain in the ear
otomastoiditis (ō-tō–*mas*-toyd-Ī-tis)	inflammation of the ear and the mastoid bone
otomycosis (ō-tō-mī-KŌ-sis)	abnormal condition of fungus in the ear (usually affects the external auditory meatus)
otopyorrhea (ō-tō-pī-ō-RĒ-a)	discharge of pus from the ear
otosclerosis (ō-tō-skle-RŌ-sis)	hardening of the ear (stapes) (caused by irregular bone development and resulting in hearing loss)
tympanitis (tim-pan-Ī-tis)	inflammation of the middle ear (also called *otitis media*) (Figure 13-3)

Practice saying each of these terms aloud. To hear the terms, access the **PRONOUNCE IT** activity for this chapter on the Student CD that accompanies this text. Or, to hear the terms and their definitions with a CD player or computer, obtain the Pronunciation CD designed for use with this text.

Learn the definitions and spellings of the disease and disorder terms by completing exercises 4, 5, and 6.

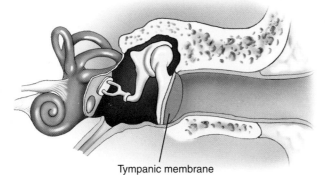

Tympanic membrane

Figure 13-3
Otitis media. Signs include bulging, perforated, reddened, or retracted tympanic membrane.

EXERCISE 4

Analyze and define the following terms.

1. otomycosis _____

2. tympanitis _____

3. otomastoiditis _____

4. otalgia _____

5. labyrinthitis _____

6. myringitis _____

7. otosclerosis _____

8. mastoiditis _____

9. otopyorrhea _____

EXERCISE 5

Build disease and disorder terms for the following definitions with the word parts you have learned.

1. inflammation of the
   tympanic membrane   _____ / _____
                            WR   S

2. discharge of pus from the ear   _____ / ___ / _____ / ___ / _____
                                       WR   CV   WR   CV   S

3. inflammation of the mastoid
   bone   _____ / _____
              WR   S

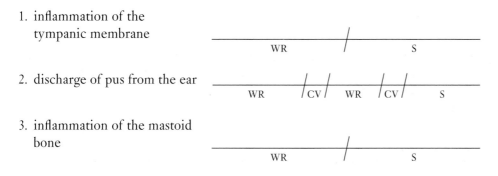

4. pain in the ear

_____ / _____
WR   S

5. hardening of the ear (stapes)

_____ / _____ / _____
WR   CV   S

6. abnormal condition of fungus in the ear

_____ / _____ / _____ / _____
WR   CV   WR   S

7. inflammation of the ear and the mastoid bone

_____ / _____ / _____ / _____
WR   CV   WR   S

8. inflammation of the labyrinth

_____ / _____
WR   S

9. inflammation of the middle ear

_____ / _____
WR   S

EXERCISE 6

Spell each of the disease and disorder terms. Have someone dictate the terms on p. 462 to you. Think about the word parts before attempting to write the word. Study any words you have spelled incorrectly.

1. _____   6. _____

2. _____   7. _____

3. _____   8. _____

4. _____   9. _____

5. _____

Disease and Disorder Terms

Not Built from Word Parts

Term	Definition
acoustic neuroma (a-KOOS-tik) (nū-RŌ-ma)	benign tumor within the auditory canal growing from the acoustic nerve. May cause hearing loss.
ceruminoma (se-roo-mi-NŌ-ma)	tumor of a gland that secretes earwax (cerumen)
Ménière disease (me-NĀR) (di-ZĒZ)	chronic disease of the inner ear characterized by dizziness and ringing in the ear and hearing loss
otitis externa (ō-TĪ-tis) (ex-TER-na)	inflammation of the outer ear (Figure 13-4)
otitis media (OM) (ō-TĪ-tis) (MĒ-dia)	inflammation of the middle ear (see Figure 13-3)

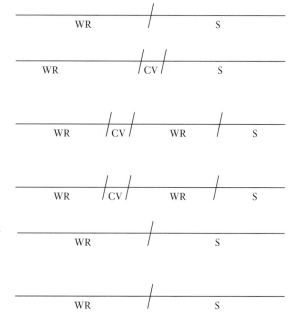

Figure 13-4
Otitis externa.

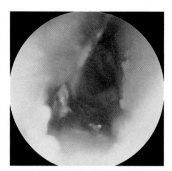

CAM TERM

Lymphatic drainage therapy is the use of gentle massage to stimulate the movement of fluid in the lymphatic system. Lymphatic drainage might be used to treat sinusitis or otitis media.

presbycusis............................ hearing impairment in old age
   (prez-bē-KŪ-sis)

tinnitus.................................. ringing in the ears
   (tin-NĪ-tus)

vertigo................................... a sense that either one's own body (subjective
   (VER-tig-ō)   vertigo) or the environment (objective vertigo)
                                        is revolving. May indicate inner ear disease.

Practice saying each of these terms aloud. To hear the terms, access the **PRONOUNCE IT** activity for this chapter on the Student CD that accompanies this text. Or, to hear the terms and their definitions with a CD player or computer, obtain the Pronunciation CD designed for use with this text.

Learn the definitions and spellings of the disease and disorder terms by completing exercises 7, 8, and 9.

EXERCISE   7

Fill in the blanks with the correct terms.

1. The patient reported that her body seemed to be revolving, or _____, and ringing in the ears, or _____.

2. A chronic ear disease characterized by dizziness, ringing in the ears, and hearing loss is called _____ disease.

3. Inflammation of the middle ear is called _____ _____.

4. _____ is the name given to a tumor of a gland that secretes earwax.

5. _____ _____ means inflammation of the outer ear.

6. A benign tumor arising from the acoustic nerve is called a(n) _____ _____.

7. _____ is hearing impairment in old age.

EXERCISE   8

Match the terms in the first column with the correct definitions in the second column.

_____ 1. vertigo
_____ 2. ceruminoma
_____ 3. tinnitus
_____ 4. Ménière disease
_____ 5. otitis externa
_____ 6. acoustic neuroma
_____ 7. otitis media
_____ 8. presbycusis

a. inflammation of the middle ear
b. tumor of a gland that secretes earwax
c. chronic ear problem characterized by vertigo, tinnitus, and hearing loss
d. benign tumor arising from the acoustic nerve
e. sense of revolving of one's own body or the environment
f. hardening of the oval window
g. ringing in the ears
h. inflammation of the outer ear
i. hearing impairment in old age

EXERCISE 9

Spell the disease and disorder terms. Have someone dictate the terms on pp. 464-465 to you. Study any words you have spelled incorrectly.

1. _____   5. _____

2. _____   6. _____

3. _____   7. _____

4. _____   8. _____

Surgical Terms

Built from Word Parts

Term	Definition
labyrinthectomy..................... (*lab*-i-rin-THEK-tō-mē)	excision of the labyrinth
mastoidectomy..................... (*mas*-toy-DEK-tō-mē)	excision of the mastoid bone
mastoidotomy..................... (*mas*-toy-DOT-ō-mē)	incision into the mastoid bone
myringoplasty..................... (mi-RING-gō-*plas*-tē)	surgical repair of the tympanic membrane
myringotomy..................... (mir-in-GOT-ō-mē)	incision into the tympanic membrane (performed to release pus or fluid and relieve pressure in the middle ear) (also called *tympanocentesis*) (Exercise Figure B)
stapedectomy..................... (stā-pe-DEK-tō-mē)	excision of the stapes. (Performed to restore hearing in cases of otosclerosis. The stapes is replaced by a prosthesis.) (Figure 13-5)
tympanoplasty..................... (tim-pan-ō-PLAS-tē)	surgical repair of the middle ear

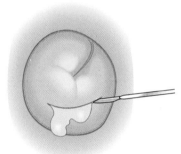

Exercise Figure B

Fill in the blanks to complete labeling of the diagram.

_____ / ___ / _____
tympanic / **cv** / **incision**
membrane

performed to release pus from the middle ear through the tympanic membrane to treat acute otitis media.

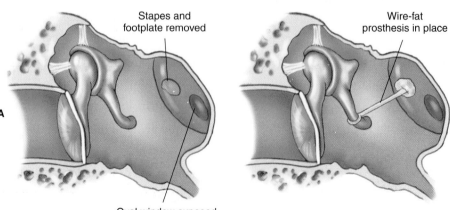

Stapes and footplate removed

Wire-fat prosthesis in place

A

B

Oval window exposed

Figure 13-5

Stapedectomy. **A,** Stapes is removed; **B,** prothesis is in place.

Practice saying each of these terms aloud. To hear the terms, access the **PRONOUNCE IT** activity for this chapter on the Student CD that accompanies this text. Or, to hear the terms and their definitions with a CD player or computer, obtain the Pronunciation CD designed for use with this text.

Learn the definitions and spellings of the surgical terms by completing exercises 10, 11, and 12.

EXERCISE   10

Analyze and define the following surgical terms.

1. mastoidectomy _____

2. myringotomy _____

3. labyrinthectomy _____

4. mastoidotomy _____

5. tympanoplasty _____

6. myringoplasty _____

7. stapedectomy _____

EXERCISE   11

Build surgical terms for the following definitions by using the word parts you have learned.

1. incision into the mastoid bone
   _____ / _____ / _____
   WR   CV   S

2. excision of the labyrinth
   _____ / _____
   WR   S

3. surgical repair of the middle ear
   _____ / _____ / _____
   WR   CV   S

4. excision of the mastoid bone
   _____ / _____
   WR   S

5. incision into the tympanic membrane
   _____ / _____ / _____
   WR   CV   S

6. surgical repair of the tympanic membrane
   _____ / _____ / _____
   WR   CV   S

7. excision of the stapes
   _____ / _____
   WR   S

EXERCISE 12

Spell each of the surgical terms. Have someone dictate the terms on p. 466 to you. Think about the word parts before attempting to write the word. Study any words you have spelled incorrectly.

1. _____   5. _____

2. _____   6. _____

3. _____   7. _____

4. _____

Diagnostic Terms

Built from Word Parts

Term	Definition
acoumeter (a-KOO-me-ter)	instrument used to measure (acuteness of) hearing
audiogram (AW-dē-ō-gram)	(graphic) record of hearing
audiometer (*aw*-dē-OM-e-ter)	instrument used to measure hearing
audiometry (*aw*-dē-OM-e-trē)	measurement of hearing (Exercise Figure C)
otoscope (Ō-tō-skōp)	instrument used for visual examination of the ear
otoscopy (ō-TOS-kō-pē)	visual examination of the ear
tympanometer (tim-pa-NOM-e-ter)	instrument used to measure middle ear function
tympanometry (tim-pa-NOM-e-trē)	measurement (movement) of the tympanic membrane

Practice saying each of these terms aloud. To hear the terms, access the **PRONOUNCE IT** activity for this chapter on the Student CD that accompanies this text. Or, to hear the terms and their definitions with a CD player or computer, obtain the Pronunciation CD designed for use with this text.

Learn the definitions and spellings of the diagnostic terms by completing exercises 13, 14, and 15.

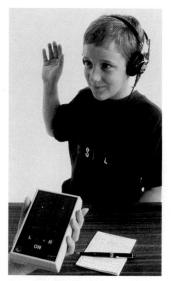

Exercise Figure C

Fill in the blanks to label this photograph showing the measurement of hearing.

_____ / _____ / _____
hearing / **cv** / **measurement**

One earphone emits a test sound while the other emits a masking noise. The patient is asked to signal when the test sound occurs.

EXERCISE 13

Analyze and define the following diagnostic terms.

1. otoscope _____

2. audiometry _____

3. audiogram _____

4. otoscopy _____

5. audiometer _____

6. tympanometry _____

7. acoumeter _____

8. tympanometer _____

EXERCISE 14

Build diagnostic terms that correspond to the following definitions by using the word parts you have learned.

1. measurement (of movement) of the tympanic membrane

　　_____ / __ / _____
　　WR　　　　　　CV　　　　　S

2. instrument used to measure hearing

　　_____ / __ / _____
　　WR　　　　　　CV　　　　　S

3. visual examination of the ear

　　_____ / __ / _____
　　WR　　　　　　CV　　　　　S

4. (graphic) record of hearing

　　_____ / __ / _____
　　WR　　　　　　CV　　　　　S

5. instrument used for visual examination of the ear

　　_____ / __ / _____
　　WR　　　　　　CV　　　　　S

6. measurement of hearing

　　_____ / __ / _____
　　WR　　　　　　CV　　　　　S

7. instrument used to measure (acuteness of) hearing

　　_____ / _____
　　　　　　WR　　　　　　S

8. instrument used to measure middle ear (function)

　　_____ / __ / _____
　　WR　　　　　　CV　　　　　S

EXERCISE 15

Spell each of the diagnostic terms. Have someone dictate the terms on p. 468 to you. Think about the word parts before attempting to write the word. Study any words you have spelled incorrectly.

1. _____　2. _____

3. _____   6. _____

4. _____   7. _____

5. _____   8. _____

Complementary Terms

Built from Word Parts

Term	Definition
audiologist................................... (aw-dē-OL-ō-jist)	one who studies and specializes in hearing
audiology .... (aw-dē-OL-ō-jē)	study of hearing
aural................................... (AW-rul)	pertaining to the ear
otologist................................... (ō-TOL-ō-jist)	physician who studies and treats diseases of the ear
otology .... (ō-TOL-ō-jē)	study of the ear (a branch of medicine that deals with diseases of the ear)
otorhinolaryngologist (ENT)............. (ō-tō-rī-nō-*lar*-in-GOL-ō-jist)	physician who studies and treats diseases of the ear, nose, and larynx (throat) (also called *otolaryngologist*)

Practice saying each of these terms aloud. To hear the terms, access the **PRONOUNCE IT** activity for this chapter on the Student CD that accompanies this text. Or, to hear the terms and their definitions with a CD player or computer, obtain the Pronunciation CD designed for use with this text.

Exercises 16, 17, and 18 will help you learn the definitions and spellings of the complementary terms related to the ear.

EXERCISE   16

Analyze and define the following complementary terms.

1. otology   _____

2. audiologist _____

3. otorhinolaryngologist _____

4. audiology   _____

5. otologist _____

6. aural   _____

EXERCISE 17

Build the complementary terms for the following definitions by using the word parts you have learned.

1. study of hearing

    _____ / ___ / _____
    WR   CV   S

2. physician who studies and
   treats diseases of the ear,
   nose, and larynx (throat)

    _____ / __ / _____ / __ / _____ / __ / __
    WR   CV   WR   CV   WR   CV   S

3. study of the ear

    _____ / ___ / _____
    WR   CV   S

4. one who studies and
   specializes in hearing

    _____ / ___ / _____
    WR   CV   S

5. physician who studies and
   treats diseases of the ear

    _____ / ___ / _____
    WR   CV   S

6. pertaining to the ear

    _____ / _____
    WR   S

EXERCISE 18

Spell each of the complementary terms. Have someone dictate the terms on p. 470 to you. Think about the word parts before attempting to write the word. Study any words you have spelled incorrectly.

1. _____   4. _____

2. _____   5. _____

3. _____   6. _____

Abbreviations

AOM	acute otitis media
EENT	eyes, ears, nose, and throat
ENT	ears, nose, throat
OM	otitis media

EXERCISE 19

Write the meaning of the following abbreviations.

1. ENT _____ _____ _____

2. EENT _____ _____ _____ _____

3. OM _____ _____

4. AOM _____ _____ _____

TABLE 13-1

Plural Endings

Greek and Latin Plural Endings

Plurals are formed in Greek and Latin terms by using the suffixes listed below. Plurals are
formed in medical language by using the English plural endings for terms originating from
English modern language; and by using Greek and Latin plural endings for terms originating
from Greek and Latin language.

Latin		Greek	
Singular	*Plural*	*Singular*	*Plural*
fimbria	fimbriae	adenoma	adenomata
thorax	thoraces	spermatozoon	spermatozoa
appendix	appendices	larynx	larynges
diverticulum	diverticula	metastasis	metastases
bronchus	bronchi		
testis	testes		

English Plural Endings

Plurals are formed in the English language by adding -s, -es, or -ies at the end of a word.

Singular	Plural
dog	dogs
fox	foxes
canary	canaries

> Alternative plural endings such as **thoraxes** or **appendixes** may be used. Both **thoraces** and **thoraxes**; and **appendices** and **appendixes** are considered correct.

EXERCISE 20 *Learn Plural Endings*

Convert the following terms, which have been introduced in previous chapters, to
plurals. Refer to the previous information and/or to Common Plural Endings for Medical
Terms listed on the inside back cover of the text.

1. thrombus _____

2. staphylococcus   _____

3. streptococcus   _____

4. alveolus   _____

5. glomerulus   _____

6. testis   _____

7. ovum   _____

8. diagnosis   _____

9. bacterium   _____

10. nucleus   _____

11. pharynx   _____

12. sarcoma   _____

13. carcinoma   _____

14. anastomosis   _____

15. prosthesis   _____

16. embolus   _____

17. prognosis   _____

18. spermatozoon   _____

19. fimbria   _____

20. thorax   _____

21. appendix   _____

EXERCISE 21   *Use Plural Endings*

Circle the correct singular or plural term to match the context of information in the sentence.

1. During a colonoscopy the gastroenterologist noted the patient had several (diverticula, diverticulum) in his transverse colon.
2. Bronchogenic carcinoma was diagnosed in the patient's left (bronchus, bronchi).
3. Bilateral orchiditis is inflammation of the (testes, testis).
4. The light brown mole with notched borders turned out to be a (melanomata, melanoma).
5. Multiple (thrombus, thrombi) were observed on the lung scan.
6. Many (diagnosis, diagnoses) of benign tumors are picked up during whole body scanning.
7. Diagnostic studies have shown (metastasis, metastases) of the patient's carcinoma of the breast to both her lungs and brain.

CHAPTER REVIEW

EXERCISE **22** *Interact with Medical Records*

Complete the progress note by writing the medical terms in the blanks. Use the list of definitions with the corresponding numbers.

University Hospital and Medical Center
4700 North Main Street • Wellness, Arizona 54321 • (987) 555-3210

PATIENT NAME: Jimmy Tohe   **CASE NUMBER:**   99665-AUD
DATE OF BIRTH: 03/04/xx   **DATE:**   09/04/xx

PROGRESS NOTE

SUBJECTIVE DATA: Jimmy Tohe is a 62-year-old Native-American male, appearing younger than his stated age. He was brought into the 1. _____ clinic by his daughter, who states that he is unable to hear what is being said to him by family members. She states that this problem has existed for at least 30 years but that it appears to be getting markedly worse. The patient states he had several episodes of ear infections as a child and young adult. He denies any 2. _____ or 3. _____ .

OBJECTIVE DATA: Temperature, 99.4. Pulse, 72. Respirations, 20. Blood pressure, 136/76. Weight, 162 pounds. Patient ambulates without difficulty. Alert and oriented ×3. 4. _____ reveals scarring of the tympanic membranes bilaterally. Auditory canals appear normal bilaterally. Patient states he is allergic to Demerol.

ASSESSMENT:
1. Severe loss of hearing bilaterally, probably caused by 5. _____ _____ as a child.
2. Recent exacerbation of hearing loss most likely attributable to 6. _____ .

PLAN:
1. Patient referred to 7. _____ for complete 8. _____ workup.

_____
Bridey McKeegan, MD

BM/mcm

---

1. abbreviation for ears, nose, and throat
2. ringing in the ears
3. a sense of ones own body or the environment revolving
4. visual examination of the ear
5. inflammation of the middle ear
6. hearing impairment in old age
7. one who studies and specializes in hearing
8. measurement of hearing

EXERCISE 23 _Interpret Medical Terms_

To test your understanding of the terms introduced in this chapter, circle the words that correctly complete the sentences. The italicized phrase is the definition of the term.

1. _Inflammation of the eardrum_ is (labyrinthitis, mastoiditis, myringitis).
2. The patient reported _ringing in the ears,_ or (tinnitus, vertigo, tympanitis).
3. The patient seeking a _specialist for his labyrinthitis_ consulted an (optometrist, audiologist, otologist).
4. The physician planned to release the pus from the middle ear by making an _incision in the tympanic membrane,_ or performing a (mastoidotomy, myringotomy, labyrinthectomy).

EXERCISE 24 _Read Medical Terms in Use_

Practice pronunciation of terms by reading the following information on acute otitis media. Use the pronunciation key following the medical term to assist you in saying the words.

Acute Otitis Media
Acute otitis media (ō-TĪ-tis) (MĒ-dia) is one of the most common pediatric infections. Most middle ear infections are caused by bacteria, and some by viruses. Symptoms include **otalgia** (ō-TAL-jē-a), **otorrhea** (ō-tō-RĒ-a), ear pulling, and irritability. The tympanic membrane will be bulging, red in color, with a thickened appearance and reduced translucency. Antibiotics may be ordered if the infection does not resolve on its own. If unresponsive to antibiotic treatment, a **myringotomy** (mir-in-GOT-ō-mē) may be performed to identify the causative pathogen, allowing for the appropriate antibiotic treatment to be prescribed.

EXERCISE 25 _Comprehend Terms in Use_

Test your comprehension of terms in the previous passage by answering T for true and F for false.

_____ 1. Inflammation of the outer ear is one of the most common pediatric infections.

_____ 2. Pain and discharge from the ear are symptoms of acute otitis media.

_____ 3. Surgical repair of the tympanic membrane may be performed to identify causative organisms.

For further practice or to evaluate what you have learned, use the Student CD that accompanies this text.

COMBINING FORMS CROSSWORD PUZZLE

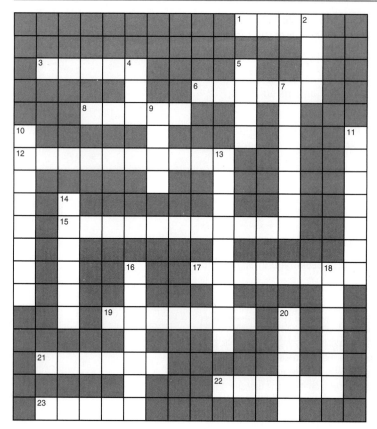

Across Clues

1. pupil
3. hearing
6. cornea
8. light
12. labyrinth
15. conjunctiva
17. mastoid
19. tear duct
21. cornea
22. retina
23. double

Down Clues

2. vision
4. ear
5. cold
7. eardrum, middle ear
9. tension
10. eyelid
11. eardrum
13. eye
14. sclera
16. stapes
18. tear
20. hearing

REVIEW OF WORD PARTS

Can you define and spell the following word parts?

Combining Forms

acou/o	mastoid/o
audi/o	myring/o
aur/i	ot/o
aur/o	staped/o
labyrinth/o	tympan/o

REVIEW OF TERMS

Can you build, analyze, define, pronounce, and spell the following terms *built from word parts?*

Diseases and Disorders

labyrinthitis
mastoiditis
myringitis
otalgia
otomastoiditis
otomycosis
otopyorrhea
otosclerosis
tympanitis

Surgical

labyrinthectomy
mastoidectomy
mastoidotomy
myringoplasty
myringotomy
stapedectomy
tympanoplasty

Diagnostic

acoumeter
audiogram
audiometer
audiometry
otoscope
otoscopy
tympanometer
tympanometry

Complementary

audiologist
audiology
aural
otologist
otology
otorhinolaryngologist (ENT)

Can you define, pronounce, and spell the following terms *not built from word parts?*

Diseases and Disorders

acoustic neuroma
ceruminoma
Ménière disease
otitis externa
otitis media (OM)
presbycusis
tinnitus
vertigo

14

Musculoskeletal System

OUTLINE

OBJECTIVES

On completion of this chapter you will be able to:

1. Identify the anatomy of the musculoskeletal system.
2. Define, pronounce, and spell types of body movements.
3. Define and spell the word parts presented in this chapter.
4. Build and analyze medical terms with word parts presented in this and previous chapters.
5. Define, pronounce, and spell the disease and disorder, diagnostic, surgical, and complementary terms for the musculoskeletal system.
6. Interpret the meanings of the abbreviations presented in this chapter.
7. Read medical documents and interpret medical terminology contained in them.

ANATOMY

The musculoskeletal system is made up of muscles, bones, and joints. The body contains 206 bones and more than 600 muscles. Joints are any place in the body at which two or more bones meet.

Function

The functions of the muscular system are movement, posture, joint stability, and heat production. The functions of the skeletal system are to provide a framework for the body, protect the soft body parts such as the brain, store calcium, and produce blood cells.

Bone Structure

Periosteum
is composed of the prefix **peri-,** meaning **surrounding,** and the word root **oste,** meaning **bone.**

Endosteum
is composed of the prefix **endo-,** meaning **within,** and the word root **oste,** meaning **bone.**

Diaphysis
comes from the Greek **diaphusis,** meaning **state of growing between.**

periosteum	outermost layer of the bone, made up of fibrous tissue (Figure 14-1)
compact bone	dense, hard layers of bone tissue that lie underneath the periosteum
cancellous (spongy) bone	contains little spaces like a sponge and is encased in the layers of compact bone
endosteum	membranous lining of the hollow cavity of the bone
diaphysis	shaft of the long bones (see Figure 14-1)

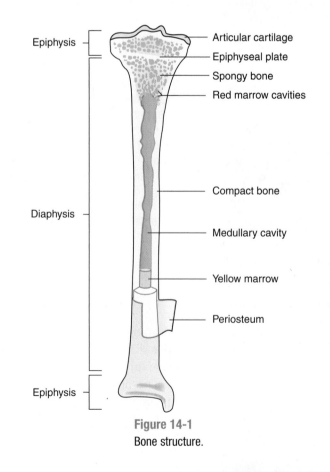

Epiphysis

Articular cartilage
Epiphyseal plate
Spongy bone
Red marrow cavities

Diaphysis

Compact bone

Medullary cavity

Yellow marrow

Periosteum

Epiphysis

Figure 14-1
Bone structure.

epiphysis (*pl.* epiphyses)	ends of the long bone
bone marrow	material found in the cavities of bones
red marrow	thick, blood-like material found in flat bones and the ends of long bones. Location of blood cell formation.
yellow marrow	soft, fatty material found in the medullary cavity of long bones

Epiphysis
has been used in the English language since the 1600s and retains the meaning given to it by a Greco-Roman physician. It means a **portion of bone attached for a time to another bone by a cartilage, but that later combines with the principal bone.** During the period of growth, the epiphysis is separated from the main portion of the bone by cartilage.

Skeletal Bones

maxilla	upper jawbone (Figure 14-2, *A*)
mandible	lower jawbone (see Figure 14-2, *A*)
vertebral column	made up of bones called *vertebrae (pl.)* or *vertebra (sing.)* through which the spinal cord runs. The vertebral column protects the spinal cord, supports the head, and provides a point of attachment for ribs and muscles (Figure 14-3).
cervical vertebrae (C1 to C7)	first set of seven bones, forming the neck
thoracic vertebrae (T1 to T12)	second set of 12 vertebrae; they articulate with the 12 pairs of ribs to form the outward curve of the spine
lumbar vertebrae (L1 to L5)	third set of five larger vertebrae, which forms the inward curve of the spine
sacrum	next five vertebrae, which fuse together to form a triangular bone positioned between the two hip bones
coccyx	four vertebrae fused together to form the tailbone (Figure 14-4)
lamina (*pl.* laminae)	part of the vertebral arch
clavicle	collarbone (see Figure 14-2, *A*)
scapula	shoulder blade (see Figure 14-2, *B*)
acromion	extension of the scapula, which forms the high point of the shoulder (Figure 14-2, *B*)
sternum	breastbone (see Figure 14-2, *A*)
xiphoid process	lower portion of the sternum
humerus	upper arm bone (see Figure 14-2, *A* and *B*)
ulna and radius	lower arm bones (see Figure 14-2, *A* and *B*)
carpal bones	wrist bones (see Figure 14-2, *A*)
metacarpal bones	hand bones (see Figure 14-2, *A*)
phalanges (*sing.* phalanx)	finger and toe bones (see Figure 14-2, *A*)
pelvic bone, hip bone	made up of three bones fused together (see Figure 14-2, *A*)
ischium	lower, rear portion on which one sits
ilium	upper, wing-shaped part on each side
pubis	anterior portion of the pelvic bone

Metacarpus
literally means **beyond the wrist.** It is composed of the prefix **meta-,** meaning **beyond,** and **carpus,** meaning **wrist.**

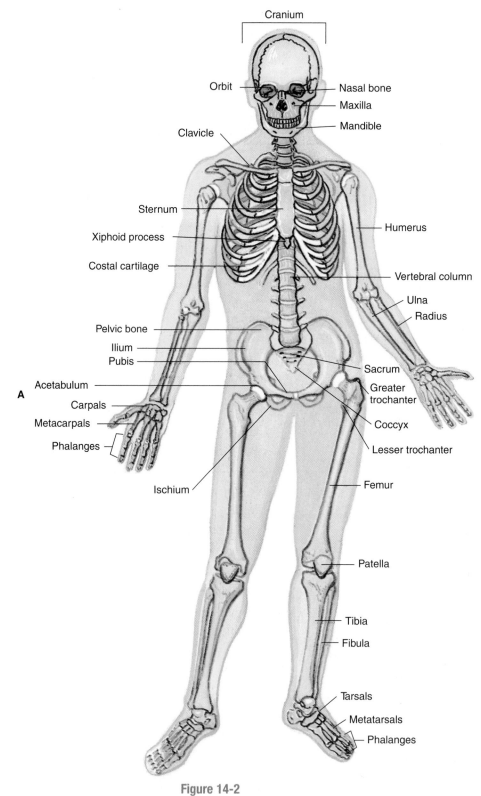

Figure 14-2
A, Anterior view of the skeleton.

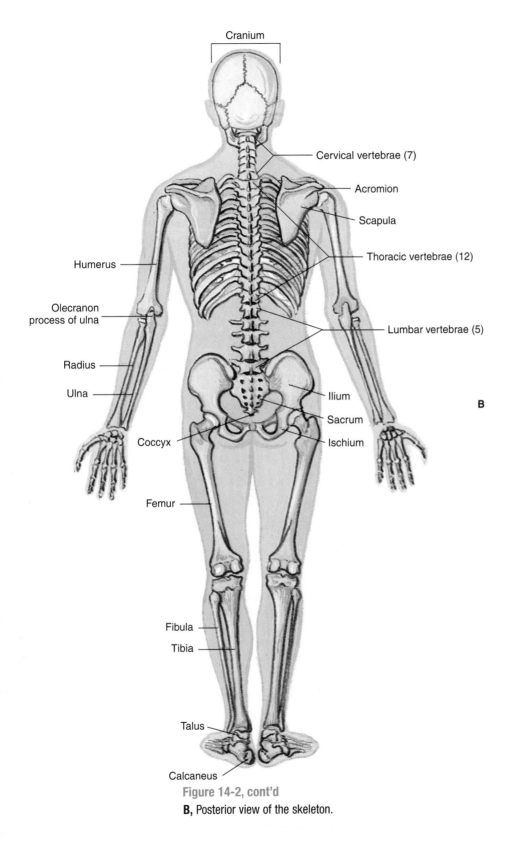

Cranium

Cervical vertebrae (7)

Acromion

Scapula

Thoracic vertebrae (12)

Humerus

Olecranon
process of ulna

Lumbar vertebrae (5)

Radius

Ulna

Ilium

Sacrum

Coccyx

Ischium

Femur

B

Fibula

Tibia

Talus

Calcaneus

Figure 14-2, cont'd
B, Posterior view of the skeleton.

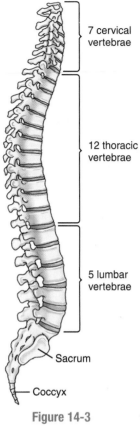

7 cervical vertebrae

12 thoracic vertebrae

5 lumbar vertebrae

Sacrum

Coccyx

Figure 14-3
Vertebral column.

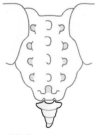

Figure 14-4

Coccyx is derived from the Greek word *cuckoo* because of its resemblance to a cuckoo's beak.

acetabulum	large socket in the pelvic bone for the head of the femur
femur	upper leg bone (see Figure 14-2, *A* and *B*)
tibia and fibula	lower leg bones (see Figure 14-2, *A* and *B*)
patella (*pl.* patellae)	kneecap (see Figure 14-2, *A*)
tarsal bones	ankle bones (see Figure 14-2, *A*)
calcaneus	heel bone (see Figure 14-2, *B*)
metatarsal bones	foot bones (see Figure 14-2, *A*)

Joints

Joints, also called *articulations,* hold our bones together and make movement possible (in most joints) (Figure 14-5).

articular cartilage	smooth layer of gristle covering the contacting surface of joints
meniscus	crescent-shaped cartilage found in the knee
intervertebral disk	cartilaginous pad found between the vertebrae in the spine
pubic symphysis	cartilaginous joint at which two pubic bones fuse together
synovia	fluid secreted by the synovial membrane and found in joint cavities
bursa (*pl.* bursae)	fluid-filled sac that allows for easy movement of one part of a joint over another
ligament	flexible, tough band of fibrous connective tissue that attaches one bone to another at a joint
tendon	band of fibrous connective tissue that attaches muscle to bone
aponeurosis	strong sheet of tissue that acts as a tendon to attach muscles to bone

Muscles

skeletal muscles (also known as *striated muscles*)	attached to bones by tendons and make body movement possible. Skeletal muscles produce action by pulling and by working in pairs. Also known as *voluntary muscles* because we have control over these muscles (Figure 14-6, *A, B,* and *C*).
smooth muscles (also known as *unstriated muscles*)	located in internal organs such as the walls of blood vessels and the digestive tract. They are also called *involuntary muscles* because they respond to impulses from the autonomic nerves and are not controlled voluntarily (see Figure 14-6, *C*).

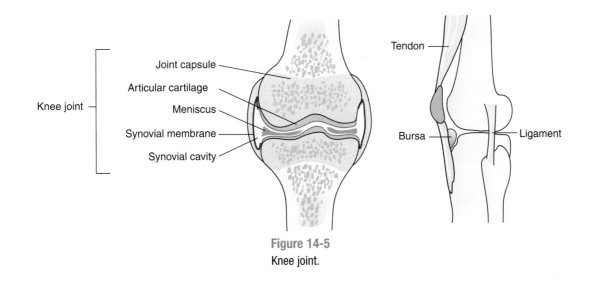

Figure 14-5
Knee joint.

cardiac muscle
(known as *myocardium*)................. forms most of the wall of the heart. Its involuntary contraction produces the heartbeat (see Figure 14-6, *C*).

Learn the anatomic terms by completing exercises 1, 2, and 3.

EXERCISE 1

Match the definitions in the first column with the correct terms in the second column.

_____ 1. shaft of a long bone   a. skeletal muscle

_____ 2. hard layer of bone tissue   b. cancellous bone

_____ 3. outermost layer of bone   c. smooth muscle

_____ 4. found in bone cavities   d. diaphysis

_____ 5. lining of the bone cavity   e. endometrium

_____ 6. end of each long bone   f. cardiac muscle

_____ 7. contains little spaces   g. epiphysis

_____ 8. produces heartbeats   h. periosteum

_____ 9. voluntary muscles   i. compact bone

_____ 10. located in internal   j. endosteum
         organs
                                     k. bone marrow

EXERCISE 2

Write the name of the bone to match the definition.

1. shoulder blade   _____

2. breastbone   _____

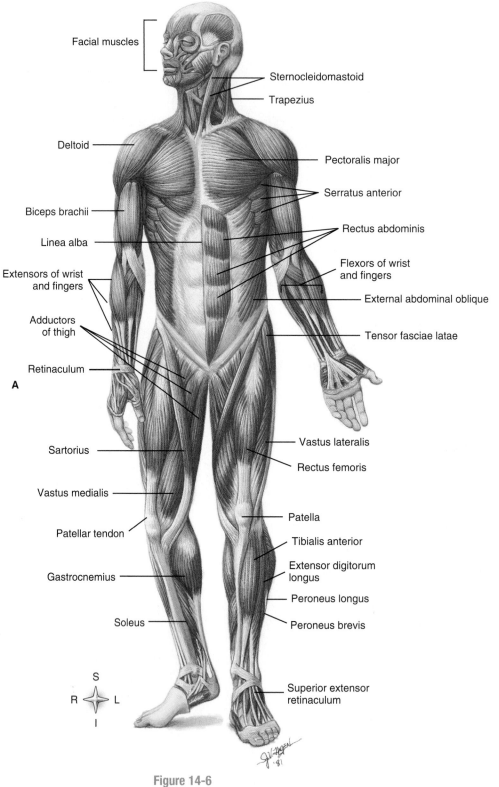

Facial muscles

Sternocleidomastoid

Trapezius

Deltoid

Pectoralis major

Serratus anterior

Biceps brachii

Rectus abdominis

Linea alba

Flexors of wrist
and fingers

Extensors of wrist
and fingers

External abdominal oblique

Adductors
of thigh

Tensor fasciae latae

Retinaculum

A

Vastus lateralis

Sartorius

Rectus femoris

Vastus medialis

Patella

Patellar tendon

Tibialis anterior

Extensor digitorum
longus

Gastrocnemius

Peroneus longus

Soleus

Peroneus brevis

S

R — L

I

Superior extensor
retinaculum

Figure 14-6

A, Anterior view of the muscular system.

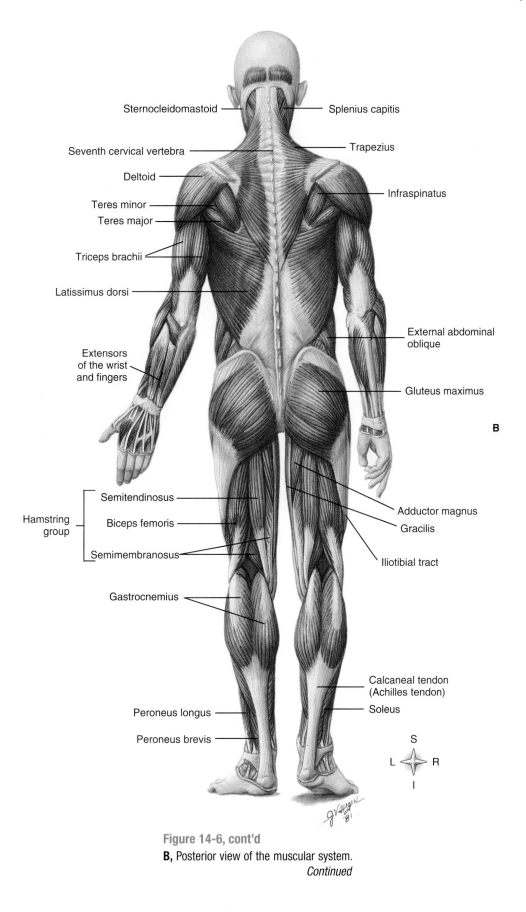

Figure 14-6, cont'd
B, Posterior view of the muscular system.
Continued

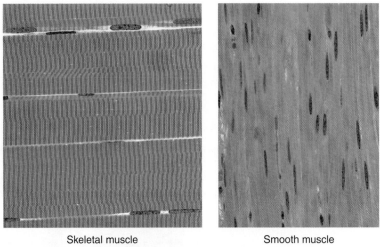

Skeletal muscle   Smooth muscle

C

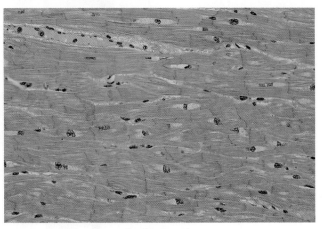

Cardiac muscle

Figure 14-6, cont'd

C, Microscopic photographs of muscle tissue.

3. lower jawbone   _____

4. collarbone   _____

5. upper arm bone   _____

6. lower arm bones   a. _____

    b. _____

7. ankle bones   _____

8. finger, toe bones   _____

9. foot bones   _____

10. hand bones   _____

11. upper leg bone   _____

12. lower leg bones   a. _____

    b. _____

13. kneecap _____

14. neck _____   _____

15. third set of vertebrae _____

16. anterior portion of the
    pelvic bone _____

17. five vertebrae fused together _____

18. lower rear portion of the
    pelvic bone _____

19. tailbone _____

20. upper, wing-shaped part of
    the pelvic bone _____

21. wrist bones _____

EXERCISE   3

Match the definitions in the first column with the correct terms in the second column.

_____ 1. attaches muscle to bone   a. acetabulum

_____ 2. fluid-filled sac   b. aponeurosis

_____ 3. smooth layer of gristle   c. bursa

_____ 4. socket in the pelvic bone   d. calcaneus

_____ 5. fluid   e. cartilage

_____ 6. heel bone   f. intervertebral disk

_____ 7. attaches bone to bone   g. lamina

_____ 8. cartilage found in the   h. ligament
          knee
                                      i. meniscus
_____ 9. pubic bone joint
                                      j. periosteum
_____ 10. acts as a tendon
                                      k. pubic symphysis
_____ 11. found between each
           vertebra   l. synovia

_____ 12. part of the arch of the   m. tendon
           vertebra

Types of Body Movements

Bones and muscles work together to produce various types of body movements. Some
are listed below (Figure 14-7).

Term	Definition
abduction.................................... (ab-DUK-shun)	movement of drawing away from the middle

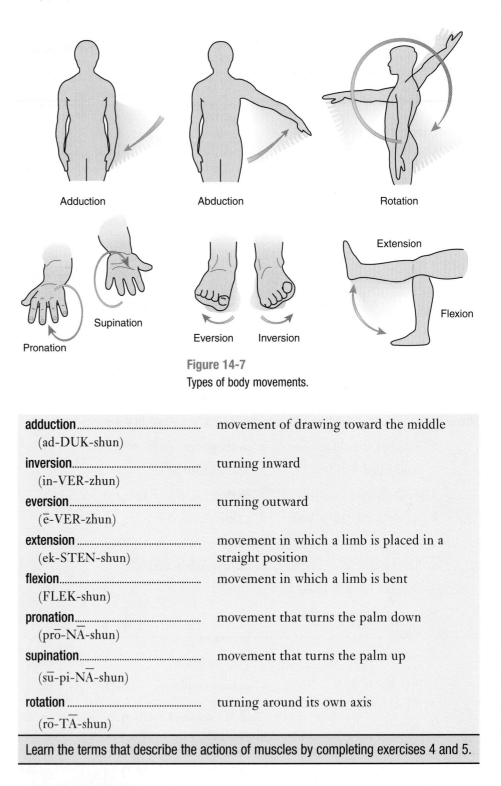

Figure 14-7
Types of body movements.

adduction .... (ad-DUK-shun)	movement of drawing toward the middle
inversion .... (in-VER-zhun)	turning inward
eversion .... (ē-VER-zhun)	turning outward
extension .... (ek-STEN-shun)	movement in which a limb is placed in a straight position
flexion .... (FLEK-shun)	movement in which a limb is bent
pronation .... (prō-NĀ-shun)	movement that turns the palm down
supination .... (sū-pi-NĀ-shun)	movement that turns the palm up
rotation .... (rō-TĀ-shun)	turning around its own axis

Learn the terms that describe the actions of muscles by completing exercises 4 and 5.

EXERCISE 4

Write the definitions of the following terms.

1. abduction _____

2. pronation _____

3. supination _____

4. rotation _____

5. extension _____

6. eversion _____

7. adduction _____

8. flexion _____

9. inversion _____

EXERCISE 5

Match the terms in the first column with the correct definitions in the second column.

_____ 1. abduction

_____ 2. adduction

_____ 3. pronation

_____ 4. rotation

_____ 5. eversion

_____ 6. extension

_____ 7. flexion

_____ 8. inversion

_____ 9. supination

a. movement in which the limb is placed in a straight position

b. movement that turns the palm up

c. turning outward

d. drawing toward the middle

e. conveying toward the center

f. turning inward

g. movement in which the limb is bent

h. drawing away from the middle

i. movement that turns the palm down

j. turning around its own axis

WORD PARTS

Combining Forms of the Musculoskeletal System

At first glance the number of word parts introduced in this chapter may seem overwhelming, but notice that many of them are names for bones already learned in the anatomic section. The definitions of the word parts include both anatomic terms and commonly used words. For example, both *carpal* and *wrist bone* are given as the definition of the combining form *carp/o*. Learn the anatomic locations and definitions of the combining forms of the musculoskeletal system by completing Exercise Figures A and B on pp. 493-494.

Combining Form	Definition
carp/o	carpals (wrist bones)
clavic/o, clavicul/o	clavicle (collarbone)

cost/o	rib
crani/o	cranium (skull)
femor/o	femur (upper leg bone)
fibul/o	fibula (lower leg bone)
humer/o	humerus (upper arm bone)
ili/o	ilium
ischi/o	ischium
lumb/o	loin, lumbar region of the spine
mandibul/o	mandible (lower jawbone)
maxill/o	maxilla (upper jawbone)
patell/o	patella (kneecap)
pelv/i, pelv/o (NOTE: both *i* and *o* may be used as the connecting vowel with *pelvis*)	pelvis, pelvic bone (also covered in Chapter 9)
phalang/o	phalanges (finger or toe bones)
pub/o	pubis
rachi/o	spine, vertebral column
radi/o	radius (lower arm bone)
sacr/o	sacrum
scapul/o	scapula (shoulder blade)
spondyl/o, vertebr/o	vertebra
stern/o	sternum (breastbone)
tars/o	tarsals (ankle bones)
tibi/o	tibia (lower leg bone)
uln/o	ulna (lower arm bone)

> **Disk**
> is from the Greek **diskos,** meaning flat plate. A variant spelling, **disc,** is also used, though chiefly in ophthalmology.

Learn the anatomic locations and definitions of the combining forms by completing exercises 6 through 9, and Exercise Figures A and B.

EXERCISE 6

Write the definitions of the following combining forms.

1. clavic/o _____

2. cost/o _____

3. crani/o _____

4. femor/o _____

5. clavicul/o _____

6. humer/o _____

7. ili/o _____

8. ischi/o _____

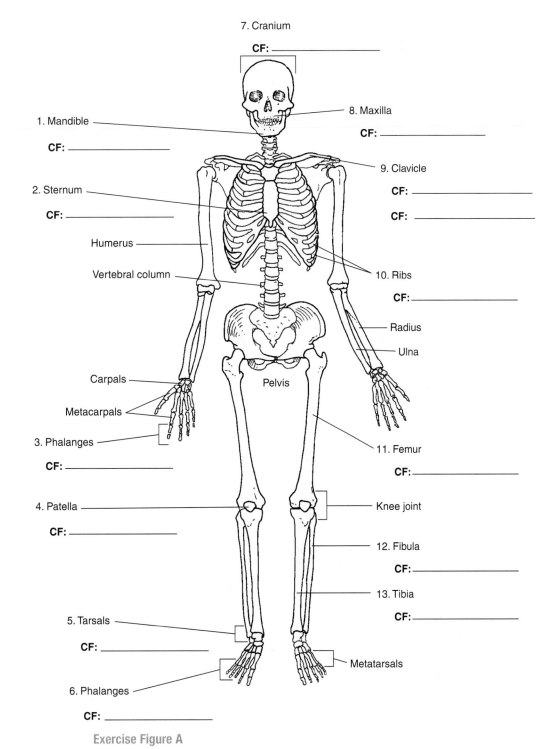

Exercise Figure A

Fill in the blanks with combining forms in this diagram of the skeleton, anterior view.

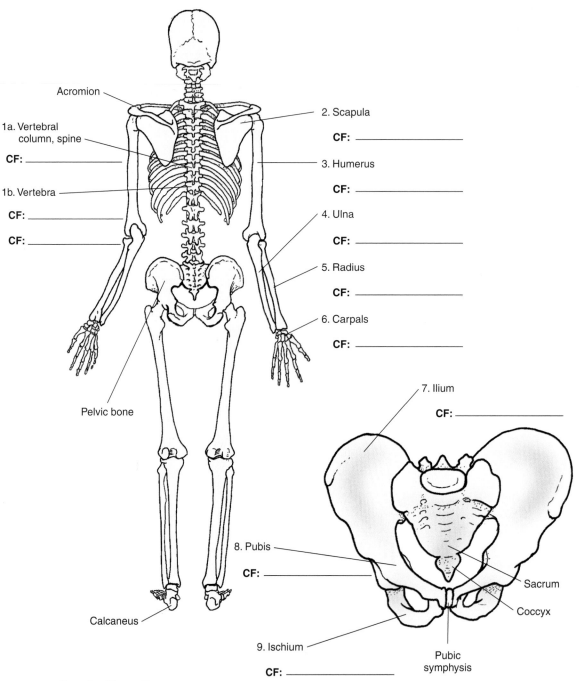

Acromion

1a. Vertebral
column, spine

CF: _____

1b. Vertebra

CF: _____

CF: _____

Pelvic bone

Calcaneus

2. Scapula

CF: _____

3. Humerus

CF: _____

4. Ulna

CF: _____

5. Radius

CF: _____

6. Carpals

CF: _____

7. Ilium

CF: _____

8. Pubis

CF: _____

9. Ischium

CF: _____

Sacrum

Coccyx

Pubic
symphysis

Exercise Figure B
Fill in the blanks with combining forms in this diagram of the skeleton, posterior view, and the pelvis.

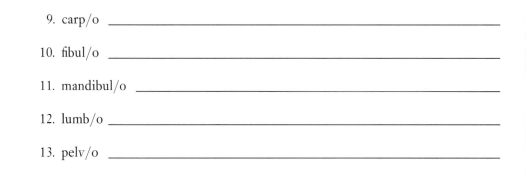

9. carp/o _____

10. fibul/o _____

11. mandibul/o _____

12. lumb/o _____

13. pelv/o _____

EXERCISE   7

Write the combining form for each of the following terms.

1. clavicle   a. _____

                         b. _____

2. rib   _____

3. cranium   _____

4. femur   _____

5. humerus   _____

6. carpals   _____

7. ischium   _____

8. fibula   _____

9. ilium   _____

10. mandible   _____

11. loin, lumbar region of the spine _____

12. pelvis, pelvic bone a. _____

                         b. _____

EXERCISE   8

Write the definitions of the following combining forms.

1. rachi/o _____

2. patell/o _____

3. spondyl/o _____

4. maxill/o _____

5. phalang/o _____

6. uln/o _____

7. radi/o _____

8. tibi/o _____

9. pub/o _____

10. tars/o _____

11. scapul/o _____

12. stern/o _____

13. vertebr/o _____

14. sacr/o _____

EXERCISE 9

Write the combining form for each of the following terms.

1. maxilla   _____

2. ulna   _____

3. radius   _____

4. tibia   _____

5. pubis   _____

6. tarsals   _____

7. vertebra   a. _____

                                 b. _____

8. sternum   _____

9. scapula   _____

10. patella   _____

11. phalanges   _____

12. sacrum   _____

13. vertebral column, spine   _____

Combining Forms for Joints

Combining Form	Definition
aponeur/o	aponeurosis
arthr/o	joint
burs/o	bursa (cavity)
chondr/o	cartilage
disk/o	intervertebral disk

menisc/o	....	meniscus (crescent)
synovi/o	....	synovia, synovial membrane
ten/o, tend/o, tendin/o	....	tendon

Learn the anatomic locations and definitions of the combining forms by completing exercises 10 and 11 and Exercise Figure C.

EXERCISE 10

Write the definitions of the following combining forms.

1. arthr/o _____

2. aponeur/o _____

3. menisc/o _____

4. tendin/o _____

5. chondr/o _____

6. ten/o _____

7. burs/o _____

8. tend/o _____

9. synovi/o _____

10. disk/o _____

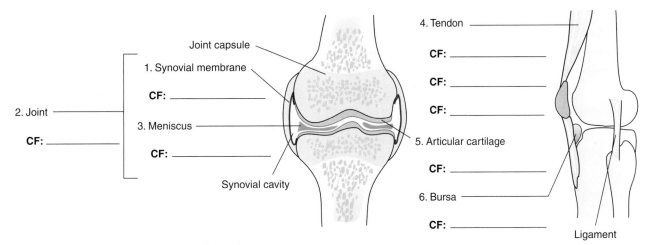

Exercise Figure C
Fill in the blanks with combining forms on this diagram of the knee joint.

EXERCISE 11

Write the combining form for each of the following terms.

1. meniscus _____

2. aponeurosis _____

3. joint _____

4. cartilage _____

5. tendon a. _____

b. _____

c. _____

6. bursa _____

7. synovia, synovial membrane _____

8. intervertebral disk _____

Combining Forms Commonly Used with Musculoskeletal System Terms

Combining Form	Definition
ankyl/o	crooked, stiff, bent
kinesi/o	movement, motion
kyph/o	hump
lamin/o	lamina (thin, flat plate or layer)
lord/o	bent forward
myel/o	bone marrow
(NOTE: *myel/o* also means *spinal cord*; see Chapter 15.)	
my/o, myos/o	muscle
(NOTE: *my/o* was introduced in Chapter 2.)	
oste/o	bone
petr/o	stone
(NOTE: *lith/o*, also a combining form for *stone*, was introduced in Chapter 6.)	
scoli/o	crooked, curved

Learn the anatomic locations and definitions of the combining forms by completing exercises 12 and 13.

EXERCISE 12

Write the definitions of the following combining forms.

1. my/o _____

2. petr/o _____

3. kinesi/o _____

4. oste/o _____

5. lamin/o _____

6. myel/o _____

7. kyph/o _____

8. ankyl/o _____

9. scoli/o _____

10. myos/o _____

11. lord/o _____

EXERCISE 13

Write the combining form for each of the following.

1. muscle   a. _____

                     b. _____

2. stone   _____

3. movement, motion _____

4. bone   _____

5. lamina   _____

6. bone marrow   _____

7. hump   _____

8. crooked, stiff, bent   _____

9. crooked, curved   _____

10. bent forward   _____

Prefixes

Prefix	Definition
inter-	between
supra-	above
sym-, syn-	together, joined

Learn the prefixes by completing exercises 14 and 15.

EXERCISE 14

Write the definition of the following prefixes.

1. supra- _____

2. sym-, syn- _____

3. inter- _____

EXERCISE 15

Write the prefix for each of the following definitions.

1. together, joined   a. _____

                       b. _____

2. between _____

3. above _____

Suffixes

Suffix	Definition
-asthenia	weakness
-clasia, -clasis, -clast	break
-desis	surgical fixation, fusion
-physis	growth
-schisis	split, fissure

Learn the suffixes by completing exercises 16 and 17.
Refer to Appendix A and Appendix B for a complete listing of word parts.

EXERCISE 16

Write the definitions of the following suffixes.

1. -physis _____

2. -clasis _____

3. -desis _____

4. -clast _____

5. -schisis _____

6. -clasia _____

7. -asthenia _____

EXERCISE 17

Write the suffix for each of the following definitions.

1. growth   _____

2. weakness   _____

3. break   a. _____

                      b. _____

                      c. _____

4. surgical fixation, fusion   _____

5. split, fissure   _____

MEDICAL TERMS

The terms you need to learn to complete this chapter are listed below. The exercises following each list will help you learn the definition and the spelling of each word.

Disease and Disorder Terms

Built from Word Parts

Term	Definition
ankylosis (an-kil-Ō-sis)	abnormal condition of stiffness (often referring to a joint, such as the result of chronic rheumatoid arthritis)
arthritis (ar-THRĪ-tis)	inflammation of a joint. (The most common forms of arthritis are rheumatoid arthritis and osteoarthritis.) (Figure 14-8)
arthrochondritis (*ar*-thrō-kon-DRĪ-tis)	inflammation of joint cartilages
bursitis (ber-SĪ-tis)	inflammation of a bursa
bursolith (BER-sō-lith)	stone in a bursa

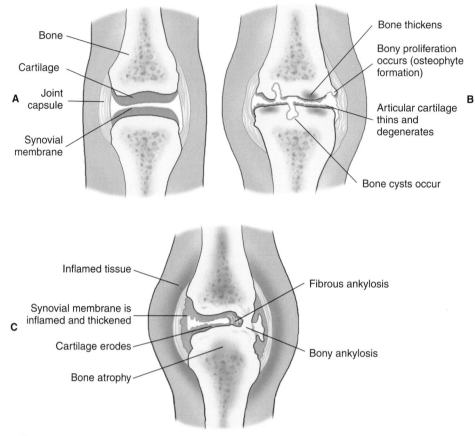

Figure 14-8

A, Normal knee joint. **B,** Osteoarthritis of the knee joint. **C,** Rheumatoid arthritis of the knee joint.

carpoptosis .... (kar-pō-TŌ-sis)	drooping wrist (wristdrop)
chondromalacia .... (kon-drō-ma-LĀ-shē-a)	softening of cartilage
cranioschisis .... (krā-nē-OS-ki-sis)	(congenital) fissure of the skull
diskitis .... (dis-KĪ-tis)	inflammation of an (intervertebral) disk
fibromyalgia .... (fī-brō-MĪ-al-jē-a)	pain in the fibrous tissues and muscles (a common condition characterized by widespread pain and stiffness of muscles, fatigue, and disturbed sleep)
kyphosis .... (kī-FŌ-sis)	abnormal condition of a hump (of the thoracic spine) (also called *hunchback* or *humpback*) (Exercise Figure D)
lordosis .... (lōr-DŌ-sis)	abnormal condition of bending forward (forward curvature of the lumbar spine) (also called *swayback*) (see Exercise Figure D)
maxillitis .... (mak-si-LĪ-tis)	inflammation of the maxilla

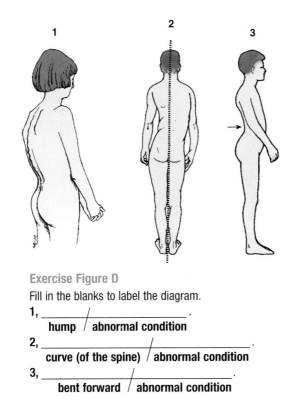

Exercise Figure D

Fill in the blanks to label the diagram.

1, _____ / _____ .
   hump / abnormal condition

2, _____ / _____ .
   curve (of the spine) / abnormal condition

3, _____ / _____ .
   bent forward / abnormal condition

meniscitis .... (*men*-i-SĪ-tis)	inflammation of a meniscus
myasthenia .... (*mī*-as-THĒ-nē-a)	muscle weakness
myeloma .... (*mī*-e-LŌ-ma)	(malignant) tumor of the bone marrow
osteitis .... (*os*-tē-Ī-tis)	inflammation of the bone
osteoarthritis (OA) .... (*os*-tē-ō-ar-THRĪ-tis)	inflammation of the bone and joint (see Figure 14-8)
osteocarcinoma .... (*os*-tē-ō-*kar*-si-NŌ-ma)	cancerous tumor of the bone
osteochondritis .... (*os*-tē-ō-kon-DRĪ-tis)	inflammation of the bone and cartilage
osteofibroma .... (*os*-tē-ō-fī-BRŌ-ma)	tumor of the bone and fibrous tissue
osteomalacia .... (*os*-tē-ō-ma-LĀ-shē-a)	softening of bones
osteomyelitis .... (*os*-tē-ō-*mī*-e-LĪ-tis)	inflammation of the bone and bone marrow
osteopetrosis .... (*os*-tē-ō-pe-TRŌ-sis)	abnormal condition of stonelike bones (marblelike bones caused by increased formation of bone)
osteosarcoma .... (os-tē-ō-sar-KŌ-ma)	malignant tumor of the bone

polymyositis	inflammation of many muscles
(*pol*-ē-mī-ō-SĪ-tis)	
rachischisis	(congenital) fissure of the vertebral column (also called *spina bifida*) (Exercise Figure C in Chapter 15)
(ra-KIS-kis-is)	
scoliosis	abnormal (lateral) curve (of the spine) (see Exercise Figure D)
(skō-lē-Ō-sis)	
spondylarthritis	inflammation of the vertebral joints
(*spon*-dil-ar-THRĪ-tis)	
synoviosarcoma	malignant tumor of the synovial membrane
(si-*nō*-vē-ō-sar-KŌ-ma)	
tendinitis	inflammation of a tendon (also spelled *tendonitis*)
(*ten*-di-NĪ-tis)	
tenodynia	pain in a tendon
(*ten*-ō-DIN-ē-a)	
tenosynovitis	inflammation of the tendon and synovial membrane
(ten-ō-sin-ō-VĪ-tis) (NOTE: the *i* in *synovi* is dropped because the suffix begins with an *i*.)	

Practice saying each of these terms aloud. To hear the terms, access the **PRONOUNCE IT** activity for this chapter on the Student CD that accompanies this text. Or, to hear the terms and their definitions with a CD player or computer, obtain the Pronunciation CD designed for use with this text.

Learn the definitions and spellings of the disease and disorder terms by completing exercises 18, 19, and 20.

EXERCISE 18

Analyze and define the following disease and disorder terms.

1. osteitis _____

2. osteomyelitis _____

3. osteopetrosis _____

4. osteomalacia _____

5. osteocarcinoma _____

6. osteochondritis _____

7. osteofibroma _____

8. arthritis _____

9. arthrochondritis _____

10. myeloma _____

11. tendinitis _____

12. tenodynia _____

13. carpoptosis _____

14. bursitis _____

15. spondylarthritis _____

16. ankylosis _____

17. kyphosis _____

18. scoliosis _____

19. cranioschisis _____

20. maxillitis _____

21. meniscitis _____

22. rachischisis _____

23. bursolith _____

24. myasthenia _____

25. osteosarcoma _____

26. chondromalacia _____

27. synoviosarcoma _____

28. tenosynovitis _____

29. polymyositis _____

30. diskitis _____

31. lordosis _____

32. osteoarthritis _____

33. fibromyalgia _____

EXERCISE 19

Build disease and disorder terms for the following definitions with the word parts you have learned.

1. cancerous tumor of the
   bone

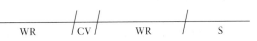

   WR   CV   WR   S

2. inflammation of the bone and cartilage

_____ /CV/ _____ / _____
WR   CV   WR   S

3. tumor of the bone and fibrous tissue

_____ /CV/ _____ / _____
WR   CV   WR   S

4. inflammation of a joint

_____ / _____
WR   S

5. inflammation of joint cartilage

_____ /CV/ _____ / _____
WR   CV   WR   S

6. tumor of the bone marrow

_____ / _____
WR   S

7. inflammation of a tendon

_____ / _____
WR   S

8. pain in a tendon

_____ / _____
WR   S

9. drooping wrist (wristdrop)

_____ /CV/ _____
WR   CV   S

10. inflammation of the bursa

_____ / _____
WR   S

11. inflammation of the vertebral joints

_____ / _____ / _____
WR   WR   S

12. abnormal condition of stiffness

_____ / _____
WR   S

13. abnormal condition of a hump (of the thoracic spine)

_____ / _____
WR   S

14. abnormal (lateral) curve of the spine

_____ / _____
WR   S

15. fissure of the skull

_____ /CV/ _____
WR   CV   S

16. inflammation of the maxilla

_____ / _____
WR   S

17. inflammation of the meniscus

_____ / _____
WR   S

18. fissure of the vertebral column

_____ / _____
WR   S

19. stone in the bursa

———————————— / ————— / ————————————
WR ———————— CV ———————————— S

20. muscle weakness

———————————————— / ————————————————
———————— WR ———————————— S

21. inflammation of the bone

———————————————— / ————————————————
———————— WR ———————————— S

22. inflammation of the bone
    and bone marrow

———————— / ————— / ———————— / ————————
WR ——— CV ———— WR ——— S

23. abnormal condition of
    stonelike bones (marblelike
    bones)

———————— / ————— / ———————— / ————————
WR ——— CV ———— WR ——— S

24. softening of bones

———————— / ————— / ————————————————
WR ———— CV ———————— S

25. inflammation of the
    tendon and synovial
    membrane

———————— / ————— / ———————— / ————————
WR ——— CV ———— WR ——— S

26. malignant tumor of the
    synovial membrane

———————— / ————— / ————————————————
WR ———— CV ———————— S

27. malignant tumor of the
    bone

———————— / ————— / ————————————————
WR ———— CV ———————— S

28. softening of cartilage

———————— / ————— / ————————————————
WR ———— CV ———————— S

29. inflammation of an (inter-
    vertebral) disk

———————————————— / ————————————————
———————— WR ———————————— S

30. inflammation of many
    muscles

———————— / ———————— / ————————————
P ————— WR ———————— S

31. abnormal condition of
    bending forward

———————————————— / ————————————————
———————— WR ———————————— S

32. inflammation of the bone
    and joint

———————— / ————— / ———————— / ————————
WR ——— CV ———— WR ——— S

33. pain in the fibrous tissues
    and muscles

———————— / ————— / ———————— / ————————
WR ——— CV ———— WR ——— S

EXERCISE **20**

Spell each of the disease and disorder terms. Have someone dictate the terms on pp. 501-504 to you. Think about the word parts before attempting to write the word. Study any words you have spelled incorrectly.

1. _____

2. _____

3. _____

4. _____

5. _____

6. _____

7. _____

8. _____

9. _____

10. _____

11. _____

12. _____

13. _____

14. _____

15. _____

16. _____

17. _____

18. _____

19. _____

20. _____

21. _____

22. _____

23. _____

24. _____

25. _____

26. _____

27. _____

28. _____

29. _____

30. _____

31. _____

32. _____

33. _____

Disease and Disorder Terms

Not Built from Word Parts

Ankylosing Spondylitis was first described in 1884 by Adolf von Strümpell (1853-1925). It became known as **Strümpell-Marie disease** after von Strümpell and French physician Pierre Marie.

Term	Definition
ankylosing spondylitis.................... (an-kil-Ō-sing) (*spon*-di-LĪ-tis)	form of arthritis that first affects the spine and adjacent structures, and that, as it progresses, causes a forward bend of the spine (also called *Strümpell-Marie arthritis* or *disease*, and *rheumatoid spondylitis*)
bunion..................................... (BUN-yun)	abnormal enlargement of the joint at the base of the great toe. It is a common problem, often hereditary or caused by poorly fitted shoes (also called *hallux valgus*) (Figure 14-9).

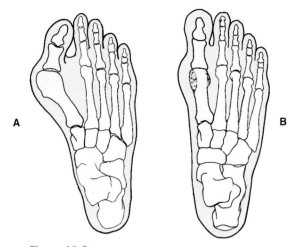

Figure 14-9
A, Right foot with a bunion. **B,** Right foot after a bunionectomy.

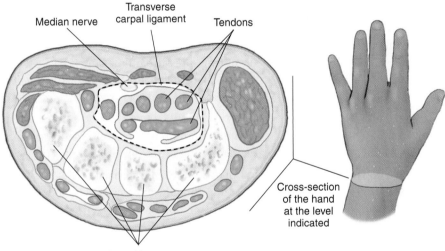

Figure 14-10
Carpal tunnel syndrome (CTS). The hand and wrist show edema, which is compressing the median nerve.

carpal tunnel syndrome (CTS)......... (KAR-pl) (TUN-el) (SIN-drŏm)	a common, painful disorder of the wrist caused by compression of a nerve (Figure 14-10)
Colles fracture....................................... (KOL-ēz) (FRA-chŭr)	a type of wrist fracture (the fracture is at the lower end of the radius, the distal fragment being displaced backward) (Figure 14-11)
exostosis... (*ex*-os-TŌ-sis)	abnormal benign growth on the surface of a bone (also called *spur*)
fracture (fx)... (FRAK-chŭr)	broken bone (Figure 14-12)
gout... (gowt)	disease in which an excessive amount of uric acid in the blood causes sodium urate crystals *(tophi)* to be deposited in the joints, especially that of the great toe (Figure 14-13)

> **Colles Fracture**
> was first described in 1814 by Irish surgeon and anatomist **Abraham Colles** (1773-1843). In 1804 Colles was appointed Professor of Anatomy and Surgery at the Irish College of Surgeons.

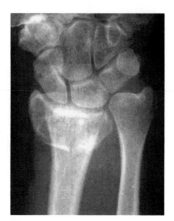

Figure 14-11
Radiograph showing a Colles fracture.

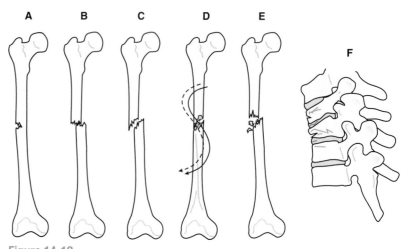

Figure 14-12

Types of fractures. **A,** Greenstick; **B,** transverse; **C,** oblique; **D,** spiral; **E,** comminuted; **F,** compression.

herniated disk......................... (HER-nē-āt-ed) (disk)	rupture of the intervertebral disk cartilage, which allows the contents to protrude through it, putting pressure on the spinal nerve roots (also called *slipped disk, ruptured disk, herniated intervertebral disk,* or *herniated nucleus pulposus* [HNP]) (Figure 14-14, *A*)
muscular dystrophy (MD)................. (MUS-kū-lar) (DIS-trō-fē)	group of hereditary diseases characterized by degeneration of muscle and weakness
myasthenia gravis (MG).................... (*mī*-as-THĒ-nē-a) (GRA-vis)	chronic disease characterized by muscle weakness and thought to be caused by a defect in the transmission of impulses from nerve to muscle cell. The face, larynx, and throat are frequently affected; no true paralysis of the muscles exists.
osteoporosis.............................. (*os*-tē-ō-po-RO-sis)	abnormal loss of bone density occurring frequently in postmenopausal women (Figure 14-15)
rheumatoid arthritis (RA).................. (RŪ-ma-toid) (ar-THRĪ-tis)	a chronic systemic disease characterized by autoimmune inflammatory changes in the connective tissue throughout the body (see Figure 14-8)

Figure 14-13
Gout.

Rotator Cuff Injuries and Repair
The rotator cuff of the shoulder stabilizes the head of the humerus during shoulder abduction (see Figure 14-7). Degenerative changes, repetitive motions, or falls can cause tears in older adults, and trauma may cause tears in young adults. Symptoms include shoulder pain and the inability to maintain abduction of the arm at the shoulder. If conservative treatments such as physical therapy, drugs, and heat/cold applications are not effective, surgical treatment, most commonly referred to as *rotator cuff repair,* is performed.

Repetitive motion syndrome is an increasingly common and somewhat controversial diagnosis in which pain develops in the hand and forearm in the course of normal work activities. Permanent injury is not common.

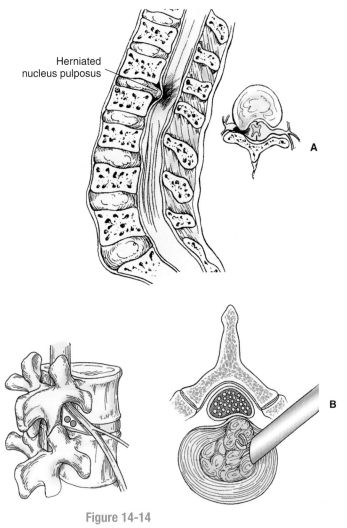

Herniated
nucleus pulposus

A

B

Figure 14-14
A, Herniated disk; **B,** diskectomy.

Practice saying each of these terms aloud. To hear the terms, access the **PRONOUNCE IT** activity for this chapter on the Student CD that accompanies this text. Or, to hear the terms and their definitions with a CD player or computer, obtain the Pronunciation CD designed for use with this text.

Learn the definitions and spellings of the disease and disorder terms by completing exercises 21, 22, and 23.

EXERCISE 21

Write the term for each of the following definitions.

1. abnormal benign growth
   on the surface of a bone   _____

2. group of hereditary diseases characterized by
   degeneration of muscle
   and weakness   _____   _____

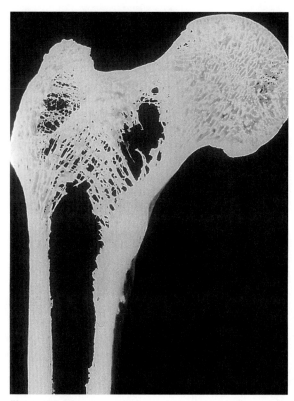

Figure 14-15
This thin section of the femur shows the loss of bone seen in patients with osteoporosis.

3. chronic disease characterized by muscle weakness and thought to be caused by a defect in the transmission of impulses from nerve to muscle cell

_____   _____

4. abnormal enlargement of the joint at the base of the great toe

_____

5. form of arthritis that first affects the spine and adjacent structures

_____   _____

6. disease in which an excessive amount of uric acid in the blood causes sodium urate crystals (tophi) to be deposited in the joints

_____

7. rupture of the intervertebral disk cartilage, which allows the contents to protrude through it, putting pressure on the spinal nerve roots

   a. _____ _____

   b. _____ _____

   c. _____ _____

   d. _____ _____ _____

8. broken bone

   _____

9. abnormal loss of bone density

   _____

10. a disorder of the wrist caused by compression of a nerve

   _____ _____ _____

11. a type of fractured wrist

   _____ _____

12. form of arthritis characterized by inflammatory changes in the connective tissue throughout the body

   _____ _____

EXERCISE 22

Write the definitions of the following terms.

1. exostosis _____

2. muscular dystrophy _____

3. myasthenia gravis _____

4. bunion _____

5. ankylosing spondylitis _____

6. osteoporosis _____

7. gout _____

8. herniated disk, slipped disk, ruptured disk _____

9. fracture _____

10. carpal tunnel syndrome _____

11. Colles fracture _____

12. rheumatoid arthritis _____

EXERCISE 23

Spell the disease and disorder terms. Have someone dictate the terms on pp. 508-510 to you. Study any words you have spelled incorrectly.

1. _____   7. _____

2. _____   8. _____

3. _____   9. _____

4. _____   10. _____

5. _____   11. _____

6. _____   12. _____

Surgical Terms

Built from Word Parts

Term	Definition
aponeurorrhaphy (*ap*-ō-nū-ROR-a-fē)	suture of an aponeurosis
arthroclasia (*ar*-thrō-KLA-zhē-a)	(surgical) breaking of a (stiff) joint
arthrodesis (*ar*-thrō-DE-sis)	surgical fixation of a joint
arthroplasty (AR-thrō-plas-tē)	surgical repair of a joint (see box on p. 516)
bursectomy (bur-SEK-tō-mē)	excision of a bursa
carpectomy (kar-PEK-tō-mē)	excision of a carpal bone
chondrectomy (kon-DREK-tō-mē)	excision of a cartilage
chondroplasty (KON-drō-plas-tē)	surgical repair of a cartilage
costectomy (kos-TEK-tō-mē)	excision of a rib
cranioplasty (KRA-nē-ō-plas-tē)	surgical repair of the skull
craniotomy (*kra*-nē-OT-ō-mē)	incision of the skull (as for surgery of the brain)
diskectomy (dis-KEK-tō-mē)	excision of an intervertebral disk (also spelled *discectomy*)

Endoscopic diskectomy is now an option for treatment of a herniated disk for some patients. It differs from open diskectomy in that there is no bone removal, no large skin incision, no large muscle dissection, and no sutures. Hospitalization is not required.

laminectomy...................................... (*lam*-i-NEK-tō-mē)	excision of a lamina (often performed to relieve pressure on the nerve roots in the lower spine caused by a herniated disk and other conditions) (see Figure 14-14, *B*)
maxillectomy...................................... (*mak*-si-LEK-tō-mē)	excision of the maxilla
meniscectomy .... (*men*-i-SEK-tō-mē)	excision of the meniscus (performed for a torn cartilage)
myorrhaphy....................................... (mī-OR-a-fē)	suture of a muscle
ostectomy.. (os-TEK-tō-mē) (NOTE: one *e* is dropped.)	excision of bone
osteoclasis.. (*os*-tē-OK-la-sis)	(surgical) breaking of a bone (to correct a deformity)
patellectomy...................................... (*pat*-e-LEK-tō-mē)	excision of the patella
phalangectomy................................... (fal-an-JEK-tō-mē)	excision of a finger or toe bone
rachiotomy .... (*ra*-kē-OT-ō-mē)	incision into the vertebral column
spondylosyndesis............................... (*spon*-di-lō-SIN-dē-sis) (NOTE: the prefix *syn-* appears in the middle of the term.)	fusing together of the vertebrae (spinal fusion)
synovectomy .... (sin-ō-VEK-tō-mē) (NOTE: the *i* in *synovi* is dropped because the suffix begins with a vowel.)	excision of the synovial membrane (of a joint)
tarsectomy .... (tar-SEK-tō-mē)	excision of (one or more) tarsal bones
tenomyoplasty.................................... (*ten*-ō-MĪ-ō-plas-tē)	surgical repair of the tendon and muscle
tenorrhaphy .... (ten-OR-a-fē)	suture of a tendon
vertebroplasty.................................... (ver-TE-brō-plas-tē)	surgical repair of the vertebra

Practice saying each of the terms aloud. To hear the terms, access the **PRONOUNCE IT** activity for this chapter on the Student CD that accompanies this text. Or, to hear the terms and their definitions with a CD player or computer, obtain the Pronunciation CD designed for use with this text.

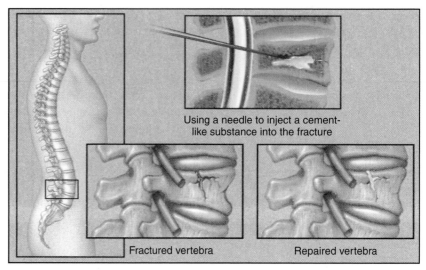

Using a needle to inject a cement-like substance into the fracture

Fractured vertebra   Repaired vertebra

Figure 14-16
Vertebroplasty involves injecting bone cement into fractured and collapsed vertebrae of the spine to seal fractures and prevent further compression.

New Procedures for Treatment of Compression Fractures Caused by Osteoporosis
Percutaneous vertebroplasty (PV) is a minimally invasive operation in which an interventional radiologist places a needle through the skin into the damaged vertebra. A special liquid cement called *polymethylmethacrylate (PMMA)* is injected into the area through the needle to fill the holes left by osteoporosis. The liquid takes 20 minutes to harden, sealing and stabilizing the fracture and relieving pain. Vertebroplasties were first performed in 1984 and are currently being performed in select health care centers in the United States (Figure 14-16).

Kyphoplasty was approved in 1998 by the Food and Drug Administration. Kyphoplasty is similar to vertebroplasty except a balloonlike device is used to expand the compressed vertebra before the cement is injected.

Palmar uniportal endoscopic carpal tunnel release, also called the *Mirza technique,* is an endoscopic technique for carpal tunnel release surgery. Previously carpal tunnel release was done with open surgery.

Types of Arthroplasties
Total hip replacement arthroplasty is indicated for degenerative joint disease or rheumatoid arthritis. The operation commonly involves replacement of the hip joint with a metallic femoral head and a plastic-coated acetabulum (Figure 14-17).

Total knee joint replacement arthroplasty is designed to replace worn surfaces of the knee joint. Various prostheses are used (see Figure 14-17).

Metatarsal arthroplasty is used to treat deformities associated with rheumatoid arthritits or hallux valgus and to treat painful or unstable joints.

Percutaneous diskectomy is a surgical procedure that uses fluoroscopy to guide insertion of a nucleotome into the affected spinal disk and remove the thick, sticky nucleus of the disk. This allows the disk to soften and contract, relieving the severe low back and leg pain.

Learn the definitions and spellings of the surgical terms by completing exercises 24, 25, and 26.

EXERCISE   24

Analyze and define the following surgical terms.

1. osteoclasis _____

2. ostectomy _____

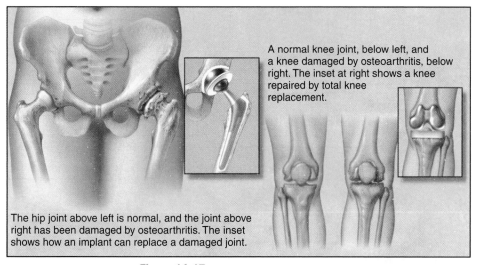

The hip joint above left is normal, and the joint above right has been damaged by osteoarthritis. The inset shows how an implant can replace a damaged joint.

A normal knee joint, below left, and a knee damaged by osteoarthritis, below right. The inset at right shows a knee repaired by total knee replacement.

Figure 14-17
Replacing joints damaged by osteoarthritis.

 3. arthroclasia _____

 4. arthrodesis _____

 5. arthroplasty _____

 6. chondrectomy _____

 7. chondroplasty _____

 8. myorrhaphy _____

 9. tenomyoplasty _____

10. tenorrhaphy _____

11. costectomy _____

12. patellectomy _____

13. aponeurorrhaphy _____

14. carpectomy _____

15. phalangectomy _____

16. meniscectomy _____

17. spondylosyndesis _____

18. laminectomy _____

19. bursectomy _____

20. craniotomy _____

21. cranioplasty _____

22. maxillectomy _____

23. rachiotomy _____

24. tarsectomy _____

25. synovectomy _____

26. diskectomy _____

27. vertebroplasty _____

EXERCISE 25

Build surgical terms for the following definitions by using the word parts you have learned.

1. (surgical) breaking of a bone (to correct a deformity)

   _____ / ___ / _____
   WR   CV   S

2. excision of bone

   _____ / _____
   WR   S

3. (surgical) breaking of a (stiff) joint

   _____ / ___ / _____
   WR   CV   S

4. surgical fixation of a joint

   _____ / ___ / _____
   WR   CV   S

5. surgical repair of a joint

   _____ / ___ / _____
   WR   CV   S

6. excision of cartilage

   _____ / _____
   WR   S

7. surgical repair of cartilage

   _____ / ___ / _____
   WR   CV   S

8. suture of a muscle

   _____ / ___ / _____
   WR   CV   S

9. surgical repair of a tendon and muscle

   _____ / ___ / ___ / ___ / _____
   WR   CV   WR   CV   S

10. suture of a tendon

    _____ / ___ / _____
    WR   CV   S

11. excision of a rib

    _____ / _____
    WR   S

12. excision of the patella

_____ / _____
WR   S

13. suture of an aponeurosis

_____ // _____
WR   CV   S

14. excision of a carpal bone

_____ / _____
WR   S

15. excision of a finger or toe bone

_____ / _____
WR   S

16. excision of a meniscus

_____ / _____
WR   S

17. fusing together of the vertebrae

_____ // _____ / _____
WR   CV   P   S

18. excision of a lamina

_____ / _____
WR   S

19. excision of a bursa

_____ / _____
WR   S

20. incision of the skull

_____ // _____
WR   CV   S

21. surgical repair of the skull

_____ // _____
WR   CV   S

22. excision of the maxilla

_____ / _____
WR   S

23. incision of the vertebral column

_____ // _____
WR   CV   S

24. excision of (one or more) tarsal bones

_____ / _____
WR   S

25. excision of the synovial membrane

_____ / _____
WR   S

26. excision of an intervertebral disk

_____ / _____
WR   S

27. surgical repair of the vertebra

_____ // _____
WR   CV   S

Spell each of the surgical terms. Have someone dictate the terms on pp. 514-515 to you. Think about the word parts before attempting to write the word. Study any words you have spelled incorrectly.

1. _____   15. _____

2. _____   16. _____

3. _____   17. _____

4. _____   18. _____

5. _____   19. _____

6. _____   20. _____

7. _____   21. _____

8. _____   22. _____

9. _____   23. _____

10. _____   24. _____

11. _____   25. _____

12. _____   26. _____

13. _____   27. _____

14. _____

Diagnostic Terms

Built from Word Parts

Term	Definition
Diagnostic Imaging	
arthrography	x-ray imaging a joint (with contrast medium).
(ar-THROG-ra-fē)	(MRI has mostly replaced arthrography as the imaging technique for the knee, wrist, hip, and shoulder. Arthrography is still used for specialized functions such as when metal is present in the body.)
Endoscopy	
arthroscopy	visual examination of a joint (Exercise
(ar-THROS-kō-pē)	Figure E)

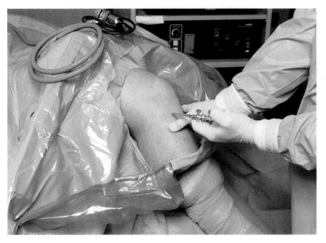

Exercise Figure E

Fill in the blanks to complete labeling of the diagram.

_____ / ___ / _____ of the knee, performed for

joint / **cv** / **visual examination**

diagnostic purposes or for surgical repair of ligaments or meniscus.

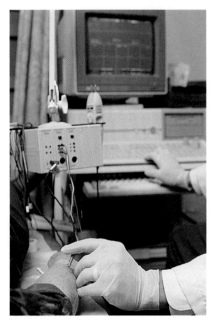

Figure 14-18

Patient having an electromyogram (EMG) of the forearm.

Other

arthrocentesis................................... surgical puncture of a joint to aspirate fluid
  (ar-thrō-sen-TĒ-sis)

electromyogram (EMG)..................... record of the (intrinsic) electrical activity in
  (ē-lek-trō-MĪ-ō-gram)   a (skeletal) muscle (Figure 14-18)

Practice saying each of these words aloud. To hear the terms, access the **PRONOUNCE IT** activity for this chapter on the Student CD that accompanies this text. Or, to hear the terms and their definitions with a CD player or computer, obtain the Pronunciation CD designed for use with this text.

Learn the definitions and spellings of the diagnostic terms by completing exercises 27, 28, and 29.

EXERCISE 27

Analyze and define the following diagnostic terms.

1. electromyogram _____

2. arthrography _____

3. arthroscopy _____

4. arthrocentesis _____

EXERCISE 28

Build diagnostic terms for the following definitions using word parts you have learned.

1. x-ray imaging of a joint

_____ / CV / _____
WR   CV   S

2. visual examination of a joint

_____ / CV / _____
WR   CV   S

3. surgical puncture of a joint to aspirate fluid

_____ / CV / _____
WR   CV   S

4. record of the electrical activity of a muscle

_____ / CV / WR / CV / _____
WR   CV   WR   CV   S

EXERCISE 29

Spell each of the diagnostic terms. Have someone dictate the terms on pp. 520-521 to you. Think about the word parts before attempting to write the word. Study any words you have spelled incorrectly.

1. _____   3. _____

2. _____   4. _____

Diagnostic Imaging Procedures

The following diagnostic imaging procedures are commonly used for diagnosing diseases, fractures, strains, and other conditions of the musculoskeletal system.

   Radiography (x-ray) of the bones and joints is used to identify fractures or tumors, monitor healing, or identify abnormal structures (see Figure 14-11).

   Computed tomography (CT) of the bones and joints gives accurate definition of bone structure and demonstrates subtle changes such as linear fractures (Figure 14-19).

   Magnetic resonance imaging (MRI) is used to evaluate the ligaments of the knee, spinal stenosis, and degenerative disk changes (Figure 14-20).

   Bone scan (nuclear medicine test) is used to detect the presence of metastatic disease of the bone and to monitor degenerative bone disease (Figure 14-21).

   Single-photon emission computed tomography (SPECT) of the bone is an even more sensitive nuclear method for detecting bone abnormalities.

   Bone densitometry is a method of determining the density of bone by radiographic techniques used to diagnose osteoporosis.

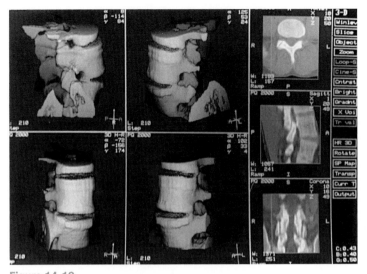

Figure 14-19
CT scan showing three-dimensional reconstruction images of the lumbar spine.

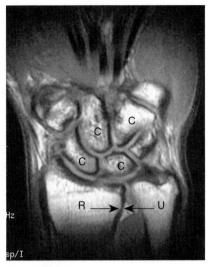

Figure 14-20
Coronal MRI scan of the wrist. Marrow within the carpal bones *(C)*, radius *(R)*, and ulna *(U)*.

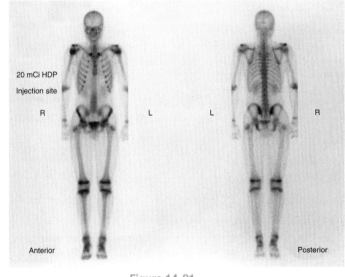

Figure 14-21
Whole body bone scan.

Complementary Terms

Built from Word Parts

Term	Definition
arthralgia (ar-THRAL-jē-a)	pain in the joint
atrophy (AT-rō-fē)	without development (wasting)
bradykinesia (brād-ē-kin-Ē-zhē-a)	slow movement

carpal (CAR-pal)	pertaining to the wrist
cranial (KRĀ-nē-al)	pertaining to the cranium
dyskinesia (dis-ki-NĒ-zhē-a)	difficult movement
dystrophy (DIS-trō-fē)	abnormal development
femoral (FEM-ō-ral)	pertaining to the femur
humeral (HŪ-mer-al)	pertaining to the humerus
hyperkinesia (*hī*-per-kin-Ē-zhē-a)	excessive movement (overactive)
hypertrophy (hī-PER-trō-fē)	excessive development
iliofemoral (*il*-ē-ō-FEM-ō-ral)	pertaining to the ilium and femur
intercostal (in-ter-KOS-tal)	pertaining to between the ribs
intervertebral (*in*-ter-VER-te-bral)	pertaining to between the vertebrae
intracranial (*in*-tra-KRĀ-nē-al)	pertaining to within the cranium
ischiofibular (*is*-kē-ō-FIB-ū-lar)	pertaining to the ischium and fibula
ischiopubic (*is*-kē-ō-PŪ-bik)	pertaining to the ischium and pubis
lumbar (LUM-bar)	pertaining to the loins (the part of the back between the thorax and pelvis)
lumbocostal (lum-bō-KOS-tal)	pertaining to the loins and the ribs
lumbosacral (lum-bō-SĀ-kral)	pertaining to the lumbar regions (loin) and the sacrum
osteoblast (OS-tē-ō-blast)	developing bone cell
osteocyte (OS-tē-ō-sīt)	bone cell
osteonecrosis (*os*-tē-ō-ne-KRŌ-sis)	abnormal death of bone (tissues)
pelvic (PEL-vik)	pertaining to the pelvis
pelvisacral (pel-vi-SĀ-kral)	pertaining to the pelvis and the sacrum
pubofemoral (*pū*-bō-FEM-ō-ral)	pertaining to the pubis and femur

sacral.............................. (SĀ-kral)	pertaining to the sacrum
sacrovertebral.............................. (sā-krō-VER-te-bral)	pertaining to the sacrum and vertebrae
sternoclavicular.............................. (*ster*-nō-kla-VIK-ū-lar)	pertaining to the sternum and clavicle
sternoid.............................. (STER-noyd)	resembling the sternum
subcostal.............................. (sub-KOS-tal)	pertaining to below the rib
submandibular.............................. (*sub*-man-DIB-ū-lar)	pertaining to below the mandible
submaxillary.............................. (sub-MAK-si-lar-ē)	pertaining to below the maxilla
subscapular.............................. (sub-SKAP-ū-lar)	pertaining to below the scapula
substernal.............................. (sub-STER-nal)	pertaining to below the sternum
suprascapular.............................. (sū-pra-SKAP-ū-lar)	pertaining to above the scapula
suprapatellar.............................. (sū-pra-pa-TEL-ar)	pertaining to above the patella
symphysis.............................. (SIM-fi-sis)	growing together
vertebrocostal.............................. (*ver*-te-brō-KOS-tal)	pertaining to the vertebrae and ribs

Practice saying each of these terms aloud. To hear the terms, access the **PRONOUNCE IT** activity for this chapter on the Student CD that accompanies this text. Or, to hear the terms and their definitions with a CD player or computer, obtain the Pronunciation CD designed for use with this text.

Exercises 30, 31, and 32 will help you learn the definitions and spellings of the complementary terms related to the musculoskeletal system.

EXERCISE 30

Analyze and define the following complementary terms.

1. symphysis _____

2. femoral _____

3. humeral _____

4. intervertebral _____

5. hyperkinesia _____

6. dyskinesia _____

7. bradykinesia _____

8. intracranial _____

9. sternoclavicular _____

10. iliofemoral _____

11. ischiofibular _____

12. submaxillary _____

13. ischiopubic _____

14. submandibular _____

15. pubofemoral _____

16. suprascapular _____

17. subcostal _____

18. vertebrocostal _____

19. subscapular _____

20. osteoblast _____

21. osteocyte _____

22. osteonecrosis _____

23. sternoid _____

24. arthralgia _____

25. carpal _____

26. lumbar _____

27. lumbocostal _____

28. lumbosacral _____

29. sacral _____

30. sacrovertebral _____

31. substernal _____

32. suprapatellar _____

33. dystrophy _____

34. atrophy _____

35. hypertrophy _____

36. intercostal _____

37. cranial _____

38. pelvic _____

39. pelvisacral _____

EXERCISE 31

Build the complementary terms for the following definitions by using the word parts you have learned.

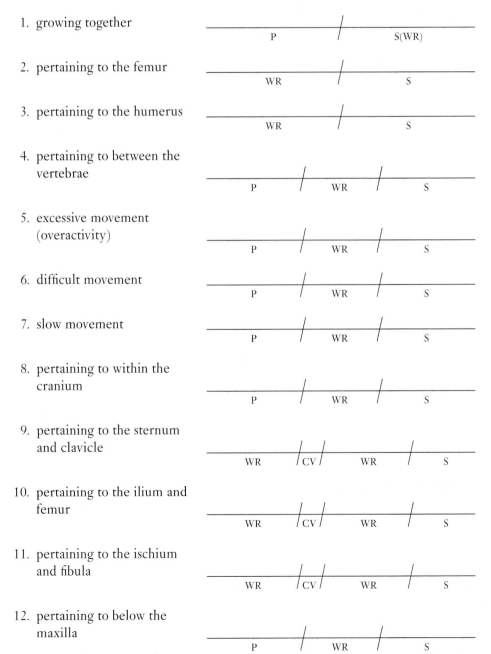

1. growing together

    P   S(WR)

2. pertaining to the femur

    WR   S

3. pertaining to the humerus

    WR   S

4. pertaining to between the vertebrae

    P   WR   S

5. excessive movement (overactivity)

    P   WR   S

6. difficult movement

    P   WR   S

7. slow movement

    P   WR   S

8. pertaining to within the cranium

    P   WR   S

9. pertaining to the sternum and clavicle

    WR   CV   WR   S

10. pertaining to the ilium and femur

    WR   CV   WR   S

11. pertaining to the ischium and fibula

    WR   CV   WR   S

12. pertaining to below the maxilla

    P   WR   S

13. pertaining to the ischium and pubis

_____ / ___ / _____ / _____
WR / CV / WR / S

14. pertaining to below the mandible

_____ / _____ / _____
P / WR / S

15. pertaining to the pubis and femur

_____ / ___ / _____ / _____
WR / CV / WR / S

16. pertaining to above the scapula

_____ / _____ / _____
P / WR / S

17. pertaining to below the rib

_____ / _____ / _____
P / WR / S

18. pertaining to the vertebrae and ribs

_____ / ___ / _____ / _____
WR / CV / WR / S

19. pertaining to below the scapula

_____ / _____ / _____
P / WR / S

20. developing bone cell

_____ / ___ / _____
WR / CV / WR

21. bone cell

_____ / ___ / _____
WR / CV / S

22. abnormal death of bone (tissues)

_____ / ___ / _____ / _____
WR / CV / WR / S

23. resembling the sternum

_____ / _____
WR / S

24. pain in the joint

_____ / _____
WR / S

25. pertaining to the wrist

_____ / _____
WR / S

26. pertaining to the sacrum

_____ / _____
WR / S

27. pertaining to the loins

_____ / _____
WR / S

28. pertaining to the sacrum and vertebrae

_____ / ___ / _____ / _____
WR / CV / WR / S

29. pertaining to the lumbar region (loin) and the sacrum

_____ / ___ / _____ / _____
WR / CV / WR / S

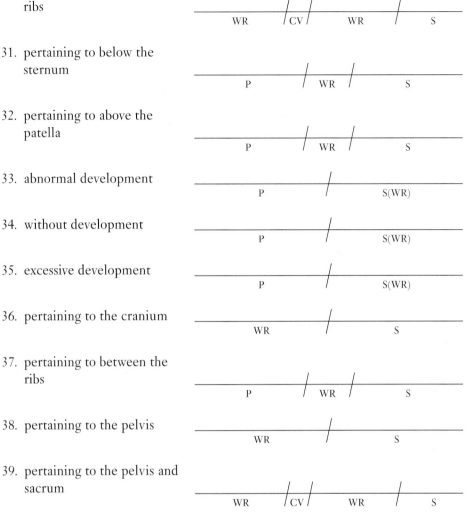

30. pertaining to the loins and ribs
_____ / ___ / _____ / ___
WR   CV   WR   S

31. pertaining to below the sternum
_____ / _____ / _____
P   WR   S

32. pertaining to above the patella
_____ / _____ / _____
P   WR   S

33. abnormal development
_____ / _____
P   S(WR)

34. without development
_____ / _____
P   S(WR)

35. excessive development
_____ / _____
P   S(WR)

36. pertaining to the cranium
_____ / _____
WR   S

37. pertaining to between the ribs
_____ / _____ / _____
P   WR   S

38. pertaining to the pelvis
_____ / _____
WR   S

39. pertaining to the pelvis and sacrum
_____ / ___ / _____ / ___
WR   CV   WR   S

EXERCISE 32

Spell each of the complementary terms. Have someone dictate the terms on pp. 523-525 to you. Think about the word parts before attempting to write the word. Study any words you have spelled incorrectly.

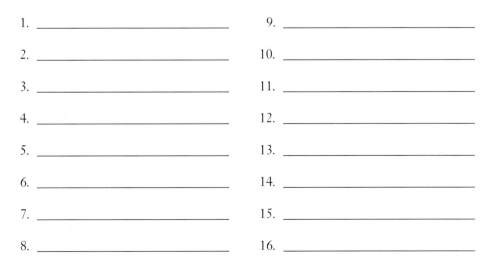

1. _____
2. _____
3. _____
4. _____
5. _____
6. _____
7. _____
8. _____
9. _____
10. _____
11. _____
12. _____
13. _____
14. _____
15. _____
16. _____

17. _____ 29. _____

18. _____ 30. _____

19. _____ 31. _____

20. _____ 32. _____

21. _____ 33. _____

22. _____ 34. _____

23. _____ 35. _____

24. _____ 36. _____

25. _____ 37. _____

26. _____ 38. _____

27. _____ 39. _____

28. _____

Complementary Terms

Not Built from Word Parts

Term	Definition
chiropodist, podiatrist (ki-ROP-ō-dist) (pō-DĪ-a-trist)	specialist in treating and diagnosing diseases and disorders of the foot, including medical and surgical treatment
chiropractic (kī-rō-PRAK-tik)	system of therapy that consists of manipulation of the vertebral column
chiropractor (kī-rō-PRAK-tor)	specialist in chiropractic
orthopedics (ortho) (or-thō-PĒ-diks)	branch of medicine dealing with the study and treatment of diseases and abnormalities of the musculoskeletal system
orthopedist (or-thō-PĒ-dist)	physician who specializes in orthopedics
orthotics (or-THOT-iks)	making and fitting of orthopedic appliances, such as arch supports, used to support, align, prevent, or correct deformities
orthotist (OR-thō-tist)	a person who specializes in orthotics
osteopath (OS-tē-ō-path)	physician who specializes in osteopathy

osteopathy... (*os*-tē-OP-a-thē)	system of medicine that uses the usual forms of diagnosis and treatment but places greater emphasis on the role of the relation between body organs and the musculoskeletal system; manipulation may be used in addition to other treatments
prosthesis (*pl.* prostheses)............... (pros-THĒ-sis)	an artificial substitute for a missing body part such as a leg, eye, or total hip replacement

Practice saying each of these terms aloud. To hear the terms, access the **PRONOUNCE IT** activity for this chapter on the Student CD that accompanies this text. Or, to hear the terms and their definitions with a CD player or computer, obtain the Pronunciation CD designed for use with this text.

Learn the definitions and spellings of the complementary terms by completing exercises 33, 34, and 35.

EXERCISE 33

Match the definitions in the first column with the correct terms in the second column. The terms in the second column may be used more than once.

_____ 1. specialist in manipulation of the vertebral column

_____ 2. branch of medicine dealing with treatment of diseases of the musculoskeletal system

_____ 3. physician who places emphasis on manipulation

_____ 4. foot specialist

_____ 5. substitute for a body part

_____ 6. system of therapy

_____ 7. system of medicine

_____ 8. making of orthopedic appliances

_____ 9. skilled in orthotics

a. chiropodist

b. chiropractic

c. chiropractor

d. osteopath

e. osteopathy

f. orthopedics

g. orthopedist

h. podiatrist

i. orthotics

j. prosthesis

k. orthotist

EXERCISE 34

Write the definitions of the following.

1. chiropractor _____

2. chiropractic _____

3. orthopedics _____

4. orthopedist _____

5. chiropodist _____

6. podiatrist _____

7. osteopath _____

8. osteopathy _____

9. orthotics _____

10. prosthesis _____

11. orthotist _____

EXERCISE 35

Spell each of the complementary terms. Have someone dictate the terms on pp. 530-531 to you. Study any words you have spelled incorrectly.

1. _____   7. _____

2. _____   8. _____

3. _____   9. _____

4. _____   10. _____

5. _____   11. _____

6. _____

Abbreviations

C1-C7	cervical vertebrae
CTS	carpal tunnel syndrome
EMG	electromyogram
fx	fracture
HNP	herniated nucleus pulposus
L1-L5	lumbar vertebrae
MD	muscular dystrophy
MG	myasthenia gravis
OA	osteoarthritis
ortho	orthopedics
RA	rheumatoid arthritis
T1-T12	thoracic vertebrae

EXERCISE 36

Write the meaning of the abbreviations in the following sentences.

1. Vertebrae make up the bones of the spinal column. **C1 to C7** _____ _____ are the first set that form the neck. The second set **T1 to T12** _____ _____ articulate with the 12 pairs of ribs that form the outward curve of the spine. **L1 to L5** _____ _____, the third set, are larger and form the inward curve of the spine.

2. Patients with **RA** _____ _____ often have obesity, muscle atrophy, and weakness because of inactivity.

3. Approximately 27% of Americans have **OA** _____; as the population ages this figure is expected to increase.

4. Acquired **MG** _____ _____ most often affects women and the onset occurs at any age. It is an acquired autoimmune disorder.

5. **EMG** _____ is used to evaluate patients with localized or diffuse muscle weakness, such as polymyositis.

6. **CTS** _____ _____ _____ is a common condition in which, for various reasons, the median nerve in the wrist becomes compressed, causing numbness and pain.

7. Nine types of **MD** _____ _____ have been identified. Because symptoms of the disease are similar to other muscular disorders, diagnosis is often difficult.

8. **HNP** _____ _____ _____ may also be referred to as slipped or ruptured disk or herniated intervertebral disk.

CHAPTER REVIEW

EXERCISE 37   *Interact with Medical Records*

Complete the operative report by writing the medical terms in the blanks. Use the list of definitions on p. 535 with the corresponding numbers.

University Hospital and Medical Center
4700 North Main Street • Wellness, Arizona 54321 • (987) 555-3210

PATIENT NAME: William McBride   **CASE NUMBER:**   10003-MKL
DATE OF BIRTH: 12/04/xx   **DATE:**   04/30/xx

OPERATIVE REPORT

HISTORY: William McBride is a 55-year-old white man who reports pain in his left knee when walking and golfing. He states that his knees have "been painful" for many years since he quit playing semiprofessional hockey, but the pain has become much more severe in the last 6 months. He was admitted to the Medical Center's Outpatient 1. _____ Center for an 2. _____ of his left knee.

PREOPERATIVE DIAGNOSIS: Degenerative 3. _____ of the left knee, with possible tear of the 4. _____ meniscus.

OPERATIVE REPORT: After induction of spinal anesthetic, the patient was positioned on the operating table, and a tourniquet was applied over the upper left thigh. After positioning the leg in a circumferential holder, the end of the table was flexed to allow the leg to hang freely. The patient's left leg was prepped and draped in the usual manner. After exsanguination of the leg with an Esmarch bandage, the tourniquet was inflated to 300 mm Hg. The knee was inspected by anterolateral and anteromedial parapatellar portholes.

FINDINGS: The synovium in the 5. _____ pouch showed moderate to severe inflammatory changes with villi formation and hyperemia. The undersurface of the patella showed loss of normal articular cartilage on the lateral patellar facet with exposed bone in that area and moderate to severe 6. _____ of the medial facet. Similar changes were noted in the intercondylar groove. In the medial compartment, the patient had smooth articular cartilage on the femur and moderate chondromalacia of the tibial plateau. The medial meniscus appeared normal with no evidence of tears and a smooth articular surface on the femoral condyle. No additional 7. _____ being identified.

The tourniquet was then released and the knee flushed with lactated Ringer solution until the bleeding slowed. The wounds were Steri-Stripped closed, a sterile bandage with an external Ace wrap applied, and the patient returned to the postoperative recovery area in stable condition. The patient tolerated the procedure well.

POSTOPERATIVE DIAGNOSIS: Degenerative arthritis with mild chondromalacia of the left knee.

Martin Spencer, DO

MS/mcm

1. branch of medicine dealing with the study and treatment of diseases and abnormalities of the musculoskeletal system
2. visual examination of a joint
3. inflammation of a joint
4. toward the middle or midline
5. pertaining to above the patella
6. softening of the cartilage
7. study of body changes caused by disease

EXERCISE 38   *Interpret Medical Terms*

To test your understanding of the terms introduced in this chapter, circle the words that correctly complete the sentences. The italicized words refer to the correct answer.

1. The medical term for *hunchback* is (kyphosis, ankylosis, scoliosis).
2. The medical term for *excision of cartilage* is (carpectomy, chondrectomy, costectomy).
3. *Difficult movement* is (hyperkinesia, bradykinesia, dyskinesia).
4. Vitamin D deficiency in adults may cause *osteomalacia,* or (muscle weakness, marblelike bones, softening of bones).
5. The *surgical breaking of a bone* to correct a deformity is called (osteoclasis, arthroclasia, osteoplasty).
6. The medical term that means *pertaining to below the rib* is (subscapular, subcostal, substernal).
7. The medical term for *growing together* is (diaphysis, epiphysis, symphysis).
8. A(n) (orthopedist, podiatrist, chiropractor) is *competent to treat* a person with a *fractured femur.*
9. (Osteoporosis, osteopetrosis, osteomyelitis) is the *abnormal loss of bone density.*
10. A common *disorder of the wrist caused by compression of a nerve* is called (lordosis, carpal tunnel syndrome, synoviosarcoma).

EXERCISE 39   *Read Medical Terms in Use*

Practice the pronunciation of terms by reading the following statements. Use the pronunciation key following the medical terms to assist you in saying the word.

1. The **orthopedist** (or-thō-PĒ-dist) recommended Mr. Jones have an **arthrodesis** (ar-thrō-DĒ-sis) to reduce pain caused from an ankle **fracture** (FRAK-chur) he sustained several years ago.
2. Mrs. Brown severed a tendon by accidentally walking through a glass patio door. A **tenorrhaphy** (ten-OR-a-fē) was performed to repair the tendon.
3. An **electromyogram** (e-lek-trō-MĪ-ō-gram) can assist the physician in diagnosing **muscular dystrophy** (MUS-kū-lar) (DIS-trō-fē). **Atrophy** (AT-rō-fē) frequently occurs in patients with this disease.
4. Adjective forms of medical terms are used by health professionals to indicate areas of the body that describe anatomic locations, areas of pain, sites of injections, locations of lesions, and so forth. Below are some examples.
   a. **cranial** (KRĀ-nē-al) laceration
   b. **intercostal** (in-ter-KOS-tal) muscles
   c. pain in the **subcostal** (sub-KOS-tal) region
   d. herniation of an **intervertebral** (in-ter-VER-te-bral) disk
   e. **intracranial** (in-tra-KRĀ-nē-al) pressure
   f. **femoral** (FEM-or-al) artery
   g. strain of the **ischiopubic** (is-kē-ō-PŪ-bik) area
   h. degenerative disease of the **sternoclavicular** (ster-nō-kla-VIK-ū-lar) joint

EXERCISE   **40**   *Comprehend Medical Terms in Use*

Test your comprehension of terms in the previous statements by circling the correct answer.

1. T   F   A specialist in treating and diagnosing disorders of the foot recommended Mr. Jones for surgical fixation of the ankle joint.
2. A record of electrical activity of muscles is used in the diagnosis of:
   a. an abnormal benign growth on the surface of the body
   b. a group of hereditary diseases involving muscular degeneration and weakness
   c. wrist fracture
   d. form of arthritis that causes a forward bend of the spine
3. Which of the following is true for statements in Exercise 39, number 4?
   a. herniation within the vertebra
   b. degenerative disease of the joint between the scapula and collarbone
   c. laceration of the wrist
   d. pain below the ribs

EXERCISE   **41**   *Use Plural Endings*

Circle the correct singular or plural term to match the context of the sentence.

1. The (epiphysis, epiphyses) are the enlarged ends of the long bone.
2. The distal (phalanx, phalanges) of the ring finger was fractured.
3. Osteoporosis was present in four lumbar (vertebrae, vertebra).
4. A (prosthesis, prostheses) was implanted in the left hip.
5. Many synovial joints contain (bursa, bursae).

For further practice or to evaluate what you have learned, use the Student CD that accompanies this text.

COMBINING FORMS CROSSWORD PUZZLE

Across Clues

1. cartilage
2. ulna
6. scapula
9. tendon
10. developing cell
12. bursa
14. clavicle
16. maxilla
18. vertebra
19. ischium
22. tibia
26. stone
28. aponeurosis
29. crooked
32. fibula
34. spine, vertebral column
35. joint

Down Clues

1. skull
3. movement, motion
4. mandible
5. pubis
7. finger or toe bone
8. hump
11. rib
13. kneecap
15. meniscus
17. ilium
20. wrist bone
21. bone marrow
23. vertebra
24. sternum
25. radius
27. bone
30. lamina
31. tarsals
33. abbreviation for rheumatoid arthritis

REVIEW OF WORD PARTS

Can you define and spell the following word parts?

Combining Forms

					Prefixes	Suffixes
ankyl/o	disk/o	lumb/o	petr/o	synovi/o	inter-	-asthenia
aponeur/o	femor/o	mandibul/o	phalang/o	tars/o	supra-	-clasia
arthr/o	fibul/o	maxill/o	pub/o	ten/o	sym-	-clasis
burs/o	humer/o	menisc/o	rachi/o	tend/o	syn-	-clast
carp/o	ili/o	my/o	radi/o	tendin/o		-desis
chondr/o	ischi/o	myel/o	sacr/o	tibi/o		-physis
clavic/o	kinesi/o	myos/o	scapul/o	uln/o		-schisis
clavicul/o	kyph/o	oste/o	scoli/o	vertebr/o		
cost/o	lamin/o	patell/o	spondyl/o			
crani/o	lord/o	pelv/i, pelv/o	stern/o			

REVIEW OF TERMS

Can you build, analyze, define, pronounce, and spell the following terms *built from word parts?*

Diseases and Disorders

ankylosis
arthritis
arthrochondritis
bursitis
bursolith
carpoptosis
chondromalacia
cranioschisis
diskitis
fibromyalgia
kyphosis
lordosis
maxillitis
meniscitis
myasthenia
myeloma
osteitis
osteoarthritis (OA)
osteocarcinoma
osteochondritis
osteofibroma
osteomalacia
osteomyelitis
osteopetrosis
osteosarcoma
polymyositis
rachischisis
scoliosis
spondylarthritis
synoviosarcoma
tendinitis
tenodynia
tenosynovitis

Surgical

aponeurorrhaphy
arthroclasia
arthrodesis
arthroplasty
bursectomy
carpectomy
chondrectomy
chondroplasty
costectomy
cranioplasty
craniotomy
diskectomy
laminectomy
maxillectomy
meniscectomy
myorrhaphy
ostectomy
osteoclasis
patellectomy
phalangectomy
rachiotomy
spondylosyndesis
synovectomy
tarsectomy
tenomyoplasty
tenorrhaphy
tenotomy
vertebroplasty

Diagnostic

arthrocentesis
arthrography
arthroscopy
electromyogram
(EMG)

Complementary

arthralgia
atrophy
bradykinesia
carpal
cranial
dyskinesia
dystrophy
femoral
humeral
hyperkinesia
hypertrophy
iliofemoral
intercostal
intervertebral
intracranial
ischiofibular
ischiopubic
lumbar
lumbocostal
lumbosacral

osteoblast
osteocyte
osteonecrosis
pelvic
pelvisacral
pubofemoral
sacral
sacrovertebral
sternoclavicular
sternoid
subcostal
submandibular
submaxillary
subscapular
substernal
suprapatellar
suprascapular
symphysis
vertebrocostal

Can you define, pronounce, and spell the following terms *not built from word parts?*

Diseases and Disorders

ankylosing spondylitis
bunion
carpal tunnel syndrome (CTS)
Colles fracture
exostosis
fracture (fx)
gout
herniated disk
muscular dystrophy (MD)
myasthenia gravis (MG)
osteoporosis
rheumatoid arthritis (RA)

Complementary

chiropodist
chiropractic
chiropractor
orthopedics (ortho)
orthopedist
orthotics
orthotist
osteopath
osteopathy
podiatrist
prosthesis

Nervous System and Common Behavioral Health Terms

OBJECTIVES

On completion of this chapter you will be able to:

1. Identify the organs and other structures of the nervous system.
2. Define and spell the word parts presented in this chapter.
3. Build and analyze medical terms with word parts presented in this and previous chapters.
4. Define, pronounce, and spell the disease and disorder, diagnostic, surgical, and complementary terms for the nervous system.
5. Define common behavioral health disorders.
6. Interpret the meaning of abbreviations presented in this chapter.
7. Read medical documents and interpret medical terminology contained in them.

ANATOMY

Function

The nervous system and the endocrine system cooperate in regulating and controlling the activities of the other body systems.

The nervous system may be divided into two parts: the *central nervous* system (CNS) and the *peripheral nervous system* (PNS) (Figures 15-1 and 15-2). The central nervous system consists of the brain and spinal cord. The peripheral nervous system is made up of cranial nerves, which carry impulses between the brain and neck and head, and spinal nerves, which carry messages between the spinal cord and abdomen, limbs, and chest.

Organs of the Central Nervous System

brain	major portion of the central nervous system (see Figure 15-2)
cerebrum	largest portion of the brain, divided into left and right hemispheres. The cerebrum controls the skeletal muscles, interprets general senses (such as temperature, pain, and touch), and contains centers for sight and hearing. Intellect, memory, and emotional reactions also take place in the cerebrum.
ventricles	spaces within the brain that contain a fluid called *cerebrospinal fluid.* The cerebrospinal fluid flows through the subarachnoid space around the brain and spinal cord.
cerebellum	located under the posterior portion of the cerebrum. Its function is to assist in the coordination of skeletal muscles and to maintain balance. (also called *hindbrain*)
brainstem	stemlike portion of the brain that connects with the spinal cord. Ten of the 12 cranial nerves originate in the brainstem.
pons	literally means *bridge.* It connects the cerebrum with the cerebellum and brainstem.
medulla oblongata	located between the pons and spinal cord. It contains centers that control respiration, heart rate, and the muscles in the blood vessel walls, which assist in determining blood pressure.
midbrain	most superior portion of the brainstem
cerebrospinal fluid (CSF)	clear, colorless fluid contained in the ventricles that flows through the subarachnoid space around the brain and spinal cord. It cushions the brain and spinal cord from shock, transports nutrients, and clears metabolic waste.
spinal cord	passes through the vertebral canal extending from the medulla oblongata to the level of the second lumbar vertebra. The spinal cord conducts nerve impulses to and from the brain and initiates reflex action to sensory information without input from the brain.

Cerebellum

was named in the third century BC by Erasistratus, who also named the cerebrum. **Cerebellum** literally means **little brain** and is the diminutive of **cerebrum,** meaning **brain.** Although it was named long ago, its function was not understood until the nineteenth century.

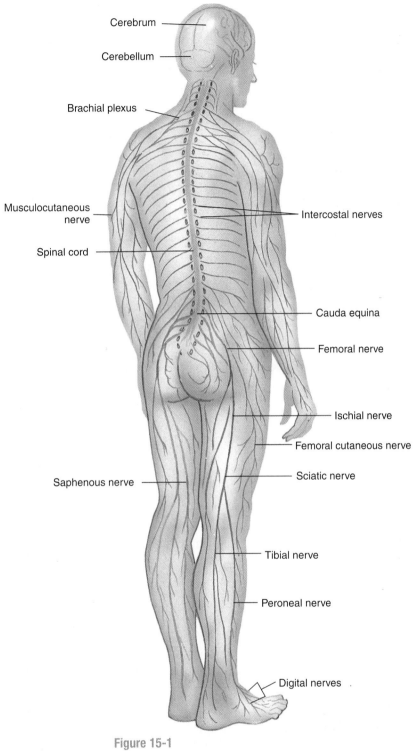

Figure 15-1
A, Simplified view of the nervous system.
Continued

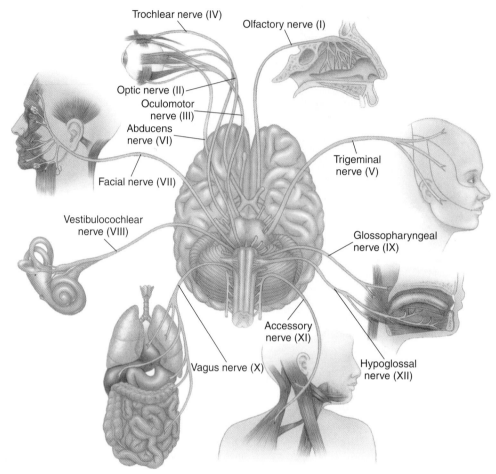

Figure 15-1, cont'd
B, Cranial nerves.

---

meninges	three layers of membrane that cover the brain and spinal cord (Figure 15-3)
dura mater	tough outer layer of the meninges
arachnoid	delicate middle layer of the meninges. The arachnoid membrane is loosely attached to the pia mater by weblike fibers, which allow for the *subarachnoid space.*
pia mater	thin inner layer of the meninges

Organs of the Peripheral Nervous System

nerve	cordlike structure that carries impulses from one part of the body to another. There are 12 pairs of cranial nerves and 31 pairs of spinal nerves (see Figures 15-1 and 15-3).
ganglion (*pl.* ganglia)	group of nerve cell bodies located outside the central nervous system

Learn the anatomic terms by completing exercises 1 and 2.

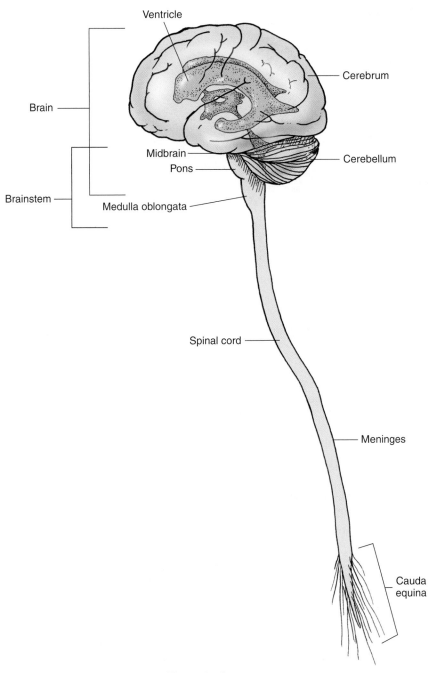

Figure 15-2
Brain and spinal cord.

EXERCISE   1

Fill in the blanks with the correct terms.

The layer of membrane that covers the brain and spinal cord is called the
(1) _____. Three layers that comprise this membrane are called
(2) _____ _____, (3) _____, and
(4) _____ _____. Below the middle layer is a space called
the (5) _____ _____ through which the (6) _____
_____ flows around the brain and spinal cord.

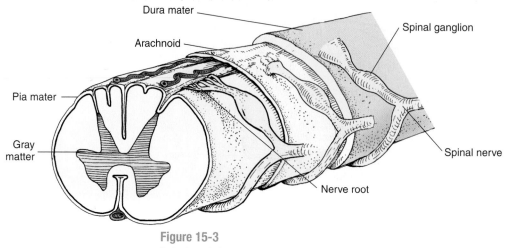

Figure 15-3
Spinal cord showing layers of meninges.

EXERCISE 2

Match the definitions in the first column with the correct terms in the second column.

_____ 1. maintains balance

_____ 2. connects the cerebrum with the cerebellum and brainstem

_____ 3. spaces within the brain

_____ 4. contains the control center for respiration

_____ 5. carries impulses from one part of the body to another

_____ 6. conducts impulses to and from the brain and initiates reflex action to sensory information

_____ 7. group of nerve cell bodies outside the central nervous system

_____ 8. colorless fluid contained in the ventricles

a. nerve

b. ganglion

c. cerebrospinal fluid

d. cerebellum

e. medulla oblongata

f. pons

g. ventricles

h. spinal cord

i. pia mater

WORD PARTS

Combining Forms of the Nervous System

Study the word parts and their definitions listed below. Completing the exercises that follow will help you learn the terms.

Combining Form	Definition
cerebell/o...	cerebellum
cerebr/o...	cerebrum, brain
dur/o	hard, dura mater
encephal/o	brain
gangli/o, ganglion/o......................................	ganglion
mening/i, mening/o... (NOTE: both *i* and *o* are used as combining vowels with *mening/*.)	meninges
myel/o .... (NOTE: *myel/o* also means *bone marrow;* see Chapter 14.)	spinal cord
neur/o.. (NOTE: *neur/o* was introduced in Chapter 2.)	nerve
radic/o, radicul/o, rhiz/o..	nerve root (proximal end of a peripheral nerve, closest to the spinal cord)

Learn the anatomic locations and meanings of the combining forms by completing exercises 3 and 4 and Exercise Figures A and B.

EXERCISE 3

Write the definitions of the following combining forms.

1. cerebell/o _____

2. neur/o _____

3. myel/o _____

4. mening/o, mening/i _____

5. encephal/o _____

6. cerebr/o _____

7. radicul/o _____

8. gangli/o _____

9. radic/o _____

10. dur/o _____

11. ganglion/o _____

12. rhiz/o _____

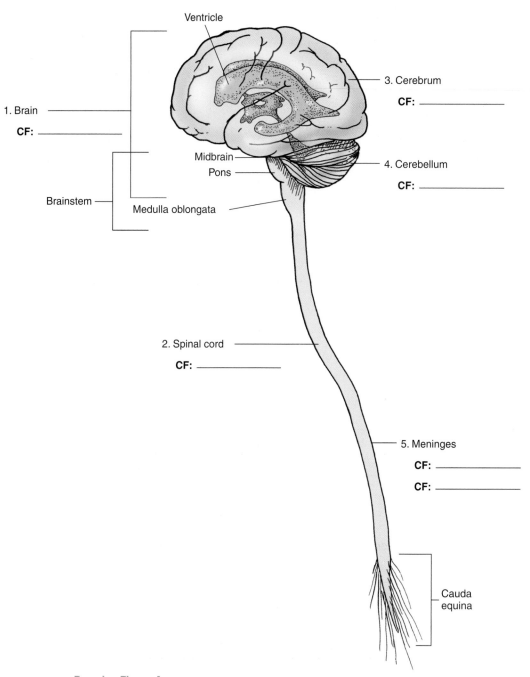

Ventricle

1. Brain

CF: —————

Brainstem

Midbrain
Pons
Medulla oblongata

3. Cerebrum

CF: —————

4. Cerebellum

CF: —————

2. Spinal cord

CF: —————

5. Meninges

CF: —————
CF: —————

Cauda
equina

Exercise Figure A
Fill in the blanks with combining forms in this diagram of the brain and spinal cord.

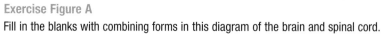

EXERCISE   4

Write the combining form for each of the following terms.

1. cerebellum   _____

2. nerve   _____

3. spinal cord   _____

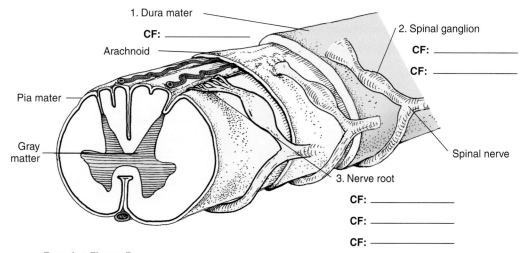

1. Dura mater

CF: _____

Arachnoid

2. Spinal ganglion

CF: _____

CF: _____

Pia mater

Gray
matter

Spinal nerve

3. Nerve root

CF: _____

CF: _____

CF: _____

Exercise Figure B
Fill in the blanks with combining forms in this diagram of the spinal cord and layers of meninges.

4. meninges   a. _____

b. _____

5. brain   _____

6. cerebrum, brain   _____

7. nerve root   a. _____

b. _____

c. _____

8. hard, dura mater   _____

9. ganglion   a. _____

b. _____

Combining Forms Commonly Used with Nervous System Terms

Combining Form	Definition
esthesi/o	sensation, sensitivity, feeling
ment/o, phren/o, psych/o	mind
mon/o	one
phas/o	speech
poli/o	gray matter
quadr/i	four

(NOTE: an *i* is the combining vowel in *quadr/i*.)

Learn the combining forms by completing exercises 5 and 6.

EXERCISE   5

Write the definitions of the following combining forms.

1. mon/o _____

2. psych/o _____

3. quadr/i _____

4. ment/o _____

5. phas/o _____

6. esthesi/o _____

7. phren/o _____

8. poli/o _____

EXERCISE   6

Write the combining form for each of the following.

1. four   _____

2. one   _____

3. mind   a. _____

                            b. _____

                            c. _____

4. speech   _____

5. gray matter   _____

6. sensation, sensitivity, feeling   _____

Prefix

Prefix	Definition
tetra-...	four

Suffixes

Suffix	Definition
-iatrist..	specialist, physician (-*logist* also means specialist)
-iatry..	treatment, specialty

-ictal	seizure, attack
-paresis	slight paralysis (*-plegia*, meaning *paralysis*, was covered in Chapter 12)

Learn the prefix and suffixes by completing exercises 7 and 8. Refer to Appendix A and Appendix B for a complete listing of word parts.

EXERCISE 7

Write the definitions of the following prefix and suffixes.

1. -paresis _____

2. -iatry _____

3. -ictal _____

4. -iatrist _____

5. tetra- _____

EXERCISE 8

Write the prefix or suffix for each of the following.

1. slight paralysis _____

2. treatment, specialty _____

3. seizure _____

4. specialist, physician _____

5. four _____

MEDICAL TERMS

The terms you need to learn to complete this chapter are listed below. The exercises following each list will help you learn the definition and spelling of each word.

Disease and Disorder Terms

Built from Word Parts

Term	Definition
cerebellitis (ser-e-bel-Ī-tis)	inflammation of the cerebellum
cerebral thrombosis (se-RĒ-bral) (throm-BŌ-sis)	abnormal condition of a clot, pertaining to the cerebrum (blood clot in a blood vessel of the brain)

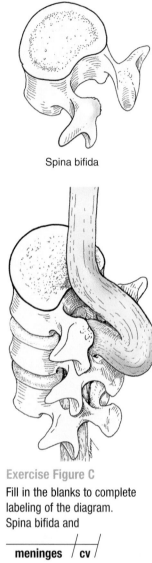

Spina bifida

Exercise Figure C

Fill in the blanks to complete labeling of the diagram. Spina bifida and

_____/ cv /_____
meninges / **cv** /

_____/ cv /_____
spinal / **cv** / **protrusion**
cord

duritis .... (dū-RĪ-tis)	inflammation of the dura mater
encephalitis .... (*en*-sef-a-LĪ-tis)	inflammation of the brain
encephalomalacia .... (en-*sef*-a-lō-ma-LĀ-shē-a)	softening of the brain
encephalomyeloradiculitis .... (en-*sef*-a-lō-*mī*-e-lō-ra-*dik*-ū- LĪ-tis)	inflammation of the brain, spinal cord, and nerve roots
gangliitis .... (*gang*-glē-Ī-tis)	inflammation of a ganglion
meningitis .... (*men*-in-JĪ-tis)	inflammation of the meninges
meningocele .... (me-NING-gō-sēl)	protrusion of the meninges (through a defect in the skull or vertebral column)
meningomyelocele .... (me-*ning*-gō-MĪ-e-lō-*sēl*)	protrusion of the meninges and spinal cord (through the vertebral column) (also called *myelomeningocele*) (Exercise Figure C)
neuralgia .... (nū-RAL-jē-a)	pain in a nerve
neurasthenia .... (*nū*-ras-THĒ-nē-a)	nerve weakness (nervous exhaustion, fatigue, and weakness)
neuritis .... (nū-RĪ-tis)	inflammation of a nerve
neuroarthropathy .... (*nū*r-ō-ar-THROP-a-thē)	disease of nerves and joints
neuroblast .... (NŪ-rō-blast)	developing nerve cell
neuroma .... (nū-RŌ-ma)	tumor made up of nerve (cells)
poliomyelitis .... (*pō*-lē-ō-*mī*-e-LĪ-tis)	inflammation of the gray matter of the spinal cord. (This infectious disease, commonly referred to as *polio*, is caused by one of three polio viruses.)
polyneuritis .... (*pol*-ē-nū-RĪ-tis)	inflammation of many nerves
radiculitis .... (ra-*dik*-ū-LĪ-tis)	inflammation of the nerve roots
rhizomeningomyelitis .... (rī-zō-me-ning-gō-mī-e- LĪ-tis)	inflammation of the nerve root, meninges, and spinal cord
subdural hematoma .... (sub-DŪ-ral) (*hēm*-a-TŌ-ma)	blood tumor, pertaining to below the dura mater (*hematoma*, literally translated, means *blood tumor*; however, a hematoma is a blood mass or collection of blood)

Practice saying each of these terms aloud. To hear the terms, access the **PRONOUNCE IT** activity for this chapter on the Student CD that accompanies this text. Or, to hear the terms and their definitions with a CD player or computer, obtain the Pronunciation CD designed for use with this text.

Learn the definitions and spellings of the disease and disorder terms by completing exercises 9, 10, and 11.

EXERCISE 9

Analyze and define the following terms.

1. neuritis _____

2. neuroma _____

3. neuralgia _____

4. neuroarthropathy _____

5. neuroblast _____

6. neurasthenia _____

7. encephalomalacia _____

8. encephalitis _____

9. encephalomyeloradiculitis _____

10. meningitis _____

11. meningocele _____

12. meningomyelocele _____

13. radiculitis _____

14. cerebellitis _____

15. gangliitis _____

16. duritis _____

17. polyneuritis _____

18. poliomyelitis _____

19. cerebral thrombosis _____

20. subdural hematoma _____

21. rhizomeningomyelitis _____

EXERCISE 10

Build disease and disorder terms for the following definitions with the word parts you have learned.

1. inflammation of the nerve

_____ / _____
WR   S

2. tumor made up of nerve (cells)

_____ / _____
WR   S

3. pain in a nerve

_____ / _____
WR   S

4. disease of nerves and joints

_____ /CV/ _____ /CV/ _____
WR   WR   S

5. developing nerve cell

_____ /CV/ _____
WR   WR

6. nerve weakness (nervous exhaustion, fatigue, and weakness)

_____ / _____
WR   S

7. softening of the brain

_____ /CV/ _____
WR   S

8. inflammation of the brain

_____ / _____
WR   S

9. inflammation of the brain, spinal cord, and nerve roots

_____ /CV/ _____ /CV/ _____ / _____
WR   WR   WR   S

10. inflammation of the meninges

_____ / _____
WR   S

11. protrusion of the meninges (through a defect in the skull or vertebral column)

_____ /CV/ _____
WR   S

12. protrusion of the meninges and spinal cord (through the vertebral column)

_____ /CV/ _____ /CV/ _____
WR   WR   S

13. inflammation of the (spinal) nerve roots

_____ / _____
WR   S

14. inflammation of the cerebellum

_____ / _____
WR   S

15. inflammation of the
    ganglion

    _____ / _____
         WR   S

16. inflammation of the dura
    mater

    _____ / _____
         WR   S

17. inflammation of many
    nerves

    _____ / _____ / _____
        P   WR   S

18. inflammation of the gray
    matter of the spinal cord

    _____ / __ / _____ / _____
       WR   CV   WR   S

19. abnormal condition of a
    clot (in) pertaining to the
    cerebrum

    _____ / _____   _____ / _____
      WR   S   WR   S

20. blood tumor (mass) per-
    taining to below the dura
    mater

    ____ / ____ / ____   _____ / _____
     P   WR   S   WR   S

21. inflammation of the nerve
    root, meninges, and spinal
    cord

    _____ / __ / _____ / __ / _____ / ____
      WR   CV   WR   CV   WR   S

EXERCISE   11

Spell each of the disease and disorder terms. Have someone dictate the terms on
pp. 551-552 to you. Think about the word parts before attempting to write the word.
Study any words you have spelled incorrectly.

1. _____   12. _____

2. _____   13. _____

3. _____   14. _____

4. _____   15. _____

5. _____   16. _____

6. _____   17. _____

7. _____   18. _____

8. _____   19. _____

9. _____   20. _____

10. _____   21. _____

11. _____

Disease and Disorder Terms

Not Built from Word Parts

Term	Definition
Alzheimer disease (AD) .... (AWLZ-*hī*-mer) (di-ZEZ)	disease characterized by early senility, confusion, loss of recognition of persons or familiar surroundings, restlessness, and impaired memory
amyotrophic lateral sclerosis (ALS).. (a-mī-ō-TROF-ik) (LAT-er-al) (skle-RO-sis)	progressive muscle atrophy caused by hardening of nerve tissue on the lateral columns of the spinal cord. Also called *Lou Gehrig disease.*
Bell palsy .... (bel) (PAWL-zē)	paralysis of muscles on one side of the face, usually a temporary condition. Symptoms include a sagging mouth on the affected side and nonclosure of the eyelid (Figure 15-4).
cerebral aneurysm .... (se-RE-bral) (AN-ū-rizm)	aneurysm in the cerebrum (aneurysm was covered in Chapter 10)
cerebral palsy (CP) .... (se-RE-bral) (PAWL-zē)	condition characterized by lack of muscle control and partial paralysis, caused by a brain defect or lesion present at birth or shortly after
cerebrovascular accident (CVA)...... (se-re-bro-VAS-kū-lar)	interruption of blood supply to the brain caused by a cerebral thrombosis, cerebral embolus, or cerebral hemorrhage. The patient may experience mild to severe paralysis. Also called *stroke,* or *brain attack* (Figure 15-5).

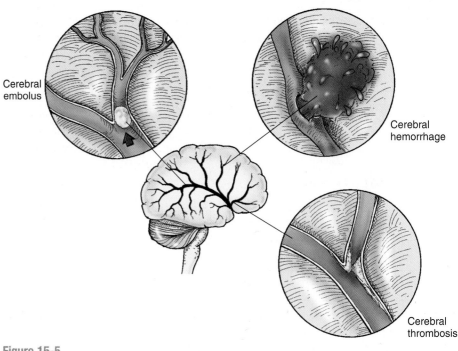

Cerebral embolus

Cerebral hemorrhage

Cerebral thrombosis

Figure 15-4
Bell palsy.

Figure 15-5
Cerebrovascular accident, which may be caused by a cerebral embolus, a cerebral thrombosis, or a cerebral hemorrhage.

Cerebrovascular accident is the most common disease of the nervous system. It is the third highest cause of death in the United States.

epilepsy	disorder in which the main symptom is recurring seizures
(EP-i-lep-sē)	
hydrocephalus	increased amount of cerebrospinal fluid in the ventricles of the brain, which can cause enlargement of the cranium
(hī-drō-SEF-a-lus)	
multiple sclerosis (MS)...............	degenerative disease characterized by sclerotic patches along the brain and spinal cord
(mul-TIP-al) (skle-RŌ-sis)	
neurosis (*pl.* neuroses)...............	emotional disorder that involves an ineffective way of coping with anxiety or inner conflict
(nū-RO-sis)	
Parkinson disease (PD)...............	chronic degenerative disease of the central nervous system. Symptoms include resting tremors of the hands and feet, rigidity, expressionless face, and shuffling gait. It usually occurs after the age of 50 years.
(PAR-kin-sun) (di-ZĒZ)	
psychosis (*pl.* psychoses)	major mental disorder characterized by extreme derangement, often with delusions and hallucinations
(sī-KO-sis)	
Reye syndrome	disease of the brain and other organs such as the liver. Affects children and adolescents. The cause is unknown, but it typically follows a viral infection.
(RI) (SIN-drōm)	
sciatica	inflammation of the sciatic nerve, causing pain that travels from the thigh through the leg to the foot and toes. Can be caused by injury, infection, arthritis, herniated disk, or from prolonged pressure on the nerve from sitting for long periods (Figure 15-6).
(sī-AT-i-ka)	
shingles	viral disease that affects the peripheral nerves and causes blisters on the skin that follow the course of the affected nerves. Also called *herpes zoster* (Figure 15-7).
(SHING-gelz)	
transient ischemic attack (TIA)	sudden deficient supply of blood to the brain lasting a short time. The symptoms may be similar to those of CVA, but with TIA the symptoms are temporary and the usual outcome is complete recovery.
(tra-SĒ-ent) (is-KEM-ik) (a-TAK)	

Epilepsy
was written about by Hippocrates, in 400 BC, in a book titled **Sacred Disease.** It was believed at one time that epilepsy was a punishment for offending the gods. The Greek **epilepsia** meant **seizure** and is derived from **epi,** meaning **upon,** and **lambaneia,** meaning **to seize.** The term literally means **seized upon** (by the gods).

Hydrocephalus
literally means **water in the head** and is made of the word parts **hydro,** meaning **water,** and **cephal,** meaning **head.** The condition was first described around AD 30 in the book **De Medicina.**

Parkinson Disease
is also called **parkinsonism, paralysis agitans,** and **shaking palsy.** Since James Parkinson, an English professor, described the disease in 1817 in his **Essay on the Shaking Palsy,** it has often been referred to as **Parkinson disease.**

Shingles
is an outbreak of the varicella virus, which also causes chickenpox. The virus enters the nervous system and remains dormant for years if the immune system does not destroy the virus after chickenpox.
Stress, medication, age, or illness can reactivate the virus, causing shingles.

Practice saying each of these terms aloud. To hear the terms, access the **PRONOUNCE IT** activity for this chapter on the Student CD that accompanies this text. Or, to hear the terms and their definitions with a CD player or computer, obtain the Pronunciation CD designed for use with this text.

Learn the definitions and spellings of the disease and disorder terms by completing exercises 12, 13 and 14.

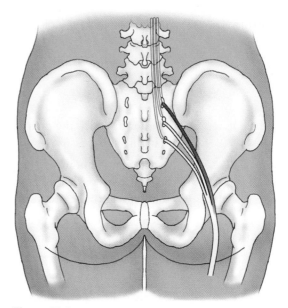

Figure 15-6
The sciatic nerve, the longest in the body, travels through the hip from the spine to the thigh and continues with branches throughout the lower leg and foot. Sciatica is the inflammation of the nerve along its course.

EXERCISE 12

Many of the disease and disorder terms include word parts you have studied in this chapter or previous chapters. To become familiar with the terms, write the definition of the italicized word part in each of the following.

1. *cerebr*ovascular accident _____

2. *psych*osis _____

3. *epi*lepsy _____

4. multiple *sclerosis* _____

5. hydro*cephalus* _____

6. *neur*osis _____

7. *cerebr*al palsy _____

EXERCISE 13

Match the diseases in the first column with the corresponding phrases in the second column.

_____ 1. psychosis

_____ 2. sciatica

_____ 3. transient ischemic
      attack

a. causes pain from the thigh to the toes

b. derangement, possibly including delusions and hallucinations

c. paralysis of muscles on one side of the face

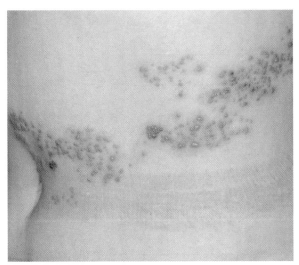

Figure 15-7
Shingles.

_____ 4. Parkinson disease

_____ 5. cerebral palsy

_____ 6. hydrocephalus

_____ 7. neurosis

_____ 8. cerebrovascular accident

_____ 9. Alzheimer disease

_____ 10. Reye syndrome

_____ 11. epilepsy

_____ 12. multiple sclerosis

_____ 13. shingles

_____ 14. amyotrophic lateral sclerosis

_____ 15. Bell palsy

_____ 16. cerebral aneurysm

d. hardened patches scattered along the brain and spinal cord

e. inability to cope with anxiety or inner conflict

f. aneurysm in the cerebrum

g. mild to severe paralysis

h. blisters on the skin

i. early senility

j. resting tremors of the hands and feet and rigidity

k. inflammation of the spinal cord

l. lack of muscle control

m. affects children and adolescents, typically after viral infections

n. deficient supply of blood to the brain

o. also called _Lou Gehrig disease_

p. increased amount of cerebrospinal fluid in the ventricles of the brain

q. recurring seizures

EXERCISE 14

Spell the disease and disorder terms. Have someone dictate the terms on pp. 556-557 to you. Study any words you have spelled incorrectly.

1. _____   3. _____

2. _____   4. _____

5. _____   11. _____

6. _____   12. _____

7. _____   13. _____

8. _____   14. _____

9. _____   15. _____

10. _____   16. _____

Surgical Terms

Built from Word Parts

Term	Definition
ganglionectomy (*gang*-glē-on-EK-tō-mē)	excision of a ganglion (also called *gangliectomy*)
neurectomy (nū-REK-tō-mē)	excision of a nerve
neurolysis (nū-ROL-i-sis)	separating a nerve (from adhesions)
neuroplasty (NŪ-rō-plas-tē)	surgical repair of a nerve
neurorrhaphy (nū-ROR-a-fē)	suture of a nerve
neurotomy (nū-ROT-ō-mē)	incision into a nerve
radicotomy, rhizotomy (*rad*-i-KOT-ō-mē) (rī-ZOT-ō-mē)	incision into a nerve root (Exercise Figure D)

Practice saying each of these terms aloud. To hear the terms, access the **PRONOUNCE IT** activity for this chapter on the Student CD that accompanies this text. Or, to hear the terms and their definitions with a CD player or computer, obtain the Pronunciation CD designed for use with this text.

Learn the definitions and spellings of the surgical terms by completing exercises 15, 16, and 17.

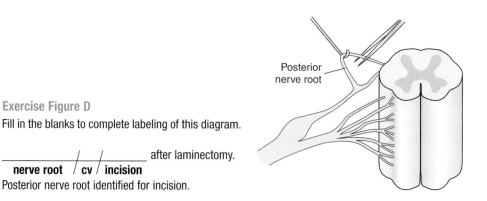

Exercise Figure D

Fill in the blanks to complete labeling of this diagram.

Posterior nerve root

_____ / _____ / _____ after laminectomy.

nerve root / **cv** / **incision**

Posterior nerve root identified for incision.

EXERCISE 15

Analyze and define the following surgical terms.

1. radicotomy _____

2. neurectomy _____

3. neurorrhaphy _____

4. ganglionectomy _____

5. neurotomy _____

6. neurolysis _____

7. neuroplasty _____

8. rhizotomy _____

EXERCISE 16

Build surgical terms for the following definitions by using the word parts you have learned.

1. incision into a nerve
   root

   a. _____ / ____ / _____
      WR   CV   S

   b. _____ / ____ / _____
      WR   CV   S

2. excision of a nerve

   _____ / _____
      WR   S

3. suture of a nerve

   _____ / ____ / _____
      WR   CV   S

4. excision of a ganglion

   _____ / _____
      WR   S

5. incision into a nerve

   _____ / ____ / _____
      WR   CV   S

6. separating a nerve
   (from adhesions)

   _____ / ____ / _____
      WR   CV   S

7. surgical repair of a
   nerve

   _____ / ____ / _____
      WR   CV   S

EXERCISE 17

Spell each of the surgical terms. Have someone dictate the terms on p. 560 to you. Think about the word parts before attempting to write the word. Study any words you have spelled incorrectly.

1. _____   5. _____

2. _____   6. _____

3. _____   7. _____

4. _____   8. _____

Diagnostic Terms

Built from Word Parts

Term	Definition
Diagnostic Imaging	
cerebral angiography .... (se-RĒ-bral) (an-jē-OG-ra-fē)	x-ray imaging of the blood vessels in the brain (after an injection of contrast medium)
CT myelography .... (mī-e-LOG-ra-fē)	process of recording (scan) the spinal cord (after an injection of a contrast agent into the subarachnoid space. Size, shape, and position of the spinal cord and nerve roots are demonstrated.) (Exercise Figure E)

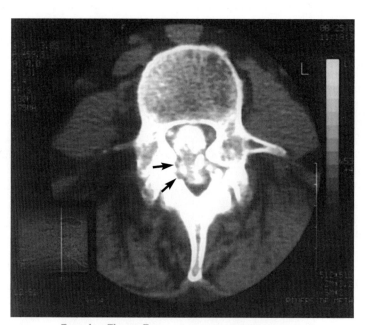

Exercise Figure E

Fill in the blanks to complete labeling of the diagram.

CT _____ / __ / _____

spinal cord / **cv** / **process of recording**

Neurodiagnostic Procedures

echoencephalography (EchoEG)..... (ek-ō-en-*sef*-a-LOG-ra-fē)	process of recording the brain (structures) by sound (also called *ultrasonography* of the brain)
electroencephalogram (EEG)............ (e-*lek*-trō-en-SEF-a-lō-gram)	record of the electrical impulses of the brain
electroencephalograph...................... (e-*lek*-trō-en-SEF-a-lō-graf)	instrument used to record the electrical impulses of the brain
electroencephalography................... (e-*lek*-trō-en-*sef*-a-LOG-ra-fē)	process of recording the electrical impulses of the brain

Practice saying each of these words aloud. To hear the terms, access the **PRONOUNCE IT** activity for this chapter on the Student CD that accompanies this text. Or, to hear the terms and their definitions with a CD player or computer, obtain the Pronunciation CD designed for use with this text.

Learn the definitions and spellings of the diagnostic terms by completing exercises 18, 19, and 20.

EXERCISE   18

Analyze and define the following diagnostic terms.

1. electroencephalogram   _____

2. electroencephalograph   _____

3. electroencephalography   _____

4. echoencephalography   _____

5. CT myelography   _____

6. cerebral angiography   _____

EXERCISE   19

Build diagnostic terms that correspond to the following definitions by using the word parts you have learned.

1. process of recording brain
   (structures) by use of sound

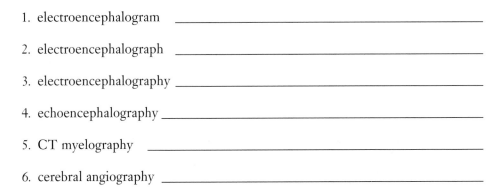

2. record of the electrical
   impulses of the brain

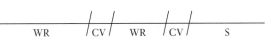

3. instrument used for recording
   the electrical impulses of the
   brain

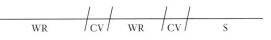

4. process of recording the electrical impulses of the brain

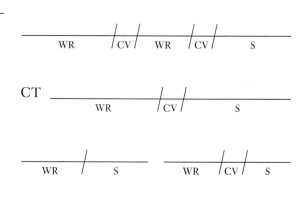
_____ /CV/ WR /CV/ S
WR

5. process of recording (scan) the spinal cord

CT _____ /CV/ _____ S
WR

6. x-ray imaging of the blood vessels in the brain

_____ / S   _____ /CV/ S
WR   WR

EXERCISE 20

Spell each of the diagnostic terms. Have someone dictate the terms on pp. 562-563 to you. Think about the word parts before attempting to write the word. Study any words you have spelled incorrectly.

1. _____   4. _____

2. _____   5. _____

3. _____   6. _____

Diagnostic Terms

Not Built from Word Parts

Term	Definition
Diagnostic Imaging	
computed tomography of the brain (CT scan)................................. (com-PŪ-td) (tō-MOG-ra-fē)	process that includes the use of a computer to produce a series of images of the tissues of the brain at any desired depth. The procedure is noninvasive, painless, and particularly useful in diagnosing brain tumors (Figures 15-8 and 15-9).
magnetic resonance imaging of the brain (MRI scan)........................ (mag-NET-ik) (re-zo-NANCE) (IM-a-jing)	a noninvasive technique that produces cross-sectional and sagittal images of soft tissues of the brain by magnetic waves. Unlike CT scan, MRI produces images without use of radiation. It is used to visualize tumors, edema, multiple sclerosis, and herniated disks (Figure 15-10).
positron emission tomography of the brain (PET scan).................... (POS-i-tron) (e-MI-shun) (tō-MOG-ra-fē)	an imaging technique with a radioactive substance that permits viewing a slice of the brain to examine blood flow and metabolic activity. Images are projected on a viewing screen (Figure 15-11).

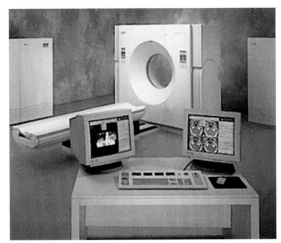

Figure 15-8
CT scanner.

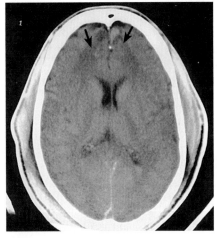

Figure 15-9
CT scan of the brain demonstrating bilateral brain contusions *(arrows)* caused by trauma.

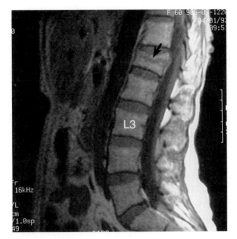

Figure 15-10
Sagittal MRI section of the lumbar spine demonstrating a compression fracture of L1 after trauma *(arrow).*

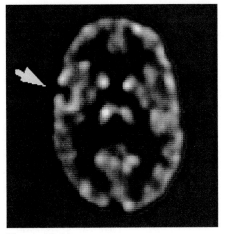

Figure 15-11
Positron emission tomography (PET) brain scan.

Neurodiagnostic Procedures

**evoked potential studies
(EP studies)**..
(ē-VOKD) (pō-TEN-shal)

a group of diagnostic tests that measure changes and responses in brain waves elicited by visual, auditory, or somatosensory stimuli. Visual evoked response (VER) is a response to visual stimuli. Auditory evoked response (AER) is a response to auditory stimuli.

Other

lumbar puncture (LP)..........................
(LUM-bar) (PUNK-chur)

insertion of a needle into the subarachnoid space usually between the third and fourth lumbar vertebrae. It is performed for many reasons, including the removal of cerebrospinal fluid for diagnostic purposes (Figure 15-12).

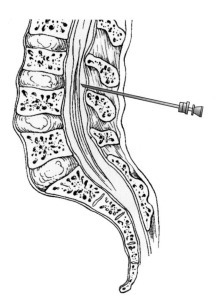

Figure 15-12
Lumbar puncture with needle in place.

The **first full-scale CT unit** for head scanning was installed in a hospital in **Wimbledon,** United Kingdom in **1971.** Its ability to provide neurological diagnostic information gained rapid recognition. The first units in the **United States** were used in **1973.** The first scanner for visualizing sections of the body other than the brain was developed in **1974** by Dr. Robert Ledly at Georgetown University Medical Center.

A **magnetic resonance imaging scanner** was first used in the **United States** in **1981.** The scanner was developed in England and installed there in 1975.

Stereotactic radiosurgery is used to treat patients with **brain tumors** or **arteriovenous malformations (AVMs).** A special frame is mounted on the patient's head. Images of the brain are produced by MRI. A high-powered computer uses the images to design a plan for high-intensity radiation that matches the exact size and shape of the tumor. Radiation is then delivered directly to the tumor only, sparing surrounding tissue.

Practice saying each of the terms aloud. To hear the terms, access the **PRONOUNCE IT** activity for this chapter on the Student CD that accompanies this text. Or, to hear the terms and their definitions with a CD player or computer, obtain the Pronunciation CD designed for use with this text.

Learn the definitions and spelling of diagnostic terms by completing exercises 21, 22, and 23.

EXERCISE 21

Fill in the blanks with the correct terms.

1. A computer is used to produce images during _____ _____ of the brain.

2. A needle is inserted into the subarachnoid space during a(n) _____ _____.

3. _____ _____ _____ produces images to examine blood flow and metabolic activity of the brain.

4. Uses magnetic waves to produce images of the brain: _____

   _____ _____.

5. Measures responses in brain waves from stimuli: _____

   _____ _____.

EXERCISE 22

Write the definitions of the following terms.

1. lumbar puncture _____

2. computed tomography of the brain   _____

3. magnetic resonance imaging _____

4. positron emission tomography of the brain   _____

5. evoked potential studies _____

EXERCISE 23

Spell each of the diagnostic terms. Have someone dictate the terms on pp. 564-565 to you. Study any words you have spelled incorrectly.

1. _____   4. _____

2. _____   5. _____

3. _____

Complementary Terms

Built from Word Parts

Term	Definition
anesthesia (*an*-es-THE-ze-a)	without (loss of) feeling or sensation
aphasia (a-FA-ze-a)	condition of without speaking (loss or impairment of the ability to speak)
cephalalgia (*sef*-el-AL-je-a)	pain in the head (headache) (also called *cephalgia*)
cerebral (se-RE-bral)	pertaining to the cerebrum
craniocerebral (*kra*-ne-o-sar-E-bral)	pertaining to the cranium and cerebrum
dysphasia (dis-FA-ze-a)	condition of difficulty speaking
encephalosclerosis (en-*sef*-a-lo-skle-RO-sis)	hardening of the brain

hemiparesis (*hem*-i-pa-RĒ-sis)	slight paralysis of half (right or left side of the body)
hemiplegia (*hem*-i-PLĒ-jē-a)	paralysis of half (right or left side of the body); (cerebrovascular accident is the most common cause of hemiplegia) (Exercise Figure F)
hyperesthesia (hī-per-es-THĒ-zē-a)	excessive sensitivity (to stimuli)
interictal (in-ter-IK-tal)	(occurring) between seizures or attacks
intracerebral (in-tra-SER-e-bral)	pertaining to within the cerebrum
monoparesis (mon-ō-pa-RĒ-sis)	slight paralysis of one (limb)
monoplegia (*mon*-ō-PLĒ-jē-a)	paralysis of one (limb)
myelomalacia (*mī*-e-lō-ma-LĀ-shē-a)	softening of the spinal cord
neuroid (NŪ-royd)	resembling a nerve
neurologist (nū-ROL-ō-jist)	physician who studies and treats diseases of the nerves (nervous system)
neurology (nū-ROL-ō-jē)	study of nerves (branch of medicine dealing with diseases of the nervous system)
panplegia (pan-PLĒ-jē-a)	total paralysis (also spelled *pamplegia*)
phrenic (FREN-ik)	pertaining to the mind
phrenopathy (fre-NOP-a-thē)	disease of the mind
postictal (pōst-IK-tal)	(occurring) after a seizure or attack
preictal (prē-IK-tal)	(occurring) before a seizure or attack
psychiatrist (sī-KĪ-a-trist)	a physician who studies and treats disorders of the mind
psychiatry (sī-KĪ-a-trē)	specialty of the mind (branch of medicine that deals with the treatment of mental disorders)
psychogenic (sī-kō-JEN-ik)	originating in the mind
psychologist (sī-KOL-ō-jist)	specialist of the mind
psychology (sī-KOL-ō-jē)	study of the mind (a profession that involves dealing with the mind and mental processes in relation to human behavior)
psychopathy (sī-KOP-a-thē)	(any) disease of the mind

Psychiatrist
a **physician** who has had **additional training** and experience in prevention, diagnosis, and treatment of mental disorders.

Clinical Psychologist
is one who has had **graduate study** in **psychology** and training in clinical psychology and who provides testing and counseling for mental and emotional disorders. A psychologist cannot prescribe medication or medical tests and treatments.

psychosomatic .... pertaining to the mind and body (interrela-
  (sī-kō-sō-MAT-ik)   tions of)
quadriplegia............................... paralysis of four (limbs) (see Exercise Figure F)
  (kwod-ri-PLĒ-jē-a)

subdural .... pertaining to below the dura mater
  (sub-DŪ-ral)

tetraplegia.................................. paralysis of four (limbs) (synonymous with
  (te-tra-PLĒ-jē-a)   *quadriplegia*) (see Exercise Figure F)

Practice saying each of these terms aloud. To hear the terms, access the **PRONOUNCE IT**
activity for this chapter on the Student CD that accompanies this text. Or, to hear the
terms and their definitions with a CD player or computer, obtain the Pronunciation CD
designed for use with this text.

Exercises 24, 25, and 26 will help you learn the definitions and spellings of the complementary terms related to the nervous system.

EXERCISE 24

Analyze and define the following complementary terms.

1. hemiplegia _____

2. tetraplegia _____

3. neurologist _____

4. neurology _____

5. neuroid _____

6. quadriplegia _____

7. cerebral _____

8. monoplegia _____

9. aphasia _____

10. dysphasia _____

11. hemiparesis _____

12. anesthesia _____

13. hyperesthesia _____

14. subdural _____

15. cephalalgia _____

16. psychosomatic _____

17. psychopathy _____

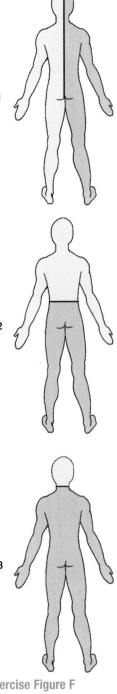

Exercise Figure F
Fill in the blanks to complete
labeling of this diagram of types
of paralysis.

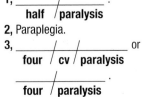

1, _____ / _____ .
      half / **paralysis**
2, Paraplegia.
3, _____ / _____ / _____ or
      four / **cv** / **paralysis**

_____ / _____ .
      four / **paralysis**

18. psychology _____

19. psychiatry _____

20. psychologist _____

21. psychogenic _____

22. phrenic _____

23. phrenopathy _____

24. craniocerebral _____

25. myelomalacia _____

26. encephalosclerosis _____

27. postictal _____

28. panplegia _____

29. interictal _____

30. monoparesis _____

31. preictal _____

32. psychiatrist _____

33. intracerebral _____

EXERCISE 25

Build the complementary terms for the following definitions by using the word parts you have learned.

1. slight paralysis of half (right
   or left side of the body) _____ / _____
                                          P   S(WR)

2. without (loss of) feeling or
   sensation _____ / _____ / _____
              P   WR   S

3. excessive sensitivity (to
   stimuli) _____ / _____ / _____
              P   WR   S

4. below the dura mater _____ / _____ / _____
              P   WR   S

5. pain in the head (headache) _____ / _____
              WR   S

6. pertaining to the mind and body (interrelations of)

_____ / ___ / _____ / ___
WR   CV   WR   S

7. (any) disease of the mind

_____ / ___ / _____
WR   CV   S

8. study of the mind

_____ / ___ / _____
WR   CV   S

9. specialty of the mind (branch of medicine that deals with the treatment of mental disorders)

_____ / _____
WR   S

10. specialist of the mind

_____ / ___ / _____
WR   CV   S

11. originating in the mind

_____ / ___ / _____
WR   CV   S

12. pertaining to the mind

_____ / _____
WR   S

13. disease of the mind

_____ / ___ / _____
WR   CV   S

14. pertaining to the cranium and cerebrum

_____ / ___ / _____ / ___
WR   CV   WR   S

15. softening of the spinal cord

_____ / ___ / _____
WR   CV   S

16. hardening of the brain

_____ / ___ / _____
WR   CV   S

17. paralysis of half (left or right side) of the body

_____ / _____
P   S(WR)

18. paralysis of four (limbs)

_____ / _____
P   S(WR)

19. physician who studies and treats diseases of the nervous system

_____ / ___ / _____
WR   CV   S

20. study of nerves (branch of medicine dealing with diseases of the nervous system)

_____ / ___ / _____
WR   CV   S

21. resembling a nerve

_____ / _____
WR   S

22. paralysis of four (limbs)

_____ / / _____
WR   CV   S

23. pertaining to the cerebrum

_____ / _____
WR   S

24. paralysis of one (limb)

_____ / / _____
WR   CV   S

25. condition of without speaking (loss or impairment of
the ability to speak)

_____ / / _____
P   WR   S

26. condition of difficulty
speaking

_____ / / _____
P   WR   S

27. (occurring) before a seizure
or attack

_____ / _____
P   S(WR)

28. slight paralysis of one (limb)

_____ / / _____
WR   CV   S

29. (occurring) after a seizure

_____ / _____
P   S(WR)

30. total paralysis

_____ / _____
P   S(WR)

31. (occurring) between
seizures or attacks

_____ / _____
P   S(WR)

32. a physician who treats
mental disorders

_____ / _____
WR   S

33. pertaining to within the
cerebrum

_____ / / _____
P   WR   S

EXERCISE 26

Spell each of the complementary terms. Have someone dictate the terms on pp. 567-569 to you. Think about the word parts before attempting to write the word. Study any words you have spelled incorrectly.

1. _____   5. _____

2. _____   6. _____

3. _____   7. _____

4. _____   8. _____

9. _____   22. _____

10. _____   23. _____

11. _____   24. _____

12. _____   25. _____

13. _____   26. _____

14. _____   27. _____

15. _____   28. _____

16. _____   29. _____

17. _____   30. _____

18. _____   31. _____

19. _____   32. _____

20. _____   33. _____

21. _____

Complementary Terms

Not Built from Word Parts

Term	Definition
afferent (AF-er-ent)	conveying toward a center (for example, afferent nerves carry impulses to the central nervous system)
ataxia (a-TAK-sē-a)	lack of muscle coordination
cognitive (COG-ni-tiv)	pertaining to the mental processes of comprehension, judgment, memory, and reason
coma (KŌ-ma)	state of profound unconsciousness
concussion (kon-KUSH-un)	jarring or shaking that results in an injury. Brain concussions are caused by slight or severe head injury; symptoms include vertigo and loss of consciousness.
conscious (KON-shus)	awake, alert, aware of one's surroundings
convulsion (kun-VUL-zhun)	sudden, involuntary contraction of a group of muscles (synonymous with *seizure*)
dementia (de-MEN-shē-a)	loss of cognitive abilities
disorientation (dis-ō-rē-en-TĀ-shun)	a state of mental confusion as to time, place, or identity

efferent.. conveying away from the center (for example,
   (EF-er-ent)   efferent nerves carry information away from
                                                the central nervous system)

gait... a manner or style of walking
   (gāt)

incoherent....................................... unable to express one's thoughts or ideas in
   (in-kō-HĒR-ent)   an orderly, intelligible manner

paraplegia....................................... paralysis from the waist down caused by
   (*par*-a-PLĒ-jē-a)   damage to the lower level of the spinal cord

seizure.. sudden attack with an involuntary series of
   (SĒ-zher)   contractions (synonymous with convulsion)

shunt.. tube implanted in the body to redirect the
   (shunt)   flow of a fluid

syncope... fainting or sudden loss of consciousness caused
   (SIN-cō-pē)   by lack of blood supply to the cerebrum

unconsciousness................................ state of being unaware of surroundings and
   (un-KON-shus-nes)   incapable of responding to stimuli as a result
                                                of injury, shock, or illness

> **Paraplegia**
> is composed of the Greek **para,** meaning **beside,** and **plegia,** meaning **paralysis.** It has been used since Hippocrates' time and at first meant paralysis of any limb or side of the body. Since the nineteenth century, it has been used to mean paralysis from the waist down.

Practice saying each of these terms aloud. To hear the terms, access the **PRONOUNCE IT** activity for this chapter on the Student CD that accompanies this text. Or, to hear the terms and their definitions with a CD player or computer, obtain the Pronunciation CD designed for use with this text.

Learn the definitions and spellings of the complementary terms by completing exercises 27, 28, and 29.

EXERCISE 27

Write the term for each of the following definitions.

1. jarring or shaking that results in an injury

   _____

2. state of being unaware of surroundings and incapable of responding to stimuli as a result of injury, shock, or illness

   _____

3. awake, alert, aware of one's surroundings

   _____

4. sudden attack with involuntary contractions

   _____

5. sudden, involuntary contraction of a group of muscles

   _____

6. tube implanted in the body to redirect the flow of a fluid

   _____

7. paralysis from the waist
   down caused by damage to
   the lower level of the spinal
   cord   _____

8. state of profound
   unconsciousness   _____

9. fainting   _____

10. lack of muscle coordination   _____

11. a manner or style of walking   _____

12. loss of cognitive abilities   _____

13. unable to express one's
    thoughts or ideas in an
    orderly, intelligible manner   _____

14. a state of mental confusion
    as to time, place, or identity   _____

15. pertaining to the mental
    processes of comprehension,
    judgment, memory, and
    reason   _____

16. conveying toward the center   _____

17. conveying away from the
    center   _____

EXERCISE 28

Write the definitions for the following terms.

1. shunt _____

2. paraplegia _____

3. coma _____

4. concussion _____

5. unconsciousness _____

6. conscious _____

7. seizure _____

8. convulsion _____

9. syncope _____

10. ataxia _____

11. dementia _____

12. gait _____

13. cognitive _____

14. disorientation _____

15. incoherent _____

16. efferent _____

17. afferent _____

EXERCISE 29

Spell each of the complementary terms. Have someone dictate the terms on pp. 573-574 to you. Study any words you have spelled incorrectly.

1. _____   10. _____

2. _____   11. _____

3. _____   12. _____

4. _____   13. _____

5. _____   14. _____

6. _____   15. _____

7. _____   16. _____

8. _____   17. _____

9. _____

Common Behavioral Health Disorders

Although the terms below are listed as behavioral health disorders, medications, physical changes, substance abuse, and illness may contribute to these conditions.

Term	Definition
anorexia nervosa (an-ō-REK-sē-a) (ner-VŌ-sa)	an eating disorder characterized by failure to maintain body weight, intensive fear of gaining weight, pronounced desire for thinness, and, in females, amenorrhea (introduced in Chapter 11)
anxiety disorder (ang-ZĪ-e-tē) (dis-OR-der)	an emotional disorder characterized by feelings of apprehension, tension, or uneasiness arising typically from the anticipation of unreal or imagined danger

attention deficit–hyperactivity disorder (ADHD) ....
(a-TEN-shun) (DEF-i-sit) (hī-PER-ac-*tiv*-i-tē)

a disorder of learning and behavioral problems characterized by marked inattention, impulsiveness, and hyperactivity

bipolar disorder.............................
(bī-PŌ-lar)
(dis-OR-der)

a major psychological disorder typified by a disturbance in mood. The disorder is manifested by manic and depressive episodes that may alternate or may occur simultaneously.

bulimia nervosa ....
(bū-LĒ-mē-a) (ner-VŌ-sa)

an eating disorder characterized by uncontrolled binge eating followed by purging (induced vomiting) (introduced in Chapter 11)

major depression ....
(mā-jor)
(dē-PRESH-un)

a mood disturbance characterized by feelings of sadness, despair, and discouragement. Depression ranges from normal feelings of sadness (resulting from and proportional to personal loss or tragedy), through dysthymia (depressive neurosis), to major depression.

obsessive-compulsive disorder (OCD)...
(ob-SES-iv-kom-PUL-siv)
(dis-OR-der)

a disorder characterized by intrusive, unwanted thoughts that result in the tendency to perform repetitive acts or rituals (compulsions), usually as a means of releasing tension or relieving anxiety.

panic attack.....................................
(PAN-ik) (a-tak)

an episode of acute anxiety, occurring unpredictably, with feelings of acute apprehension, dyspnea, dizziness, sweating, and/or chest pain

phobia ....
(FŌ-bē-a)

a marked and persistent fear that is excessive or unreasonable cued by the presence or anticipation of a specific situation or object

pica..
(PĪ-ka)

compulsive eating of nonnutritive substances such as clay or ice. This condition is often a result of an iron deficiency. When iron deficiency is the cause of pica the condition will disappear in 1 or 2 weeks when treated with iron therapy.

posttraumatic stress disorder (PTSD)...
(pōst-tra-MAT-ik)
(stes) (dis-OR-der)

a disorder characterized by an acute emotional response to a traumatic event or severe emotional stress such as an airplane crash, repeated physical or emotional trauma, or military combat. Symptoms include anxiety, sleep disturbance, difficulty concentrating, and depression.

schizophrenia..................................
(skiz-ō-FRĒ-nē-a)

any one of a large group of psychotic disorders characterized by gross distortions of reality, disturbance of language and communication, withdrawal from social interaction, and the disorganization and fragmentation of thought, perception, and emotional reaction.

✿ CAM TERM

Craniosacral therapy is the use of gentle manual pressure applied to the skull and spine to affect the meninges and cerebrospinal fluid. Craniosacral therapy is used extensively, with a high rate of success, to treat attention deficit–hyperactivity disorder (ADHD).

| somatoform disorders........................ | physical symptoms for which no known |
| (sō-MAT-ō-form) | physical cause exists. |

Refer to Appendix I for a more complete list of psychiatric terms.
Practice saying the terms aloud. To hear the terms, access the **PRONOUNCE IT** activity for this chapter on the Student CD that accompanies this text. Or, to hear the terms and their definitions with a CD player or computer, obtain the Pronunciation CD designed for use with this text.

Learn the definitions and spellings of common psychiatric disorder terms by completing exercises 30 and 31.

EXERCISE 30

Match the definitions in the first column with the correct terms in the second column.

_____ 1. manifested by manic and depressive episodes

_____ 2. an episode of acute anxiety

_____ 3. characterized by feelings of apprehension and tension

_____ 4. a disorder of learning and behavioral problems

_____ 5. a mood disturbance characterized by feelings of sadness, despair, and discouragement

_____ 6. a marked and persistent fear that is excessive or unreasonable

_____ 7. binge eating followed by purging

_____ 8. physical symptoms for which no known physical cause exists

_____ 9. eating of nonnutritive substances, such as ice

_____ 10. failure to maintain body weight

_____ 11. characterized by gross distortions of reality and disturbance of language and communication

a. phobia

b. anxiety disorder

c. attention deficit–hyperactivity disorder

d. somatoform disorders

e. schizophrenia

f. anorexia nervosa

g. bulimia nervosa

h. pica

i. bipolar disorder

j. major depression

k. obsessive-compulsive disorder

l. posttraumatic stress disorder

m. panic attack

_____ 12. acute emotional
response to a traumatic
event

_____ 13. intrusive unwanted
thoughts that result in
rituals and/or repetitive
acts

EXERCISE 31

Spell each of the psychiatric terms. Have someone dictate the terms on pp. 576-578 to you. Study any words you have spelled incorrectly.

1. _____   8. _____

2. _____   9. _____

3. _____   10. _____

4. _____   11. _____

5. _____   12. _____

6. _____   13. _____

7. _____

Abbreviations

AD	Alzheimer disease
ADHD	attention deficit–hyperactivity disorder
ALS	amyotrophic lateral sclerosis
CNS	central nervous system
CP	cerebral palsy
CSF	cerebrospinal fluid
CVA	cerebrovascular accident
EchoEG	echoencephalography
EEG	electroencephalogram
EP studies	evoked potential studies
LP	lumbar puncture
MRI scan	magnetic resonance imaging scan
MS	multiple sclerosis
OCD	obsessive-compulsive disorder
PD	Parkinson disease
PET scan	positron emission tomography scan
PNS	peripheral nervous system
PTSD	posttraumatic stress disorder
TIA	transient ischemic attack

EXERCISE 32

Write the meaning of the abbreviations in the following sentences.

1. Diagnostic tests used to diagnose patients with diseases of the nervous system include **EchoEG** _____, **EEG** _____, **MRI scan** _____ _____ _____, **PET scan** _____ _____ _____, **EP studies** _____ _____, and **LP** _____ _____.

2. Diseases that affect the nervous system are **AD** _____ _____, **ALS** _____ _____ _____, **CP** _____ _____, **MS** _____ _____, and **PD** _____ _____.

3. **CVA** _____ _____ is the disruption of normal blood supply to the brain. It often occurs suddenly. Because of this, Hippocrates used the term *apoplexy,* which literally means *struck down,* to describe the condition. The term *stroke,* which is still commonly used to describe CVA, grew out of the term *apoplexy,* meaning *struck down* or *stroke.* The term *brain attack* is a fairly new term used to signify that a stroke is in progress and an emergency situation exists. An ischemic stroke, which is caused by a thrombosis or embolus, is frequently preceded by a **TIA** _____ _____ _____.

4. The examination of **CSF** _____ _____ may assist in the diagnosis of cerebral hemorrhage, meningitis, encephalitis, and other diseases.

5. Three common psychiatric disorders are **PTSD,** _____ _____ _____, **OCD** _____ _____ _____, and **ADHD** _____ _____ _____ _____.

6. The nervous system may be divided into the **CNS** _____ _____ _____, and the **PNS** _____ _____ _____.

CHAPTER REVIEW

EXERCISE **33** *Interact with Medical Records*

Complete the progress note by writing the medical terms in the blanks. Use the list of definitions with the corresponding numbers.

University Hospital and Medical Center
4700 North Main Street • Wellness, Arizona 54321 • (987) 555-3210

PATIENT NAME: Eldon Drake   **CASE NUMBER:** 71086-NUR
DATE OF BIRTH: 08/12/xx   **DATE OF ADMISSION:** 01/02/xx

PROGRESS NOTE

HISTORY: Eldon Drake is an 85-year-old white man who was admitted to the hospital on 01/02/xx for fever and confusion. Mr. Drake was in his usual state of good health until 3 days before admission, when he began to show signs of confusion and 1. _____ accompanied by a fever of 38.5. His fever continued, and he showed a steady decline in 2. _____ function. He developed expressive 3. _____.

OBJECTIVE FINDINGS: On physical examination the patient was 4. _____ and alert but disoriented to time and place. Blood pressure was 160/80. Pulse, 96. Respirations, 20. Temperature 38.8. There were no focal neurologic deficits. Chest x-ray, urinalysis, and blood cultures were negative. A 5. _____ consultation was obtained. 6. _____ _____ _____ of the brain was performed, which disclosed 7. _____. An 8. _____ was markedly abnormal for his age.

TREATMENT SUMMARY: The patient was given acyclovir intravenous infusion. On the second hospital day, the patient developed a generalized 9. _____. He was placed on intravenous Dilantin and Lorazepam. He later lapsed into a semicomatose state. He responded to tactile and verbal stimuli but was completely 10. _____. A nasogastric tube was placed, and enteral feedings were begun. After 14 days of IV acyclovir, the patient slowly began to improve and by the third week of his illness, he was talking normally and taking nourishment. He is expected to make a complete recovery.

Rashid Magolot, MD

RM/mcm

---

1. a state of mental confusion as to time, place, or identity
2. pertaining to the mental processes of comprehension, judgment, memory, and reason
3. loss of the ability to speak
4. awake, alert, and aware of one's surroundings
5. study of nerves (branch of medicine dealing with diseases of the nervous system)
6. noninvasive technique that produces cross-sectional and sagittal images of the brain by magnetic waves
7. inflammation of the brain
8. record of electrical impulses of the brain
9. sudden attack with involuntary series of contractions
10. unable to express one's thoughts or ideas in an orderly, intelligible manner

EXERCISE 34 *Interpret Medical Terms*

To test your understanding of the terms introduced in this chapter, circle the words that correctly complete the sentences. The italicized words refer to the correct answer.

1. *Tetraplegia* is synonymous with (paraplegia, monoplegia, hemiplegia, quadriplegia).
2. The *inability to speak* or (aphagia, aphasia, dysphasia, dysphagia) may be an after-effect of cerebrovascular accident.
3. A symptom of brain concussion that may cause a patient to be *unaware of his or her surroundings* and *unable to respond to stimuli* is (subconscious, unconscious, convulsive).
4. The newborn had *meninges protruding through a defect in his skull,* or a (meningocele, myelomeningocele, myelomalacia).
5. *The branch of medicine that deals with the treatment of mental disorders* is (neurology, psychology, psychiatry).
6. *Multiple sclerosis* is a disease of the nervous system and generally occurs in young adults. It is characterized by (seizures, hardened patches along the brain and spinal cord, muscular tremors).
7. *The process of recording of electrical impulses of the brain,* or (echoencephalogram, electroencephalogram, electroencephalograph, electroencephalography), is used to study brain function and is valuable for diagnosing epilepsy, tumors, and other brain diseases.
8. Cerebral *thrombosis,* or abnormal condition of (a) (blood clot, infection, hardened patches), may cause a stroke.
9. The patient was admitted to the neurology unit of the hospital with a diagnosis of cerebrovascular accident. The physician ordered *a diagnostic procedure to examine blood flow and metabolic activity* or (computed tomography, positron emission tomography, magnetic resonance imaging).
10. The patient was diagnosed with (ganglion, ganglia) on both wrists.

EXERCISE 35 *Read Medical Terms in Use*

Practice pronunciation of terms by reading the following document. Use the pronunciation key following the medical term to assist you in saying the word.

A 78-year-old right-handed man presented to the Emergency Department with a right **hemiparesis** (*hem*-i-pa-RĒ-sis), expressive **aphasia** (a-FĀ-zē-a), and no apparent **cognitive** (COG-ni-tiv) decline. He has a history of hypertension and 2 years ago had a **transient ischemic** (is-KĒM-ik) **attack.** A **computed tomography** (tō-MOG-ra-fē) scan of the brain was negative for an **intracerebral** (in-tra-SER-e-bral) hemorrhage. A **neurologist** (nū-ROL-ō-jist) was consulted. She confirmed the diagnosis of a **cerebrovascular** (se-rē-brō-VAS-kū-lar) **accident** after **magnetic resonance imaging** (mag-NET-ik) (re-zo-NANCE) (IM-a-jing) of the brain demonstrated an ischemic area of the left **cerebral** (se-RĒ-bral) cortex.

EXERCISE 36   *Comprehend Medical Terms in Use*

Test your comprehension of terms in the previous medical document by circling the correct answer.

1. While in the emergency department the patient had:
   a. inability to swallow and paralysis from the waist down
   b. inability to speak and slight paralysis of the right side of the body
   c. inability to swallow and slight paralysis of the right side of the body
   d. inability to speak and paralysis from the waist down
2. T   F   A diagnosis of stroke was made after an MRI of the brain was performed.
3. The patient had a history of:
   a. sudden deficient supply of blood to the brain
   b. sudden loss of consciousness
   c. slight paralysis of one side
   d. a clot in the cerebrum

COMBINING FORMS CROSSWORD PUZZLE

Across Clues

2. mind
4. cerebellum
6. abbreviation for diabetes insipidus
7. abbreviation for undetermined origin
8. brain
13. nerve root
14. mind
15. ganglion
16. speech

Down Clues

1. four
2. spinal cord
3. gray matter
5. sensation
6. dura mater
9. cerebrum
10. meninges
11. one
12. mind

REVIEW OF WORD PARTS

Can you define and spell the following word parts?

Combining Forms

cerebell/o	myel/o
cerebr/o	neur/o
dur/o	phas/o
encephal/o	phren/o
esthesi/o	poli/o
gangli/o	psych/o
ganglion/o	quadr/i
mening/i	radic/o
mening/o	radicul/o
ment/o	rhiz/o
mon/o	

Prefix

tetra-

Suffixes

-iatrist
-iatry
-ictal
-paresis

REVIEW OF TERMS

Can you build, analyze, define, pronounce, and spell the following terms *built from word parts?*

Diseases and Disorders

cerebellitis
cerebral thrombosis
duritis
encephalitis
encephalomalacia
encephalomyeloradiculitis
gangliitis
meningitis
meningocele
meningomyelocele
neuralgia
neurasthenia
neuritis
neuroarthropathy
neuroblast
neuroma
poliomyelitis
polyneuritis
radiculitis
rhizomeningomyelitis
subdural hematoma

Surgical

ganglionectomy
neurectomy
neurolysis
neuroplasty
neurorrhaphy
neurotomy
radicotomy
rhizotomy

Diagnostic

cerebral angiography
CT myelography
echoencephalography
    (EchoEG)
electroencephalogram
    (EEG)
electroencephalograph
electroencephalography

Complementary

anesthesia
aphasia
cephalalgia
cerebral
craniocerebral
dysphasia
encephalosclerosis
hemiparesis
hemiplegia
hyperesthesia
interictal
intracerebral
monoparesis
monoplegia
myelomalacia
neuroid
neurologist
neurology
panplegia
phrenic
phrenopathy
postictal
preictal
psychiatrist
psychiatry
psychogenic
psychologist
psychology
psychopathy
psychosomatic
quadriplegia
subdural
tetraplegia

Can you define, pronounce, and spell the following terms *not built from word parts?*

Diseases and Disorders

Alzheimer disease (AD)
amyotrophic lateral
  sclerosis (ALS)
Bell palsy
cerebral aneurysm
cerebral palsy (CP)
cerebrovascular accident
  (CVA)
epilepsy
hydrocephalus
multiple sclerosis (MS)
neurosis
Parkinson disease (PD)
psychosis
Reye syndrome
sciatica
shingles
transient ischemic attack
  (TIA)

Diagnostic

computed tomography
  of the brain (CT)
evoked potential
  studies (EP)
lumbar puncture (LP)
magnetic resonance
  imaging (MRI)
positron emission
  tomography of the
  brain (PET)

Complementary

afferent
ataxia
cognitive
coma
concussion
conscious
convulsion
dementia
disorientation
efferent
gait
incoherent
paraplegia
seizure
shunt
syncope
unconsciousness

Common Behavioral Health Disorders

anorexia nervosa
anxiety disorder
attention deficit–
  hyperactivity disorder
  (ADHD)
bipolar disorder
bulimia nervosa
major depression
obsessive-compulsive
  disorder (OCD)
panic attack
phobia
pica
posttraumatic stress
  disorder (PTSD)
schizophrenia
somatoform disorders

16

Endocrine System

OUTLINE

OBJECTIVES

On completion of this chapter you will be able to:

1. Identify the organs and other structures of the endocrine system.
2. Define and spell the word parts presented in this chapter.
3. Build and analyze medical terms with word parts presented in this and previous chapters.
4. Define, pronounce, and spell the disease and disorder, diagnostic, surgical, and complementary terms for the endocrine system.
5. Interpret the meaning of the abbreviations presented in this chapter.
6. Read medical documents and interpret medical terminology contained in them.

ANATOMY

Function

The function of the endocrine system is to regulate body activities through the use of chemical messengers called *hormones,* which when released into the bloodstream influence metabolic activities, growth, and development (Figure 16-1). The nervous system also regulates body activities but does so through electrical impulses and activation of glandular secretions. *Hormones* secreted by the *endocrine glands* that make up the endocrine system go directly into the bloodstream and are transported throughout the body. They are referred to as *ductless glands* because they do not have ducts to carry their secretions. In contrast, the *exocrine* or *duct glands* have ducts that carry their secretions from the producing gland to other parts of the body. An example is the parotid gland, which produces saliva that flows through the parotid duct into the mouth. Only those terms related to the major endocrine glands—pituitary, thyroid, parathyroids, adrenals, and the islets of Langerhans in the pancreas—are presented in this chapter. The thymus and the male and female sex glands were discussed in previous chapters.

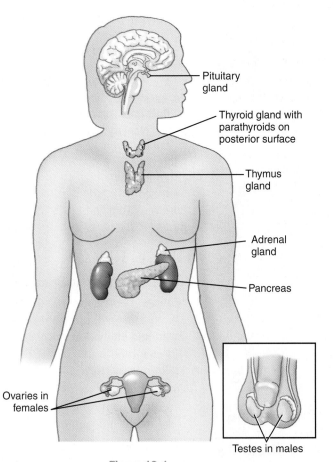

Figure 16-1
The endocrine system.

Endocrine Glands

pituitary gland, hypophysis cerebri	approximately the size of a pea and located at the base of the brain. The pituitary is divided into two lobes (Figure 16-2).
anterior lobe or adenohypophysis	produces and secretes the following hormones:
growth hormone (GH)	regulates the growth of the body
adrenocorticotropic hormone (ACTH)	stimulates the adrenal cortex
thyroid-stimulating hormone (TSH)	stimulates the thyroid gland
gonadotropic hormones	affect the male and female reproductive systems
follicle-stimulating hormone (FSH), luteinizing hormone (LH)	regulate development, growth, and function of the ovaries and testes
prolactin or lactogenic hormone (PRL)	promotes development of glandular tissue during pregnancy and produces milk after birth of an infant
posterior lobe or neurohypophysis	stores and releases antidiuretic hormone and oxytocin
antidiuretic hormone (ADH)	stimulates the kidney to reabsorb water
oxytocin	stimulates uterine contractions during labor and postpartum
hypothalamus	located near the pituitary gland in the brain. The hypothalamus secretes "releasing" hormone that functions to stimulate or inhibit the release of pituitary gland hormones.
thyroid gland	largest endocrine gland. It is located in the neck below the larynx and comprises bilateral lobes connected by an isthmus (see Figure 16-2). The thyroid gland secretes the hormones triiodothyronine (T_3) and thyroxine (T_4), which require iodine for their production. Thyroxine is necessary for body cell metabolism.
parathyroid glands	four small bodies lying directly behind the thyroid (see Figure 16-2). Parathormone (PTH), the hormone produced by the glands, helps maintain the level of calcium in the blood.

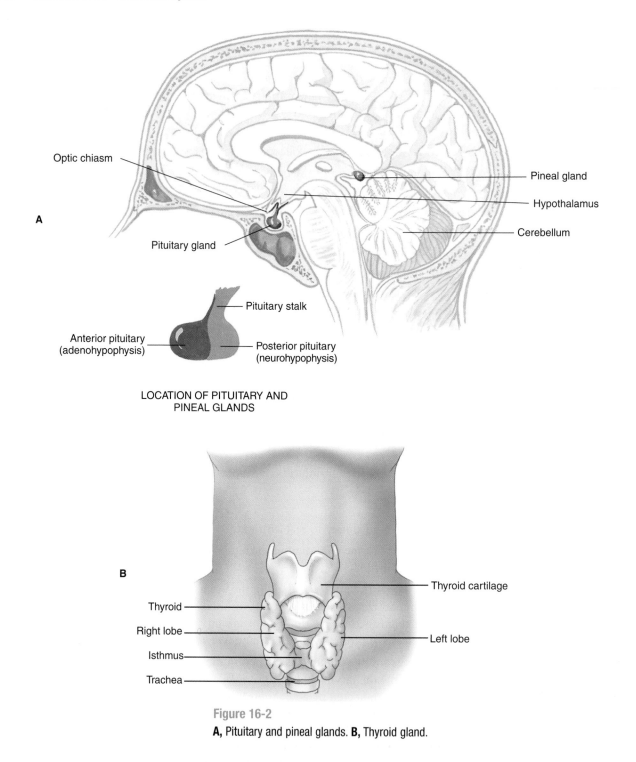

LOCATION OF PITUITARY AND
PINEAL GLANDS

Figure 16-2

A, Pituitary and pineal glands. **B,** Thyroid gland.

islets of Langerhans .... clusters of endocrine tissue found throughout the pancreas, made up of different cell types that secrete various hormones, including insulin and glucagon. Nonendocrine cells found throughout the pancreas perform nonendocrine functions such as digestion (Figure 16-3).

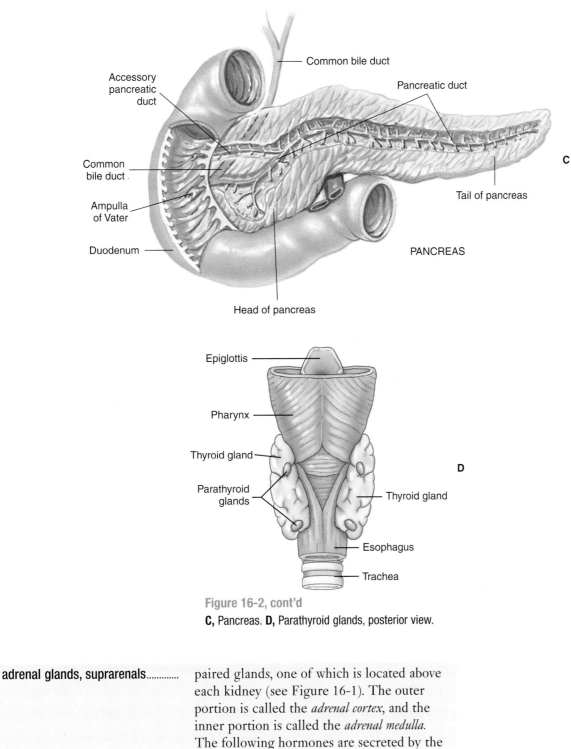

Common bile duct

Accessory
pancreatic
duct

Pancreatic duct

Common
bile duct

C

Ampulla
of Vater

Tail of pancreas

Duodenum

PANCREAS

Head of pancreas

Epiglottis

Pharynx

Thyroid gland

D

Parathyroid
glands

Thyroid gland

Esophagus

Trachea

Figure 16-2, cont'd
C, Pancreas. **D,** Parathyroid glands, posterior view.

adrenal glands, suprarenals............	paired glands, one of which is located above each kidney (see Figure 16-1). The outer portion is called the *adrenal cortex*, and the inner portion is called the *adrenal medulla*. The following hormones are secreted by the adrenal glands:
cortisol.................................	secreted by the cortex. It aids the body during stress by increasing glucose levels to provide energy (also called *hydrocortisone*)
aldosterone.............................	secreted by the cortex. Electrolytes (mineral salts) that are necessary for normal body function are regulated by this hormone.

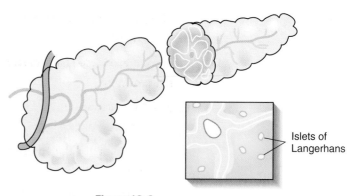

Figure 16-3
Pancreas, with islets of Langerhans.

| epinephrine (adrenaline), norepinephrine (noradrenaline) ... | secreted by the medulla. These hormones help the body to deal with stress by increasing the blood pressure, heartbeat, and respirations. |

Learn the anatomic terms by completing exercises 1 and 2.

EXERCISE 1

Match the terms in the first column with the correct definitions in the second column.

_____ 1. adrenal cortex

_____ 2. adrenal glands

_____ 3. adrenaline

_____ 4. adrenal medulla

_____ 5. adrenocorticotropic hormone

_____ 6. adenohypophysis

_____ 7. aldosterone

a. hormone that stimulates the adrenal cortex

b. tissue that secretes cortisol and aldosterone

c. anterior lobe of pituitary that secretes growth hormone and thyroid-stimulating hormone

d. another name for epinephrine

e. assists in regulating body electrolytes

f. another name for norepinephrine

g. located above each kidney

h. secretes epinephrine and norepinephrine

EXERCISE 2

Match the terms in the first column with the correct phrases in the second column.

_____ 1. antidiuretic hormone

_____ 2. islets of Langerhans

_____ 3. neurohypophysis

_____ 4. parathyroid glands

a. portions of the pancreas that secrete insulin

b. glands that maintain the blood calcium level

_____ 5. pituitary gland

_____ 6. thyroid gland

c. gland located in the neck that secretes thyroxine

d. hormone secreted by posterior lobe of the pituitary

e. gland that stores and releases antidiuretic hormone and oxytocin

f. another name for the anterior lobe of the pituitary

g. gland located at the base of the brain

WORD PARTS

Combining Forms of the Endocrine System

Study the word parts and their definitions listed below. Completing the exercises that follow will help you learn the terms.

Combining Form	Definition
aden/o (NOTE: *aden/o* was introduced in Chapter 2.)	gland
adren/o, adrenal/o	adrenal glands
cortic/o	cortex (the outer layer of a body organ)
endocrin/o	endocrine
parathyroid/o	parathyroid glands
thyroid/o, thyr/o	thyroid gland

Learn the anatomic locations and meanings of the combining forms by completing exercises 3 and 4 and Exercise Figures A and B.

EXERCISE   3

Write the definitions of the following combining forms.

1. cortic/o _____

2. adren/o _____

3. parathyroid/o _____

4. thyroid/o _____

5. adrenal/o _____

6. thyr/o _____

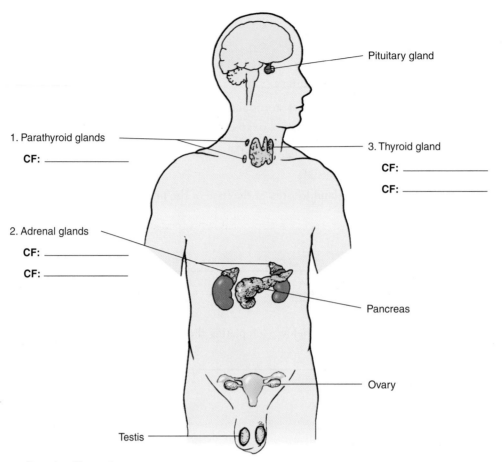

Pituitary gland

1. Parathyroid glands

CF: _____

3. Thyroid gland

CF: _____

CF: _____

2. Adrenal glands

CF: _____

CF: _____

Pancreas

Ovary

Testis

Exercise Figure A
Fill in the blanks with combining forms in this diagram of the endocrine glands in the human body.

7. endocrin/o _____

8. aden/o _____

EXERCISE 4

Write the combining form for each of the following terms.

1. adrenal gland
   a. _____
   b. _____

2. thyroid gland
   a. _____
   b. _____

3. endocrine _____

4. cortex _____

5. parathyroid gland _____

6. gland _____

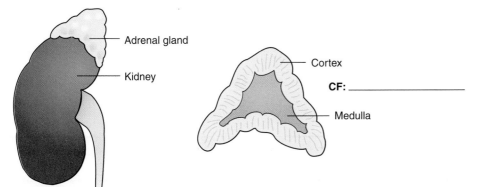

Exercise Figure B
Fill in the blank with the combining form in this diagram of adrenal glands (with transverse cross-sectional view).

Combining Forms Commonly Used with Endocrine System Terms

Combining Form	Definition
acr/o	extremities, height
calc/i	calcium
(NOTE: The combining vowel is *i*.)	
dips/o	thirst
kal/i	potassium
(NOTE: the combining vowel is *i*.)	
natr/o	sodium

Learn the combining forms by completing exercises 5 and 6.

EXERCISE 5

Write the definitions of the following combining forms.

1. dips/o _____

2. kal/i _____

3. calc/i _____

4. acr/o _____

5. natr/o _____

EXERCISE 6

Write the combining form for each of the following.

1. extremities, height   _____

2. calcium   _____

3. thirst _____

4. potassium _____

5. sodium _____

Suffix

Suffix	Definition
-drome	run, running

Learn the suffix by completing exercises 7 and 8. Refer to Appendix A and Appendix B for a complete list of word parts.

EXERCISE 7

Write the definition of the following word part.

1. -drome _____

EXERCISE 8

Write the suffix for the following.

1. run, running _____

MEDICAL TERMS

The terms you need to learn to complete this chapter are listed below. The exercises following each list will help you learn the definition and spelling of each word.

Disease and Disorder Terms

Built from Word Parts

Term	Definition
acromegaly .... (*ak*-rō-MEG-a-lē)	enlargement of the extremities (and bones of the face, hands, and feet caused by excessive production of the growth hormone by the pituitary gland after puberty) (Exercise Figure C)
adenitis .... (ad-e-NI-tis)	inflammation of a gland
adenodynia .... (*ad*-e-nō-DIN-ē-a)	pain in a gland
adenomalacia .... (*ad*-e-nō-ma-LĀ-shē-a)	abnormal softening of a gland
adenomegaly .... (*ad*-e-nō-MEG-a-lē)	enlargement of a gland

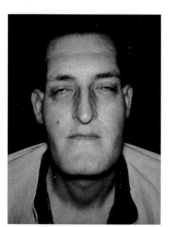

Exercise Figure C

Fill in the blanks to complete labeling of this photograph.

_____ / __cv__
extremities

_____ , a metabolic
enlargement

disorder characterized by marked enlargement of the bones of the face and extremities.

adenosis................................... (ad-e-NŌ-sis)	abnormal condition of a gland
adrenalitis............................... (ad-rēn-al-Ī-tis)	inflammation of the adrenal gland
adrenomegaly.......................... (ad-rēn-ō-MEG-a-lē)	enlargement (of one or both) of the adrenal glands
hypercalcemia.......................... (hī-per-kal-SĒ-mē-a)	excessive calcium (Ca) in the blood
hyperglycemia.......................... (hī-per-glī-SĒ-mē-a)	excessive sugar in the blood
hyperkalemia............................ (hī-per-ka-LĒ-mē-a)	excessive potassium (K) in the blood
hyperthyroidism....................... (hī-per-THĪ-royd-izm)	state of excessive thyroid gland activity (characterized by excessive secretion of thyroid hormones)
hypocalcemia........................... (hī-pō-kal-SĒ-mē-a)	deficient level of calcium in the blood
hypoglycemia........................... (hī-pō-glī-SĒ-mē-a)	deficient level of sugar in the blood
hypokalemia............................. (hī-pō-ka-LĒ-mē-a)	deficient level of potassium in the blood
hyponatremia........................... (hī-pō-na-TRĒ-mē-a)	deficient level of sodium (Na) in the blood
hypothyroidism........................ (hī-pō-THĪ-royd-izm)	state of deficient thyroid gland activity (characterized by decreased secretion of thyroid hormones)
parathyroidoma........................ (par-a-THĪ-roy-dō-ma)	tumor of a parathyroid gland
thyroiditis............................... (thī-roy-DĪ-tis)	inflammation of the thyroid gland

Practice saying each of these terms aloud. To hear the terms, access the **PRONOUNCE IT** activity for this chapter on the Student CD that accompanies this text. Or, to hear the terms and their definitions with a CD player or computer, obtain the Pronunciation CD designed for use with this text.

Learn the definitions and spellings of the disease and disorder terms by completing exercises 9, 10, and 11.

EXERCISE   9

Analyze and define the following terms.

1. adrenalitis _____

2. hypocalcemia _____

3. hyperthyroidism _____

4. hyperkalemia _____

5. hyperglycemia _____

6. adrenomegaly _____

7. adenomegaly _____

8. hypothyroidism _____

9. hypokalemia _____

10. adenitis _____

11. parathyroidoma _____

12. acromegaly _____

13. adenodynia _____

14. hypoglycemia _____

15. hypercalcemia _____

16. adenomalacia _____

17. hyponatremia _____

18. adenosis _____

19. thyroiditis _____

EXERCISE 10

Build disease and disorder terms for the following definitions with the word parts you have learned.

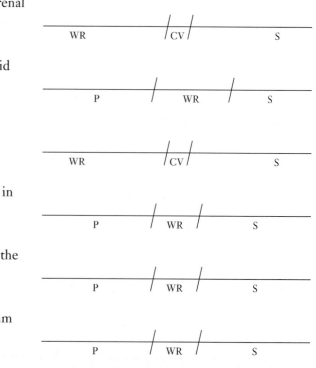

1. enlargement of the adrenal gland

   WR / CV / S

2. state of deficient thyroid gland activity

   P / WR / S

3. enlargement of the extremities

   WR / CV / S

4. deficient level of sugar in the blood

   P / WR / S

5. excessive potassium in the blood

   P / WR / S

6. deficient level of calcium in the blood

   P / WR / S

7. state of excessive production of the thyroid gland

_____ / _____ / _____
P   WR   S

8. abnormal softening of a gland

_____ / _____ / _____
WR   CV   S

9. excessive calcium in the blood

_____ / _____ / _____
P   WR   S

10. pain in a gland

_____ / _____
WR   S

11. tumor of a parathyroid

_____ / _____
WR   S

12. excessive sugar in the blood

_____ / _____ / _____
P   WR   S

13. abnormal condition of a gland

_____ / _____
WR   S

14. deficient level of potassium in the blood

_____ / _____ / _____
P   WR   S

15. inflammation of the adrenal gland

_____ / _____
WR   S

16. enlargement of a gland

_____ / _____ / _____
WR   CV   S

17. deficient level of sodium in the blood

_____ / _____ / _____
P   WR   S

18. inflammation of a gland

_____ / _____
WR   S

19. inflammation of the thyroid gland

_____ / _____
WR   S

EXERCISE 11

Spell each of the disease and disorder terms. Have someone dictate the terms on pp. 596-597 to you. Think about the word parts before attempting to write the word. Study any words you have spelled incorrectly.

1. _____   3. _____

2. _____   4. _____

5. _____   13. _____

6. _____   14. _____

7. _____   15. _____

8. _____   16. _____

9. _____   17. _____

10. _____   18. _____

11. _____   19. _____

12. _____

Disease and Disorder Terms

Not Built from Word Parts

Term	Definition
acidosis .... (*as*-i-DŌ-sis)	condition brought about by an abnormal accumulation of acid products of metabolism, seen frequently in uncontrolled diabetes mellitus (see discussion of diabetes mellitus that follows)
Addison disease .... (AD-i-sun) (di-ZĒZ)	chronic syndrome resulting from a deficiency in the hormonal secretion of the adrenal cortex. Symptoms may include weakness, darkening of skin, loss of appetite, depression, and other emotional problems.
cretinism .... (KRĒ-tin-izm)	condition caused by congenital absence or atrophy (wasting away) of the thyroid gland, resulting in hypothyroidism. The disease is characterized by puffy features, mental deficiency, large tongue, and dwarfism.
Cushing syndrome .... (KOOSH-ing) (SIN-drōm)	group of symptoms attributed to the excessive production of cortisol by the adrenal cortices (*pl.* of cortex). This syndrome may be the result of a pituitary tumor. Symptoms include abnormally pigmented skin, "moon face," pads of fat on the chest and abdomen, "buffalo hump" (fat on the upper back), and wasting away of muscle (Figure 16-4).
diabetes insipidus (DI) .... (dī-a-BĒ-tēz) (in-SIP-i-dus)	result of decreased secretion of antidiuretic hormone by the posterior lobe of the pituitary gland. Symptoms include excessive thirst *(polydipsia)* and large amounts of urine *(polyuria)* and sodium being excreted from the body.

Addison Disease
was named in **1855** for **Thomas Addison,** an English physician and pathologist. He described the disease as a "morbid state with feeble heart action, anemia, irritability of the stomach, and a peculiar change in the color of the skin."

Cushing Syndrome
was named for an American neurosurgeon, **Harvey Williams Cushing** (1869-1939), after he described adrenocortical hyperfunction.

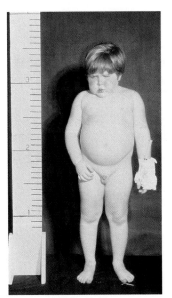

Figure 16-4
Cushing syndrome.

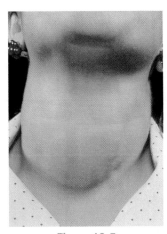

Figure 16-5
Goiter.

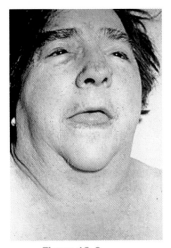

Figure 16-6
Myxedema.

diabetes mellitus (DM)......................
(dī-a-BĒ-tēz) (mel-LĪ-tus)

chronic disease involving a disorder of carbohydrate metabolism. Diabetes mellitus is caused by underactivity of the islets of Langerhans in the pancreas, which results in insufficient production of insulin. When the disease is not controlled or is untreated, the patient may develop ketosis, acidosis, and finally coma.

gigantism......................
(jī-GAN-tizm)

condition brought about by overproduction of growth hormone by the pituitary gland before puberty

goiter......................
(GOY-ter)

enlargement of the thyroid gland (Figure 16-5)

Graves disease......................
(grāvz) (di-ZĒZ)

a disorder of the thyroid gland characterized by the presence of hyperthyroidism, goiter, and exophthalmos

ketosis......................
(kē-TŌ-sis)

condition resulting from uncontrolled diabetes mellitus, in which the body has an abnormal concentration of ketone bodies (compounds that are a normal product of fat metabolism)

myxedema......................
(mik-se-DĒ-ma)

condition resulting from a deficiency of the thyroid hormone thyroxine. A severe form of hypothyroidism in an adult. Symptoms include puffiness of the face and hands, coarse and thickened skin, enlarged tongue, slow speech, and anemia (Figure 16-6).

tetany......................
(TET-a-nē)

condition affecting nerves causing muscle spasms as a result of low amounts of calcium in the blood caused by a deficiency of the parathyroid hormone

---

Gigantism and Acromegaly
are both caused by overproduction of growth hormone. **Gigantism** occurs before puberty and before the growing ends of the bones have closed. If untreated, an individual may reach 8 feet tall in adulthood.

Acromegaly occurs after puberty. The bones most affected are those in the hands, feet, and jaw.

Insufficient production of growth hormone in children is one cause of **dwarfism**, or underdevelopment of the body. In adulthood, a dwarf may be as small as 2.5 feet tall.

Goiter
may be caused by Graves disease, thyroiditis, or a thyroid nodule, which is a lump on the thyroid gland. Goiter is a general term for the enlargement of the thyroid gland.

Because of early medical intervention and because iodine is in table salt and many foods, goiter is rare in the United States today.

Hypothyroidism
is the state of deficient thyroid gland activity, resulting in the decreased production of the thyroid hormone called thyroxine. A severe form of hypothyroidism in adults is called **myxedema** and in children is called **cretinism**.

thyrotoxicosis.............................	a condition caused by excessive thyroid
(*thī*-rō-*tok*-si-KŌ-sis)	hormones

Practice saying each of these terms aloud. To hear the terms, access the **PRONOUNCE IT** activity for this chapter on the Student CD that accompanies this text. Or, to hear the terms and their definitions with a CD player or computer, obtain the Pronunciation CD designed for use with this text.

Learn the definitions and spellings of the disease and disorder terms by completing exercises 12, 13, and 14.

Diabetes Mellitus

Two major forms of diabetes mellitus are **type 1,** previously called *insulin-dependent diabetes mellitus (IDDM)* or *juvenile-onset diabetes,* and **type 2,** previously called *noninsulin-dependent diabetes mellitus (NIDDM)* or *adult-onset diabetes (AODM).*

Type 1 diabetes mellitus

Cause	the beta cells of the pancreas that produce insulin are destroyed and eventually no insulin is produced
Characteristics	abrupt onset, occurs primarily in childhood or adolescence. Patients often are thin.
Symptoms	polyuria, polydipsia, weight loss, and hyperglycemia
Treatment	insulin injections and diet

Type 2 diabetes mellitus

Cause	resistance of body cells to the action of insulin and also a decrease in insulin secretion
Characteristics	slow onset, usually occurs in middle-aged or elderly adults. Many patients are obese.
Symptoms	fatigue, blurred vision, thirst, and hyperglycemia. May have neural or vascular complications.
Treatment	oral hypoglycemics or insulin and diet

Long-term complications of both types of diabetes mellitus include diabetic neuropathy, diabetic nephropathy, diabetic retinopathy, and atherosclerosis.

EXERCISE 12

Match the terms in the first column with the correct definitions in the second column.

_____ 1. acidosis

_____ 2. Addison disease

_____ 3. cretinism

_____ 4. Cushing syndrome

_____ 5. diabetes insipidus

_____ 6. diabetes mellitus

_____ 7. gigantism

_____ 8. goiter

_____ 9. ketosis

_____ 10. myxedema

_____ 11. tetany

a. results from a deficiency in the hormonal secretion of the adrenal cortex

b. attributed to the excessive production of cortisol

c. caused by underactivity of the islets of Langerhans

d. abnormal accumulation of acid products of metabolism

e. enlargement of the thyroid gland

f. results from low blood calcium

g. caused by excessive thyroid hormones

_____ 12. thyrotoxicosis

_____ 13. Graves disease

h. result of a decreased amount of anti-diuretic hormone

i. caused by deficiency of the thyroid hormone

j. caused by a wasting away of the thyroid gland

k. abnormal concentration of compounds resulting from fat metabolism

l. caused by overproduction of the pituitary growth hormone

m. caused by an excessive amount of parathormone

n. characterized by hyperthyroidism, goiter, and exophthalmos

EXERCISE 13

Write the name of the endocrine gland responsible for each of the following conditions.

1. myxedema _____

2. tetany _____

3. ketosis _____

4. gigantism _____

5. goiter _____

6. Addison disease _____

7. diabetes mellitus _____

8. cretinism _____

9. acidosis _____

10. Cushing syndrome _____

11. diabetes insipidus _____

12. Graves disease _____

13. thyrotoxicosis _____

EXERCISE 14

Spell the disease and disorder terms. Have someone dictate the terms on pp. 600-603 to you. Study any words you have spelled incorrectly.

1. _____   8. _____

2. _____   9. _____

3. _____   10. _____

4. _____   11. _____

5. _____   12. _____

6. _____   13. _____

7. _____

Surgical Terms

Built from Word Parts

Term	Definition
adenectomy .... (*ad*-en-EK-tō-mē)	excision of a gland
adrenalectomy .... (ad-*rē*-nal-EK-tō-mē)	excision of an adrenal gland
parathyroidectomy .... (*par*-a-*thī*-royd-EK-tō-mē)	excision of a parathyroid gland
thyroidectomy .... (*thī*-royd-EK-tō-mē)	excision of the thyroid gland
thyroidotomy .... (*thī*-royd-OT-ō-mē)	incision of the thyroid gland
thyroparathyroidectomy .... (*thī*-rō-par-a-*thī*-royd-EK-tō-mē)	excision of the thyroid and parathyroid glands

Practice saying each of these terms aloud. To hear the terms, access the **PRONOUNCE IT** activity for this chapter on the Student CD that accompanies this text. Or, to hear the terms and their definitions with a CD player or computer, obtain the Pronunciation CD designed for use with this text.

Learn the definitions and spellings of the surgical terms by completing exercises 15, 16, and 17.

EXERCISE 15

Analyze and define the following surgical terms.

1. thyroidotomy _____

2. adrenalectomy _____

3. thyroparathyroidectomy _____

4. thyroidectomy   _____

5. parathyroidectomy _____

6. adenectomy_____

EXERCISE   16

Build surgical terms for the following definitions by using the word parts you have learned.

1. excision of the thyroid gland   _____/_____
   <small>WR   S</small>

2. excision of the thyroid and
   parathyroid glands   _____/__/_____/_____
   <small>WR   CV   WR   S</small>

3. excision of the adrenal gland   _____/_____
   <small>WR   S</small>

4. excision of a parathyroid
   gland   _____/_____
   <small>WR   S</small>

5. incision of the thyroid gland   _____/__/_____
   <small>WR   CV   S</small>

6. excision of a gland   _____/_____
   <small>WR   S</small>

EXERCISE   17

Spell each of the surgical terms. Have someone dictate the terms on p. 604 to you. Think about the word parts before attempting to write the word. Study any words you have spelled incorrectly.

1. _____   4. _____

2. _____   5. _____

3. _____   6. _____

Diagnostic Terms

Not Built from Word Parts

Term	Definition
Diagnostic Imaging	
radioactive iodine uptake test (RAIU).......................... (rā-dē-ō-AK-tiv) (Ī-ō-dīn)	a nuclear medicine scan that measures thyroid function. Radioactive iodine is given to the patient orally, after which its uptake into the thyroid gland is measured.

thyroid scan................................ a nuclear medicine test that shows the size,
    (THĪ-royd) shape, and position of the thyroid gland. The
patient is given a radioactive substance to
visualize the thyroid gland. An image is recorded as the scanner is passed over the neck
area. Used to detect tumors and nodules.

Laboratory

fasting blood sugar (FBS)................ a blood test to determine the amount of glucose (sugar) in the blood after fasting for 8 to
10 hours. Elevation indicates diabetes mellitus.

thyroid-stimulating hormone
level (TSH) (thyrotropin).................... a blood test that measures the amount of
    (THĪ-royd) thyroid-stimulating hormone in the blood. Used
to diagnose hyperthyroidism and to monitor
patients on thyroid replacement therapy.

thyroxine level (T₄)............................ a blood study that gives the direct measure-
    (thī-ROK-sin) ment of the amount of thyroxine in the pa-
tient's blood. A greater-than-normal amount
indicates hyperthyroidism; a less-than-normal
amount indicates hypothyroidism.

Ultrasound and **computed tomography (CT scanning)** are also used to diagnose various other conditions
of the endocrine system. Examples are CT of the adrenal glands and thyroid ultrasonography.

Practice saying each of the terms aloud. To hear the terms, access the **PRONOUNCE IT**
activity for this chapter on the Student CD that accompanies this text. Or, to hear the
terms and their definitions with a CD player or computer, obtain the Pronunciation CD
designed for use with this text.

To learn the definition and spelling of diagnostic terms complete exercises 18, 19,
and 20.

EXERCISE 18

Match the terms in the first column with their correct definitions in the second column.

_____ 1. fasting blood sugar

_____ 2. thyroid scan

_____ 3. thyroxine level

_____ 4. radioactive iodine
uptake

_____ 5. thyroid-stimulating
hormone level

a. a nuclear medicine test used to determine the size, shape, and position of the
thyroid gland

b. determines the amount of glucose in the
blood

c. used to determine hypernatremia

d. uses radioactive iodine to measure thyroid function

e. used to diagnose hyperthyroidism and to
monitor thyroid replacement therapy

f. measures the amount of thyroxine in the
blood

EXERCISE   19

Write the name of the procedure that measures each of the following.

1. thyroid function

   _____

2. amount of glucose in the
   blood

   _____

3. amount of thyroid-stimulating
   hormone in the blood

   _____

4. amount of thyroxine in the
   blood

   _____

5. size, shape, and position of
   the thyroid gland

   _____

EXERCISE   20

Spell each of the diagnostic terms. Have someone dictate the terms on pp. 605-606 to you. Study any words you have spelled incorrectly.

1. _____   4. _____

2. _____   5. _____

3. _____

Complementary Terms

Built from Word Parts

Term	Definition
adrenocorticohyperplasia................ (a-drē-nō-kōr-ti-kō-hī-per-PLA-zhē-a) (NOTE: *hyper,* a prefix, appears within this word.)	excessive development of the adrenal cortex
adrenopathy.............................. (*ad*-rēn-OP-a-thē)	disease of the adrenal gland
calcipenia .... (kal-si-PĒ-nē-a)	deficiency of calcium (also called *hypocalcemia*)
cortical.................................. (KŌR-ti-kal)	pertaining to the cortex
corticoid .... (KŌR-ti-koyd)	resembling the cortex
endocrinologist........................ (en-dō-kri-NOL-ō-jist)	a physician who studies and treats diseases of the endocrine system
endocrinology .... (en-dō-kri-NOL-ō-jē)	the study of the endocrine (system) (a branch of medicine dealing with diseases of the endocrine system)

endocrinopathy .... (en-dō-kri-NOP-a-thē)	(any) disease of the endocrine system
euthyroid .... (ū-THĪ-royd)	resembling a normal (functioning) thyroid gland
polydipsia .... (*pol-ē*-DIP-sē-a)	abnormal state of much thirst
syndrome .... (SIN-drōm)	(set of symptoms that) run (occur) together

Practice saying each of these terms aloud. To hear the terms, access the **PRONOUNCE IT** activity for this chapter on the Student CD that accompanies this text. Or, to hear the terms and their definitions with a CD player or computer, obtain the Pronunciation CD designed for use with this text.

Learn the definitions and spellings of the complementary terms by completing exercises 21, 22, and 23.

EXERCISE 21

Analyze and define the following complementary terms.

1. corticoid _____

2. syndrome _____

3. adrenopathy _____

4. endocrinologist _____

5. polydipsia _____

6. calcipenia _____

7. endocrinopathy _____

8. adrenocorticohyperplasia _____

9. euthyroid _____

10. cortical _____

11. endocrinology _____

EXERCISE 22

Build the complementary terms for the following definitions by using the word parts you have learned.

1. (any) disease of the endocrine system

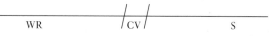

WR   CV   S

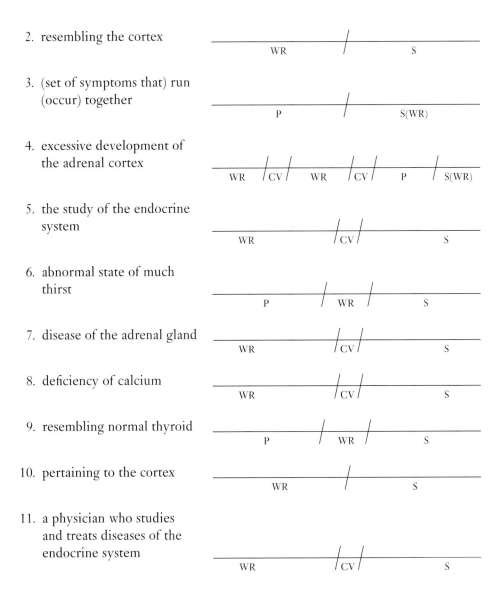

2. resembling the cortex

⎯⎯⎯⎯⎯⎯⎯⎯ / ⎯⎯⎯⎯⎯⎯⎯⎯
WR   S

3. (set of symptoms that) run
   (occur) together

⎯⎯⎯⎯⎯⎯⎯⎯ / ⎯⎯⎯⎯⎯⎯⎯⎯
P   S(WR)

4. excessive development of
   the adrenal cortex

⎯⎯ / CV / ⎯⎯ / CV / ⎯⎯ / ⎯⎯
WR   WR   P   S(WR)

5. the study of the endocrine
   system

⎯⎯⎯⎯ / CV / ⎯⎯⎯⎯
WR   S

6. abnormal state of much
   thirst

⎯⎯ / ⎯⎯ / ⎯⎯
P   WR   S

7. disease of the adrenal gland

⎯⎯ / CV / ⎯⎯
WR   S

8. deficiency of calcium

⎯⎯ / CV / ⎯⎯
WR   S

9. resembling normal thyroid

⎯⎯ / ⎯⎯ / ⎯⎯
P   WR   S

10. pertaining to the cortex

⎯⎯⎯⎯ / ⎯⎯⎯⎯
WR   S

11. a physician who studies
    and treats diseases of the
    endocrine system

⎯⎯ / CV / ⎯⎯
WR   S

EXERCISE 23

Spell each of the complementary terms. Have someone dictate the terms on pp. 607-608 to you. Think about the word parts before attempting to write the word. Study any words you have spelled incorrectly.

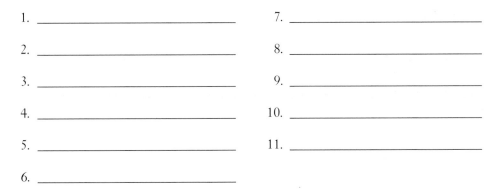

1. _____   7. _____

2. _____   8. _____

3. _____   9. _____

4. _____   10. _____

5. _____   11. _____

6. _____

Complementary Terms

Not Built from Word Parts

Term	Definition
exophthalmos (ek-sof-THAL-mos)	abnormal protrusion of the eyeball (Figure 16-7)
hormone (HOR-mōn)	a chemical substance secreted by an endocrine gland that is carried in the blood to a target tissue
isthmus (IS-mus)	narrow strip of tissue connecting two large parts in the body, such as the isthmus that connects the two lobes of the thyroid gland (see Figure 16-2, *B*)
metabolism (me-TAB-ō-lizm)	sum total of all the chemical processes that take place in a living organism

> **Exophthalmos**
> is derived from the Greek **ex,** meaning **outward,** and **ophthalmos,** meaning **eye.** Protrusion of the eyeball is sometimes a symptom of Graves disease, first described by Dr. Robert Graves, an Irish physician, in 1835.

Practice saying each of these terms aloud. To hear the terms, access the **PRONOUNCE IT** activity for this chapter on the Student CD that accompanies this text. Or, to hear the terms and their definitions with a CD player or computer, obtain the Pronunciation CD designed for use with this text.

Learn the definitions and spellings of the complementary terms by completing exercises 24, 25, and 26.

EXERCISE 24

Fill in the blanks with the correct terms.

1. The total of all the chemical processes that take place in a living organism is called its _____.

2. A chemical substance secreted by an endocrine gland is called a(n) _____.

3. A narrow strip of tissue connecting larger parts in the body is called a(n) _____.

4. Abnormal protrusion of the eyeball is called _____.

EXERCISE 25

Write the definitions of the following terms.

1. isthmus _____

2. metabolism _____

3. hormone _____

4. exophthalmos _____

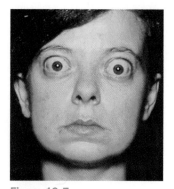

Figure 16-7
Abnormal protrusion of eyeballs, exophthalmos, a characteristic of thyroid disease.

EXERCISE 26

Spell each of the complementary terms. Have someone dictate the terms on p. 610 to you. Study any words you have spelled incorrectly.

1. _____   3. _____

2. _____   4. _____

Abbreviations

DI..	diabetes insipidus
DM	diabetes mellitus
FBS..	fasting blood sugar
RAIU..	radioactive iodine uptake
T_4	thyroxine level

EXERCISE 27

Write the meaning of the following abbreviations.

1. RAIU _____ _____ _____

2. FBS _____ _____ _____

3. DM _____ _____

4. DI _____ _____

5. T_4 _____ _____

EXERCISE 28 *Interact with Medical Records*

Complete the history and physical by writing the medical terms in the blanks. Use the list of definitions on p. 613 with the corresponding numbers.

University Hospital and Medical Center
4700 North Main Street • Wellness, Arizona 54321 • (987) 555-3210

PATIENT NAME: Jane Nelson   **CASE NUMBER:** 021286-END
DATE OF BIRTH: 05/21/xx   **DATE:** 06/20/xx

HISTORY AND PHYSICAL

CHIEF COMPLAINT: Jane Nelson is a 53-year-old white woman presenting with an episode of syncope at work, complaining of excessive urination and thirst and fatigue for approximately 1 month.

HISTORY OF PRESENT ILLNESS: For the past 4 weeks she has been having 1. _____ and 2. _____ , drinking 3 to 4 quarts of water daily for the past 10 days. This has also resulted in nocturia, getting up two to three times a night to void. She denies anorexia, nausea, vomiting, 3. _____ , or any abdominal pain.

MEDICAL HISTORY: No known allergies. No previous hospitalizations. She does not smoke or drink. She has had no recent illness.

FAMILY HISTORY: Mother died of a 4. _____ _____ at age 78. Father is still living at the age of 85, but has had 5. _____ _____ for 20 years. She has two brothers, both in good health, and no sisters.

SOCIAL HISTORY: Unmarried without children. She does not smoke and uses alcohol rarely.

REVIEW OF SYSTEMS: She denies fever, chills, headache, palpitations, chest pain, or edema.

PHYSICAL EXAM: Temperature, 98.9. Pulse, 80. Respirations, 24. Her blood pressure is 125/80. Her weight is 143 pounds, down 10 pounds since her last routine visit 3 months ago. **HEENT:** Normal. **CHEST:** Clear to auscultation and percussion. **HEART:** Normal S1 and S2. No S3 or S4. No murmurs, lifts, heaves, or thrills. Regular rhythm. **ABDOMEN:** Soft, nontender, bowel sounds normal, without evidence of organomegaly. **RECTAL:** Unremarkable. **EXTREMITIES:** No 6. _____ , clubbing, or edema. Pedal pulses are intact.
NEUROLOGIC: Alert and oriented to time, person, and place. Cranial nerves II through XII are grossly intact.

LABORATORY FINDINGS: Random blood sugar was discovered to be greater than 600 mg/dl. Urinalysis showed moderate ketonuria. Guaiac was negative.

ASSESSMENT: Diabetic 7. _____ , most likely caused by type 2 diabetes mellitus.

PLAN: Administer IV fluids and insulin. Schedule 8. _____ consult for this afternoon for complete diagnosis and treatment.

Christina Kraemer, MD

CK/mcm

1. excessive urine
2. excessive thirst
3. vomiting of blood
4. interruption of blood supply to the brain caused by cerebral thrombosis, cerebral embolism, or cerebral hemorrhage
5. chronic disease involving disorder of carbohydrate metabolism caused by underactivity of islets of Langerhans in the pancreas, which results in insufficient production of insulin
6. abnormal condition of blue (bluish discoloration of skin) caused by inadequate supply of oxygen in the blood
7. abnormal concentration of ketone bodies
8. study of the endocrine system

EXERCISE 29 *Interpret Medical Terms*

To test your understanding of the terms introduced in this chapter, circle the words that correctly complete the sentences. The italicized words refer to the correct answer.

1. A patient who has an *enlargement of the thyroid gland* has (myxedema, tetany, goiter).
2. A condition that results from *uncontrolled diabetes mellitus* is (calcipenia, ketosis, tetany).
3. *Addison disease* is caused by an *underfunctioning* of the (adrenal, pituitary, thyroid) gland.
4. *Decreased secretion* of (ACTH, antidiuretic hormone, TSH) may cause diabetes insipidus.
5. *Cushing syndrome* is caused by (overactivity, underactivity) of the *adrenal cortices*.
6. A *wasting away of the thyroid gland* may result in (cretinism, myxedema, tetany).
7. The term that means *pain in a gland* is (adenomalacia, adenomegaly, adenodynia).

EXERCISE 30 *Read Medical Terms in Use*

Practice pronunciation of the terms by reading the following medical document. Use the pronunciation key following the medical terms to assist you.

A 55-year-old female patient presented to her doctor because of a 10-pound weight gain, fatigue, hair loss, dry skin, and cold intolerance. She was referred to an **endocrinologist** (en-dō-kri-NOL-ō-jist), who established a diagnosis of **hypothyroidism** (hī-pō-THĪ-royd-izm) after test results indicated an elevated **thyroid** (THĪ-royd)-**stimulating hormone** (TSH) level and a low **thyroxine** (thī-ROX-sin) level. Thyroid hormone therapy was prescribed. Approximately 20 years ago she was diagnosed with Graves disease characterized by hyperthyroidism, **exophthalmos** (ek-sof-THAL-mos), fatigue, irritability, weight loss, and **goiter** (GOY-ter). At this time she had an increased **radioactive iodine** (ra-dē-ō-ak-tiv) (Ī-ō-dīn) **uptake** (RAIU). Treatment included a thyroidectomy (*thī*-royd-EK-tō-mē) with subsequent thyroid hormone therapy. She remained in a **euthyroid** (ū-THĪ-royd) state until she stopped taking the medication 6 months ago. Consequently she became hypothyroid and could easily have developed **myxedema** (*mik*-se-DĒ-ma) if she had not sought treatment.

EXERCISE 31 *Comprehend Medical Terms in Use*

Test your comprehension of terms in the previous medical document by circling the correct answer.

1. On a recent visit to the endocrinologist the patient was diagnosed with:
   a. a state of deficient thyroid gland activity
   b. an enlargement of the thyroid gland
   c. a state of excessive thyroid gland activity
   d. Graves disease

2. After a thyroidectomy the patient remained in a state resembling a:
   a. stressed thyroid gland
   b. normal thyroid gland
   c. hyperactive thyroid gland
   d. hypoactive thyroid gland
3. The patient's earlier diagnosis of Graves disease was characterized by:
   a. thirst, excessive thyroid activity, protruding eyes
   b. protruding eyes, spasms, excessive thyroid activity
   c. excessive thyroid activity, enlargement of the thyroid gland, protruding eyes
   d. enlargement of the extremities, excessive thyroid activities, protruding eyes
4. What type of diagnostic procedure was used to assist in diagnosing hypothyroidism?
   a. computed tomography
   b. nuclear medicine
   c. ultrasound
   d. blood test

For further practice or to evaluate what you have learned, use the Student CD that accompanies this text.

WORD PARTS CROSSWORD PUZZLE

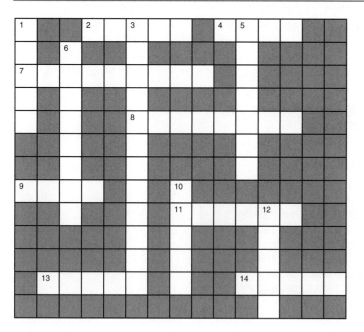

Across Clues
2. thirst
4. extremities, height
7. endocrine
8. thyroid gland
9. potassium
11. adrenal glands
13. thyroid gland
14. run, running

Down Clues
1. gland
3. parathyroid glands
5. cortex
6. adrenal glands
10. calcium
12. sodium

REVIEW OF WORD PARTS

Can you define and spell the following word parts?

Combining Forms

acr/o	endocrin/o
aden/o	kal/i
adren/o	natr/o
adrenal/o	parathyroid/o
calc/i	thyr/o
cortic/o	thyroid/o
dips/o	

Suffix

-drome

REVIEW OF TERMS

Can you build, analyze, define, pronounce, and spell the following terms *built from word parts?*

Diseases and Disorders

acromegaly	hyperglycemia
adenitis	hyperkalemia
adenodynia	hyperthyroidism
adenomalacia	hypocalcemia
adenomegaly	hypoglycemia
adenosis	hypokalemia
adrenalitis	hyponatremia
adrenomegaly	hypothyroidism
hypercalcemia	parathyroidoma
	thyroiditis

Surgical

adenectomy
adrenalectomy
parathyroidectomy
thyroidectomy
thyroidotomy
thyroparathyroidectomy

Complementary

adrenocorticohyperplasia
adrenopathy
calcipenia
cortical
corticoid
endocrinologist
endocrinology
endocrinopathy
euthyroid
polydipsia
syndrome

Can you define, pronounce, and spell the following terms *not built from word parts?*

Diseases and Disorders	Diagnostic	Complementary
acidosis	fasting blood sugar (FBS)	hormone
Addison disease	radioactive iodine uptake (RAIU)	isthmus
cretinism	thyroid scan	metabolism
Cushing syndrome	thyroid-stimulating hormone	exophthalmos
diabetes insipidus (DI)	level (TSH)	
diabetes mellitus (DM)	thyroxine level (T$_4$)	
gigantism		
goiter		
Graves disease		
ketosis		
myxedema		
tetany		
thyrotoxicosis		

APPENDIX A

Combining Forms, Prefixes, and Suffixes Alphabetized According to Word Part

Combining Forms	Definition	Chapter
abdomin/o	abdomen, abdominal cavity	11
acou/o	hearing	13
acr/o	extremities, height	16
aden/o	gland	2, 16
adenoid/o	adenoids	5
adrenal/o	adrenal gland	16
adren/o	adrenal gland	16
albumin/o	albumin	6
alveol/o	alveolus	5
amni/o	amnion	9
amnion/o	amnion	9
andr/o	male	7
angi/o	vessel	10
ankyl/o	crooked, stiff, bent	14
an/o	anus	11
anter/o	front	3
antr/o	antrum	11
aort/o	aorta	10
aponeur/o	aponeurosis	14
appendic/o	appendix	11
arche/o	first, beginning	8
arteri/o	artery	10
arthr/o	joint	14
atel/o	imperfect, incomplete	5
ather/o	yellowish, fatty plaque	10
atri/o	atrium	10
aur/i	ear	13
aur/o	ear	13
aut/o	self	4
azot/o	urea, nitrogen	6
balan/o	glans penis	7
bi/o	life	4
blast/o	developing cell	6
blephar/o	eyelid	12
bronch/i	bronchus	5
bronch/o	bronchus	5
burs/o	bursa (cavity)	14
calc/i	calcium	16
cancer/o	cancer	2
capn/o	carbon dioxide	5
carcin/o	cancer	2
cardi/o	heart	10

Combining Forms	Definition	Chapter
carp/o	carpals (wrist bones)	14
caud/o	tail (downward)	3
cec/o	cecum	11
celi/o	abdomen (abdominal cavity)	11
cephal/o	head	3, 9
cerebell/o	cerebellum	15
cerebr/o	cerebrum, brain	15
cervic/o	cervix	8
cheil/o	lip	11
chlor/o	green	2
cholangi/o	bile duct	11
chol/e	gall, bile	11
choledoch/o	common bile duct	11
chondr/o	cartilage	14
chori/o	chorion	9
chrom/o	color	2
clavic/o	clavicle (collarbone)	14
clavicul/o	clavicle (collarbone)	14
col/o	colon	11
colon/o	colon	11
colp/o	vagina	8
coni/o	dust	4
conjunctiv/o	conjunctiva	12
core/o	pupil	12
corne/o	cornea	12
cor/o	pupil	12
cortic/o	cortex (outer layer of body organ)	16
cost/o	rib	14
crani/o	cranium (skull)	14
cry/o	cold	12
crypt/o	hidden	4
culd/o	cul-de-sac	8
cutane/o	skin	4
cyan/o	blue	2
cyst/o	bladder, sac	6
cyt/o	cell	2
dacry/o	tear, tear duct	12
dermat/o	skin	4
derm/o	skin	4
diaphragmat/o	diaphragm	5
dipl/o	two, double	12
dips/o	thirst	16
disk/o	intervertebral disk	14
dist/o	away (from the point of attachment of a body part)	3
diverticul/o	diverticulum	11
dors/o	back	3
duoden/o	duodenum	11
dur/o	hard, dura mater	15
ech/o	sound	10
electr/o	electricity, electrical activity	10

Combining Forms	Definition	Chapter
embry/o	embryo, to be full	9
encephal/o	brain	15
endocrin/o	endocrine	16
enter/o	intestine	11
epididym/o	epididymis	7
epiglott/o	epiglottis	5
episi/o	vulva	8
epitheli/o	epithelium	2
erythr/o	red	2
esophag/o	esophagus	9, 11
esthesi/o	sensation, sensitivity, feeling	15
eti/o	cause (of disease)	2
femor/o	femur (upper leg bone)	14
fet/i	fetus, unborn child	9
fet/o	fetus, unborn child	9
fibr/o	fiber	2
fibul/o	fibula (lower leg bone)	14
gangli/o	ganglion	15
ganglion/o	ganglion	15
gastr/o	stomach	11
gingiv/o	gum	11
glomerul/o	glomerulus	6
gloss/o	tongue	11
glyc/o	sugar	6
glycos/o	sugar	6
gno/o	knowledge	2
gravid/o	pregnancy	9
gynec/o	woman	8
gyn/o	woman	8
hemat/o	blood	5
hem/o	blood	5
hepat/o	liver	11
herni/o	hernia	11
heter/o	other	4
hidr/o	sweat	4
hist/o	tissue	2
humer/o	humerus (upper arm bone)	14
hydr/o	water	6
hymen/o	hymen	8
hyster/o	uterus	8
iatr/o	medicine, physician, treatment	2
ile/o	ileum	11
ili/o	ilium	14
infer/o	below	3
irid/o	iris	12
iri/o	iris	12
ischi/o	ischium	14
isch/o	deficiency, blockage	10
jejun/o	jejunum	11
kal/i	potassium	16
kary/o	nucleus	2

Combining Forms	Definition	Chapter
kerat/o	cornea	12
kerat/o	horny tissue, hard	4
kinesi/o	movement, motion	14
kyph/o	hump	14
labyrinth/o	labyrinth, inner ear	13
lacrim/o	tear duct, tear	12
lact/o	milk	9
lamin/o	lamina (thin, flat plate or layer)	14
lapar/o	abdomen, abdominal cavity	11
laryng/o	larynx	5
later/o	side	3
lei/o	smooth	2
leuk/o	white	2
lingu/o	tongue	11
lip/o	fat	2
lith/o	stone, calculus	6
lob/o	lobe	5
lord/o	bent forward	14
lumb/o	loin (or lumbar region of the spine)	14
lymph/o	lymph, lymph gland	10
mamm/o	breast	8
mandibul/o	mandible (lower jawbone)	14
mast/o	breast	8
mastoid/o	mastoid	13
maxill/o	maxilla (upper jawbone)	14
meat/o	meatus (opening)	6
melan/o	black	2
mening/i	meninges	15
mening/o	meninges	15
menisc/o	meniscus (crescent)	14
men/o	menstruation	8
ment/o	mind	15
metr/i	uterus	8
metr/o	uterus	8
mon/o	one	15
muc/o	mucus	5
myc/o	fungus	4
myel/o	bone marrow	14
myel/o	spinal cord	15
my/o	muscle	2, 14
myos/o	muscle	14
myring/o	eardrum	13
nas/o	nose	5
nat/o	birth	9
necr/o	death (cells, body)	4
nephr/o	kidney	6
neur/o	nerve	2, 15
noct/i	night	6
ocul/o	eye	12
olig/o	scanty, few	6
omphal/o	umbilicus, navel	9

Combining Forms	Definition	Chapter
onc/o	tumor	2
onych/o	nail	4
oophor/o	ovary	8
ophthalm/o	eye	12
opt/o	vision	12
orchid/o	testis, testicle	7
orchi/o	testis, testicle	7
orch/o	testis, testicle	7
organ/o	organ	2
or/o	mouth	11
orth/o	straight	5
oste/o	bone	14
ot/o	ear	13
ox/i	oxygen	5
ox/o	oxygen	5
pachy/o	thick	4
palat/o	palate	11
pancreat/o	pancreas	11
parathyroid/o	parathyroid gland	16
par/o	bear, give birth to, labor	9
part/o	bear, give birth to, labor	9
patell/o	patella (kneecap)	14
path/o	disease	2
pelv/i	pelvis, pelvic bone	9, 14
pelv/o	pelvis, pelvic bone	9, 14
perine/o	perineum	8
peritone/o	peritoneum	11
petr/o	stone	14
phalang/o	phalanx (finger or toe bone)	14
pharyng/o	pharynx	5
phas/o	speech	15
phleb/o	vein	10
phot/o	light	12
phren/o	mind	15
plasm/o	plasma	10
pleur/o	pleura	5
pneumat/o	lung, air	5
pneum/o	lung, air	5
pneumon/o	lung, air	5
poli/o	gray matter	15
polyp/o	polyp, small growth	11
poster/o	back, behind	3
prim/i	first	9
proct/o	rectum	11
prostat/o	prostate gland	7
proxim/o	near (the point of attachment of a body part)	3
pseud/o	false	9
psych/o	mind	15
pub/o	pubis	14
puerper/o	childbirth	9
pulmon/o	lung	5

Combining Forms	Definition	Chapter
pupill/o	pupil	12
pyel/o	renal pelvis	6
pylor/o	pylorus (pyloric sphincter)	9, 11
py/o	pus	5
quadr/i	four	15
rachi/o	spinal or vertebral column	14
radic/o	nerve root	15
radicul/o	nerve root	15
radi/o	radius (lower arm bone)	14
rect/o	rectum	11
ren/o	kidney	6
retin/o	retina	12
rhabd/o	rod-shaped, striated	2
rhin/o	nose	5
rhiz/o	nerve root	15
rhytid/o	wrinkles	4
sacr/o	sacrum	14
salping/o	fallopian (uterine) tube	8
sarc/o	flesh, connective tissue	2
scapul/o	scapula (shoulder bone)	14
scler/o	sclera	12
scoli/o	crooked, curved	14
seb/o	sebum (oil)	4
sept/o	septum	5
sial/o	saliva	11
sigmoid/o	sigmoid	11
sinus/o	sinus	5
somat/o	body	2
somn/o	sleep	5
son/o	sound	6
spermat/o	spermatozoan, sperm	7
sperm/o	spermatozoan, sperm	7
spir/o	breathe, breathing	5
splen/o	spleen	10
spondyl/o	vertebra	14
staped/o	stapes (middle ear bone)	13
staphyl/o	grapelike clusters	4
stern/o	sternum (breastbone)	14
stomat/o	mouth	11
strept/o	twisted chains	4
super/o	above	3
synovi/o	synovia, synovial membrane	14
system/o	system	2
tars/o	tarsals (ankle bones)	14
tendin/o	tendon	14
tend/o	tendon	14
ten/o	tendon	14
test/o	testis, testicle	7
therm/o	heat	10
thorac/o	thorax (chest)	5
thromb/o	clot	10

Combining Forms	Definition	Chapter
thym/o	thymus gland	10
thyroid/o	thyroid gland	16
thyr/o	thyroid gland	16
tibi/o	tibia (lower leg bone)	14
tom/o	cut, section	6
ton/o	tension, pressure	12
tonsill/o	tonsil	5
trache/o	trachea	5
trachel/o	cervix	8
trich/o	hair	4
tympan/o	eardrum, middle ear	13
uln/o	ulna (lower arm bone)	14
ungu/o	nail	4
ureter/o	ureter	6
urethr/o	urethra	6
ur/o	urine, urinary tract	6
urin/o	urine, urinary tract	6
uter/o	uterus	8
uvul/o	uvula	11
vagin/o	vagina	8
valv/o	valve	10
valvul/o	valve	10
vas/o	vessel, duct	7
ven/o	vein	10
ventricul/o	ventricle	10
ventr/o	belly, front	3
vertebr/o	vertebra	14
vesic/o	bladder, sac	6
vesicul/o	seminal vesicles	7
viscer/o	internal organs	2
vulv/o	vulva	8
xanth/o	yellow	2
xer/o	dry	4

Prefix	Definition	Chapter
a-	without, absence of	5
an-	without, absence of	5
ante-	before	9
bi-	two	3, 12
bin-	two	12
brady-	slow	10
dia-	through, complete	2
dys-	difficult, labored, painful, abnormal	2
endo-	within	5
epi-	on, upon, over	4
eu-	normal, good	5
hemi-	half	11
hyper-	above, excessive	2
hypo-	below, incomplete, deficient	2
inter-	between	14
intra-	within	4

Prefix	Definition	Chapter
meta-	after, beyond, change	2
micro-	small	9
multi-	many	9
neo-	new	2
nulli-	none	9
pan-	all, total	5
para-	beside, beyond, around	4
per-	through	4
peri-	surrounding (outer)	8
poly-	many, much	5
post-	after	9
pre-	before	9
pro-	before	2
sub-	under, below	4
supra-	above	14
sym-	together, joined	14
syn-	together, joined	14
tachy-	fast, rapid	10
tetra-	four	15
trans-	through, across, beyond	7
uni-	one	3

Suffix	Definition	Chapter
-a	no meaning	9
-ac	pertaining to	10
-ad	toward	3
-al	pertaining to	2
-algia	pain	5
-amnios	amniotic fluid, amnion	9
-apheresis	removal	10
-ar	pertaining to	5
-ary	pertaining to	5
-asthenia	weakness	14
-atresia	absence of a normal body opening, occlusion, closure	8
-cele	hernia, protrusion	5
-centesis	surgical puncture to aspirate fluid	5
-clasia	break	14
-clasis	break	14
-clast	break	14
-coccus (*pl.* cocci)	berry-shaped (a form of bacterium)	4
-crit	to separate	10
-cyesis	pregnancy	9
-cyte	cell	2
-desis	surgical fixation, fusion	14
-drome	run, running	16
-eal	pertaining to	5
-ectasis	stretching out, dilatation, expansion	5
-ectomy	excision, surgical removal	4
-emia	blood condition	5
-esis	condition	6

Suffix	Definition	Chapter
-gen	substance or agent that produces or causes	2
-genesis	origin, cause	2
-genic	producing, originating, causing	2
-gram	record, x-ray image	5
-graph	instrument used to record	10
-graphy	process of recording, x-ray imaging	5
-ia	condition of diseased or abnormal state	4
-ial	pertaining to	8
-iasis	condition	6
-iatrist	specialist, physician	15
-iatry	treatment, specialty	15
-ic	pertaining to	2
-ictal	seizure, attack	15
-ior	pertaining to	3
-is	no meaning	9
-ism	state of	7
-itis	inflammation	4
-logist	one who studies and treats, specialist, physician	2
-logy	study of	2
-lysis	loosening, dissolution, separating	6
-malacia	softening	4
-megaly	enlargement	6
-meter	instrument used to measure	5
-metry	measurement	5
-odynia	pain	10
-oid	resembling	2
-oma	tumor, swelling	2
-opia	vision (condition)	12
-opsy	view of, viewing	4
-osis	abnormal condition (means *increase* when used with blood cell word roots)	2
-ous	pertaining to	2
-oxia	oxygen	5
-paresis	slight paralysis	15
-partum	childbirth, labor	9
-pathy	disease	2
-penia	abnormal reduction in number	10
-pepsia	digestion	11
-pexy	surgical fixation, suspension	5
-phagia	eating, swallowing	4
-phobia	abnormal fear of or aversion to specific things	12
-phonia	sound or voice	5
-physis	growth	14
-plasia	condition of formation, development, growth	2
-plasm	growth, substance, formation	2
-plasty	surgical repair	4
-plegia	paralysis	12
-pnea	breathing	5
-poiesis	formation	10

Suffix	Definition	Chapter
-ptosis	dropping, sagging, prolapse	6
-rrhagia	rapid flow of blood	5
-rrhaphy	suturing, repairing	6
-rrhea	flow, excessive discharge	4
-rrhexis	rupture	9
-salpinx	fallopian tube	8
-sarcoma	malignant tumor	2
-schisis	split, fissure	14
-sclerosis	hardening	10
-scope	instrument used for visual examination	5
-scopic	pertaining to visual examination	5
-scopy	visual examination	5
-sis	state of	2
-spasm	sudden, involuntary muscle contraction	5
-stasis	control, stop, standing	2
-stenosis	constriction or narrowing	5
-stomy	creation of an artificial opening	5
-thorax	chest	5
-tocia	birth, labor	9
-tome	instrument used to cut	4
-tomy	cut into or incision	5
-tripsy	surgical crushing	6
-trophy	nourishment, development	6
-uria	urine, urination	6
-um	no meaning	9
-us	no meaning	10

Combining Forms, Prefixes, and Suffixes Alphabetized According to Definition

Definition	Combining Form	Chapter
abdomen	abdomin/o	11
abdomen	lapar/o	11
abdomen (abdominal cavity)	celi/o	11
above	super/o	3
adenoids	adenoid/o	5
adrenal gland	adren/o	16
adrenal gland	adrenal/o	16
albumin	albumin/o	6
alveolus	alveol/o	5
amnion	amni/o	9
amnion	amnion/o	9
antrum	antr/o	11
anus	an/o	11
aorta	aort/o	10
aponeurosis	aponeur/o	14
appendix	appendic/o	11
artery	arteri/o	10
atrium	atri/o	10
away (from the point of attachment of a body part)	dist/o	3
back	dors/o	3
back, behind	poster/o	3
bear, give birth to, labor, childbirth	part/o	9
bear, give birth to, labor, childbirth	par/o	9
belly, front	ventr/o	3
below	infer/o	3
bent forward	lord/o	14
bile duct	cholangi/o	11
birth	nat/o	9
black	melan/o	2
bladder, sac	cyst/o	6
bladder, sac	vesic/o	6
blood	hemat/o	5
blood	hem/o	5
blue	cyan/o	2
body	somat/o	2
bone	oste/o	14
bone marrow	myel/o	14
brain	encephal/o	15
breast	mamm/o	8
breast	mast/o	8
breathe, breathing	spir/o	5

Definition	Combining Form	Chapter
bronchus	bronch/o	5
bursa (cavity)	burs/o	14
calcium	calc/i	16
cancer	cancer/o	2
cancer	carcin/o	2
carbon dioxide	capn/o	5
carpus (wrist bone)	carp/o	14
cartilage	chondr/o	14
cause (of disease)	eti/o	2
cecum	cec/o	11
cell	cyt/o	2
cerebellum	cerebell/o	15
cerebrum, brain	cerebr/o	15
cervix	cervic/o, trachel/o	8
childbirth	puerper/o	9
chorion	chori/o	9
clavicle (collarbone)	clavic/o	14
clavicle (collarbone)	clavicul/o	14
clot	thromb/o	10
cold	cry/o	12
colon	col/o, colon/o	11
color	chrom/o	2
common bile duct	choledoch/o	11
conjunctiva	conjunctiv/o	12
cornea	corne/o	12
cornea	kerat/o	12
cortex	cortic/o	16
cranium, skull	crani/o	14
crooked, curved	scoli/o	14
crooked, stiff, bent	ankyl/o	14
cul-de-sac	culd/o	8
cut, section	tom/o	6
death (cells, body)	necr/o	4
deficiency, blockage	isch/o	10
developing cell	blast/o	6
diaphragm	diaphragmat/o	5
disease	path/o	2
diverticulum	diverticul/o	11
dry	xer/o	4
duodenum	duoden/o	11
dust	coni/o	4
ear	ot/o	13
ear	aur/i, aur/o	13
eardrum	myring/o	13
eardrum, middle ear	tympan/o	13
electricity, electrical activity	electr/o	10
embryo, to be full	embry/o	9
endocrine	endocrin/o	16
epididymis	epididym/o	7
epiglottis	epiglott/o	5
epithelium	epitheli/o	2

Definition	Combining Form	Chapter
esophagus	esophag/o	9, 11
extremities, height	acr/o	16
eye	ophthalm/o	12
eye	ocul/o	12
eyelid	blephar/o	12
fallopian tube	salping/o	8
false	pseud/o	9
fat	lip/o	2
femur (upper leg bone)	femor/o	14
fetus, unborn child	fet/o, fet/i	9
fiber	fibr/o	2
fibula (lower leg bone)	fibul/o	14
first	prim/i	9
first, beginning	arche/o	8
flesh, connective tissue	sarc/o	2
four	quadr/i	15
fungus	myc/o	3
gall, bile	chol/e	11
ganglion	gangli/o	15
ganglion	ganglion/o	15
gland	aden/o	2, 16
glans penis	balan/o	7
glomerulus	glomerul/o	6
grapelike clusters	staphyl/o	4
gray matter	poli/o	15
green	chlor/o	2
gum	gingiv/o	11
hair	trich/o	4
hard, dura mater	dur/o	15
head	cephal/o	9
hearing	audi/o	13
hearing	acou/o	13
heart	cardi/o	10
heat	therm/o	10
hernia	herni/o	11
hidden	crypt/o	4
horny tissue, hard	kerat/o	4
humerus (upper arm bone)	humer/o	14
hump	kyph/o	14
hymen	hymen/o	8
ileum	ile/o	11
ilium	ili/o	14
imperfect, incomplete	atel/o	5
inner ear	labyrinth/o	13
internal organs	viscer/o	2
intervertebral disk	disk/o	14
intestine	enter/o	11
iris	irid/o	12
iris	iri/o	12
ischium	ischi/o	14
jejunum	jejun/o	11

Definition	Combining Form	Chapter
joint	arthr/o	14
kidney	nephr/o	6
kidney	ren/o	6
knowledge	gno/o	2
labyrinth	labyrinth/o	13
lamina (thin flat plate or layer)	lamin/o	14
larynx	laryng/o	5
life	bi/o	4
light	phot/o	12
lip	cheil/o	11
liver	hepat/o	11
lobe	lob/o	5
lung	pulmon/o	5
lung, air	pneumat/o	5
lung, air	pneum/o	5
lung, air	pneumon/o	5
lymph, lymph gland	lymph/o	10
male	andr/o	7
mandible (lower jaw bone)	mandibul/o	14
mastoid	mastoid/o	13
maxilla (upper jaw bone)	maxill/o	14
meatus (opening)	meat/o	6
medicine (treatment)	iatr/o	2
meninges	mening/o, mening/i	15
meniscus (crescent)	menisc/o	14
menstruation	men/o	8
middle	medi/o	3
mind	ment/o	15
mind	psych/o	15
mind	phren/o	15
mouth	or/o	11
mouth	stomat/o	11
movement, motion	kinesi/o	14
mucus	muc/o	5
muscle	my/o	2, 14
muscle	myos/o	14
nail	ungu/o	4
nail	onych/o	4
near (the point of attachment of a body part)	proxim/o	3
nerve	neur/o	2, 15
nerve root	radicul/o	15
nerve root	radic/o	15
nerve root	rhiz/o	15
night	noct/i	6
nose	rhin/o	5
nose	nas/o	5
nucleus	kary/o	2
one	mon/o	15
organ	organ/o	2
other	heter/o	4

Definition	Combining Form	Chapter
ovary	oophor/o	8
oxygen	ox/o, ox/i	5
palate	palat/o	11
pancreas	pancreat/o	11
parathyroid gland	parathyroid/o	16
patella (kneecap)	patell/o	14
pelvis, pelvic bone	pelv/i, pelv/o	14
perineum	perine/o	8
peritoneum	peritone/o	11
phalanx (finger or toe)	phalang/o	14
pharynx	pharyng/o	5
physician (treatment)	iatr/o	2
plasma	plasm/o	10
pleura	pleur/o	5
potassium	kal/i	16
pregnancy	gravid/o	9
prostate gland	prostat/o	7
pubis	pub/o	14
pupil	core/o, cor/o	12
pupil	pupill/o	12
pus	py/o	5
pylorus, pyloric sphincter	pylor/o	9, 11
radius (lower arm bone)	radi/o	14
rectum	proct/o	11
rectum	rect/o	11
red	erythr/o	2
renal pelvis	pyel/o	6
retina	retin/o	12
rib	cost/o	14
rod-shaped, striated	rhabd/o	2
sacrum	sacr/o	14
saliva	sial/o	11
scanty, few	olig/o	6
scapula (shoulder blade)	scapul/o	14
sclera	scler/o	12
sebum (oil)	seb/o	4
self	aut/o	4
seminal vesicles	vesicul/o	7
sensation, sensitivity, feeling	esthesi/o	14
septum	sept/o	5
side	later/o	3
sigmoid	sigmoid/o	11
sinus	sinus/o	5
skin	cutane/o	4
skin	dermat/o	4
skin	derm/o	4
sleep	somn/o	5
small growth	polyp/o	11
smooth	lei/o	2
sound	son/o	6
sound	ech/o	10

Definition	Combining Form	Chapter
speech	phas/o	15
spermatozoa, sperm	sperm/o	7
spermatozoa, sperm	spermat/o	7
spinal cord	myel/o	15
spleen	splen/o	10
stapes	staped/o	13
sternum (breast bone)	stern/o	14
stomach	gastr/o	11
stone	petr/o	14
stone, calculus	lith/o	6
straight	orth/o	5
sugar	glycos/o	6
sugar	glyc/o	6
sweat	hidr/o	4
synovia, synovial membrane	synovi/o	14
system	system/o	2
tail (downward)	caud/o	3
tarsus (ankle bone)	tars/o	14
tear duct, tear	lacrim/o	12
tear, tear duct	dacry/o	12
tendon	ten/o	14
tendon	tendin/o	14
tendon	tend/o	14
tension, pressure	ton/o	12
testis, testicle	orch/o	7
testis, testicle	test/o	7
testis, testicle	orchi/o	7
testis, testicle	orchid/o	7
thick	pachy/o	4
thirst	dips/o	16
thorax (chest)	thorac/o	5
thymus gland	thym/o	10
thyroid gland	thyroid/o	16
thyroid gland	thyr/o	16
tibia (lower leg bone)	tibi/o	14
tissue	hist/o	2
tongue	lingu/o	11
tongue	gloss/o	11
tonsils	tonsill/o	5
trachea	trache/o	5
tumor	onc/o	2
twisted chains	strept/o	4
two, double	dipl/o	12
ulna (lower arm bone)	uln/o	14
umbilicus, navel	omphal/o	9
urea, nitrogen	azot/o	6
ureter	ureter/o	6
urethra	urethr/o	6
urinary bladder	vesic/o, cyst/o	6
urine, urinary tract	urin/o	6
urine, urinary tract	ur/o	6

Definition	Combining Form	Chapter
uterus	uter/o	8
uterus	metr/o, metr/i	8
uterus	hyster/o	8
uvula	uvul/o	11
vagina	vagin/o	8
vagina	colp/o	8
valve	valv/o	10
valve	valvul/o	10
vein	phleb/o	10
vein	ven/o	10
ventricle	ventricul/o	10
vertebra	vertebr/o	14
vertebral or spinal column	rachi/o	14
vessel	angi/o	10
vessel, duct	vas/o	7
vision	opt/o	12
vulva	vulv/o	8
vulva	episi/o	8
water	hydr/o	6
white	leuk/o	2
woman	gyn/o	8
woman	gynec/o	8
wrinkles	rhytid/o	4
yellow	xanth/o	2
yellowish, fatty plaque	ather/o	10

Definition	Prefix	Chapter
above	supra-	14
above, excessive	hyper-	2
after	post-	9
after, beyond, change	meta-	2
all, total	pan-	5
before	ante-, pre-	9
before	pro-	2
below, incomplete, deficient	hypo-	2
beside, beyond, around	para-	4
between	inter-	14
difficult, labored, painful, abnormal	dys-	2
fast, rapid	tachy-	10
four	tetra-, quadri-	14
half	hemi-	11
many	multi-	9
many, much	poly-	5
new	neo-	2
none	nulli-	9
normal	eu-	5
on, upon, over	epi-	4
one	uni-	3
outside, outward	ex-, exo-	16
slow	brady-	10
small	micro-	9

Definition	Suffix	Chapter
growth	-physis	14
growth, substance, formation	-plasm	2
hardening	-sclerosis	10
hernia, protrusion	-cele	5
inflammation	-itis	4
instrument used for visual examination	-scope	5
instrument used to measure	-meter	5
instrument used to cut	-tome	4
instrument used to record	-graph	10
labor	-partum	9
loosening, dissolution, separating	-lysis	6
malignant tumor	-sarcoma	2
measurement	-metry	5
nourishment, development	-trophy	6
one who studies and treats (specialist, physician)	-logist	2
origin, cause	-genesis	2
oxygen	-oxia	5
pain	-odynia	10
pain	-algia	5
paralysis	-plegia	12
pertaining to	-ac	10
pertaining to	-ous	2, 6
pertaining to	-ar	5
pertaining to	-ic	2
pertaining to	-ial	8
pertaining to	-ior	3
pertaining to	-eal	5
pertaining to	-ary	5
pertaining to	-al	2
pertaining to sound or voice	-phonia	5
pertaining to visual examination	-scopic	5
physician, specialist	-iatrist	15
pregnancy	-cyesis	9
process of recording, x-ray imaging	-graphy	5
producing, originating, causing	-genic	2
rapid flow of blood	-rrhagia	5
record, x-ray image	-gram	5
removal	-apheresis	10
resembling	-oid	2
run, running	-drome	16
rupture	-rrhexis	9
seizure, attack	-ictal	15
slight paralysis	-paresis	15
softening	-malacia	4
split, fissure	-schisis	14
state of	-ism	7
state of	-sis	2
stretching out, dilation, expansion	-ectasis	5
study of	-logy	2

Additional Combining Forms, Prefixes, and Suffixes

The following word parts were not included in the text. They are listed here for your easy reference. *As you discover word parts not included in this list, add them to the space provided at the end of Appendix C.*

Combining Form	Definition
acanth/o	thorny, spiny
acetabul/o	acetabulum (hip socket)
actin/o	ray, radius
aer/o	air, gas
algesi/o	pain
ambly/o	dull, dim
amyl/o	starch
anis/o	unequal, dissimilar
arteriol/o	arteriole (small artery)
articul/o	joint
axill/o	armpit
bacteri/o	bacteria
bil/i	bile
brachi/o	arm
bucc/o	cheek
cerumin/o	cerumen (earwax)
chir/o	hand
dactyl/o	fingers or toes
dent/i	tooth
dextr/o	right
diaphor/o	sweat
dynam/o	power, strength
ectop/o	located away from usual place
emmetr/o	a normal measure
faci/o	face
ger/o	old age, aged
geront/o	old age, aged
gluc/o	sweetness, sugar
gnath/o	jaw
gon/o	seed
home/o	sameness, unchanging
hom/o	same
hypn/o	sleep
ichthy/o	fish
immun/o	immune
is/o	equal, same
kin/e	movement
labi/o	lips
macr/o	abnormal largeness

Combining Form	Definition
morph/o	form, shape
myelon/o	spinal cord
narc/o	stupor
nyct/o	night
nyctal/o	night
oo/o	egg, ovum
ov/i	egg
ov/o	egg
papill/o	nipple
pector/o	chest
ped/o	child, foot
phac/o	lens of the eye
phak/o	lens of the eye
physi/o	nature
pod/o	foot
poikil/o	varied, irregular
pyr/o	fever, heat
tars/o	edge of the eyelid, tarsal (instep of foot)
top/o	place
toxic/o	poison

Prefix	Definition
ab-	from, away from
ana-	up, again, backward
anti-	against
apo-	upon
cata-	down
con-	together
contra-	against
de-	from, down from, lack of
dis-	to undo, free from
ecto-	outside, outer
eso-	inward
ex-	outside, outward
exo-	outside, outward
extra-	outside of, beyond
in-	in, into, not
infra-	under, below
mal-	bad

Prefix	Definition
meso-	middle
re-	back
retro-	back, behind
semi-	half
tri-	three
ultra-	beyond, excess

Suffix	Definition
-agra	excessive pain
-ase	enzyme
-cidal	killing
-clysis	irrigating, washing
-crine	separate, secrete
-ectopia	displacement
-emesis	vomiting
-er	one who
-ician	one who

Suffix	Definition
-lepsy	seizure
-lytic	destroy, reduce
-mania	madness, insane desire
-morph	form, shape
-odia	smell
-opia	vision
-philia	love
-phily	love
-phoria	feeling
-porosis	passage
-prandial	meal
-praxia	in front of, before
-ptysis	spitting
-sepsis	infection
-stalsis	contraction
-ule	little

Record additional word parts below that you have discovered:

APPENDIX D

Abbreviations

These abbreviations are written as they appear most commonly in the medical and health care environment. Some may also appear in both capital and small letters and with or without periods.

Common Medical Abbreviations	Definitions
ab	abortion
abd	abdomen
ABE	acute bacterial endocarditis
ABGs	arterial blood gases
a.c.	before meals
ACS	acute cardiac syndrome
ACTH	adrenocorticotropic hormone
AD	Alzheimer disease
ADH	antidiuretic hormone
ADL	activities of daily living
ad lib	as desired
Adm	admission
AFB	acid-fast bacillus
Afib	atrial fibrillation
AHD	arteriosclerotic heart disease
AI	aortic insufficiency
AICD	automatic implantable cardioverter defibrillator
AIDS	acquired immune deficiency syndrome
AKA	above-knee amputation
ALB	albumin
alk phos	alkaline phosphatase
ALL	acute lymphocytic leukemia
ALS	amyotrophic lateral sclerosis
AM	between midnight and noon
AMA	against medical advice; American Medical Association
amb	ambulate, ambulatory
AMI	acute myocardial infarction

Common Medical Abbreviations	Definitions
AML	acute myelocytic leukemia
amp	ampule
amt	amount
ant	anterior
AODM	adult-onset diabetes mellitus
AOM	acute otitis media
AP	anteroposterior; angina pectoris
A&P	auscultation and percussion; anterior and posterior colporrhaphy
ARDS	adult respiratory distress syndrome
ARM	artificial rupture of membranes
ARMD	age-related macular degeneration
ASA	aspirin
ASCVD	arteriosclerotic cardiovascular disease
ASD	atrial septal defect
ASHD	arteriosclerotic heart disease
Ast	astigmatism
as tol	as tolerated
AUL	acute undifferentiated leukemia
AV	arteriovenous
AVR	aortic valve replacement
ax	axillary
BA	bronchial asthma
BBB	bundle branch block
BE	barium enema
b.id.	twice a day
BK	below knee
BKA	below-knee amputation

Common Medical Abbreviations	Definitions
BM	bowel movement
BOM	bilateral otitis media
BP	blood pressure
BPH	benign prostatic hyperplasia
BR	bedrest
BRP	bathroom privileges
BS	blood sugar; bowel sounds; breath sounds
BSO	bilateral salpingo-oophorectomy
BUN	blood urea nitrogen
Bx	biopsy
$\bar{c}$	with
C.	Celsius
C_1-C_7	cervical vertebrae
Ca.	calcium
CA	cancer; carcinoma
CABG	coronary artery bypass graft
CAD	coronary artery disease
CAL	calorie
CAP	capsule
CAPD	continuous ambulatory peritoneal dialysis
cath	catheterization
CBC	complete blood count
CBR	complete bed rest
CBS	chronic brain syndrome
CC	chief complaint or colony count
CCU	coronary care unit
CDH	congenital dislocation of the hip
CEA	carcinoembryonic embryonic antigen
CF	cystic fibrosis
CHB	complete heart block
CHD	coronary heart disease
CHF	congestive heart failure
CHO	carbohydrate
chemo	chemotherapy
chol	cholesterol
CI	coronary insufficiency
circ	circumcision
CIS	carcinoma in situ
Cl	chloride
CLD	chronic liver disease
CLL	chronic lymphocytic leukemia

Common Medical Abbreviations	Definitions
cl liq	clear liquid
cm	centimeter
CML	chronic myelogenous leukemia
CNS	central nervous system
c/o	complains of
CO	carbon monoxide
CO_2	carbon dioxide
COB	coordination of benefits
COLD	chronic obstructive lung disease
comp	compound
cond	condition
COPD	chronic obstructive pulmonary disease
CP	cerebral palsy
CPAP	continuous positive airway pressure
CPD	cephalopelvic disproportion
CPK	creatine phosphokinase
CPN	chronic pyelonephritis
CPR	cardiopulmonary resuscitation
CRD	chronic respiratory disease
creat	creatinine
CRF	chronic renal failure
C&S	culture and sensitivity
C/S, CS, C-section	cesarean section
CSF	cerebrospinal fluid
CT	computed tomography
CTS	carpal tunnel syndrome
Cu	copper
CVA	cerebrovascular accident
CVP	central venous pressure
Cx	cervix
CXR	chest x-ray
DAT	diet as tolerated
D&C	dilation and curettage
del	delivery
DI	diabetes insipidus
DIC	diffuse intravascular coagulation
diff	differential (part of complete blood count)
disch	discharge
DLE	discoid lupus erythematosus
DM	diabetes mellitus

Common Medical Abbreviations	Definitions
DNA	deoxyribonucleic acid
DOA	dead on arrival
DOB	date of birth
Dr.	dram
DRG	diagnosis-related group
DSA	digital subtraction angiography
DVT	deep vein thrombosis
DW	distilled water
D/W	dextrose in water
Dx	diagnosis
E	enema
EBL	estimated blood loss
ECG	electrocardiogram
echo	echocardiogram
Echo EG	echoencephalography
ECT	electroconvulsive therapy
ED	emergency department
EDD	estimated date of delivery
EEG	electroencephalogram
EENT	eyes, ears, nose, and throat
EGD	esophagogastroduo-denoscopy
EKG	electrocardiogram
elix	elixir
EM	emmetropia
EMG	electromyogram
ENG	electronystagmography
ENT	ears, nose, and throat
EP	ectopic pregnancy
EP studies	evoked potential studies
ERCP	endoscopic retrograde cholangiopancreatography
ERT	estrogen replacement therapy
ESR	erythrocyte sedimentation rate
ESRD	end-stage renal disease
ESWL	extracorporeal shock-wave lithotripsy
etio	etiology
exam	examination
ext	extract; external
F	Fahrenheit
FBD	fibrocystic breast disease
FBS	fasting blood sugar
Fe	iron
FHT	fetal heart tones

Common Medical Abbreviations	Definitions
flu	influenza
FOB	fecal occult blood
Fr	French (catheter size)
FSH	follicle-stimulating hormone
FTT	failure to thrive
FUO	fever of undetermined origin
Fx	fracture
g	gram
GC	gonorrhea
GERD	gastroesophageal reflux disease
GI	gastrointestinal
GSW	gunshot wound
gtt	drops
GTT	glucose tolerance test
GU	genitourinary
Gyn	gynecology
h	hour
H	hypodermic
HAART	highly active antiretroviral therapy
HB	heart block
HCVD	hypertensive cardiovascular disease
HD	hemodialysis
HHD	hypertensive heart disease
H&H	hemoglobin and hematocrit
HCl	hydrochloric acid
HCO_3	bicarbonate
Hct	hematocrit
Hg	mercury
hgb	hemoglobin
HIV	human immunodeficiency virus
HMD	hyaline membrane disease
HNP	herniated nucleus pulposus
H_2O	water
H_2O_2	hydrogen peroxide (hydrogen dioxide)
HOB	head of bed
H&P	history and physical examination
H. pylori	*Helicobacter pylori*

Common Medical Abbreviations	Definitions
HRT	hormone replacement therapy
ht	height
HTN	hypertension
Hx	history
hypo	hypodermic
IBS	irritable bowel syndrome
ICD	implantable cardiac defibrillator
ICU	intensive care unit
IDDM	insulin-dependent diabetes mellitus
I&D	incision and drainage
IHD	ischemic heart disease
IM	intramuscular
inf	inferior
INR	international normalized ratio
I&O	intake and output
IPG	impedance plethysmography
IPPB	intermittent positive pressure breathing
irrig	irrigation
isol	isolation
IUD	intrauterine device
IV	intravenous
IVC	intravenous cholangiogram
IVP	intravenous pyelogram
K	potassium
KCl	potassium chloride
kg	kilogram
KO	keep open
KUB	kidney, ureter, bladder (x-ray)
KVO	keep vein open
L	liter
L_1-L_5	lumbar vertebrae
lab	laboratory
lac	laceration
LAP	laparotomy
lat	lateral
L&D	labor and delivery
LDH	lactic dehydrogenase
LE	lupus erythematosus
lg	large
LLL	left lower lobe
LLQ	left lower quadrant
LMP	last menstrual period

Common Medical Abbreviations	Definitions
LNMP	last normal menstrual period
LOC	loss of consciousness, level of consciousness
LP	lumbar puncture
LPN	licensed practical nurse
LR	lactated Ringer (IV solution)
lt	left
LTB	laryngotracheobronchitis
LUL	left upper lobe
LUQ	left upper quadrant
mcg	microgram
MCH	mean corpuscular hemoglobin
MCV	mean corpuscular volume
MD	muscular dystrophy
mEq	milliequivalent
mets	metastasis
mg	milligram
MG	myasthenia gravis
MI	myocardial infarction
ml	milliliter
mm	millimeter
MM	multiple myeloma
MOM	milk of magnesia
MR	may repeat
MRCP	magnetic resonance cholangiopancreatography
MRSA	methicillin-resistant *Staphylococcus aureus*
MS	multiple sclerosis
MVP	mitral valve prolapse
Na	sodium
NaCl	sodium chloride (salt)
NAS	no added salt
NB	newborn
neg	negative
neuro	neurology
NG	nasogastric
NICU	neurological intensive care unit; neonatal intensive care unit
NIDDM	non-insulin-dependent diabetes mellitus
NIVA	noninvasive vascular assessment
noc	night
noct	night
NPO	nothing by mouth

Common Medical Abbreviations | Definitions

Common Medical Abbreviations	Definitions
NS	normal saline
NSR	normal sinus rhythm
N&V	nausea and vomiting
NVS	neurovital signs
O$_2$	oxygen
OB	obstetrics
OD	right eye; overdose
oint.	ointment
OM	otitis media
OOB	out of bed
OP	outpatient
Ophth	ophthalmic
OR	operating room
Ortho	orthopedics
OS	left eye
OSA	obstructive sleep apnea
OT	occupational therapy
OTC	over-the-counter drugs
oto	otology
OU	both eyes; each eye
oz	ounce
$\bar{p}$	after
P	phosphorus
PA	physician's assistant or posteroanterior
PAC	premature atrial contractions
PAD	peripheral arterial disease
PAT	paroxysmal atrial tachycardia
pc	after meals
PCP	*Pneumocystis carinii*
PCU	progressive care unit
PCV	packed cell volume
PD	Parkinson disease
PDA	patent ductus arteriosus
PDR	*Physicians' Desk Reference*
PE	pulmonary embolism
Peds	pediatrics
PEEP	positive end expiratory pressure
PEG	percutaneous endoscopic gastrostomy
per	by
PERRLA	pupils equal, round, reactive to light and accommodation
PET scan	positron emission tomography scan

Common Medical Abbreviations	Definitions
PFTs	pulmonary function tests
PICC	peripherally inserted central catheter
PICU	pediatric intensive care unit
PID	pelvic inflammatory disease
PKU	phenylketonuria
PM	between noon and midnight
PMS	premenstrual syndrome
PNS	peripheral nervous system
po	orally; postoperative; phone order
post-op	postoperatively
PP	postpartum or postprandial (after meals)
PPD	purified protein derivative
pr	per rectum
PRBC	packed red blood cells
pre-op	preoperatively
PRN	as needed
PSA	prostate specific antigen
pt	patient; pint
PT	physical therapy
PT	prothrombin time
PTCA	percutaneous transluminal coronary angioplasty
PTT	partial thromboplastin time
PUL	percutaneous ultrasound lithotripsy
PVC	premature ventricular contractions
PVD	peripheral vascular disease
Px	prognosis
q	every
q_h	every (number) hour (e.g., q2h)
qid	four times per day
qn	every night
qt	quart
R	rectal
RA	rheumatoid arthritis
RAD	reactive airway disease

Common Medical Abbreviations | Definitions

Common Medical Abbreviations	Definitions
RAIU	radioactive iodine uptake
RBC	red blood cell count
RDS	respiratory distress syndrome
reg	regular
REM	rapid eye movement
resp	respirations
RHD	rheumatic heart disease
RLL	right lower lobe
RLQ	right lower quadrant
RN	registered nurse
R/O	rule out
ROM	range of motion
RR	recovery room
rt	right; routine
RT	respiratory therapy
RUL	right upper lobe
Rx	prescription
RXT	radiation therapy
$\bar{s}$	without
SAB	spontaneous abortion
SARS	severe acute respiratory syndrome
SBE	subacute bacterial endocarditis; self breast examination
SHG	sonohystogram
SICU	surgical intensive care unit
SIDS	sudden infant death syndrome
SLE	systemic lupus erythematosus
SMAC	sequential multiple analysis computer
SMR	submucous resection
SO	salpingo-oophorectomy
SPECT	single-photon emission computed tomography
ss	one-half
SSE	soapsuds enema
STAPH or staph	staphylococcus
stat	immediately
STD	sexually transmitted disease
STREP or strep	streptococcus
subling	sublingual
subq	subcutaneously
sup	superior

Common Medical Abbreviations | Definitions

Common Medical Abbreviations	Definitions
supp	suppository
surg	surgical
SVD	spontaneous vaginal delivery
SVN	small-volume nebulizer
SWL	shock wave lithotripsy
T_1-T_{12}	thoracic vertebrae
T_4	thyroxine
tab	tablet
TAB	therapeutic abortion
T&A	tonsillectomy and adenoidectomy
TAH	total abdominal hysterectomy
TAH-BSO	total abdominal hysterectomy-bilateral salpingo-oophorectomy
TAT	tetanus antitoxin
TB	tuberculosis
TCDB	turn, cough, deep breathe
TCT	thrombin clotting time
TEE	transesophageal echocardiogram
temp	temperature
THA	total hip arthroplasty
TIA	transient ischemic attack
tid	three times per day
tinct	tincture
TKA	total knee arthroplasty
TPN	total parenteral nutrition
tr	tincture
trach	tracheostomy
TSH	thyroid-stimulating hormone
TSS	toxic shock syndrome
TUIP	transurethral incision of the prostate
TULIP	transurethral laser incision of the prostate
TUMP	transurethral microwave thermotherapy
TURP	transurethral resection of the prostate
TVH	total vaginal hysterectomy
TVS	transvaginal sonography
TWE	tap water enema
Tx	treatment

Common Medical Abbreviations | Definitions

Common Medical Abbreviations	Definitions
UA	urinalysis
UGI	upper gastrointestinal
UGISBFT	upper gastrointestinal, small bowel follow through
UNG	ointment
UPPP	uvulopalatopharyngoplasty
URI	upper respiratory infection
US	ultrasound
UTI	urinary tract infection
UV	ultraviolet
UVR	ultraviolet radiation
vag	vaginal
VATS	video-assisted thoracic surgery
VBAC	vaginal birth after cesarean section

Common Medical Abbreviations	Definitions
VCUG	voiding cystourethrogram
VD	venereal disease
VDRL	Venereal Disease Research Laboratory
VLAP	visual ablation of the prostate
VPS	ventilation/perfusion scanning
VS	vital signs
WA	while awake
WBC	white blood cell count
W/C	wheelchair
wt	weight
XRT	radiotherapy; radiation therapy

APPENDIX E

Pharmacology Terms

Term	Definition
abortifacient	a drug that causes uterine muscles to contract with subsequent abortion of the fetus
absorption	the process in which a drug is taken up into the body, organ, tissue, or cell
adrenergic agonist	a drug that stimulates aspects of the sympathetic nervous system
adverse drug reaction (ADR)	any harmful or unintended reaction to a drug administered at a normal dose
aggregation inhibitor	a drug that stops platelets from bonding together
aldosterone receptor antagonist (ARA)	a drug that prevents reabsorption of water and sodium; used in chronic heart failure to minimize edema
amebicide	an agent that kills amoebas
ampoule (or ampule)	a small, sterile glass or plastic container that usually holds a single dose of a solution to be administered parenterally
analgesic	a drug that relieves pain. A *narcotic analgesic* is used for severe pain but can result in dependence and tolerance. A *nonnarcotic analgesic* is used for mild to moderate pain and is less likely to cause dependence and tolerance.
androgen	natural and synthetic hormones involved in male reproduction and secondary gender attributes
anesthetic	a drug that causes numbness or a loss of feeling that can be used locally or systemically; often used systemically to put a patient "to sleep" during extensive procedures
angiotensin receptor blocker (ARB) (also called *angiotensin II antagonist*)	a drug that blocks the angiotensin molecule from binding to its receptors throughout the body to reduce high blood pressure
angiotensin converting enzyme inhibitor (ACEI or ACE inhibitor)	a drug that blocks a step in the renin-angiotensin system to prevent the formation of angiotensin, which is a major contributor to high blood pressure
antacid	a drug that neutralizes acid in the stomach
antiadrenergic agent	a drug that blocks adrenergic receptors to reduce sympathetic nervous system activity in the body
antiandrogen	a drug that blocks the effects of androgen hormones in the body
antianginal	a drug that relieves the chest pain paroxysms caused by lack of oxygen delivery to the heart; typically involves vasodilation
antiarrhythmic	a drug that treats abnormal heart rhythm
antiarthritic	a drug that is used in the treatment of arthritis
antibacterial	a drug that targets bacteria to kill or halt growth or replication
antibiotic	a drug that targets microorganisms to kill or halt growth or replication
anticholinergic	a drug that blocks the action of acetylcholine and therefore opposes the parasympathetic nervous system

Term	Definition
anticholinesterase	a drug that prevents the breakdown of acetylcholine to yield a cholinergic or parasympathetic effect
anticoagulant	a drug that prevents blood clotting and coagulation
anticonvulsant	a drug that reduces the incidence and severity of seizures and convulsions (may also be referred to as an antiepileptic drug)
antidepressant	a drug used to treat mental depression
antidiabetic	a drug that treats diabetes mellitus by controlling glucose levels in the blood
antidiarrheal	a drug that treats diarrhea by increasing water absorption, decreasing muscle contraction of the intestines, altering electrolyte exchange, or absorbing toxins or microorganisms
antiemetic	a drug that reduces or prevents nausea and vomiting
antiestrogen	a drug used to block the action of estrogen hormones in the body
antifungal	a drug that targets fungus to kill or halt growth or replication
antiglaucoma	a drug that treats glaucoma of the eye
antigout	a drug that opposes the buildup of uric acid crystals in the joints to prevent and treat gout attacks
antihistamine	a drug that treats allergic and hypersensitivity reactions by blocking histamine
antihyperlipidemic	a drug used to treat high cholesterol by affecting low-density lipoprotein, high-density lipoprotein, total cholesterol, and/or triglyceride levels, which are collectively called lipids
antihypertensive	a drug that lowers blood pressure
anti-inflammatory	a drug that reduces inflammation
antimicrobial	a drug that targets microorganisms to kill or halt growth or replication
antimigraine	a drug that treats migraines and other similar types of headaches
antineoplastic agent	a drug used to destroy or halt the rapid replication of cancer cells
antiparkinsonian agent	a drug that treats Parkinson disease and parkinsonism by elevating the levels of dopamine in the brain
antiplatelet	a drug that prevents platelet formation or causes platelet destruction
antipsoriatic	a drug that treats psoriasis
antipsychotic	a drug that treats psychosis disorders by inducing a calming or tranquilizing effect and/or by adjusting neurotransmitter levels in the brain
antipyretic	a drug that reduces fever
antirheumatic	a drug that prevents or relieves rheumatism by affecting the immune system
antiseptic	a chemical agent that can safely be applied to external tissues to halt the growth of microorganisms
antispasmodic	a drug that prevents or relieves muscle spasms
antithrombin	a drug that prevents fibrin production, thereby reducing blood coagulation
antithyroid agent	a drug that counters hyperthyroidism by reducing the production of thyroid hormones
antitussive	a drug that suppresses coughing
antiviral	a drug that targets viruses to kill or halt growth or replication
anxiolytic	a drug that relieves anxiety
astringent	an agent that reduces inflammation and irritation and provides a protective barrier on mucosa and skin by contracting the surface tissue
bactericidal	the designation for an antimicrobial agent that kills or destroys bacteria

Term	Definition
bacteriostatic	the designation for an antimicrobial agent that halts the growth or replication of bacteria but does not destroy them
barbiturates	a class of drugs used to produce relaxation and sleep
beta-blocker	a drug that inhibits beta-adrenergic receptors; mostly used to lower blood pressure
bioavailability	the percentage of administered drug that is available to affect the body and target site(s) after absorption, metabolism, and other factors
bile acid sequestrant	a type of antihyperlipidemic drug used to lower high cholesterol levels by increasing the excretion of bile acid
birth control (BC)	exogenous hormones to prevent pregnancy
bisphosphonates	drugs that bind to bone matrix to treat osteoporosis
benzodiazepine (BZD)	a drug that binds to receptors in the brain to calm and sedate the central nervous system
cardiac glycoside	a drug that treats abnormal heart rhythm and improves contractility of the heart in congestive heart failure
calcium channel blocker (CCB)	a drug that regulates the entry of calcium into muscle cells of the heart and blood vessels to lower blood pressure
capsule (cap)	a small, digestible container (usually made of gelatin) used to hold a dose of medication for oral administration
central nervous system (CNS) stimulant	excites the central nervous system; can be used for many brain disorders
chemical name	the exact designation of the chemical structure of a drug
chemotherapy	the treatment of infection, cancer, and other diseases with chemical agents. *Chemo* is the term commonly used for the medication treatments cancer patients receive.
cholinergic	an agent that acts like acetylcholine to activate the parasympathetic nervous system
colony-stimulating factor	aids in the replication of blood cells in the bone marrow
COMT inhibitor (catechol-o-methyltransferase inhibitor)	an agent that prevents the breakdown of compounds that COMT degrades; used primarily to treat Parkinson disease
contraindications	factors that prohibit administration of a drug
controlled substance	a drug that has been identified as having the potential for abuse or addiction and is designated as schedule I, II, III, IV, or V under the Controlled Substance Act
corticosteroid	a drug that mimics hormones produced by the adrenal glands and has anti-inflammatory and immunosuppressive effects
cream	a water-based, semisolid preparation that usually contains a drug and is applied topically to external parts of the body
decongestant	a drug that breaks up nasal and head congestion
deterrent	an agent that aids in curbing behavioral impulses
disease modifying antirheumatic drug (DMARD)	a drug that slows the progression of rheumatoid arthritis
disinfectant	a chemical agent that can be applied to inanimate objects to destroy microorganisms
distribution	the uptake pattern of drug molecules by various tissues throughout the body

Term	Definition
diuretic	a drug that promotes the formation and excretion of urine to reduce the volume of extracellular fluid; commonly referred to as a "water pill"
dopaminergic	a drug that acts like dopamine; mostly used to treat Parkinson disease by increasing dopamine-dependent activity in the brain
dose	the amount of a drug or other substance to be administered at one time
drug	any substance taken by mouth; injected into a muscle, the skin, a blood vessel, or a cavity of the body; or applied topically to treat, cure, prevent, or diagnose a disease or condition
drug-drug interaction	a modification of the effect of a drug when administered with another drug; food can also interact with a drug to cause a modification of the drug's effect
elimination	the removal of a substance from the body by any route, including the kidneys, liver, lungs, and sweat glands
elixir	a liquid containing sweeteners, flavorings, water, and/or alcohol in which an oral medication may be dispersed
emulsion	a stable mixture that contains one component suspended within another component that it can not normally dissolve in or mix with
enema	a liquid agent that is administered rectally to clear the contents of the bowel
enteral	the use of oral ingestion as a mode of drug administration
epidural	injection of a drug into the epidural space of the spine
estrogens	natural and synthetic hormones that are involved in female reproduction and secondary gender characteristics
expectorant	a drug that breaks up the mucus in the lungs so that it can be expelled
fibrates	a type of antihyperlipidemic drug that raises HDL levels and lowers total cholesterol, LDL, and triglyceride levels
Food and Drug Administration (FDA)	a federal agency responsible for the enforcement of federal regulations regarding the manufacturing and distribution of food, drugs, and cosmetics as protection against the sale of impure or dangerous substances
formulary	a listing of drugs and drug information used by health practitioners within an institution to prescribe treatment that is medically appropriate
gastrointestinal (GI) stimulant	a drug that causes the muscles of the stomach and GI tract to contract and move the contents along
generic name	the official, established nonproprietary name assigned to a drug
gonadotropin-releasing hormone	a drug that causes the release of gonadotropins, which are hormones that stimulate the gonads (ovary or testis) and control reproductive activity
hemostatic	a drug that stops bleeding or hemorrhaging
histamine H_2 antagonist	a drug that counters an allergic reaction by blocking histamine from binding its H_2 receptors
hormone replacement therapy	a regimen that mimics the body's normal levels of female hormones when they are no longer produced; typically used during menopause

Term	Definition
hypoglycemic	a drug that lowers blood sugar
hypnotics	a class of drugs used to induce sleep; may also be used as sedatives
immunomodulator	a drug that influences the function of the immune system by either suppressing or enhancing it
immunosuppressant	a drug that reduces the ability of the immune system to function; used in autoimmune diseases and to prepare a patient for an organ transplant
infusion	the prolonged administration of a fluid substance directly into a vein, artery, or under the skin where the flow rate is driven by gravity or a mechanical pump
inhalation	a method of drug administration that involves the breathing in of a spray, vapor, or powder
inhaled corticosteroid	a drug that provides an anti-inflammatory effect directly to the lungs
injection	the introduction of a substance into the body by using a needle
intramuscular (IM)	the administration of a medication into a muscle
intrathecal	the administration of a drug into the subarachnoid space of the meninges in the spine
intrauterine device (IUD)	a hormone-containing device that is inserted directly in the vagina or uterus to prevent pregnancy
intravenous (IV)	the administration of a medication directly into a vein
keratolytic	an agent that augments the shedding of the top layer of dead skin
laxative	a drug that aids the evacuation of the bowels
leukotriene receptor antagonist	a drug that blocks late-stage regulators of allergic and hypersensitivity reactions
mechanism of action	the means by which a drug exerts a desired effect
metabolism	the chemical changes that a drug or other substance undergoes in the body
miotic	an agent that contracts the pupil
mood stabilizer	a drug that balances neurotransmitters in the brain to prevent periods of either mania or depression in bipolar patients
mucolytic	a drug that breaks up the mucus in the lungs so that it can be expelled
muscle relaxant	a drug that reduces muscle contractility to relieve tension- or spasm-induced pain
mydriatic	an agent that dilates the pupil
narcotics	a class of drugs that have opiumlike effects to cause drowsiness, pain relief, and sedation. These drugs can be habit forming and are considered controlled substances.
neuroleptic	a drug that reduces abnormal psychomotor activities in psychotic patients
neuromuscular blocking agents (NMBA)	a drug that blocks all nerve stimulation of the skeletal muscles to cause paralysis
nitrates	a drug that dilates the blood vessels
nonsteroidal anti-inflammatory drug (NSAID)	a drug that reduces pain, inflammation, and fever
ointment	an oil-based, semisolid preparation that usually contains a drug and is applied topically to external parts of the body

Term	Definition
ophthalmic	an agent that is intended to be used in the eye
oral	the administration of a medication by mouth
oral contraceptive	exogenous hormones taken by mouth to prevent pregnancy
over-the-counter (OTC) drugs (also called *nonprescription drugs*)	drugs that may be purchased without a prescription
ovulation stimulant	a drug that enhances the release of an egg from the ovary to promote pregnancy
oxytocic hormones	a drug that stimulates the uterine muscles to contract, thereby inducing labor in a pregnant woman
parasympatholytic	an agent that blocks the actions of the parasympathetic nervous system
parasympathomimetic	an agent that enhances the actions of the parasympathetic nervous system
parenteral	a drug or agent that is administered into the body by an injection, thereby bypassing the digestive tract
pediculicide	an agent that kills lice
pharmaceutical	a drug used for medicinal purposes
pharmacist	a person formally trained to formulate and dispense medications
pharmacodynamics	the study of the actions of a drug on the body
pharmacogenomics	the study of the correlation between genetics and response to a drug
pharmacokinetics	the study of the actions of the body on a drug
pharmacology	the study of the preparation, properties, uses, and actions of drugs
pharmacy	a place for preparing and dispensing drugs
phosphodiesterase inhibitor	a drug that blocks the inactivation of cyclic adenosine monophosphate either to increase cardiac output or to increase vasodilation in the penis
placebo	an inactive substance, prescribed as if it were an effective dose of a needed medication
pregnancy category	a level of risk the FDA assigns a drug based on documented problems with the use of that drug during pregnancy. The risk categories from safest to most harmful are A, B, C, D, and X.
prescription	an order for medication, therapy, or a therapeutic device given by a properly authorized person to a person properly authorized to dispense or perform the order for the specified patient
preservative	a substance included in some parenterals and topicals used to prevent the growth of microorganisms in the product
progestins	synthetic or natural hormones that are involved in female reproduction and secondary sex characteristics
proton pump inhibitor (PPI)	a drug that blocks acid production in the stomach
radiopharmaceutical	a drug with a radioactive component; used for diagnosis or treatment
retinoid	a derivative of vitamin A that regulates the growth of epithelial cells; often used to treat acne
route of administration	any one of the ways in which a drug or agent may be given to a patient
scabicide	an agent that kills scabies
sedative	a drug that depresses the central nervous system to calm a patient
side effect	any reaction or result from a medication other than what was intended
smoking cessation agent	a drug that helps the patient quit smoking; may be a behavioral deterrent or a nicotine substitute

Term	Definition
solution	a homogenous mixture of one or more substances dissolved into another substance
statins	a class of drugs used to treat dyslipidemia that work by inhibiting 3-hydroxy-3-methylglutaryl coenzyme A reductase
subcutaneous (SC, SQ)	the introduction of a medication into the tissue just beneath the skin
sublingual tablet	a form of drug that dissolves under the tongue
suppository	a topical form of drug that is inserted into the rectum, vagina, or penis
suspension	a liquid in which particles of a solid are dispersed, but not dissolved, and in which the dispersal is maintained by stirring or shaking the mixture
sympatholytic	an agent that blocks the actions of the sympathetic nervous system
sympathomimetic	an agent that enhances the actions of the sympathetic nervous system
tablet	a small, solid dosage form of a medication
thrombolytic	a drug that dissolves blood clots
thyroid hormone	a drug that mimics natural thyroid hormone to regulate metabolism and endocrine functions
topical	a dosage form of a medication that is applied directly to an external area of the body
toxicity	the level at which a drug's concentration within the body produces serious adverse effects
trade name	a proprietary name assigned to a drug by its manufacturer that is registered as part of the drug's identity
tranquilizer	a drug that reduces anxiety or agitation
transdermal	a method of applying a drug to unbroken skin so that it is continuously absorbed through the skin to produce a systemic effect. A transdermal patch is a drug delivery system that controls the rate of absorption through the skin.
tricyclic antidepressants (TCAs)	a class of drugs used to treat depression
triptans	a class of drugs used to treat migraine headaches by reversing blood vessel dilation in the brain
United States Pharmacopeia (USP)	a compendium, recognized officially by the federal Food, Drug, and Cosmetic Act, that contains descriptions, uses, strengths, and standards of purity for selected drugs and for all their dosage forms
urinary alkalinizer	an agent that increases the urine pH to make it more basic
vaginal ring	a device containing estrogens and progestins that is inserted in the vagina to prevent pregnancy
vasodilator	a drug that expands blood vessels to lower blood pressure
vasopressin (also called *antidiuretic hormone* or *ADH*)	a drug that contracts blood vessels to retain water and increase blood pressure
vasopressor (also called *vasoconstrictor*)	a drug that contracts blood vessels to raise blood pressure
vitamin	an organic compound essential in small quantities for normal physiologic and metabolic functioning

Reference to Time

ac	before meals	qh	every hour
ad lib	as desired	qhs	every night at bedtime
am	morning	qid	four times a day
atc	around the clock	qod	every other day
bid	twice a day	q2h, q3h, etc.	every 2 hours, every
pc	after meals		3 hours, etc.
pm	afternoon	stat	immediately
prn	as needed	tid	three times a day
q	every	wa	while awake

Reference to Formulation

cap	capsule	oint, ung	ointment
CR	controlled release	pulv	pulvule
crm	cream	sol	solution
DR	delayed release	SR	sustained release
ER	extended release	supp	suppository
MDI	metered-dose inhaler	susp	suspension
ODT	orally disintegrating tablet	tab	tablet

Reference to Dosage

cm	centimeter	mg	milligram
dr	dram	mL, ml	milliliter
Gm, g, gm	gram	oz	ounce
gr	grain	qs	of sufficient quantity
gtt, gtts	drop, drops	ss	one half
inh	inhalation	tbsp, T	tablespoon, tablespoonful
kg	kilogram	tsp, t	teaspoon, teaspoonful
L	liter		
lb	pound		
mcg	microgram		
mEq	milliequivalent		

Reference to Administration

ID	intradermal	OS	left eye
IM	intramuscular	OU	both eyes
IN	intranasal	PO	by mouth
IV	intravenous	subQ	subcutaneous
IVB	intravenous bolus		
IVP	intravenous push		
IVPB	intravenous piggy back		
OD	right eye		

Others

⊚	with	NKDA	no known drug allergies
s̄	without	NS	normal saline
D5W	5% dextrose in water		

Health Care Delivery/Managed Care Terms

Term	Definition
accepting assignment	providers of medical services agreeing that the receipt of payment from Medicare for a professional service will constitute full payment for that service
accreditation	a formal recognition that an organization conforms to a set of industry-specific, qualifying standards
Accreditation Association for Ambulatory Health Care (AAAHC)	an organization that offers accreditation for ambulatory care organizations
activities of daily living (ADL)	activities performed as part of a person's daily routine of self-care
actual charge	the amount a health care practitioner or other health care provider actually bills a patient for a particular medical service or procedure; may differ from the customary and prevailing charge in that geographic area
acute care	level of health care, generally provided in hospitals or emergency departments, for sudden, serious illnesses or trauma
administrative costs	the costs assumed by a managed care plan for administrative services
advance directive	a legal document stating a patient's wishes regarding continuation or withdrawal of treatment to be used if the patient loses decision-making abilities
allowable charge	charges for services rendered or supplies furnished by a health care provider that qualify as covered expenses under a health plan and are reimbursable under their payment formula
alternative delivery system	all forms of health care delivery systems other than traditional fee-for-service indemnity health care
alternative medicine	nontraditional medicines and medical treatments, sometimes combined with traditional types of medicine, aimed at treating or preventing illness or disease
ambulatory setting	environment in which health care services are provided on an outpatient basis
ancillary care	health care services performed by clinical personnel other than physicians and nurses
appeal process	a mechanism by which patients, practitioners, or providers may request a reconsideration of a decision made by a medical review board
assignment of benefits	the patient signs an agreement instructing the insurance company to make payment directly to the provider who renders care
attending physician	the physician in charge of the patient's care
attrition rate	the disenrollment of members from a health maintenance organization (HMO), expressed as a percentage of total plan enrollment
basic health services	benefits that all federally qualified HMOs must offer as defined in the federal HMO regulations

Term	Definition
benefit period	the time period for which a person is eligible for covered benefits under a health insurance policy
benefit schedule	a summary of covered services, limitations, and applicable copayments provided to a covered group of individuals
board certified	physicians or other health care professionals who have passed an examination by a medical specialty board and have now been certified by that board as a specialist in that area
board eligible	a physician or other health care professional who is eligible to take a specialty board examination after having completed the required schooling, training, or practice
brand name drug	a registered trademark name given to a specific product by its initial manufacturer
capitation	a per-member, monthly payment to a provider that covers contracted health care services and is paid in advance of its delivery. It exists for a specific length of time regardless of the number of times a member uses the service.
carve out	a health benefit that is removed from a larger benefit package and is contracted for separately by a managed care organization
case management	the process in which a health care professional supervises the administration of medical and ancillary services to a patient
case mix	the number, frequency, and severity of hospital admissions or managed care services used
catastrophic health insurance	health insurance that provides protection and benefits to cover the high cost of treating severe or lengthy illnesses and disabilities
Center for Medicare and Medicaid Services (CMS)	formerly the *Health Care Financing Administration* (HCFA); the federal agency responsible for administering the Medicare and Medicaid programs.
chronic disease	longstanding, persistent, noncurable disease or health condition that requires ongoing surveillance and care
claim	a notification or request for payment to an insurance or managed care company from either a provider or covered person who has received medical services
coinsurance	the percentage of the costs of medical services paid by the patient
concurrent review	a screening method by which a health care provider reviews the performance of a procedure or a hospital admission to assess its necessity
Consolidated Omnibus Budget Reconciliation Act (COBRA)	a law that requires employers to offer continued health insurance coverage to employees who have had their health insurance terminated
copayment	a nominal fee charged to HMO members for each medical visit or prescription filled
cosmetic surgery	surgery for the sole purpose of improving appearance
cost-effectiveness	the cost of a drug or procedure compared with the health care benefits resulting from it; usually considered as a ratio
cost sharing	provisions of a health insurance policy that require the insured to pay some portion of their covered medical expenses.
cost shifting	the redistribution of payment sources. When one payer obtains a discount and the providers of care increase the costs to another payer to make up the difference.

Term	Definition
current procedural terminology (CPT-4)	standardized system of terminology and coding developed by the American Medical Association and used for describing and reporting medical services and procedures
custodial care	unskilled care given for the primary purpose of meeting personal needs, such as bathing and dressing
deductible	a fixed amount of health care dollars a person must pay before payment from an insurer begins
diagnosis-related groups (DRG)	a classification system used to determine payments from Medicare based on assigning a standard flat rate to major diagnostic categories. This flat rate is paid to hospitals regardless of the full cost of the services provided.
direct costs	costs fully attributable to the provision of specific health care services
durable medical equipment (DME)	equipment used to serve a medical purpose that can withstand repeated use and is appropriate for use in the home (e.g., wheelchair)
electronic medical record	technology in which medical records are stored on computer rather than in paper files
employee assistance programs	employer-sponsored counseling services for employees and their dependents to solve workplace and personal problems
Employee Retirement Income Security Act of 1974 (ERISA)	a law that mandates reporting and disclosure requirements for health plans
evidence of insurability (EOI)	any statement or proof of a person's physical or mental condition that affects his or her eligibility for insurance coverage
exclusive provider organizations (EPO, EPA)	a preferred provider arrangement by which patient members of a health care plan must choose from a list of selected health care providers
explanation of benefits (EOB)	a statement issued to members by their health care plan listing services provided, dollars covered by benefits, and amounts not covered by insurance that members must pay
Family Medical Leave Act (FMLA)	federal law requiring employers to provide 12 weeks of unpaid sick leave per year to employees with qualifying medical circumstances
fee for service (FFS)	traditional provider reimbursement by which a patient receives a bill from a physician that includes all professional services performed
first dollar coverage	a type of insurance plan in which no deductible exists and the insurer pays the full amount of the provided services
formulary	the panel or list of drugs chosen by a hospital or managed care organization that is available to be used by physicians for their patients
gatekeeper	a primary care physician in an HMO who is the initial provider of health care and who controls and authorizes referrals to other specialists as needed
generic drug	a drug known by the common name of its main substance, instead of the brand name given by its initial manufacturer
Health Care Financing Administration (HCFA)	former name for the federal agency responsible for administering Medicare and Medicaid. Now called *Center for Medicare and Medicaid Services.*

Term	Definition
health care power of attorney..........	a type of advance directive in which a patient appoints another individual to make treatment decisions in the event the patient loses decision-making abilities
Health Insurance Portability and Accountability Act of 1996 (HIPAA) .	the act that provides for the privacy and confidentiality of medical records, limits exclusions for preexisting conditions, prohibits discrimination against employees based on their health status, and guarantees renewability of insurance to all employers
health maintenance organization (HMO)...............	an organization that provides the delivery of hospital, physician, and other health care services to an enrolled population for a fixed sum of money, paid in advance, for a specified period
health maintenance organization staff model............	the purest form of managed care in which physicians are employees of the HMO and work in clinical facilities managed by the HMO. The physicians do not practice on a traditional fee-for-service basis and do not have their own private practice.
health maintenance organization group model	the HMO contracts with an established physician group that is paid a fixed amount per patient to provide specific medical services. These physicians do not have traditional fee-for-service patients.
health maintenance organization individual practice association (IPA) model......................	the managed care organization contracts with independent physicians who work in their own private offices and see fee-for-service patients as well as HMO enrollees. They are paid by capitation for the HMO patients, and the physician assumes the responsibility for keeping the treatment cost low.
health maintenance organization point-of-service model..............	sometimes referred to as an *open-ended HMO;* the patient can receive care either within the HMO network or by going outside to a physician not contracting with the HMO. Patients decide where they wish to go at the time the service is needed, knowing fuller insurance coverage is provided if they stay within the HMO physician network.
home health care....................	medical care administered at a patient's residence by a health care professional
hospice care	a philosophy of care provided to terminally ill persons that focuses on pain relief, counseling, and dying with dignity
hospital alliance.....................	a group of hospitals that have joined together to improve their competitive positions and buying powers
hospitalist	a physician, usually a specialist, who practices exclusively in hospitals, has no outpatient responsibilities, and usually cares for the admitted patients of other physicians
ICD-10-CM........................	International Classification of Diseases, 10th Edition, Clinical Modification. A listing of diagnoses and identifying codes used by physicians for reporting medical services involving disease and injuries. This coding provides a uniform language for the submission of insurance claim forms.
indemnity insurance.................	traditional fee-for-service medical plan under which patients are billed for each medical service performed

Term	Definition
Individual Practice Association (IPA)...	an HMO model in which the health plan contracts with an organized group of physicians to provide care to HMO members from their private offices
inpatient care	admission to a hospital, for at least 24 hours, under the care of a physician
JCAHO	*Joint Commission on Accreditation of Health Care Organizations.* A private, not-for-profit organization that evaluates and accredits hospitals and other health care organizations using established standards of practice.
living will	a type of advance directive containing a patient's wishes regarding continuation or withdrawal of treatment if the patient loses decision-making abilities
long-term care	a multilevel care system providing care to elderly, chronically ill, or disabled persons in various types of facilities and at different levels of professional skill
managed health care	the use of a planned and systematic approach to providing health care, with the goal of offering quality care at the lowest possible cost
management services organization	a company that provides practice management, administrative, and support services to individual physician offices in lieu of the medical office handling their own matters
mandated benefits	health care benefits that health care plans are required by state or federal law to provide to members
Medicaid benefits	an entitlement program run by both the state and federal governments designed to provide health care coverage to patients who cannot afford to pay for private health insurance
medical savings accounts	a health care savings account in which individuals can accumulate contributions to pay for unreimbursed medical expenses
Medicare	an entitlement program run by the federal government by which people age 65 and older or persons deemed disabled for a prescribed period of time receive health care insurance. Part A covers hospitalization and Part B covers outpatient and physician services.
Medicare supplement	a private health insurance plan available to Medicare-eligible persons to cover the cost of medical care not covered by Medicare
national health insurance	a proposal to make the U.S. government the single insurer and payer for all health care
nonparticipating provider	a health care provider who has not contracted with an insurance company or HMO to provide health care
open access	arrangement that allows members to see participating providers, usually specialists, without referral from a primary physician gatekeeper
open enrollment	a period during which a managed care organization allows persons not previously enrolled to apply for plan membership
out of network	providers who do not participate in the network of a managed care organization. HMO members usually have to pay for their own out-of-network services.
out-of-pocket costs	the share of health services costs paid by the individual enrollee
outpatient care	the provision of health care services outside a hospital setting
over-the-counter (OTC) drug	a drug that does not require a prescription under federal or state law and that may be sold directly to customers
participating physician	a physician who has entered into an agreement with a health insurance plan to provide medical services to its members

Term	Definition
physician assistant	a health care professional who provides basic health care services to patients under the supervision of a physician
physician extender	health care professionals who help extend the availability of health services by substituting for physicians in performing basic medical services. A physician assistant is a physician extender.
Physicians Current Procedural Terminology (CPT)	a guide used for the billing and payment of physicians' services
Physicians' Desk Reference (PDR)	an annual compilation and publication of information concerning prescription drugs and diagnostic products, published primarily for physicians and widely used as a reference document
physician-hospital organization (PHO)	an organization owned by both a hospital and its medical staff of physicians that contracts with HMOs and assumes responsibility for providing health care services to an identified group of individuals
point of service (POS)	a form of managed care, often called an open-ended HMO or PPO, in which members are encouraged to stay in the existing network of providers but have free choice, at a higher price, of other physicians and hospitals outside the network
portability	continuous access to health insurance coverage even if a change in an individual's personal status occurs, such as employment loss or divorce
preauthorization	approval of specific services by a health insurance or managed care organization before a member receives these services
preexisting condition	illnesses or medical problems present before an individual obtains an insurance policy
preferred providers	physicians, hospitals, and other health care providers who contract to provide health care services to persons covered by a particular health plan
primary care physician (PCP)	sometimes referred to as *gatekeepers,* these general practitioners are the first physicians to see a patient for an illness
prospective payment	payment that is received before care is actually needed or rendered. It gives providers an incentive to use fewer resources because they get to keep the difference between what is prepaid and what is actually used.
provider	any licensed or approved supplier of medical services
reimbursement	payment to a medical provider in exchange for the performance of medical services
respite care	short-term, temporary custodial care that allows a family member to be briefly relieved from caring for a dependent individual
risk	the probability of loss, from expenditure for medical services for a defined patient population
Stark laws	federal laws passed in 1989 that prohibit physicians from referring patients to clinical laboratories and other health care entities in which physicians have a financial interest
third-party payer	an organization that pays for health care expenses
usual, customary, and reasonable (UCR)	the amount a managed care or health insurance company will pay for a given procedure or service calculated on the most frequent charge for the same service in a given area
utilization management	a process for measuring the optimal use of medical resources, based on medical necessity and cost-effectiveness

Term	Definition
utilization review (UR)	a systematic, retrospective review designed to determine the medical necessity and economic appropriateness of medical services performed
waiting period	the period between the start of employment and enrollment in a health insurance program and the date when an individual becomes eligible for insurance coverage and the payment of medical services

Additional Health Care Delivery/Managed Care Abbreviations and Acronyms

Abbreviation/Acronym	Definition
AAAHC	Accreditation Association for Ambulatory Health Care
AAPPO	American Association of Preferred Provider Associations
ADS	alternative delivery system
ALOS	average length of stay
AMCPA	American Managed Care Pharmacy Association
AMCRA	American Managed Care and Review Association
APT	admission per thousand
CEA	cost-effective analysis
CHO	comprehensive health organization
COB	coordination of insurance benefits
CQI	continuous quality improvement
DME	durable medical equipment
DOI	Department of Insurance
DOS	date of service
EAP	Employee Assistance Program
EOB	explanation of benefits
EOI	evidence of insurability
FP	family practice
HBO	health benefits organization
LOS	length of stay
LTC	long-term care
MCO	managed care organization
MGMA	Medical Group Management Association
OTC	over the counter
PCN	primary care network
PCP	primary care physician
PMPM	per member, per month
POS	point of service
PPO	preferred provider organization
PPS	prospective payment system
UCR	usual, reasonable, and customary
UR	utilization review

Complementary and Alternative Medicine Therapies

Term	Definition
acupressure	the digital stimulation of anatomic pressure points on the body to preserve and restore health
acupuncture	the ancient practice of inserting very thin needles into acupoints just under the skin to treat disease, increase immune response, or relieve pain
Alexander technique	the use of movement and exercises to affect physiologic structure, posture, movement, and breathing
apiotherapy	the medicinal use of honeybee venom to treat inflammatory and degenerative diseases
applied kinesiology	noninvasive manipulative treatments to stimulate or relax key muscles to attempt to resolve health problems
aromatherapy	the therapeutic use of essential concentrated oils expressed from aromatic herbs, flowers, and trees. Both the aroma and external skin applications are used as therapy in treating infections, immune deficiencies, and stress.
autosuggestion	a mild form of self-hypnosis in which an individual sits quietly, breathes deeply, and relaxes oneself to a desired state
Ayurvedic medicine	a centuries' old system of alternative medicine that includes herbs, aromatherapy, music therapy, massage, and yoga. It places equal emphasis on mind, body, and spirit in achieving the harmony of wellness.
balneotherapy	the use of baths in the treatment of disease
biofeedback	the use of learned self-control of physiologic responses by using electronic devices to demonstrate signals from the body
chelation therapy	the use of oral and intravenous agents and exercise to prevent, halt, or reverse arterial disease
clay therapy	the use of the mineral composition of clay, both internally and externally, as an elixir or a poultice
colon therapy	cleansing of the intestine to remove waste matter that interferes with healthy function and the proper assimilation and absorption of nutrients
craniosacral therapy	the use of gentle manual pressure applied to the skull and spine to treat a range of conditions from headache to spinal cord disorders and to improve overall body functioning
cupping	application of a glass vessel to the skin from which air has been exhausted by heat to create suction that draws blood to the surface, producing counterirritation
energy medicine	diagnostic screening devices to measure various electromagnetic frequencies emitted by the body to detect imbalances causing illness
environmental medicine	exploration of the role of diet and environmental allergens in influencing health and illness
enzyme therapy	plant and pancreatic enzymes ingested by mouth to improve digestion and the absorption of essential nutrients

Term	Definition
fasting	an abstinence from eating to relieve the body of the task of digestion, allowing the system to eliminate toxins to promote wellness
Feldenkrais method	the use of specific gentle body movements to increase ease and range of motion and improve flexibility and coordination
flower remedies	essences isolated from flowers that directly affect a person's emotional state to facilitate psychologic and physiologic well-being
glandular therapy	treatment of disease with natural or synthetic hormones
guided imagery	the use of focused concentration on formed mental images as suggested by a facilitator
herbal therapy	the use of herbal remedies to promote health or healing
homeopathy	a system of medical treatment based on the theory that certain diseases can be cured by giving small doses of drugs that in a healthy person would produce symptoms similar to those of the disease and stimulate the body to fight the disease
hydrotherapy	the use of hot or cold water, ice, and steam, both internally and externally, to maintain and restore health
hypnotherapy	the use of the power of suggestion and a state of altered consciousness involving focused attention to promote wellness
intravenous nutrition	administration of nutrients through a peripheral vein
juice therapy	conversion of vegetables and fruits into consumable therapeutic liquids to nourish and replenish the body in times of stress or illness
Kegel exercises	the tightening and release of vaginopelvic muscles in intervals to improve muscular tone
light therapy	the therapeutic use of ultraviolet, colored, and laser lights to reestablish the body's natural rhythm and reduce pain, depression, and other health conditions
lymphatic drainage therapy	the use of gentle massage to stimulate the movement of fluid in the lymphatic system
magnetic field therapy	application of magnets or magnetic devices to eliminate pain, facilitate the healing of bones, and counter the effects of stress
manipulation	a joint mobilization technique sometimes involving a rapid thrust or the stretching of a joint
massage therapy	the manual manipulation of soft tissue incorporating stroking, kneading, and percussion motions to increase blood supply, relax muscle fibers, and relieve tension
meditation	a mental activity focusing attention on a single activity such as breathing, an image, or a sound to calm and still the mind and stay pleasantly anchored in the present. Used to identify and control reactions to stress situations.
meridian	one of several pathways in the body believed to conduct energy between the surface and internal organs
moxibustion	similar to acupuncture and acupressure, but instead of needling or pressing the acupoint, a particular herb is ignited and burned on or near that point on the skin
music therapy	the use of music within a therapeutic relationship to address physical, emotional, cognitive, and social needs of individuals
naturopathic medicine	an array of healing practices based on the patient's individual needs and using the body's inherent ability to heal. It focuses on treating the underlying causes of disease with nontoxic therapies to restore the body's natural balance and health.

Term	Definition
neurolinguistic programming	activities aimed at helping individuals detect and reprogram unconscious patterns of thought and behavior that are negatively affecting their health or recovery from illness
osteopathy	a form of physical medicine that helps restore the structural balance of the musculoskeletal system by using joint manipulation, physical therapy, and postural reeducation. An osteopathic physician (DO) practices similar to an allopathic physician (MD).
oxygen therapy	the use of oxygen in various forms to promote healing and destroy disease-producing organisms in the body. Oxygen may be inhaled, ingested, inserted in body orifices, given intravenously, or absorbed through the skin.
phytotherapeutics	the use of plant extracts in the maintenance of health or the treatment of disease
prayer therapy	meditation to a higher power with a request for healing
Qigong	self-learned physical activities that combine movement, meditation, and breath regulation to enhance the flow of the body's energy, improve blood circulation, and enhance immune system responses
reflexology	when certain points or reflex areas on the hands, face, and feet are pressed, invisible nerve currents bring nerve energy to specific organs
Reiki	a deeply relaxing ancient spiritual massage technique in which the client lies on a table and energy is transferred through the practitioner placing hands in a sequence of standardized positions on the client's body
rolfing	practitioner uses hands to stretch and loosen connective tissue, allowing the client's muscles and joints to move more freely
rotation diet	a diet plan in which a person does not eat a given food more than once in a certain number of days
shiatsu	treatment using the noninvasive touch and pressure of finger, hand, and foot techniques to release physical and emotional tension. Involves extensive soft-tissue manipulation and both active and passive exercises.
therapeutic touch	the use of a technique that was developed in the nursing community in which the hands, usually held 2-6 inches above the body, are used to facilitate the healing process
vibrational massage therapy	a form of massage on joints and other body structures to relieve tension and stress
vitamin therapy	the use of nutrition, through diet and supplements, to decrease the incidence of disease and symptoms
watsu	a form of aquatic bodywork that takes place in chest-high warm water and involves both a series of flowing dance-like movements and a body massage by a watsu practitioner
yoga	a self-learned series of practices that use physical posture, breathing exercises, and meditation to reduce stress, lower blood pressure, regulate heart rate, reduce the aging process, and restore mind/body unity

Behavioral Health Terms

The following list of behavioral health terms is in addition to those included in Chapter 15 and is not meant to be inclusive but is designed to give the student an overview of the medical language used on a behavioral health unit.

Term	Definition
abstract thinking	a stage in the development of cognitive thought in which one has the ability to understand relationships and to categorize objects based on their essential characteristics. Abstract thinking requires flexibility, adaptability, and the use of concepts and generalizations.
acting out	indirect expression of feeling through behavior that attracts the attention of others and may be dangerous or destructive behaviors expressing unconscious conflict
adaptation	the process of changing to achieve equilibrium between an individual and the environment
adjustment disorder	a maladaptive reaction to an identifiable, transient stressful situation
affect	the outward expression of a subjectively experienced feeling state. *Blunted* affect is characterized by a severe reduction in the intensity of expression; *flat* affect refers to a loss of expression; *inappropriate* affect describes a discordance between emotional expression and the content of speech; affect is *labile* when it is characterized by marked variability.
akathisia	motor restlessness that is one of the possible complications of treatment with antipsychotic medications
amnesia	loss of memory or inability to recall past experiences usually as a consequence of physical illness, injury, or psychologic trauma
antisocial personality	a disorder characterized by repetitive failure to abide by social and legal norms and to accept responsibility for one's own behavior
apraxia	impairment of the ability to execute purposeful movements, even though adequate muscle strength, comprehension, and coordination are present
autism	a mental disorder, the features of which include onset during infancy or childhood, preoccupation with subjective mental activity, inability to interact socially, impaired communication, and repetitive body movements
behavior modification	a type of psychotherapy, based on principles of learning, which seeks to change maladaptive, observable behavior by substituting a new set of responses by the use of techniques such as reward and reinforcement
body language	a form of nonverbal communication; expression of a physical, mental, or emotional state by body position or movement
borderline personality disorder	a pervasive personality pattern, the features of which include instability of self-image, interpersonal relationships, and mood

Term	Definition
chemical dependence	a cluster of cognitive, behavioral, and physiologic symptoms that indicate impaired control of psychoactive substance use and continued use of the substance (often in large amounts) despite adverse consequences
cognition	the mental process characterized by knowing, thinking, learning, and judging
commitment	involuntary hospital admission for treatment of psychiatric illness, usually sought after a patient has been deemed a danger to self or others
confabulation	the fabrication of experiences or situations, often in a detailed and plausible way, to fill in and cover up gaps in memory
coping mechanism	the factors that enable an individual to regain emotional equilibrium after a stressful experience
cue	a stimulus that determines or may prompt the nature of a person's response
defense mechanism	an unconscious, intrapsychic reaction that offers protection to the self from a stressful situation. Examples of defense mechanisms are denial, displacement, isolation, projection, reaction formation, repression, substitution, and rationalization.
deinstitutionalization	transfer to a community setting of a patient who has been hospitalized for an extended period
delusion	a persistent false belief that is held despite evidence to the contrary. A delusion may be persecutory, grandiose, jealous, or somatic in nature.
dementia	a progressive, cognitive organic mental disorder characterized by chronic personality disintegration, confusion, disorientation, deterioration of intellectual capacity and function, and impaired memory, judgment, and control of impulses
developmental disorders	a disturbance in the acquisition of cognitive, language, motor, or social skills believed to be normally acquired by a certain age. Developmental disorders have an onset during childhood and tend to be chronic in nature.
disorientation	a state of mental confusion characterized by inadequate or incorrect perceptions of place, time, or identity. Disorientation may occur in organic mental disorders, in drug and alcohol intoxication, and after severe stress.
dyskinesia	distortion of voluntary movements; involuntary muscular activity such as tic spasms or myoclonus.
dysphoria	a disorder of affect characterized by sadness and anguish
electroconvulsive therapy (ECT)	the induction of a brief convulsion by passing electric current through the brain for the treatment of affective disorders
euphoria	a feeling of well-being or elation. An exaggerated or abnormal sense of well-being commonly is seen during the manic stages of bipolar disorder, in some forms of schizophrenia, in organic mental disorders, and in toxic and drug-induced states.
flight of ideas	a continuous stream of talk marked by a rapid and abrupt shift from one topic to another, each subject not related to the preceding one or stimulated by environmental circumstances. The condition is frequently a symptom of acute manic states or schizophrenia.

Term	Definition
gender identity disorder	a condition characterized by a persistent discomfort and sense of inappropriateness concerning one's anatomic sex and identification with the opposite sex
grandiose self	an exaggerated belief of one's importance or identity
group therapy	the application of psychotherapeutic techniques within a small group of people who experience similar difficulties. Generally, a group leader (facilitator) directs the discussion of problems in an attempt to promote individual psychologic growth and favorable behavioral change.
hallucination	a sensory perception that does not result from external stimuli, which occurs in the waking state with a continual belief that the origin of the perception is external rather than internal
insanity	a severe mental disorder; a legal rather than a medical term denoting a condition that is so severe as to interfere with the capability of functioning within the legal limits of society
learning disabled (LD)	a disorder characterized by the inadequate development, usually in children of normal or above-average intelligence, of specific academic, language, speech, and motor skills. The disorder is not the result of demonstrable physical or neurologic disorders or deficient educational opportunities.
loose association	a disturbance of thinking in which the expressed ideas appear to lack any logical sequence or relationship to one another
magical thinking	a belief that merely thinking about an event in the external world can cause it to occur or be true
maladaptive behavior	behavior that does not adjust to the environment or situation and interferes with mental health
malingering	the willful, deliberate, and fraudulent feigning or exaggeration of the symptoms of an illness
manic depressive illness (MDI)	a mood disturbance characterized by alternating attacks of mania (expansiveness, elation, and agitation) and depression, as in bipolar disorder
mental retardation (MR)	a disorder characterized by below-average general intellectual function
mental status examination (MSE)	a diagnostic procedure in which a trained interviewer asks a set of standard questions to evaluate a person's psychologic competence
neurosis	any one of the group of mental disorders characterized by anxiety symptoms and in which reality testing is intact (in contrast to psychosis)
paranoid disorder	any of a large group of mental disorders characterized by an impaired sense of reality and persistent delusions
personality disorder	a disruption in relatedness manifested in any of a large group of mental disorders. Symptoms of personality disorder include rigid, inflexible, and maladaptive behavior patterns that impair a person's ability to function in society and interpersonal relationships.
psychoanalysis	a branch of psychiatry, founded by Sigmund Freud, from which developed a system of psychotherapy based on the concepts of a dynamic unconscious
psychologic tests	any of a group of standardized tests designed to measure characteristics such as intelligence, aptitudes, and personality traits

Term	Definition
psychopharmacology	the scientific study of the drug effects on mental or behavioral activities
psychosis	any major mental disorder of organic or emotional origin characterized by a gross impairment in reality testing
psychotherapy	any of a large number of methods of treating mental and emotional disorders by psychologic techniques rather than by physical means
seasonal affective disorder (SAD)	a mood disorder associated with the decrease in sunlight during the autumn and winter and the effect of the lessened exposure on melatonin secretion. Symptoms include lethargy, depression, social withdrawal, and work difficulties.
substance abuse	the overindulgence in and dependence on a stimulant, depressant, or other chemical substance, leading to effects that are detrimental to the individual's physical or mental health or the welfare of others
therapeutic community	use of a treatment setting as a community, with the immediate aim of full participation of all clients and the eventual goal of preparing clients for life outside the treatment setting
tolerance	the need for increasing amounts of a psychoactive substance to achieve the same level of intoxication or desired effect
transference	an unconscious mechanism in which feelings and attitudes originally associated with important people and events in one's early life are attributed to others in current interpersonal relationships
withdrawal	the avoidance of social interaction; also, the occurrence of specific physical symptoms when intake of a psychoactive substance is reduced or discontinued

Additional Psychiatry Abbreviations

Abbreviation	Definition
AWOL	absent without leave/unauthorized
COT	court-ordered treatment
DSM	*Diagnostic and Statistical Manual*
DTO	danger to others
DTS	danger to self
EE	expressed emotion
EPS	extrapyramidal symptoms
GD	gravely disabled
GEI	guilty except insane
NGRI	not guilty by reason of insanity
PAD	persistently acutely disabled
RTC	residential treatment center
RTC	return to clinic
RTU	restricted to unit
S	seclusion
SMI	seriously mentally ill
S&R	seclusion and restraint
TO	time out
UALRU	unauthorized leave return urgent

APPENDIX I

Clinical Research Terms

Term	Definition
accrual	enrollment of eligible subject volunteers into a clinical trial
adjuvant treatment	secondary treatment that is given after all visible disease has been removed by a primary treatment
adverse drug reaction	all noxious and unintended responses to a medicinal product related to any dose with a reasonable possibility of a causal relation
adverse effect	an undesirable and unintended, although not necessarily unexpected, result of therapy or other intervention
adverse event	any untoward medical occurrence in a patient who does not necessarily have a causal relation with the treatment. An adverse event can be any unfavorable and unintended sign, symptom, or disease temporally associated with the use of an investigational product.
adverse reaction	an unwanted effect caused by the administration of a medicinal product. Onset may be sudden or develop over time.
arm (study arm, treatment arm, control arm)	any of the treatment groups in a randomized clinical trial. Most clinical trials have 2 or more "arms."
baseline	information gathered at the beginning of a study from which variations found in the study are measured
Belmont Report	document issued in 1979 by the National Commission for the Protection of Human Subjects of Biomedical and Behavioral Research, which established an ethical framework for clinical research activities in the United States
bias	when a point of view prevents impartial judgment on issues relating to the subject of that point of view. Bias in clinical trials is controlled by blinding and randomization.
bioavailability	the rate and extent to which the active drug ingredient or therapeutic intervention is absorbed or is otherwise available to the treatment site in the body
bioequivalence	scientific means of comparing generic and brand-name drugs, or similar drugs from different sources, such as different suppliers, different delivery systems, and different batches
biologic	any therapeutic serum, toxin, antitoxin, blood products, tissues, or analogous microbial product applicable to the prevention, treatment, or cure of diseases or injuries
biotechnology	the manipulation of biologic organisms to make products that benefit human beings. Biotechnology contributes to such diverse areas as food production, waste disposal, mining, and medicine.
blind(ing)	a procedure in which one or more parties involved in a clinical trial is kept unaware of the subject-specific treatment assignments. Single blinding refers to the subject being unaware; double blinding refers to the subject, investigator, and the research team being unaware of the treatment assignments; and triple blind is when the subject, research team, and data analysts are unaware of the treatment assignments for each subject.

Term	Definition
case control study	a study comparing persons with a given condition or disease (the cases) and persons without the condition or disease (the controls) with respect to antecedent factors
case report (or record) form	a printed, optical, or electronic document designed to record all the protocol-required information to be reported to the sponsor on each trial subject
class I, II, III medical devices	classification by the FDA of medical devices according to potential risks or hazards
clinical investigator (also known as *principal investigator*)	an advanced degreed person in charge of carrying out a clinical trial's protocol. Usually an MD, PhD, Pharm D, nurse practitioner, or other postgraduate medical/health care professional.
clinical research coordinator (CRC)	person who handles much of the administrative and operational responsibilities of a clinical trial, acts as a liaison between research site and trial sponsor, and ensures all data, records, and regulatory documents are accurate and complete
clinical trial	a research study in human beings intended to determine if new drugs, medical devices, therapies, or interventions are safe and effective; to identify any adverse reactions; and to study absorption, distribution, metabolism, and excretion of an investigational product
cohort	a group of subjects with one or more similar characteristics
compassionate use	a method of providing experimental products before final FDA approval for use in human beings. This procedure is used with very sick patients who have no other treatment options and generally requires sponsor and/or FDA approval.
conflict of interest	the situation in which an individual or organization may find it difficult to make unbiased statements or actions
contract research organization (CRO)	a company with whom a drug or device manufacturer or sponsor contracts to perform clinical trial–related activities. CROs may develop protocols, recruit subjects, collect and analyze data, and/or prepare documents for FDA approval applications.
control group (or subjects)	one group of study subjects that are given either a standard treatment or a placebo but do not get the experimental product.
crossover study	a type of clinical trial in which each subject experiences, at different times, both the experimental and control therapy
cross-sectional study	a study that examines data at one particular point in time, such as "everybody in a class on January 1" or "all 10-year-old children in a city" and does not consider within-subject effects
database	data stored in computer form for retrieval, processing, and/or analysis
data safety monitoring board	an independent committee that reviews study data while a clinical trial is in progress to ensure that subjects are not exposed to undue risks
Declaration of Helsinki	guidelines adopted in 1964 by the Eighteenth World Medical Assembly (Helsinki, Finland) and revised in 2000 by the Fifty-Second World Medical Assembly for physicians conducting biomedical research. This declaration outlines clinical trial procedures required to ensure patient safety, consent, and ethics committee reviews in human subjects.

Term	Definition
demographic data	characteristics of subjects, such as age, sex, marital status, family history of the disease or condition, and other characteristics relevant to the study
dependent variables	outcomes that are measured in an experiment. The dependent variables are expected to change as a result of an experimental intervention in the independent variable(s).
device	an instrument, apparatus, implement, machine, invention, implant, in vitro reagent, or other article intended for use in the diagnosis, treatment, or prevention of disease. A device is intended to affect the structure of function of the body, but it does not function through chemical action within or on the body.
diary cards (or journals)	subjects record data, such as frequency and severity of symptoms and responses, during a clinical trial
double-blind study	when neither the subject nor the study staff knows which participants are receiving the experimental product and which are receiving a placebo
drug-drug interaction	a modification of the effect of a drug when administered with another drug. The effect may be an increase or a decrease in the action of either substance, or it may be an adverse effect that is not normally associated with either drug.
efficacy	the maximum ability of a drug or treatment to produce a desired result regardless of dosage
eligibility	criteria that must be met before subject entry into a research study
end point	overall outcome that the protocol is designed to evaluate. Common end points are severe toxicity, disease progression, or death. The stopping point in time in a clinical study.
epidemiology	the branch of medical science that deals with the study of incidence and distribution and control of a disease in a population
ethnographic research	the study of people and their culture that involves observation of and interaction with the persons or group being studied in the group's own environment, often for long periods
evidence-based medicine	an approach to practicing medicine that involves consideration of clinical trial results that are relevant to the disease or condition being treated when making decisions about how to treat patients
exclusion criteria	a list of criteria, any one of which excludes a potential subject from participation in a study
experimental (study)	term used to denote a therapy (drug, device, procedure) that is unproven or not yet scientifically validated regarding safety and efficacy
factorial design	a study that compares two or more different sets of interventions, such as drug A versus placebo A and drug B verses placebo B. Subjects are randomly assigned to one of four groups that allows investigation of both drugs in the same study and to investigate the question of whether drugs A and B show any interaction.
510K medical device	a new medical device that is considered substantially equivalent to a device that is already being legally marketed. The term refers to the section in the Food, Drug & Cosmetic Act that describes premarket notification for these types of devices.

Term	Definition
Food and Drug Administration (FDA)..	a U.S. Department of Health and Human Services agency responsible for ensuring the safety and effectiveness of all drugs, biologics, vaccines, medical devices, blood supply, and specimen banks
FDA Form 1572.....................	Statement of Investigator form that must be completed and signed by the investigator to indicate his or her agreement to abide by U.S. federal regulation and the study protocol during the course of a clinical trial conducted under an Investigational New Drug application
gene	the fundamental physical and functional unit of heredity, which carries information from one generation to the next; a segment of DNA composed of a transcribed region and a regulatory sequence that makes transcription possible
gene therapy.......................	treatment that alters gene(s) within cells that are removed, replaced, or altered to produce new proteins that change the function of the cells
genetic engineering	the alteration of an organism's genetic, or hereditary, material to eliminate undesirable characteristics or to produce desirable new ones. Genetic engineering is used to increase plant and animal food production; to help dispose of industrial wastes; and to diagnose disease, improve medical treatment, and produce vaccines and other useful drugs.
genetics	the study of the function and behavior of genes
genome	the total genetic material of an organism; an organism's complete set of DNA sequences
genomics..........................	the study of gene structure and the relations between gene structure and biologic function in organisms
good clinical practice (GCP)	a standard for the design, conduct, performance, monitoring, auditing, recording, analyses, and reporting of clinical trials that provides assurance that the data and reported results are credible and accurate, and that the rights, integrity, and confidentiality of trial subjects are protected
historic controls.....................	control subjects (followed at some time in the past or for whom data are available through records) who are used for comparison with subjects being treated concurrently. The study is considered historically controlled when the present condition of subjects is compared with their own condition on a prior regimen or treatment.
human subjects	individuals whose physiologic or behavioral characteristics and responses are studied in a research project. Under federal regulations, human subjects are defined as living individual(s) about whom an investigator conducting research obtains (1) data through intervention or interaction with the individual or (2) identifiable private information.
hypothesis.........................	a supposition or assumption advanced as a basis for reasoning or argument, or as a guide to experimental investigation
International Conference on Harmonization (ICH)...............	a set of international guidelines developed jointly by regulatory authorities and industry to govern the conduct of clinical trials in many countries; to register new medicinal products, and to be in conformance with good clinical practice

Term	Definition
independent variables	the conditions of an experiment that are systematically manipulated by the investigator
informed consent form (ICF)	the process of learning the key facts about a clinical trial before deciding whether to participate. The informed consent form is a document that describes the rights of the study participants and includes details about the study, such as its purpose, duration, required procedures, and key contacts.
institutional review board (IRB)	an independent oversight committee of medical, scientific, and nonscientific members whose responsibility it is to ensure that a clinical trial is ethical and that the rights of study participants are protected. All biomedical and behavioral research studies with human subjects in the United States must be initially approved before they begin and periodically reviewed by an IRB. An IRB may be specific to an institution or independent, without an affiliation. Also known as *ethics review committees.*
investigational device exemptions (IDE)	exemptions from certain regulations found in the Medical Device Amendments that allow shipment of unapproved devices for use in clinical investigations
investigational new drug or device (product)	a drug or device permitted by the FDA to be tested in human beings but not yet determined to be safe and effective for a particular use in the general population and not yet licensed for marketing
(principal) investigator	a person responsible for the conduct of a clinical trial at the trial site(s)
investigator brochure	a compilation of the clinical and nonclinical data for the investigational product that is relevant to the study of the investigational product in human subjects
in vitro	literally, "in glass" or "test tube"; used to refer to processes that are carried out outside the living body, usually in the laboratory
in vivo	literally, "in the living body"; processes, such as the absorption of a drug by the human body, carried out in the living body rather than in a laboratory
legally authorized representative (LAR)	an individual or juridical or other body authorized under applicable law to consent, on behalf of a prospective subject, to the subject's participation in a research study
longitudinal study	a study that observes and measures the same subjects over a long period
maximum tolerated dose (MTD)	highest drug dose determined to produce the maximum desired effect with the least toxicity
medical device	a diagnostic or therapeutic article that does not achieve any of its principal intended purposes through chemical action within or on the body
meta-analysis	a statistical process for pooling data from many clinical trials and summarizing them through formal statistical means

Term	Definition
minimal risk	the probability and magnitude of harm or discomfort anticipated in the research that are not greater in and of themselves than those ordinarily encountered in daily life or during the performance of routine physician or psychologic examinations or tests. An institutional review board determines if a study qualifies for a minimal risk status that may affect the conduct of the study and the informed consent process.
monitor	person employed by the sponsor or contract research organization who is responsible for determining that a trial is being conducted in accordance with the protocol. Also called *clinical research associates*. Duties include helping plan and initiate a trial, assessing trial conduct at site(s), and auditing case report forms and regulatory documents.
new drug application (NDA)	an application to the FDA for a license to market a new drug in the United States
Nuremberg Code	code of ethics for conducting human medical research set forth in 1947
Office of Human Research Protections (OHRP)	a federal agency under the Department of Health and Human Services to help ensure the protection of human subjects in clinical research. OHRP issues "assurances" and supervises compliance with regulatory requirements by research institutions receiving federal funding. OHRP also provides initiatives on ethical issues in clinical research and coordinates interaction among federal agencies dealing with human subject research.
off-label use	a drug prescribed for conditions other than those approved by the FDA
open-label study	a study in which subjects and investigators know which product each subject is receiving. No blinding occurs.
orphan drugs	an FDA category that refers to medications used to treat diseases and conditions that occur rarely
outcome	the ultimate result of a medical test or treatment given to a patient or subject
parallel study design	a study design in which subject are randomly assigned to one of two or more treatment groups and each group is given a specific treatment for the entire study
participant	human volunteer who agrees to participate in a research study. Also called *subject*.
peer review	clinical trial reviewed by experts for scientific merit, participant safety, and ethical considerations
pharmacoeconomics	branch of economics that applies cost-benefit, cost-effectiveness, cost-minimization, and cost-utility analyses to compare the economics of different pharmaceutical products or to compare drug therapy to other treatments
pharmacogenetics	the study of the way drugs interact with genetic makeup or the genetic response to a drug
pharmacokinetics	the processes in a living organism of absorption, distribution, metabolism, and excretion of a drug or vaccine

Term	Definition
phase I trials	initial studies to determine the metabolism and pharmacologic actions of drugs in human beings, the side effects associated with increasing dose, and early evidence of effectiveness. May include healthy participants.
phase II trials	controlled clinical studies conducted to evaluate the effectiveness of the drug for a particular indication in patients with the disease or condition under study and to determine the common short-term side effects and risks
phase III trials	expanded controlled and uncontrolled trials after preliminary evidence suggesting effectiveness of the experimental product has been obtained. Intended to gather additional information to evaluate the overall benefit-risk relation of the product and provide an adequate basis for FDA labeling.
phase IV trials	postmarketing studies to delineate additional information, including the drug's risks, benefits, and optimal use
pilot study	a small study for helping design a study, test a study's procedures, develop questionnaires, and formulate practical arrangements, that is, how long do various activities take? Do subjects understand the survey questions as intended?
placebo	an inactive pill, liquid, or powder that has no treatment value. In clinical trials, experimental treatments are often compared with placebos to assess the treatment's effectiveness.
placebo-controlled study	a method of investigation of drugs in which an inactive substance (the placebo) is given to one group and the drug being tested is given to another group. The results obtained from both groups are then compared to see if the investigational treatment is more effective in treating the condition under study.
placebo effect	a physical or emotional change, occurring after an inactive substance is taken or administered, that is not the result of any special property of the substance
preclinical studies	the testing of experimental products in the test tube, in the laboratory, or in animals, or the testing that occurs before trials in human beings may be carried out
prevention study	study to find better ways to prevent disease in people who have never had the disease or to prevent a disease from returning
prospective studies	observing events looking forward in time, in the future, or that have not yet occurred
protocol	a formal design or plan of an experiment or research activity that includes study methodology, subject eligibility, treatment regimen, and analysis methods
protocol deviation	something that happens within a study and that does not fully conform to what was described in the protocol
qualitative variable	data that cannot be measured numerically, such as race or sex
quantitative variable	data that can be measured numerically, such as blood pressure
quasiexperimental study	a study that lacks the random assignment of subjects to treatment groups
random sample	a sample from a population in which every individual in the population has the same probability of being chosen
randomization	the process of assigning trial subjects to treatment or control groups by using an element of chance to determine the assignments to reduce bias

Term	Definition
research	a systematic investigation designed to develop or contribute to generalizable knowledge
retrospective studies	research that reviews many forms of records from the past or by obtaining information about past events elicited through interviews or surveys
risk-benefit ratio	the actual or potential risks to subjects versus the potential benefits. Risks can be physical, psychologic, social, or economic.
sample size	the number of subjects to be enrolled in each treatment group; expressed as "n"
schema	a diagrammatic overview (table of events) of a protocol from registration to the end of the trial
serious adverse event (SAE)	any untoward medical occurrence that at any dose results in death, is life-threatening, requires inpatient hospitalization or prolongation of existing hospitalization, results in persistent or significant disability/incapacity, or is a congenital anomaly/birth defect
sham treatment	an inactive device or device/procedure that mimics the actual device and can be used as a placebo in a clinical trial
single-blind study	a study in which one party, either the investigator or participant, is unaware of what medication the subject is taking
source documents	original subject/patient documents, data, and records, such as laboratory results, hospital records, recorded data from automated instruments, microfilm, radiographs, subject diaries, pharmacy dispensing records, and photographic negatives
sponsor (of a clinical trial)	an individual, agency, organization, academic institution, or company that plans, initiates, and takes responsibility for a clinical study. Usually a drug or medical device manufacturer, foundations, state/federal agencies, researchers, and academic medical centers.
standard operating procedures (SOPs)	detailed, written instructions to achieve uniformity of the performance of specific functions and/or operations
treatment group (arm)	group in the subject pool that is receiving active investigational drug or product or treatment intervention
variable	an item of data for which values are to be obtained for the research study
voluntary	free of coercion, duress, or undue inducement. In a clinical trial, refers to a subject's decision to participate.
washout period	a period during a clinical trial when the trial subjects receive no active medication to eliminate the effect of previous medication(s) the subject may have been taking
withdraw	in a research study, to end a subject's participation before he or she reaches the designated study end point

Nutritional Terms

Term	Definition
amino acid	building block of protein that can be essential (must be consumed) or nonessential (made by the body); provides 4 calories per gram
body mass index (BMI)	a tool to measure the degree of undernutrition or overnutrition; equals weight in kilograms divided by height in meters squared
calorie	a measure of the energy contained in a food
carbohydrate	a simple or complex compound made up of carbon, oxygen, and hydrogen; provides 4 calories per gram
carbohydrate counting	a method used to control blood sugars by diet for those with diabetes; often used with patients on insulin pumps
cholesterol	waxy substance made in the body or taken in by diet; found only in animal products
diet technician	a nutrition professional who has an associate's degree and has completed formal training along with passing a national board exam
dietary reference intake (DRI)	a guide to the amount of nutrients needed to prevent disease and reduce the risk of diet-related diseases
enteral nutrition	provision of nutrients through a tube into the gastrointestinal tract
fat	glycerol molecule made up of carbon, oxygen, and hydrogen with fatty acids attached; provides 9 calories per gram
fiber	materials in food that cannot be digested by the body; found mainly in plants
glucose	simplest form of carbohydrate, commonly referred to as *blood sugar*; equivalent to dextrose
hydrogenation	process of changing a liquid fat to a solid fat
macronutrients	carbohydrate, fat, or protein
malnutrition	inadequacy or abundance of one or more nutrients leading to compromised health
metabolism	the sum of all chemical and physical changes in the body
micronutrients	vitamins or minerals
minerals	inorganic substances occurring in nature that are essential for normal function and development of body systems
monounsaturated fat	a fatty acid chain with one double bond, such as olive oil and canola oil; research has shown them to be a healthy type of fat
omega-3 fatty acids	unsaturated fatty acid found in fish that must be consumed (essential fatty acid); it is associated with decreased risk of heart disease and named for the position of the first double bond
parenteral nutrition	the provision of nutrients administered through the vein
phytochemical	plant-based food components that are nonnutritive (do not provide calories) and are linked to prevention of disease
pica	a craving or intake of nonfood substances such as dirt or laundry starch
polyunsaturated fat	a fatty acid chain that contains two or more double bonds; examples include corn oil and sunflower oil

Term	Definition
prebiotics	a nondigestible food ingredient that may benefit the gastrointestinal tract by providing fuel for the growth of healthy bacteria
probiotics	live microbes that may assist in maintaining or restoring gastrointestinal health; derived from a Greek term meaning "for life"
protein	a chain of amino acids that is the body's only source of nitrogen; made up of carbon, hydrogen, oxygen, and sometimes sulfur; provides 4 calories per gram
recommended dietary allowance (RDA)	nutrient recommendations to maintain good health; prepared by the Food and Nutrition Board; based on research
registered dietitian	a nutrition professional who has completed a bachelor's degree and an internship program and has passed a national board exam; manages food and nutrition to promote health
saturated fat	a fatty acid chain with no double bonds mostly found in animal foods (e.g., lard); high intake is associated with increased risk of heart disease
therapeutic diet	a diet plan prescribed by a physician or dietitian for a disorder or disease; the diet may be altered for a specific nutrient or the percentage of macronutrients
trans fat	a substance created through the process of hydrogenation whose structure contains an unusual double bond; a high intake is associated with a higher risk of cardiovascular disease
triglyceride	a glycerol molecule with three fatty acids attached; it can increase in the blood with a diet high in simple carbohydrates or alcohol
unsaturated fat	a fatty acid chain that contains one or more double bonds
vegan	a person who consumes a diet consisting of only plant foods
vitamins	organic substances classified as fat or water soluble that have specific biochemical functions essential for normal metabolism; provided by the diet

ANSWERS

ANSWERS TO CHAPTER 1 EXERCISES

Exercise Figures

Exercise Figure A oste/o/arthr/itis

Exercise 1

1. b 2. a 3. d 4. e 5. c

Exercise 2

1. *F*, a medical term may begin with the word root and have no prefix.
2. *F*, if the suffix begins with a vowel, the combining vowel is usually not used.
3. *T*
4. *T*
5. *F*, *o* is the combining vowel most often used.
6. *T*
7. *F*, a combining vowel is used between two word roots or between a word root and a suffix to ease pronunciation.
8. *F*, a combining form is a word root with a combining vowel attached and is not one of the four word parts.
9. *T*

Exercise 3

1. WR S
   arthr/itis
   inflammation of the joint

2. WR S
   hepat/itis
   inflammation of the liver

3. P WR S
   sub/hepat/ic
   pertaining to under the liver

4. P WR S
   intra/ven/ous
   pertaining to within the vein

5. WR CV S
   arthr/o/pathy
        CF
   disease of the joint

6. WR S
   oste/itis
   inflammation of the bone

Exercise 4

1. arthr/itis
2. hepat/ic
3. sub/hepat/ic
4. intra/ven/ous

5. oste/itis
6. hepat/itis
7. oste/o/arthr/o/pathy

ANSWERS TO CHAPTER 2 EXERCISES

Exercise Figures

Exercise Figure

A. 1. cyt/o
   2. hist/o
   3. organ/o
   4. system/o

Exercise Figure

B. 1. neur/o
   2. sarc/o
   3. epitheli/o
   4. my/o

Exercise Figure

C. 1. carcin/oma
   2. melan/oma
   3. sarc/oma
   4. rhabd/o/my/o/sarcoma

Exercise Figure D. hyper/plasia

Exercise Figure

E. 1. erythr/o/cyte
   2. leuk/o/cyte

Exercise 1

1. h   6. f
2. e   7. c
3. d   8. a
4. k   9. b
5. g   10. j

Exercise 2

1. h   5. g
2. b   6. a
3. c   7. f
4. e

Exercise 3

1. flesh, connective   7. muscle
   tissue   8. nerve
2. fat   9. organ
3. nucleus   10. system
4. internal organs   11. epithelium
5. cell   12. fiber
6. tissue   13. gland

Exercise 4

1. viscer/o   8. my/o
2. epitheli/o   9. lip/o
3. organ/o   10. system/o
4. kary/o   11. sarc/o
5. cyt/o   12. fibr/o
6. hist/o   13. aden/o
7. neur/o

Exercise 5

1. tumor, mass
2. cancer
3. cause (of disease)
4. disease
5. body
6. cancer
7. rod-shaped, striated
8. smooth
9. knowledge
10. physician, medicine

Exercise 6

1. path/o   5. somat/o
2. onc/o   6. lei/o
3. eti/o   7. rhabd/o
4. a. cancer/o   8. gno/o
   b. carcin/o   9. iatr/o

Exercise 7

1. blue   5. color
2. red   6. black
3. white   7. green
4. yellow

Exercise 8

1. cyan/o   5. xanth/o
2. erythr/o   6. chrom/o
3. leuk/o   7. chlor/o
4. melan/o

Exercise 9

1. new
2. above, excessive
3. after, beyond, change
4. below, incomplete, deficient
5. difficult, labored, painful, abnormal
6. through, complete
7. before

Exercise 10

1. neo-   5. dys-
2. hyper-   6. dia-
3. hypo-   7. pro-
4. meta-

Exercise 11

1. i	9. p
2. l	10. c
3. e	11. n
4. f	12. k
5. g	13. q
6. j	14. m
7. h	15. a
8. b	16. o

Exercise 12

1. specialist, physician
2. disease
3. study of
4. pertaining to
5. control, stop, standing
6. cell
7. abnormal condition
8. pertaining to
9. a growth, a substance, a formation
10. pertaining to
11. condition of formation, development, growth
12. resembling
13. substance or agent that produces or causes
14. producing, originating, causing
15. tumor, swelling
16. origin, cause
17. malignant tumor
18. state of

Exercise 13

1. WR S
   sarc/oma
   tumor composed of connective tissue

2. WR S
   melan/oma
   black tumor

3. WR S
   epitheli/oma
   tumor composed of epithelium

4. WR S
   lip/oma
   tumor composed of fat

5. P S(WR)
   neo/plasm
   new growth

6. WR S
   my/oma
   tumor composed of muscle

7. WR S
   neur/oma
   tumor composed of nerve

8. WR S
   carcin/oma
   cancerous tumor

9. WR CV WR S
   melan/o/carcin/oma
        CF
   cancerous black tumor

10. WR CV WR CV S
    rhabd/o/my/o/sarcoma
        CF   CF
    malignant tumor of striated muscle

11. WR CV WR S
    lei/o/my/oma
        CF
    tumor of smooth muscle

12. WR CV WR S
    rhabd/o/my/oma
         CF
    tumor of striated muscle

13. WR S
    fibr/oma
    tumor composed of fiber (fibrous tissue)

14. WR CV S
    lip/o/sarcoma
        CF
    malignant tumor composed of fat

15. WR CV S
    fibr/o/sarcoma
         CF
    malignant tumor composed of fiber (fibrous tissue)

16. WR S
    aden/oma
    tumor composed of glandular tissue

17. WR CV WR S
    aden/o/carcin/oma
        CF
    cancerous tumor composed of glandular tissue

18. WR S
    chlor/oma
    tumor of green color

Exercise 14

1. melan/oma
2. carcin/oma
3. neo/plasm
4. epitheli/oma
5. sarc/oma
6. melan/o/carcin/oma
7. neur/oma
8. my/oma
9. rhabd/o/my/o/sarcoma
10. lei/o/my/oma
11. rhabd/o/my/oma
12. lei/o/my/o/sarcoma
13. lip/o/sarcoma
14. fibr/oma
15. fibr/o/sarcoma
16. aden/oma
17. aden/o/carcin/oma
18. chlor/oma

Exercise 15

Spelling exercise; see text, p. 28.

Exercise 16

1. not malignant, nonrecurrent, favorable for recovery
2. tending to become progressively worse and to cause death, as in cancer
3. improvement or absence of signs of disease
4. pertaining to disease of unknown origin
5. response to injury or destruction of tissue; signs are redness, swelling, heat, and pain
6. treatment of cancer with drugs
7. treatment of cancer with radioactive substance, such as x-ray or radiation
8. enclosed in a capsule, as in benign tumors
9. within a glass, observable within a test tube
10. within the living body
11. cancer in the early stage before invading the surrounding tissue
12. increase in the severity of a disease or its symptoms

Exercise 17

Spelling exercise; see text, p. 31.

Exercise 18

1. WR CV S
   cyt/o/logy
       CF
   study of cells

2. WR CV S
   hist/o/logy
        CF
   study of tissue

3. WR CV S
   path/o/logy
        CF
   study of disease

4. WR CV S
   path/o/logist
        CF
   a physician who studies diseases

5. WR S
   viscer/al
   pertaining to internal organs

6. P S(WR)
   meta/stasis
   beyond control (transfer of disease)

7. WR CV   S
    <u>onc</u>/<u>o</u>/genic
       CF
    causing tumors

8. WR CV   S
    <u>onc</u>/<u>o</u>/logy
       CF
    study of tumors

9. WR CV   S
    <u>kary</u>/<u>o</u>/cyte
       CF
    cell with a nucleus

10. P   S(WR)
    neo/pathy
    new disease

11. WR CV   S
    <u>kary</u>/<u>o</u>/plasm
       CF
    substance of a nucleus

12. WR CV   S
    <u>cyt</u>/<u>o</u>/genic
       CF
    producing cells

13. WR   S
    system/ic
    pertaining to a (body) system

14. WR   S
    cancer/ous
    pertaining to cancer

15. WR CV   S
    <u>cyt</u>/<u>o</u>/plasm
       CF
    cell substance

16. WR CV   S
    <u>carcin</u>/<u>o</u>/genic
       CF
    producing cancer

17. WR   S
    somat/ic
    pertaining to the body

18. WR CV   S
    <u>somat</u>/<u>o</u>/genic
       CF
    originating in the body

19. WR CV   S
    <u>somat</u>/<u>o</u>/plasm
       CF
    body substance

20. WR CV   S
    <u>somat</u>/<u>o</u>/pathy
       CF
    disease of the body

21. WR   S
    neur/oid
    resembling a nerve

22. WR CV   S
    <u>my</u>/<u>o</u>/pathy
       CF
    disease of the muscle

23. WR CV   S
    <u>erythr</u>/<u>o</u>/cyte
       CF
    red (blood) cell

24. WR CV   S
    <u>leuk</u>/<u>o</u>/cyte
       CF
    white (blood) cell

25. WR   S
    cyan/osis
    abnormal condition of blue (bluish
    discoloration of the skin)

26. WR   S
    epitheli/al
    pertaining to epithelium

27. WR S
    lip/oid
    resembling fat

28. WR CV S
    <u>eti</u>/<u>o</u>/logy
       CF
    study of causes (of disease)

29. WR   S
    xanth/osis
    abnormal condition of yellow

30. WR CV WR   S
    <u>xanth</u>/<u>o</u>/chrom/ic
       CF
    pertaining to yellow color

31. P   S(WR)
    hyper/plasia
    excessive development (of cells)

32. WR CV WR S
    <u>erythr</u>/<u>o</u>/cyt/osis
       CF
    increase in the number of red (blood)
    cells

33. WR CV WR S
    <u>leuk</u>/<u>o</u>/cyt/osis
       CF
    increase in the number of white
    (blood) cells

34. WR CV S
    <u>carcin</u>/<u>o</u>/gen
       CF
    substance that causes cancer

35.   P   S(WR)
    hypo/plasia
    incomplete development (of an organ
    or tissue)

36. WR S
    cyt/oid
    resembling a cell

37. WR CV   S
    <u>onc</u>/<u>o</u>/logist
       CF
    physician who studies and treats
    tumors

38.   P   S(WR)
    dys/plasia
    abnormal development

39. WR CV   S
    <u>path</u>/<u>o</u>/genic
       CF
    producing disease

40. P WR S
    pro/gno/sis
    state of before knowledge

41. P WR S
    dia/gno/sis
    state of complete knowledge

42. WR CV   S
    <u>iatr</u>/<u>o</u>/genic
       CF
    produced by a physician

43. WR CV   S
    <u>iatr</u>/<u>o</u>/logy
       CF
    study of medicine

Exercise 19

1. cyt/o/plasm
2. xanth/o/chrom/ic
3. meta/stasis
4. neo/pathy
5. eti/o/logy
6. kary/o/plasm
7. onc/o/logy
8. path/o/logy
9. somat/ic
10. path/o/logist
11. my/o/pathy
12. somat/o/plasm
13. xanth/osis
14. viscer/al
15. onc/o/genic
16. somat/o/genic
17. somat/o/pathy
18. erythr/o/cyte
19. neur/oid
20. system/ic
21. leuk/o/cyte
22. kary/o/cyte

23. lip/oid
24. cancer/ous
25. cyt/o/logy
26. hyper/plasia
27. cyt/oid
28. epitheli/al
29. cyan/osis
30. carcin/o/genic
31. path/o/genic
32. hist/o/logy
33. erythr/o/cyt/osis
34. hypo/plasia
35. leuk/o/cyt/osis
36. carcin/o/gen
37. onc/o/logist
38. dys/plasia
39. iatr/o/logy
40. dia/gno/sis
41. iatr/o/genic
42. pro/gno/sis

Exercise 20
Spelling exercise; see text, pp. 39-40.

Exercise 21
diagnosis; carcinoma; metastasis; prognosis; red blood cell; white blood cell; chemotherapy; radiation therapy

Exercise 22
1. chemotherapy
2. adenocarcinoma
3. pathology
4. malignant
5. radiation therapy
6. cyanosis
7. metastasis

Exercise 23
1. sarcoma, malignant
2. erythrocytosis
3. visceral
4. lipoma, nonrecurrent
5. carcinogenic
6. causes of disease
7. neoplasm
8. somatogenic
9. myopathy
10. dysplasia
11. iatrogenic
12. melanoma, pathology, prognosis
13. in vivo
14. liposarcoma
15. DNA

Exercise 24 Reading Exercise

Exercise 25
1. *F*, "no evidence of metastasis" (transfer of disease from one organ to another) means the cancer has not spread to surrounding organs.
2. *T*
3. *F*, prognosis means "prediction of the outcome of disease"; diagnosis means "identifying a disease."
4. *T*
5. *F*, an oncologist treats patients with cancer; a pathologist studies body changes caused by disease usually from a specimen in a laboratory setting.

Answers

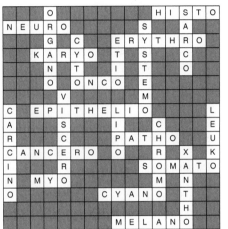

ANSWERS TO CHAPTER 3 EXERCISES
Exercise Figures
Exercise Figure
A. 1. cephal/o
2. anter/o
3. ventr/o
4. dors/o
5. poster/o
6. caud/o
7. super/o
8. later/o
9. medi/o
10. proxim/o
11. dist/o
12. infer/o

Exercise Figure
B. 1. poster/o/anter/ior
2. anter/o/poster/ior

Exercise Figure
C. 1. coronal or frontal plane
2. transverse
3. midsagittal plane

Exercise Figure
D. 1. umbilical
2. epigastric
3. hypogastric
4. hypochondriac
5. lumbar
6. iliac

Exercise Figure
E. 1. right upper quadrant (RUQ)
2. left upper quadrant (LUQ)
3. right lower quadrant (RLQ)
4. left lower quadrant (LLQ)

Exercise 1
1. belly (front)
2. head (upward)
3. side
4. middle
5. below
6. near (point of attachment of a body part)
7. above
8. away (from the point of attachment of a body part)
9. back
10. tail (downward)
11. front
12. back, behind

Exercise 2
1. later/o
2. super/o
3. cephal/o
4. dist/o
5. anter/o
6. medi/o
7. dors/o
8. ventr/o
9. caud/o
10. infer/o
11. poster/o
12. proxim/o

Exercise 3
1. c   2. b   3. d   4. a

Exercise 4
1. pertaining to   3. two
2. toward   4. one

Exercise 5
1. WR   S
   cephal/ad
   toward the head

2. WR   S
   cephal/ic
   pertaining to the head

3. WR   S
caud/al
pertaining to the tail

4. WR   S
anter/ior
pertaining to the front

5. WR   S
poster/ior
pertaining to the back

6. WR   S
dors/al
pertaining to the back

7. WR   S
super/ior
pertaining to above

8. WR   S
infer/ior
pertaining to below

9. WR   S
proxim/al
pertaining to near

10. WR   S
dist/al
pertaining to away

11. WR   S
later/al
pertaining to a side

12. WR   S
medi/al
pertaining to the middle

13. WR   S
medi/ad
toward the middle

14. WR   S
ventr/al
pertaining to the belly (front)

15. WR CV WR   S
poster/o/anter/ior
    CF
pertaining to the back and to the front

16. P   WR   S
uni/later/al
pertaining to one side

17. WR CV WR   S
medi/o/later/al
    CF
pertaining to the middle and to the side

18. WR CV WR   S
anter/o/poster/ior
    CF
pertaining to the front and to the back

19. P   WR   S
bi/later/al
pertaining to two sides

Exercise 6
1. cephal/ad
2. cephal/ic
3. caud/al
4. anter/ior
5. poster/ior, dors/al
6. super/ior
7. infer/ior
8. proxim/al
9. dist/al
10. later/al
11. medi/al
12. medi/ad
13. ventr/al
14. poster/o/anter/ior
15. medi/o/later/al
16. uni/later/al
17. anter/o/poster/ior
18. bi/later/al

Exercise 7
Spelling exercise; see text, p. 53.

Exercise 8
1. transverse
2. midsagittal
3. coronal or frontal
4. sagittal

Exercise 9
Spelling exercise; see text, p. 57.

Exercise 10
1. iliac
2. epigastric
3. hypogastric
4. hypochondriac
5. umbilical
6. lumbar

Exercise 11
1. b 2. d 3. a 4. e 5. c 6. g

Exercise 12
Spelling exercise; see text, p. 59.

Exercise 13
See answers to Exercise Figure E.

Exercise 14
Spelling exercise; see text, p. 61.

Exercise 15
1. superior
2. anterior
3. inferior
4. posteroanterior
5. anteroposterior
6. medial
7. lateral

Exercise 16
1. anteroposterior
2. lateral
3. posterior
4. medial
5. anterior

Exercise 17
1. distal
2. anterior
3. superior
4. anteroposterior; frontal (or coronal)
5. epigastric
6. lateral; sagittal
7. bilateral

Exercise 18 Reading Exercise

Exercise 19
1. *F,* "unilateral" means one side; "bilateral" means two sides. The right lumbar region is to the right of the umbilical region.
2. *T*
3. *T*

Answers

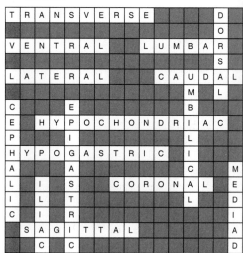

ANSWERS TO CHAPTER 4 EXERCISES
Exercise Figures
Exercise Figure
A. 1. horny tissue: kerat/o
2. sweat: hidr/o
3. hair: trich/o
4. skin: cutane/o, dermat/o, derm/o
5. sebum: seb/o

Exercise Figure B. nail: onych/o, ungu/o

Exercise Figure C. par/onych/ia

Exercise Figure D. staphyl/o/cocci

Exercise Figure E. strept/o/cocci

Exercise 1
1. c 2. d 3. g 4. b
5. f 6. h 7. a

Exercise 2
1. sweat
2. skin
3. nail
4. hair
5. horny tissue, hard
6. skin
7. sebum (oil)
8. nail
9. skin

Exercise 3
1. trich/o
2. hidr/o
3. a. onych/o
   b. ungu/o
4. seb/o
5. a. derm/o
   b. dermat/o
   c. cutane/o
6. kerat/o

Exercise 4
1. death
2. grapelike clusters
3. hidden
4. thick
5. dust
6. fungus
7. life
8. other
9. twisted chains
10. dry
11. self
12. wrinkles

Exercise 5
1. myc/o
2. necr/o
3. heter/o
4. xer/o
5. pachy/o
6. strept/o
7. rhytid/o
8. staphyl/o
9. aut/o
10. crypt/o
11. coni/o
12. bi/o

Exercise 6
1. under, below
2. beside, beyond, around
3. on, upon, over
4. within
5. through

Exercise 7
1. intra-
2. sub-
3. epi-
4. para-
5. per-

Exercise 8
1. c
2. e
3. a
4. j
5. i
6. h
7. d
8. b
9. f
10. k

Exercise 9
1. surgical repair
2. excision or surgical removal
3. softening

4. inflammation
5. instrument used to cut
6. eating, swallowing
7. excessive discharge, flow
8. berry-shaped
9. view of, viewing
10. diseased or abnormal state, condition of

Exercise 10
1. WR CV WR S
   dermat/o/coni/osis
          CF
   abnormal condition of the skin caused by dust

2. WR WR S
   hidr/aden/itis
   inflammation of the sweat glands

3. WR S
   dermat/itis
   inflammation of the skin

4. WR WR S
   pachy/derm/a
   thickening of the skin

5. WR CV S
   onych/o/malacia
         CF
   softening of the nails

6. WR CV WR S
   trich/o/myc/osis
         CF
   abnormal condition of a fungus in the hair

7. WR CV WR S
   dermat/o/fibr/oma
          CF
   fibrous tumor of the skin

8. P WR S
   par/onych/ia
   diseased state around the nail

9. WR CV WR S
   onych/o/crypt/osis
         CF
   abnormal condition of a hidden nail

10. WR CV S
    seb/o/rrhea
        CF
    excessive discharge of sebum

11. WR CV S
    onych/o/phagia
          CF
    eating the nails, nail biting

12. WR CV WR S
    xer/o/derm/a
        CF
    dry skin

13. WR CV WR S
    lei/o/derm/ia
        CF
    condition of smooth skin

Exercise 11
1. pachy/derm/a
2. onych/o/myc/osis
3. seb/o/rrhea
4. dermat/itis
5. dermat/o/fibr/oma
6. onych/o/malacia
7. hidr/aden/itis
8. onych/o/crypt/osis
9. dermat/o/coni/osis
10. onych/o/phagia
11. par/onych/ia
12. xer/o/derm/a
13. lei/o/derm/ia

Exercise 12
Spelling exercise; see text, p. 79.

Exercise 13
1. systemic lupus erythematosus
2. abscess
3. fissure
4. abrasion
5. psoriasis
6. herpes
7. pediculosis
8. tinea
9. contusion
10. gangrene
11. lesion
12. Kaposi sarcoma
13. actinic keratosis
14. carbuncle
15. acne
16. laceration
17. furuncle
18. squamous cell
19. cellulitis
20. impetigo
21. eczema
22. scabies
23. urticaria
24. basal cell
25. scleroderma
26. candidiasis
27. shingles

Exercise 14
1. f
2. j
3. g
4. l
5. m
6. c
7. i
8. k
9. e
10. b
11. h
12. a
13. d

Exercise 15
1. d
2. i
3. f
4. h
5. l
6. k
7. c
8. a
9. m
10. e
11. b
12. g
13. j
14. n

Exercise 16
Spelling exercise; see text, pp. 85-86.

Exercise 17

1. WR   S
rhytid/ectomy
excision of wrinkles

2. WR S
bi/opsy
view of life (removal of living tissue)

3. WR CV WR CV S
dermat/o/aut/o/plasty
    CF   CF
surgical repair using one's own skin (for the skin graft)

4. WR   S
onych/ectomy
excision of a nail

5. WR CV S
rhytid/o/plasty
    CF
surgical repair of wrinkles

6. WR CV WR CV S
dermat/o/heter/o/plasty
    CF   CF
surgical repair using skin from others (for the skin graft)

Exercise 18

1. rhytid/ectomy
2. bi/opsy
3. dermat/o/heter/o/plasty
4. onych/ectomy
5. rhytid/o/plasty
6. dermat/o/plasty

Exercise 19

Spelling exercise; see text, p. 88.

Exercise 20

1. WR   S
ungu/al
pertaining to the nail

2. WR   S
derma/tome
instrument used to cut skin

3. WR CV S
strept/o/coccus
    CF
berry-shaped (bacteria) in twisted chains

4. P   WR   S
hypo/derm/ic
pertaining to under the skin

5. WR CV S
dermat/o/logy
    CF
study of the skin

6. P   WR   S
sub/cutane/ous
pertaining to under the skin

7. WR CV S
staphyl/o/coccus
    CF
berry-shaped (bacteria) in grapelike clusters

8. WR CV S
kerat/o/genic
   CF
originating in horny tissue

9. WR CV S
dermat/o/logist
    CF
physician who studies and treats skin (diseases)

10. WR   S
necr/osis
abnormal condition of death

11. P WR   S
epi/derm/al
pertaining to upon the skin

12. WR CV WR S
xanth/o/derm/a
    CF
yellow skin

13. WR CV WR S
erythr/o/derm/a
    CF
red skin

14. WR CV WR S
leuk/o/derm/a
    CF
white skin

15. P   WR   S
per/cutane/ous
pertaining to through the skin

Exercise 21

1. dermat/o/logy
2. necr/osis
3. derma/tome
4. ungu/al
5. staphyl/o/cocci
6. dermat/o/logist
7. intra/derm/al
8. epi/derm/al
9. sub/cutane/ous, hypo/derm/ic
10. strept/o/cocci
11. kerat/o/genic
12. leuk/o/derm/a
13. erythr/o/derm/a
14. xanth/o/derm/a
15. per/cutane/ous

Exercise 22

Spelling exercise; see text, p. 92.

Exercise 23

1. cicatrix	17. pruritus
2. diaphoresis	18. erythema
3. emollient	19. purpura
4. verruca	20. nevus
5. macule	21. debridement
6. jaundice	22. alopecia
7. leukoplakia	23. allergy
8. petechiae	24. papule
9. ulcer	25. wheal
10. keloid	26. pustule
11. pallor	27. vesicle
12. ecchymosis	28. dermabrasion
13. albino	29. virus
14. nodule	30. induration
15. adipose	31. edema
16. cyst	32. cytomegalovirus

Exercise 24

1. m	9. g
2. o	10. d
3. h	11. b
4. a	12. f
5. j	13. k
6. e	14. c
7. n	15. q
8. l	16. i

Exercise 25

1. g	9. e
2. d	10. f
3. j	11. o
4. a	12. c
5. l	13. h
6. k	14. i
7. n	15. m
8. b	16. q

Exercise 26

Spelling exercise; see text, pp. 99-100.

Exercise 27

1. basal cell carcinoma
2. cytomegalovirus
3. systemic lupus erythematosus
4. squamous cell carcinoma
5. biopsy
6. subcutaneous
7. staphylococcus
8. streptococcus

Exercise 28

1. dermatology
2. nevus
3. medial
4. actinic keratosis
5. eczema
6. lesion

7. superior
8. pathology
9. biopsy
10. basal cell carcinoma

Exercise 29
1. contusion
2. staphylococci
3. xeroderma
4. intradermal
5. softening of the nails
6. petechiae
7. diaphoresis
8. trichomycosis
9. vesicle
10. dermatoheteroplasty
11. induration
12. xanthoderma
13. smooth

Exercise 30 Reading Exercise

Exercise 31
1. b
2. *F,* acne is the condition described in the sentence.
3. d

Answers

ANSWERS TO CHAPTER 5 EXERCISES
Exercise Figures
Exercise Figure
A. 1. adenoids: adenoid/o
   2. pharynx: pharyng/o
   3. lung: pneum/o, pneumat/o, pneumon/o, pulmon/o
   4. bronchus: bronch/i, bronch/o
   5. alveolus: alveol/o
   6. sinus: sinus/o
   7. nose: nas/o, rhin/o
   8. tonsils: tonsill/o
   9. epiglottis: epiglott/o
   10. larynx: laryng/o
   11. trachea: trache/o

12. pleura: pleur/o
13. lobe: lob/o
14. diaphragm: diaphragmat/o

Exercise Figure B. bronch/i/ectasis

Exercise Figure C. pneum/o/thorax

Exercise Figure D. adenoid/ectomy, aden/o/tome

Exercise Figure E. thorac/o/centesis

Exercise Figure F. trache/o/stomy

Exercise Figure G. bronch/o/scopy, bronch/o/scope

Exercise Figure H. endo/trache/al, laryng/o/scope

Exercise 1
1. h   5. f
2. a   6. d
3. g   7. e
4. c   8. b

Exercise 2
1. nasal septum   5. diaphragm
2. epiglottis   6. mediastinum
3. bronchioles   7. tonsils
4. nose

Exercise 3
1. larynx   11. thorax (chest)
2. bronchus   12. adenoids
3. pleura   13. pharynx
4. air, lung   14. nose
5. tonsil   15. sinus
6. lung   16. lobe
7. diaphragm   17. epiglottis
8. trachea   18. air, lung
9. alveolus   19. nose
10. air, lung   20. septum

Exercise 4
1. a. nas/o   9. diaphragmat/o
   b. rhin/o   10. sinus/o
2. laryng/o   11. thorac/o
3. a. pneum/o   12. alveol/o
   b. pneumat/o   13. pharyng/o
   c. pneumon/o   14. a. bronch/o
4. pulmon/o   b. bronch/i
5. tonsill/o   15. lob/o
6. trache/o   16. epiglott/o
7. adenoid/o   17. sept/o
8. pleur/o

Exercise 5
1. oxygen
2. breathe, breathing

3. mucus
4. imperfect, incomplete
5. straight
6. pus
7. blood
8. sleep
9. carbon dioxide

Exercise 6
1. spir/o   5. py/o
2. a. ox/o   6. muc/o
   b. ox/i   7. a. hem/o
3. atel/o   b. hemat/o
4. orth/o   8. somn/o

Exercise 7
1. within   3. all, total
2. without,   4. normal, good
   absence of   5. many, much

Exercise 8
1. endo-   4. pan-
2. eu-   5. poly-
3. a. a-
   b. an-

Exercise 9
1. k   7. a
2. f   8. l
3. g   9. h
4. c   10. d
5. b   11. e
6. j

Exercise 10
1. c   7. j
2. f   8. b
3. a   9. l
4. i   10. g
5. k   11. d
6. e   12. h

Exercise 11
1. chest
2. pertaining to
3. constriction, narrowing
4. hernia, protrusion
5. creation of an artificial opening
6. surgical fixation or suspension
7. instrument used to measure
8. sudden, involuntary muscle contraction
9. pain
10. visual examination
11. surgical puncture to aspirate fluid
12. cut into, incision
13. instrument used for visual examination
14. rapid flow of blood
15. stretching out, dilatation, expansion
16. record, x-ray image
17. breathing

18. process of recording, x-ray imaging
19. measurement
20. blood condition
21. oxygen
22. sound or voice
23. pertaining to visual examination

Exercise 12

1.   WR   S
   pleur/itis
   inflammation of the pleura

2. WR CV   WR   S
   nas/o/pharyng/itis
     CF
   inflammation of the nose and pharynx

3.   WR CV   S
   pneum/o/thorax
     CF
   air in the chest

4.   P   WR   S
   pan/sinus/itis
   inflammation of all sinuses

5.   WR   S
   atel/ectasis
   incomplete expansion (or collapsed lung)

6. WR CV WR   S
   rhin/o/myc/osis
     CF
   abnormal condition of fungus in the nose

7.   WR CV   S
   trache/o/stenosis
     CF
   narrowing of the trachea

8.   WR   S
   epiglott/itis
   inflammation of the epiglottis

9.   WR   S
   thorac/algia
   pain in the chest

10.   WR   S P S(WR)
   pulmon/ary neo/plasm
   pertaining to (in) the lung new growth (tumor)

11.   WR CV   S
   bronch/i/ectasis
     CF
   dilation of the bronchi

12.   WR   S
   tonsill/itis
   inflammation of the tonsils

13.   WR CV WR   S
   pneum/o/coni/osis
     CF
   abnormal condition of dust in the lungs

14.   WR CV WR   S
   bronch/o/pneumon/ia
     CF
   diseased state of bronchi and lungs

15.   WR   S
   pneumon/itis
   inflammation of the lung

16.   WR   S
   laryng/itis
   inflammation of the larynx

17.   WR CV S
   pneumat/o/cele
     CF
   hernia of the lung

18. WR CV S
   py/o/thorax
    CF
   pus in the chest (pleural space)

19.   WR CV   S
   rhin/o/rrhagia
     CF
   rapid flow of blood from the nose

20.   WR   S
   bronch/itis
   inflammation of the bronchi

21.   WR   S
   pharyng/itis
   inflammation of the pharynx

22.   WR   S
   trache/itis
   inflammation of the trachea

23.   WR CV WR CV WR   S
   laryng/o/trache/o/bronch/itis
     CF   CF
   inflammation of the larynx, trachea, and bronchi

24.   WR   S
   adenoid/itis
   inflammation of the adenoids

25. WR CV S
   hem/o/thorax
    CF
   blood in the chest (pleural space)

26. WR S WR   S
   lob/ar pneumon/ia
   pertaining to the lobe, diseased state of a lung

27.   WR   S
   rhin/itis
   inflammation of the nose

28.   WR CV S   WR   S
   bronch/o/genic carcin/oma
     CF
   cancerous tumor originating in a bronchus

29.   WR   S
   pneumon/ia
   diseased state of the lung

Exercise 13

1. thorac/algia
2. rhin/o/myc/osis
3. pneumat/o/cele
4. pulmon/ary neo/plasm
5. laryng/itis
6. atel/ectasis
7. adenoid/itis
8. laryng/o/trache/o/bronch/itis
9. bronch/i/ectasis
10. pleur/itis (or pleurisy)
11. pneum/o/coni/osis
12. pneumon/itis
13. pan/sinus/itis
14. trache/o/stenosis
15. nas/o/pharyng/itis
16. py/o/thorax
17. epiglott/itis
18. diaphragmat/o/cele
19. pneum/o/thorax
20. bronch/o/pneumon/ia
21. rhin/o/rrhagia
22. pharyng/itis
23. hem/o/thorax
24. trache/itis
25. bronch/itis
26. lob/ar pneumon/ia
27. rhin/itis
28. bronch/o/genic carcin/oma
29. pneumon/ia

Exercise 14
Spelling exercise; see text, pp. 122-123.

Exercise 15

1. emphysema
2. pleural effusion
3. cor pulmonale
4. coccidioidomycosis
5. cystic fibrosis
6. influenza
7. chronic obstructive pulmonary disease
8. pertussis
9. croup
10. asthma
11. pulmonary edema
12. upper respiratory infection
13. pulmonary embolism
14. epistaxis
15. Legionnaire disease
16. *Pneumocystis carinii* pneumonia

17. deviated septum
18. obstructive sleep apnea
19. tuberculosis
20. adult respiratory distress syndrome

Exercise 16

1. d	6. c
2. j	7. a
3. h	8. e
4. f	9. b
5. g	10. i

Exercise 17

1. d	6. h
2. b	7. i
3. c	8. g
4. e	9. j
5. f	10. a

Exercise 18

Spelling exercise; see text pp. 128-129.

Exercise 19

1. WR CV S
trache/o/tomy
  CF
incision of the trachea

2. WR CV S
laryng/o/stomy
  CF
creation of an artificial opening into
the larynx

3. WR S
adenoid/ectomy
excision of the adenoids

4. WR CV S
rhin/o/plasty
  CF
surgical repair of the nose

5. WR CV S
aden/o/tome
  CF
surgical instrument used to cut the
adenoids

6. WR CV S
trache/o/stomy
  CF
creation of an artificial opening into
the trachea

7. WR CV S
sinus/o/tomy
  CF
incision of a sinus

8. WR CV S
laryng/o/plasty
  CF
surgical repair of the larynx

9. WR CV WR CV S
pneum/o/bronch/o/tomy
  CF   CF
incision of lung and bronchus

10. WR CV S
bronch/o/plasty
  CF
surgical repair of a bronchus

11. WR S
lob/ectomy
excision of a lobe (of the lung)

12. WR CV WR CV S
laryng/o/trache/o/tomy
  CF   CF
incision of larynx and trachea

13. WR CV S
trache/o/plasty
  CF
surgical repair of the trachea

14. WR CV S
thorac/o/tomy
  CF
incision into the chest cavity

15. WR S
laryng/ectomy
excision of the larynx

16. WR CV S
thorac/o/centesis
  CF
surgical puncture to aspirate fluid
from the chest cavity

17. WR S
tonsill/ectomy
excision of the tonsils

18. WR CV S
pleur/o/pexy
  CF
surgical fixation of the pleura

19. WR CV S
sept/o/plasty
  CF
surgical repair of the septum

20. WR CV S
sept/o/tomy
  CF
incision into the septum

Exercise 20

1. trache/o/plasty
2. laryng/o/trache/o/tomy
3. aden/o/tome
4. thorac/o/tomy
5. trache/o/stomy
6. tonsill/ectomy
7. trache/o/tomy
8. bronch/o/plasty

9. laryng/ectomy
10. rhin/o/plasty
11. sinus/o/tomy
12. thorac/o/centesis or thora/centesis
13. adenoid/ectomy
14. laryng/o/plasty
15. lob/ectomy
16. pneum/o/bronch/o/tomy
17. laryng/o/stomy
18. pneumon/ectomy
19. sept/o/tomy
20. sept/o/plasty

Exercise 21

Spelling exercise; see text, pp. 133-134.

Exercise 22

1. WR CV S
spir/o/meter
  CF
instrument used to measure breathing

2. WR CV S
laryng/o/scope
  CF
instrument used for visual
examination of the larynx

3. WR CV S
capn/o/meter
  CF
instrument used to measure carbon
dioxide

4. WR CV S
spir/o/metry
  CF
measurement of breathing

5. WR CV S
ox/i/meter
  CF
instrument used to measure oxygen

6. WR CV S
laryng/o/scopy
  CF
visual examination of the larynx

7. WR CV S
bronch/o/scope
  CF
instrument used for visual
examination of the bronchi

8. WR CV S
thorac/o/scope
  CF
instrument used for visual
examination of the thorax

9. P S(WR)
endo/scope
instrument used for visual
examination of a hollow organ or
body cavity

10. WR CV S
 thorac/o/scopy
     CF
 visual examination of the thorax

11. P   S(WR)
 endo/scopic
 pertaining to visual examination of a
 hollow organ or body cavity

12. P   S(WR)
 endo/scopy
 visual examination of a hollow organ
 or body cavity

13. P   WR CV   S
 poly/somn/o/graphy
        CF
 process of recording many (tests)
 during sleep

Exercise 23
1. laryng/o/scopy
2. spir/o/meter
3. capn/o/meter
4. laryng/o/scope
5. bronch/o/scopy
6. spir/o/metry
7. bronch/o/scope
8. endo/scopy
9. thorac/o/scope
10. endo/scope
11. thorac/o/scopy
12. endo/scopic
13. poly/somn/o/graphy

Exercise 24
Spelling exercise; see text, p. 140.

Exercise 25
1. ventilation-perfusion scanning
2. chest computed tomography
3. chest x-ray
4. arterial blood gases
5. pulse oximetry
6. acid-fast bacilli smear
7. pulmonary function tests
8. PPD skin test

Exercise 26
1. f	5. b
2. e	6. c
3. a	7. h
4. d	8. g

Exercise 27
Spelling exercise; see text, p. 142.

Exercise 28
1. WR   S
 laryng/eal
 pertaining to the larynx

2. P S(WR)
 eu/pnea
 normal breathing

3. WR   S
 muc/oid
 resembling mucus

4. P S(WR)
 a/pnea
 absence of breathing

5. P S(WR)
 hyp/oxia
 deficient oxygen (to tissues)

6. WR CV   S
 laryng/o/spasm
     CF
 spasmodic contraction of the larynx

7. P   WR   S
 endo/trache/al
 pertaining to within the trachea

8. P S(WR)
 an/oxia
 absence of oxygen

9. P   S(WR)
 dys/phonia
 difficulty in speaking (voice)

10. WR CV WR   S
 bronch/o/alveol/ar
     CF
 pertaining to the bronchi and alveoli

11. P S(WR)
 dys/pnea
 difficult breathing

12. P   WR   S
 hypo/capn/ia
 condition of deficient in carbon
 dioxide (in the blood)

13. WR CV   S
 bronch/o/spasm
     CF
 spasmodic contraction in the
 bronchus(i)

14. WR CV S
 orth/o/pnea
     CF
 able to breathe only in a straight
 position

15. P   S(WR)
 hyper/pnea
 excessive breathing

16. P WR   S
 a/capn/ia
 condition of absence of carbon
 dioxide (in the blood)

17. P S(WR)
 hypo/pnea
 deficient breathing

18. P WR   S
 hyp/ox/emia
 deficient oxygen in the blood

19. P S(WR)
 a/phonia
 absence of voice

20. WR CV S
 rhin/o/rrhea
     CF
 discharge from the nose

21. WR   S
 thorac/ic
 pertaining to the chest

22. WR   S
 muc/ous
 pertaining to mucus

23. WR CV   WR   S
 nas/o/pharyng/eal
     CF
 pertaining to the nose and pharynx

24.   WR   S
 diaphragmat/ic
 pertaining to the diaphragm

25. P   WR   S
 intra/pleur/al
 pertaining to within the pleura

26. WR   S
 pulmon/ary
 pertaining to the lungs

Exercise 29
1. hyp/oxia
2. muc/oid
3. orth/o/pnea
4. endo/trache/al
5. an/oxia
6. dys/pnea
7. laryng/eal
8. hyper/capn/ia
9. eu/pnea
10. a/phonia
11. laryng/o/spasm
12. hypo/capn/ia
13. nas/o/pharyng/eal
14. diaphragmat/ic
15. a/pnea
16. hyp/ox/emia
17. hyper/pnea
18. bronch/o/spasm
19. hypo/pnea
20. a/capn/ia
21. dys/phonia
22. rhin/o/rrhea

23. muc/ous
24. thorac/ic
25. intra/pleur/al
26. pulmon/ary

Exercise 30
Spelling exercise; see text, pp. 147-148.

Exercise 31
1. hyperventilation
2. nebulizer
3. bronchodilator
4. ventilator
5. asphyxia
6. sputum
7. aspirate
8. airway
9. hiccup (hiccough)
10. cough
11. mucopurulent
12. hypoventilation
13. nosocomial
14. paroxysm
15. patent
16. bronchoconstrictor
17. mucus

Exercise 32
1. b	5. a
2. h	6. d
3. c	7. g
4. i	8. f

Exercise 33
1. e	6. a
2. h	7. b
3. i	8. d
4. c	9. f
5. j	

Exercise 34
Spelling exercise; see text, p. 151.

Exercise 35
1. chronic obstructive pulmonary disease; pulmonary function tests, chest x-ray, arterial blood gases, computed tomography
2. ventilation-perfusion scanning; pulmonary embolism
3. left upper lobe; left lower lobe; right upper lobe, right middle lobe, right lower lobe
4. acid-fast bacilli; tuberculosis
5. polysomnography; obstructive sleep apnea
6. *Pneumocystis carinii* pneumonia
7. oxygen; carbon dioxide

Exercise 36
1. adult respiratory distress syndrome
2. cystic fibrosis
3. influenza
4. laryngotracheobronchitis
5. upper respiratory infection

Exercise 37
1. cough
2. dyspnea
3. pulmonary
4. chest x-ray
5. bronchoscopy
6. arterial blood gases
7. hypoxemia
8. bronchogenic carcinoma
9. pulmonary function tests
10. thoracic

Exercise 38
1. epistaxis
2. laryngoplasty
3. orthopnea
4. arterial blood gases, hypoxia
5. thoracalgia
6. hyperventilation
7. nebulizer
8. hemothorax
9. pulmonary embolism
10. coccidioidomycosis
11. chest x-ray, nosocomial
12. PPD skin test

Exercise 39 Reading Exercise

Exercise 40
1. *T*
2. *F,* "hypoxemia" means deficient oxygen in the blood; "hypercapnia" means excessive carbon dioxide in the blood.
3. *T*
4. *F,* "bronchitis" means inflammation of the bronchi

Answers

ANSWERS TO CHAPTER 6 EXERCISES
Exercise Figures
Exercise Figure
A. 1. kidney: nephr/o, ren/o
2. meatus: meat/o
3. ureter: ureter/o
4. bladder: cyst/o, vesic/o
5. urethra: urethr/o

Exercise Figure
B. 1. renal pelvis: pyel/o
2. glomerulus: glomerul/o

Exercise Figure C. cyst/o/lith

Exercise Figure D. cyst/o/stomy

Exercise Figure E. lith/o/tripsy

Exercise Figure F. nephr/o/stomy

Exercise Figure G. pyel/o/lith/o/tomy

Exercise Figure H. ureter/o/stomy

Exercise Figure I. ur/o/gram

Exercise Figure J. urin/o/meter

Exercise Figure K. urin/ary

Exercise 1
1. g	5. a
2. d	6. b
3. f	7. e
4. c	

Exercise 2
1. glomerulus	6. sac, bladder
2. sac, bladder	7. urethra
3. kidney	8. kidney
4. renal pelvis	9. meatus
5. ureter	

Exercise 3
1. a. nephr/o	4. pyel/o
b. ren/o	5. glomerul/o
2. a. cyst/o	6. urethr/o
b. vesic/o	7. meat/o
3. ureter/o	

Exercise 4
1. water	8. sound
2. urea, nitrogen	9. sugar
3. night	10. developing cell, germ cell
4. stone, calculus	
5. cut, section	11. scanty, few
6. albumin	12. urine, urinary tract
7. urine, urinary tract	13. sugar

Exercise 5
1. a. glyc/o
   b. glycos/o
2. son/o
3. a. urin/o
   b. ur/o
4. hydr/o
5. blast/o
6. tom/o
7. albumin/o
8. noct/i
9. azot/o
10. lith/o
11. olig/o

Exercise 6
1. c
2. i
3. d
4. f
5. g
6. e
7. a
8. b

Exercise 7
1. suturing, repairing
2. loosening, dissolution, separating
3. condition
4. nourishment, development
5. urine, urination
6. enlargement
7. drooping, sagging, prolapse
8. surgical crushing

Exercise 8
1. WR   S
    nephr/oma
    tumor of the kidney

2. WR CV WR
    cyst/o/lith
        CF
    stone in the bladder

3. WR CV WR S
    nephr/o/lith/iasis
        CF
    condition of stone(s) in the kidney

4. WR   S
    ur/emia
    condition of urine (urea) in the blood

5. WR CV   S
    nephr/o/ptosis
        CF
    drooping kidney

6. WR CV   S
    cyst/o/cele
        CF
    protrusion of the bladder

7. WR CV   P   S
    nephr/o/hyper/trophy
        CF
    excessive development of the kidney

8. WR   S
    cyst/itis
    inflammation of the bladder

9. WR   S
    pyel/itis
    inflammation of the renal pelvis

10. WR CV S
    ureter/o/cele
        CF
    protrusion of a ureter

11. WR CV WR   S
    hydr/o/nephr/osis
        CF
    abnormal condition of water in the kidney

12. WR CV   S
    nephr/o/megaly
        CF
    enlargement of a kidney

13. WR CV WR   S
    ureter/o/lith/iasis
        CF
    condition of stone(s) in the ureters

14. WR CV WR   S
    pyel/o/nephr/itis
        CF
    inflammation of the renal pelvis and the kidney

15. WR   S
    ureter/itis
    inflammation of a ureter

16. WR   S
    nephr/itis
    inflammation of a kidney

17. WR CV WR   S
    urethr/o/cyst/itis
        CF
    inflammation of the urethra and bladder

18. WR CV   S
    ureter/o/stenosis
        CF
    narrowing of the ureter

19. WR CV WR   S
    nephr/o/blast/oma
        CF
    kidney tumor containing developing cell (tissue)

Exercise 9
1. nephr/o/megaly
2. cyst/itis
3. nephr/o/hyper/trophy
4. urethr/o/cyst/itis
5. cyst/o/cele
6. hydr/o/nephr/osis
7. cyst/o/lith
8. glomerul/o/nephr/itis
9. nephr/oma
10. nephr/o/ptosis
11. nephr/itis
12. nephr/o/lith/iasis
13. ureter/o/cele
14. pyel/itis
15. ur/emia
16. ureter/o/stenosis
17. pyel/o/nephr/itis
18. ureter/o/lith/iasis
19. nephr/o/blast/oma

Exercise 10
Spelling exercise; see text, p. 172.

Exercise 11
1. renal calculi
2. urinary retention
3. polycystic kidney disease
4. hypospadias
5. renal hypertension
6. urinary suppression
7. epispadias
8. urinary tract infection
9. sepsis

Exercise 12
1. c
2. f
3. d
4. h
5. a
6. e
7. b
8. g
9. i

Exercise 13
Spelling exercise; see text, p. 174.

Exercise 14
1. WR CV S
    vesic/o/tomy
        CF
    incision of the bladder

2. WR CV   S
    cyst/o/tomy
        CF
    incision of the bladder

3. WR CV   S
    nephr/o/stomy
        CF
    creation of an artificial opening into the kidney

4. WR CV   S
    nephr/o/lysis
        CF
    separating the kidney

5. WR   S
    cyst/ectomy
    excision of the bladder

6. WR CV WR CV S
pyel/o/lith/o/tomy
　　CF　　CF
incision of the renal pelvis to remove
a stone

7. WR CV S
nephr/o/pexy
　　CF
surgical fixation of the kidney

8. WR CV WR CV S
cyst/o/lith/o/tomy
　　CF　　CF
incision of the bladder to remove a
stone

9. WR S
nephr/ectomy
excision of a kidney

10. WR S
ureter/ectomy
excision of a ureter

11. WR CV S
cyst/o/stomy
　　CF
creation of an artificial opening into
the bladder

12. WR CV S
pyel/o/plasty
　　CF
surgical repair of the renal pelvis

13. WR CV S
cyst/o/rrhaphy
　　CF
suturing of the bladder

14. WR CV S
meat/o/tomy
　　CF
incision of the meatus

15. WR CV S
lith/o/tripsy
　　CF
surgical crushing of a stone

16. WR CV S
urethr/o/plasty
　　CF
surgical repair of the urethra

17. WR CV WR S
vesic/o/urethr/al suspension
　　CF
suspension pertaining to the urethra
and bladder

18. WR CV WR CV WR CV S
nephr/o/pyel/o/lith/o/tomy
　　CF　　CF　　CF
incision through the kidney into the
renal pelvis to remove a stone

Exercise 15

1. urethr/o/tomy
2. nephr/ectomy
3. pyel/o/lith/o/tomy
4. cyst/o/rrhaphy
5. nephr/o/lysis
6. nephr/o/stomy
7. urethr/o/plasty
8. cyst/ectomy
9. meat/o/tomy
10. a. cyst/o/tomy
    b. vesic/o/tomy
11. pyel/o/plasty
12. ureter/ectomy
13. nephr/o/pexy
14. cyst/o/lith/o/tomy
15. lith/o/tripsy
16. vesic/o/urethr/al suspension
17. cyst/o/stomy
18. nephr/o/pyel/o/lith/o/tomy

Exercise 16
Spelling exercise; see text, pp. 178-179.

Exercise 17
1. renal transplant
2. fulguration
3. extracorporeal shock wave lithotripsy

Exercise 18
1. b 2. a 3. d

Exercise 19
Spelling exercise; see text, p. 180.

Exercise 20

1. WR CV WR CV S
cyst/o/urethr/o/graphy
　　CF　　　CF
x-ray imaging of the bladder and the
urethra

2. WR CV S
meat/o/scope
　　CF
instrument used for visual
examination of a meatus

3. WR CV S
cyst/o/graphy
　　CF
x-ray imaging of the bladder

4. WR CV S
urethr/o/scope
　　CF
instrument used for visual
examination of the urethra

5. WR CV WR CV S
nephr/o/son/o/graphy
　　CF　　CF
process of recording the kidney with
sound

6. WR CV S
cyst/o/scope
　　CF
instrument used for visual
examination of the bladder

7. WR CV WR CV S
nephr/o/tom/o/gram
　　CF　　CF
(sectional) x-ray image of the kidney

8. WR CV S
cyst/o/gram
　　CF
x-ray image of the bladder

9. WR CV S
meat/o/scopy
　　CF
visual examination of the meatus

10. WR CV S
nephr/o/gram
　　CF
x-ray image of the kidney

11. WR CV S
cyst/o/scopy
　　CF
visual examination of the bladder

12. WR CV S
nephr/o/graphy
　　CF
x-ray imaging of the kidney

13. WR CV S
urin/o/meter
　　CF
instrument used to measure (specific
gravity) urine

14. 　　　　　WR CV S
(intravenous) ur/o/gram
　　　　　　CF
x-ray image of the urinary tract with
contrast medium injected intravenously

15. 　　　　　WR CV S
retrograde ur/o/gram
　　　　　　CF
x-ray image of the urinary tract (contrast
medium injected in a direction opposite
from normal through the urethra)

16. WR CV S
    <u>ren</u>/o/gram
    CF
    (graphic) record of the kidney

17. WR CV S
    <u>nephr</u>/o/scopy
    CF
    visual examination of the kidney

Exercise 21
1. cyst/o/scopy
2. nephr/o/tom/o/gram
3. intravenous ur/o/gram
4. meat/o/scope
5. urethr/o/scope
6. nephr/o/son/o/graphy
7. cyst/o/gram
8. meat/o/scopy
9. cyst/o/scope
10. voiding cyst/o/urethr/o/graphy
11. cyst/o/graphy
12. nephr/o/gram
13. urin/o/meter
14. ren/o/gram
15. nephr/o/graphy
16. retrograde ur/o/gram
17. nephr/o/scopy

Exercise 22
Spelling exercise; see text, pp. 185-186.

Exercise 23
1. KUB
2. specific gravity
3. blood urea nitrogen
4. urinalysis
5. creatinine

Exercise 24
1. c 2. b 3. d 4. a 5. f

Exercise 25
Spelling exercise; see text, p. 187.

Exercise 26
1. WR S
   noct/uria
   night urination

2. WRCV S
   <u>ur</u>/o/logist
   CF
   physician who studies and treats
   (diseases of) the urinary tract

3. WR S
   olig/uria
   scanty urine

4. WR S
   azot/emia
   (excessive) urea and nitrogenous
   substances in the blood

5. WR S
   hemat/uria
   blood in the urine

6. WR CV S
   <u>ur</u>/o/logy
   CF
   study of the urinary tract

7. P S(WR)
   poly/uria
   much (excessive) urine

8. WR S
   albumin/uria
   albumin in the urine

9. P S(WR)
   an/uria
   absence of urine

10. P WR S
    di/ur/esis
    condition of urine passing through
    (increased excretion of urine)

11. WR S
    py/uria
    pus in the urine

12. WR S
    urin/ary
    pertaining to urine

13. WR S
    glycos/uria
    sugar in the urine

14. WR S
    meat/al
    pertaining to the meatus

15. P S(WR)
    dys/uria
    difficult or painful urination

16. WR CV S
    <u>nephr</u>/o/logy
    CF
    study of the kidney

17. WR CV S
    <u>nephr</u>/o/logist
    CF
    physician who studies and treats
    diseases of the kidney

Exercise 27
1. noct/uria
2. olig/uria
3. py/uria
4. ur/o/logist
5. poly/uria
6. azot/emia
7. urin/ary
8. hemat/uria
9. ur/o/logy
10. di/ur/esis
11. an/uria
12. glycos/uria
13. dys/uria
14. albumin/uria
15. meat/al
16. nephr/o/logy
17. nephr/o/logist

Exercise 28
Spelling exercise; see text, pp. 190-191.

Exercise 29
1. urinal
2. hemodialysis
3. distended
4. catheter
5. incontinence
6. urinary
   catheterization
7. peritoneal dialysis
8. evacuate
   waste
   material
9. stricture
10. diuretic
11. enuresis
12. micturate
13. urodynamics

Exercise 30
1. e   5. d
2. g   6. c
3. f   7. h
4. a

Exercise 31
1. a   4. b
2. e   5. f
3. g   6. c

Exercise 32
Spelling exercise; see text, p. 194.

Exercise 33
1. intravenous urogram; voiding
   cystourethrogram
2. specific gravity; urinalysis
3. blood urea nitrogen
4. extracorporeal shock wave lithotripsy
5. catheterization; urinary tract infection
6. hemodialysis

Exercise 34
1. nephrolithiasis
2. urology
3. hematuria
4. KUB
5. calculi
6. cystoscopy
7. urogram
8. nephropyelolithotomy
9. catheter
10. voiding

Exercise 35
1. nephroptosis
2. ureterolithiasis
3. sepsis
4. polyuria
5. nephropexy
6. urinary
   suppression
7. cystogram
8. enuresis
9. urinary tract
   infection
10. urinalysis

Exercise 36 Reading Exercise

Exercise 37
1. b   2. d   3. a

Answers

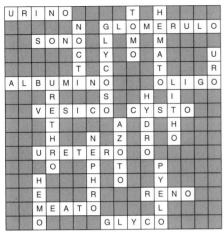

ANSWERS TO CHAPTER 7 EXERCISES

Exercise Figures

Exercise Figure

A. 1. vas, or ductus, deferens: vas/o
2. glans penis: balan/o
3. seminal vesicle: vesicul/o
4. prostate gland: prostat/o
5. epididymis: epididym/o
6. testis: orchid/o, orchi/o, orch/o, test/o

Exercise Figure B. balan/itis

Exercise Figure C. crypt/orchid/ism

Exercise Figure D. vas/ectomy

Exercise 1

1. c   9. b
2. i   10. n
3. e   11. h
4. k   12. p
5. f   13. d
6. a   14. j
7. l   15. m
8. g

Exercise 2

1. testis, testicle   6. seminal vesicle
2. vessel, duct   7. testis, testicle
3. glans penis   8. epididymis
4. prostate gland   9. testis, testicle
5. testis, testicle

Exercise 3

1. vas/o   6. a. orchid/o
2. prostat/o   b. orchi/o
3. balan/o   c. orch/o
4. vesicul/o   d. test/o
5. epididym/o

Exercise 4

1. sperm   3. sperm
2. male

Exercise 5

1. a. sperm/o   2. andr/o
   b. spermat/o

Exercise 6

1. state of
2. through, across, beyond

Exercise 7

1.   WR CV WR
   prostat/o/lith
        CF
   stone in the prostate gland

2.   WR   S
   balan/itis
   inflammation of the glans penis

3. a. WR   S
     orch/itis

   b. WR   S
     orchid/itis

   c. WR   S
     test/itis
     inflammation of the testis

4.   WR CV WR   S
   prostat/o/vesicul/itis
        CF
   inflammation of the prostate gland
   and seminal vesicles

5.   WR CV WR   S
   prostat/o/cyst/itis
        CF
   inflammation of the prostate gland
   and bladder

6.   WR   WR   S
   orchi/epididym/itis
   inflammation of the testis and
   epididymis

7.   WR CV   S
   prostat/o/rrhea
        CF
   excessive discharge from the prostate
   gland

8.   WR   S
   epididym/itis
   inflammation of the epididymis

9.   WR   S P   S(WR)
   (benign) prostat/ic hyper/plasia
   (nonmalignant) excessive development
   pertaining to the prostate gland

10. WR   WR   S
   crypt/orchid/ism
   state of hidden testis

11. WR CV   S
   balan/o/rrhea
        CF
   excessive discharge from the glans
   penis

12. WR   S
   prostat/itis
   inflammation of the prostate gland

13. P   WR   S
   an/orch/ism
   state of absence of testis

Exercise 8

1. prostat/o/cyst/itis
2. prostat/o/lith
3. a. orchid/itis
   b. orch/itis
   c. test/itis
4. (benign) prostat/ic hyper/plasia
5. crypt/orchid/ism
6. prostat/o/vesicul/itis
7. an/orch/ism
8. prostat/itis
9. orchi/epididym/itis
10. balan/o/rrhea
11. epididym/itis
12. balan/itis
13. prostat/o/rrhea

Exercise 9
Spelling exercise; see text, p. 211.

Exercise 10

1. testicular   5. prostate cancer
   carcinoma   6. erectile
2. phimosis   dysfunction
3. varicocele   7. priapism
4. hydrocele   8. testicular torsion

Exercise 11

1. d   5. a
2. c   6. f
3. e   7. i
4. b   8. h

Exercise 12
Spelling exercise; see text, pp. 214-215.

Exercise 13

1.   WR   S
   vas/ectomy
   excision of a duct

2.   WR CV WR CV   S
   prostat/o/cyst/o/tomy
        CF   CF
   incision into the prostate gland and
   bladder

3. a. WR CV S

orchid/o/tomy

CF

   b. WR CV S

orchi/o/tomy

CF

incision into a testis

4. WR S

epididym/ectomy

excision of an epididymis

5. a. WR CV S

orchid/o/pexy

CF

   b. WR CV S

orchi/o/pexy

CF

surgical fixation of a testicle

6. WR CV WR S

prostat/o/vesicul/ectomy

CF

excision of the prostate gland and
seminal vesicles

7. WR CV S

orchi/o/plasty

CF

surgical repair of testis

8. WR S

vesicul/ectomy

excision of the seminal vesicle(s)

9. WR S

prostat/ectomy

excision of the prostate gland

10. WR CV S

balan/o/plasty

CF

surgical repair of the glans penis

11. WR CV WR CV S

vas/o/vas/o/stomy

CF CF

creation of an artificial opening
between ducts

12. a. WR S

orchid/ectomy

   b. WR S

orchi/ectomy

excision of the testis

13. WR CV WR CV S

prostat/o/lith/o/tomy

CF CF

incision into prostate gland to remove
a stone

Exercise 14

1. a. orchid/ectomy
   b. orchi/ectomy
2. balan/o/plasty
3. prostat/o/cyst/o/tomy
4. vesicul/ectomy
5. prostat/o/lith/o/tomy
6. a. orchid/o/tomy
   b. orchi/o/tomy
7. epididym/ectomy
8. orchi/o/plasty
9. prostat/ectomy
10. vas/ectomy
11. prostat/o/vesicul/ectomy
12. a. orchid/o/pexy
    b. orchi/o/pexy
13. vas/o/vas/o/stomy

Exercise 15

Spelling exercise; see text, p. 218.

Exercise 16

1. suprapubic prostatectomy
2. circumcision
3. penile implant
4. hydrocelectomy
5. transurethral microwave thermotherapy
6. transurethral incision of the prostate
   gland
7. transurethral resection (of the) prostate
   gland

Exercise 17

Spelling exercise; see text, p. 221.

Exercise 18

1. digital rectal exam
2. prostate-specific antigen
3. transrectal ultrasound

Exercise 19

Spelling exercise; see text, p. 222.

Exercise 20

1. WR CV WR S

olig/o/sperm/ia

CF

condition of scanty sperm

2. WR CV S

andr/o/pathy

CF

diseases of the male

3. WR CV S

spermat/o/lysis

CF

dissolution of sperm

Exercise 21

1. spermat/o/lysis   3. olig/o/sperm/ia
2. andr/o/pathy

Exercise 22

Spelling exercise; see text, p. 223.

Exercise 23

1. period when secondary sex
   characteristics develop and the ability
   to sexually reproduce begins
2. climax of sexual stimulation
3. contagious, inflammatory venereal
   disease
4. person who is attracted to a member
   of the same sex
5. sexual intercourse between male and
   female
6. contagious venereal disease caused by
   the *herpesvirus hominis* type 2
7. person who is attracted to a member
   of the opposite sex
8. infectious venereal disease having
   lesions that can affect any organ or
   tissue
9. ejection of semen from the male
   urethra
10. male and female sex glands
11. a disease transmitted during sexual
    intercourse
12. process rendering an individual
    unable to produce offspring
13. an STD causing growths on the male
    and female genitalia
14. a disease transmitted by exchange of
    body fluids during the sexual act,
    reuse of contaminated needles, or
    contaminated blood transfusions
15. STD caused by a one-cell organism,
    Trichomonas; it affects the
    genitourinary system
16. introduction of semen into the vagina
    by artificial means
17. one of the more prevalent STDs;
    caused by bacterium, *Chlamydia
    trachomatis*
18. a cover for the penis worn during
    coitus
19. an artificial replacement of an absent
    body part
20. a type of retrovirus that causes AIDS

Exercise 24

1. g	6. i
2. e	7. c
3. h	8. b
4. a	9. j
5. d	10. f

Exercise 25

1. f	6. b
2. a	7. i
3. h	8. e
4. d	9. g
5. j	10. c

Exercise 26
Spelling exercise; see text, pp. 227-228.

Exercise 27
1. digital rectal exam benign prostatic hyperplasia transurethral resection of the prostate transurethral microwave thermotherapy transurethral incision of the prostate
2. acquired immunodeficiency syndrome; sexually transmitted disease; human immunodeficiency virus; human papilloma virus
3. prostate-specific antigen

Exercise 28
1. nocturia
2. hematuria
3. urinary
4. benign prostatic hyperplasia
5. urology

Exercise 29
1. balanorrhea
2. prepuce
3. heterosexual
4. phimosis
5. orchidopexy
6. prosthesis
7. transurethral microwave thermotherapy

Exercise 30 Reading Exercise

Exercise 31
1. a
2. c
3. d

Answers

ANSWERS TO CHAPTER 8 EXERCISES
Exercise Figures
Exercise Figure

A. 1. ovary: oophor/o
2. uterus: hyster/o, metr/o (metr/i), uter/o
3. fallopian, or uterine, tube: salping/o
4. cervix: cervic/o, trachel/o
5. vagina: colp/o, vagin/o
6. hymen: hymen/o

Exercise Figure
B. 1. vulva: episi/o, vulv/o
2. perineum: perine/o

Exercise Figure C. salping/itis

Exercise Figure D. hyster/o/ptosis

Exercise Figure E. vesic/o/vagin/al

Exercise Figure F. *1,* hyster/o/salping/o/oophor/ectomy; *2,* salping/o/oophor/ectomy; *3,* salping/o/oophor/ectomy; *4,* hyster/ectomy

Exercise Figure G. *1,* cyst/o/cele

Exercise Figure H. hyster/o/salping/o/gram

Exercise Figure I. *1,* culd/o/centesis; *2,* culd/o/scopy

Exercise 1
1. c
2. f
3. g
4. b
5. d
6. e
7. h
8. a
9. i

Exercise 2
1. b
2. c
3. d
4. k
5. e
6. f
7. g
8. l
9. i
10. j
11. h

Exercise 3
1. vagina
2. ovary
3. uterus
4. uterus
5. hymen
6. uterus
7. menstruation
8. vulva
9. cervix
10. vagina
11. woman
12. breast
13. perineum
14. fallopian tube
15. vulva
16. breast
17. beginning, first
18. cul-de-sac
19. woman
20. cervix

Exercise 4
1. a. episi/o
   b. vulv/o
2. a. mamm/o
   b. mast/o
3. men/o
4. oophor/o
5. salping/o
6. perine/o
7. a. vagin/o
   b. colp/o
8. a. uter/o
   b. metr/i, metr/o
   c. hyster/o
9. a. gynec/o
   b. gyn/o
10. hymen/o
11. culd/o
12. a. cervic/o
    b. trachel/o
13. arche/o

Exercise 5
1. -salpinx
2. -ial
3. peri-
4. -atresia

Exercise 6
1. fallopian tube
2. surrounding
3. pertaining to
4. absence of a normal body opening, occlusion, closure

Exercise 7
1. WR   S
   colp/itis
   inflammation of the vagina

2. WR   S
   cervic/itis
   inflammation of the cervix

3. WR CV   S
   hydr/o/salpinx
     CF
   water in the fallopian tube

4. WR CV   S
   hemat/o/salpinx
     CF
   blood in the fallopian tube

5. WR CV   S
   metr/o/rrhea
     CF
   excessive discharge from the uterus

6. WR   S
   oophor/itis
   inflammation of the ovary

7. WR   S
   Bartholin aden/itis
   inflammation of (Bartholin) gland

8. WR CV WR   S
   vulv/o/vagin/itis
     CF
   inflammation of the vulva and vagina

9. WR CV   S
   salping/o/cele
     CF
   hernia of the fallopian tube

10. WR CV WR CV   S
    men/o/metr/o/rrhagia
      CF   CF
    rapid flow of blood from the uterus at menstruation (and between menstrual cycles)

11. P   WR CV   S
    a/men/o/rrhea
        CF
    absence of menstrual discharge

12. P   WR CV   S
     dys/<u>men/o</u>/rrhea
              CF
     painful menstrual discharge

13. WR   S
     mast/itis
     inflammation of the breast

14. P   WR   S
     peri/metr/itis
     inflammation surrounding the uterus
     (outer layer)

15. WR CV WR   S
     <u>my/o</u>/metr/itis
        CF
     inflammation of the uterine muscle

16. P   WR   S
     endo/metr/itis
     inflammation of the inner (lining) of
     the uterus

17. P   WR   S
     endo/cervic/itis
     inflammation of the inner (lining) of
     the cervix

18. WR CV   S
     <u>py/o</u>/salpinx
        CF
     pus in the fallopian tube

19. WR   S
     hyster/atresia
     closure of the uterus (uterine cavity)

20. WR   S
     salping/itis
     inflammation of the fallopian tube

21. WR   S
     vagin/itis
     inflammation of the vagina

Exercise 8
1. mast/itis
2. metr/o/rrhea
3. salping/itis
4. vulv/o/vagin/itis
5. a/men/o/rrhea
6. cervic/itis
7. (Bartholin) aden/itis
8. hydr/o/salpinx
9. dys/men/o/rrhea
10. hemat/o/salpinx
11. a. colp/itis
    b. vagin/itis
12. men/o/metr/o/rrhagia
13. oophor/itis
14. salping/o/cele
15. peri/metr/itis
16. endo/metr/itis
17. endo/cervic/itis

18. my/o/metr/itis
19. py/o/salpinx
20. hyster/atresia

Exercise 9
Spelling exercise; see text, p. 245.

Exercise 10
1. downward placement of the uterus in
   the vagina
2. inflammation of the female pelvic
   organs
3. abnormal opening between the
   bladder and vagina
4. benign fibroid tumor of the uterine
   muscle
5. abnormal condition in which
   endometrial tissue grows in various
   areas of the pelvic cavity
6. growth of endometrium into the
   muscular portion of the uterus
7. a severe illness characterized by high
   fever, vomiting, diarrhea, and myalgia
8. a disorder characterized by one or
   more benign cysts
9. malignant tumor of the ovary
10. malignant tumor of the breast
11. malignant tumor of the cervix
12. malignant tumor of the endometrium

Exercise 11
1. vesicovaginal fistula
2. fibroid tumor
3. pelvic inflammatory disease
4. prolapsed uterus
5. endometriosis
6. adenomyosis
7. toxic shock syndrome
8. fibrocystic breast disease
9. breast cancer
10. endometrial cancer
11. ovarian cancer
12. cervical cancer

Exercise 12
Spelling exercise; see text, p. 249.

Exercise 13
1. WR CV   S
    <u>colp/o</u>/rrhaphy
        CF
    suture of the vagina

2. WR CV   S
    <u>colp/o</u>/plasty
        CF
    surgical repair of the vagina

3. WR CV   S
    <u>episi/o</u>/rrhaphy
        CF
    suture of the vulva (tear)

4.   WR CV   S
     <u>hymen/o</u>/tomy
          CF
     incision of the hymen

5.   WR CV   S
     <u>hyster/o</u>/pexy
          CF
     surgical fixation of the uterus

6.   WR   S
     vulv/ectomy
     excision of the vulva

7.   WR CV   S
     <u>perine/o</u>/rrhaphy
          CF
     suture of the perineum (tear)

8.   WR CV   S
     <u>salping/o</u>/stomy
          CF
     creation of an artificial opening in the
     fallopian tube

9.   WR CV   WR   S
     <u>salping/o</u>/oophor/ectomy
          CF
     excision of the fallopian tube and
     ovary

10.   WR   S
      oophor/ectomy
      excision of the ovary

11. WR   S
     mast/ectomy
     surgical removal of a breast

12. WR   S
     salping/ectomy
     excision of a fallopian tube

13. WR   S
     cervic/ectomy
     excision of the cervix

14. WR CV WR CV   S
     <u>colp/o</u>/<u>perine/o</u>/rrhaphy
         CF   CF
     suture of the vagina and perineum

15. WR CV WR CV   S
     <u>episi/o</u>/<u>perine/o</u>/plasty
         CF   CF
     surgical repair of the vulva and
     perineum

16. WR   S
     hymen/ectomy
     excision of the hymen

17.   WR CV WR CV WR   S
      <u>hyster/o</u>/<u>salping/o</u>/oophor/ectomy
           CF   CF
      excision of the uterus, fallopian tubes,
      and ovaries

18. WR   S
hyster/ectomy
excision of the uterus

19.   WR CV   S
<u>mamm/o</u>/plasty
     CF
surgical repair of the breast

20.   WR CV   S
<u>mamm/o</u>/tome
     CF
instrument used to cut breast (tissue)

21.   WR CV   S
<u>trachel/o</u>/rrhaphy
    CF
suture of the cervix

22.   WR   S
trachel/ectomy
excision of the cervix

Exercise 14

1. colp/o/rrhaphy
2. cervic/ectomy
3. episi/o/rrhaphy
4. episi/o/perine/o/plasty
5. colp/o/plasty
6. colp/o/perine/o/rrhaphy
7. hyster/o/salping/o/oophor/ectomy
8. hyster/o/pexy
9. hymen/ectomy
10. hymen/o/tomy
11. hyster/ectomy
12. oophor/ectomy
13. mast/ectomy
14. salping/ectomy
15. perine/o/rrhaphy
16. salping/o/oophor/ectomy
17. salping/o/stomy
18. vulv/ectomy
19. mamm/o/plasty
20. mamm/o/tome
21. trachel/o/rrhaphy
22. trachel/ectomy

Exercise 15

Spelling exercise; see text, p. 254.

Exercise 16

1. laparoscopy (sterilization) and tubal ligation
2. anterior and posterior colporrhaphy (A&P repair)
3. dilation and curettage
4. stereotactic breast biopsy
5. myomectomy
6. endometrial ablation
7. cryosurgery
8. conization
9. sentinel lymph node biopsy

Exercise 17

1. c   6. f
2. a   7. c
3. a   8. c
4. b   9. g
5. c   10. c

Exercise 18

Spelling exercise; see text, p. 259.

Exercise 19

1.   WR CV   S
<u>colp/o</u>/scopy
    CF
visual examination of the vagina

2.   WR CV   S
<u>mamm/o</u>/gram
     CF
x-ray image of the breast

3.   WR CV   S
<u>colp/o</u>/scope
    CF
instrument used for visual examination of the vagina

4.   WR CV   S
<u>hyster/o</u>/scopy
     CF
visual examination of the uterus

5.   WR CV WR CV   S
<u>hyster/o</u>/<u>salping/o</u>/gram
    CF   CF
x-ray image of the uterus and fallopian tubes

6.   WR CV   S
<u>culd/o</u>/scope
    CF
instrument used for visual examination of the Douglas cul-de-sac

7.   WR CV   S
<u>culd/o</u>/scopy
    CF
visual examination of the Douglas cul-de-sac

8.   WR CV   S
<u>culd/o</u>/centesis
    CF
surgical puncture to remove fluid from the Douglas cul-de-sac

9.   WR CV   S
<u>mamm/o</u>/graphy
     CF
x-ray imaging the breast

10.   WR CV   S
<u>hyster/o</u>/scope
     CF
instrument used for visual examination of the uterus

11. WR CV WR CV   S
<u>son/o</u>/<u>hyster/o</u>/graphy
  CF   CF
process of recording the uterus by sound

Exercise 20

1. hyster/o/salping/o/gram
2. colp/o/scopy
3. colp/o/scope
4. hyster/o/scopy
5. mamm/o/gram
6. culd/o/scope
7. culd/o/scopy
8. culd/o/centesis
9. hyster/o/scope
10. mamm/o/graphy
11. son/o/hyster/o/graphy

Exercise 21

Spelling exercise; see text, p. 264.

Exercise 22

1. cytological study of cervical and vaginal secretions used to determine the presence of abnormal or cancerous cells
2. an ultrasound procedure that obtains images of the ovaries, uterus, cervix, and uterine tubes
3. a blood test used to detect and monitor treatment of ovarian cancer

Exercise 23

1. Pap smear
2. CA-125
3. transvaginal sonography

Exercise 24

Spelling exercise; see text, p. 266.

Exercise 25

1.   WR CV   S
<u>gynec/o</u>/logist
    CF
a physician who studies and treats diseases of women

2.   WR CV   S
<u>gynec/o</u>/logy
    CF
study of women (branch of medicine dealing with diseases of the female reproductive system)

3.   WR CV WR   S
<u>vulv/o</u>/vagin/al
    CF
pertaining to the vulva and vagina

4.   WR   S
mast/algia
pain in the breast

5. WR   WR
men/arche
beginning of menstruation

6. WR CV   S
leuk/o/rrhea
   CF
white discharge (from the vagina)

7. WR CV WR CV   S
olig/o/men/o/rrhea
   CF   CF
scanty menstrual flow

8. WR CV WR   S
gyn/o/path/ic
   CF
pertaining to disease of women

9. WR CV   S
mast/o/ptosis
   CF
sagging breast

10. WR   S
vagin/al
pertaining to the vagina

Exercise 26
1. olig/o/men/o/rrhea
2. leuk/o/rrhea
3. men/arche
4. mast/algia
5. vulv/o/vagin/al
6. gynec/o/logist
7. gynec/o/logy
8. mast/o/ptosis
9. gyn/o/path/ic
10. vagin/al

Exercise 27
Spelling exercise; see text, p. 268.

Exercise 28
1. cessation of menstruation
2. painful intercourse
3. abnormal passageway between two organs or between an internal organ and the body surface
4. a syndrome involving physical and emotional symptoms occurring during the 10 days before menstruation
5. instrument for opening a body cavity to allow for visual inspection
6. replacement of hormones in the treatment of menopause

Exercise 29
1. fistula
2. dyspareunia
3. menopause
4. premenstrual syndrome
5. speculum
6. estrogen replacement therapy

Exercise 30
Spelling exercise; see text, p. 270.

Exercise 31
1. anterior and posterior colporrhaphy
2. total abdominal hysterectomy and bilateral salpingo-oophorectomy; estrogen replacement therapy
3. sonohysterogram and transvaginal sonography
4. total vaginal hysterectomy
5. dilation and curettage; cervix
6. fibrocystic breast disease
7. pelvic inflammatory disease; gynecology
8. premenstrual syndrome

Exercise 32
1. mammography
2. carcinoma
3. hysterectomy
4. adenomyosis
5. endometriosis
6. ERT
7. stereotactic breast biopsy
8. induration
9. necrosis
10. hyperplasia

Exercise 33
1. dysmenorrhea
2. endometritis
3. fallopian tube
4. suture of the vulva
5. mammoplasty
6. uterus, fallopian tubes, and ovaries
7. hematosalpinx
8. endometriosis
9. speculum
10. TSS

Exercise 34 Reading Exercise

Exercise 35
1. b
2. *T*
3. *T*
4. d

Answers

Exercise Figures
Exercise Figure
A. 1. umbilicus: omphal/o
2. fetus: fet/o, fet/i
3. amnion: amni/o, amnion/o
4. chorion: chori/o

Exercise Figure B. salping/o/cyesis

Exercise Figure C. omphal/o/cele

Exercise Figure D. amni/o/centesis

Exercise 1
1. gamete; ovulation; fertilization; zygote; gestation
2. embryo; fetus
3. amniotic; chorion; amnion; amniotic

Exercise 2
1. fetus, unborn child
2. milk
3. give birth to, bear, labor, childbirth
4. umbilicus, navel
5. amnion, amniotic fluid
6. childbirth
7. pregnancy
8. birth
9. chorion
10. embryo, to be full

Exercise 3
1. lact/o
2. fet/o, feti/i
3. chori/o
4. a. amni/o
   b. amnion/o
5. puerper/o
6. a. par/o
   b. part/o
7. gravid/o
8. embry/o
9. nat/o
10. omphal/o

Exercise 4
1. first
2. pylorus
3. head
4. esophagus
5. false
6. pelvic bone, pelvis

Exercise 5
1. cephal/o
2. pylor/o
3. pseud/o
4. esophag/o
5. prim/i
6. pelv/i, pelv/o

Exercise 6
1. after
2. many
3. none
4. small
5. before
6. before

Exercise 7
1. nulli-
2. micro-
3. multi-
4. a. ante-
   b. pre-
5. post-

Exercise 8
1. rupture
2. birth, labor
3. pregnancy
4. childbirth, labor
5. amnion, amniotic fluid

Exercise 9
1. -tocia
2. -rrhexis
3. -partum
4. -cyesis
5. -amnios

Exercise 10
1. WR CV WR S
   chori/o/amnion/itis
       CF
   inflammation of the chorion and amnion

2. WR CV WR S
   chori/o/carcin/oma
       CF
   cancerous tumor of the chorion

3. P S(WR)
   dys/tocia
   difficult labor

4. WR S
   amnion/itis
   inflammation of the amnion

5. WR CV S
   hyster/o/rrhexis
        CF
   rupture of the uterus

6. WR CV S
   embry/o/tocia
       CF
   birth of an embryo, abortion

7. WR CV S
   salping/o/cyesis
        CF
   pregnancy in a fallopian tube (ectopic pregnancy)

8. WR CV WR S
   olig/o/hydr/amnios
       CF
   scanty amnion water (less than the normal amount of amniotic fluid)

9. P WR S
   poly/hydr/amnios
   much amnion water (more than the normal amount of amniotic fluid)

Exercise 11
1. chori/o/carcin/oma
2. amnion/itis
3. chori/o/amnion/itis
4. embry/o/tocia
5. dys/tocia
6. hyster/o/rrhexis

7. salping/o/cyesis
8. olig/o/hydr/amnios
9. poly/hydr/amnios

Exercise 12
Spelling exercise; see text, p. 287.

Exercise 13
1. premature separation of the placenta from the uterine wall
2. termination of pregnancy by the expulsion from the uterus of an embryo
3. abnormally low implantation of the placenta on the uterine wall
4. severe complication and progression of preeclampsia
5. pregnancy occurring outside the uterus
6. abnormal condition, encountered during pregnancy or shortly after delivery, of high blood pressure, edema, and proteinuria

Exercise 14
1. abruptio placentae
2. eclampsia
3. abortion
4. ectopic pregnancy
5. placenta previa
6. preeclampsia

Exercise 15
Spelling exercise; see text, p. 290.

Exercise 16
1. WR S
   pylor/ic stenosis
   narrowing pertaining to the pyloric sphincter

2. WR CV S
   omphal/o/cele
        CF
   hernia at the umbilicus

3. WR S
   omphal/itis
   inflammation of the umbilicus

4. P WR S
   micro/cephal/us
   (fetus with a very) small head

5. WR CV WR S
   trache/o/esophag/eal fistula
        CF
   abnormal passageway (between) pertaining to the esophagus and the trachea

Exercise 17
1. omphal/o/cele
2. micro/cephal/us
3. pylor/ic stenosis
4. trache/o/esophag/eal fistula
5. omphal/itis

Exercise 18
Spelling exercise; see text, p. 291.

Exercise 19
1. f 2. c 3. a 4. d 5. b 6. g 7. e

Exercise 20
Spelling exercise; see text, p. 293.

Exercise 21
1. WR CV S
   episi/o/tomy
       CF
   incision of the vulva (perineum)

2. WR CV S
   amni/o/tomy
       CF
   incision into the amnion (rupture of the fetal membrane to induce labor)

3. WR CV S
   amni/o/scope
       CF
   instrument for visual examination of amniotic fluid (and fetus)

4. WR S WR CV S
   pelv/ic son/o/graphy
            CF
   pertaining to the pelvis, process of recording sound

5. WR CV S
   amni/o/centesis
       CF
   surgical puncture to aspirate amniotic fluid

6. WR CV S
   amni/o/scopy
       CF
   visual examination of amniotic fluid (and fetus)

Exercise 22
1. amni/o/tomy
2. episi/o/tomy
3. amni/o/scopy
4. amni/o/centesis
5. amni/o/scope
6. pelv/ic son/o/graphy

Exercise 23
Spelling exercise; see text, p. 295.

Exercise 24
1. WR S
   puerper/a
   childbirth

2. WR CV S
   amni/o/rrhexis
       CF
   rupture of the amnion

3. P   WR   S
   ante/part/um
   before childbirth

4. WR CV   S
   pseud/o/cyesis
     CF
   false pregnancy

5. P   WR S
   pre/nat/al
   pertaining to before birth

6. WR S
   lact/ic
   pertaining to milk

7. WR CV   S
   lact/o/rrhea
     CF
   (spontaneous) discharge of milk

8. WR CV   S
   amni/o/rrhea
     CF
   discharge (escape) of amniotic fluid

9. P   WR S
   multi/par/a
   many births

10. WR CV   S
   embry/o/genic
     CF
   producing an embryo

11. WR   S
   embry/oid
   resembling an embryo

12. WR S
   fet/al
   pertaining to the fetus

13. WR   S
   gravid/a
   pregnant (woman)

14. WR CV WR   S
   amni/o/chori/al
     CF
   pertaining to the amnion and chorion

15. P   WR   S
   multi/gravid/a
   many pregnancies

16. WR CV   S
   lact/o/genic
     CF
   producing milk (by stimulation)

17. WR   S
   nat/al
   pertaining to birth

18. WR CV WR   S
   gravid/o/puerper/al
      CF
   pertaining to pregnancy and
   childbirth

19. P   WR CV S
   neo/nat/o/logy
      CF
   study of the newborn

20. P   WR S
   nulli/par/a
   no births

21. WR S
   par/a
   birth

22. WR CV WR   S
   prim/i/gravid/a
     CF
   first pregnancy

23. P   WR   S
   post/part/um
   after childbirth

24. P   WR S
   neo/nat/e
   new birth (an infant from birth to
   4 weeks of age, synonymous with
   newborn)

25. WR CV WR S
   prim/i/par/a
     CF
   first birth

26. WR   S
   puerper/al
   pertaining to (immediately after)
   childbirth

27. P   WR   S
   nulli/gravid/a
   no pregnancies

28. P   WR   S
   intra/part/um
   within (during) labor and childbirth

29. P   WR S
   post/nat/al
   pertaining to after birth

30. P   WR CV   S
   neo/nat/o/logist
      CF
   physician who studies and treats
   disorders of the newborn

Exercise 25

1. amni/o/chori/al
2. ante/part/um
3. embry/o/genic
4. fet/al
5. pre/nat/al
6. lact/ic
7. lact/o/rrhea
8. amni/o/rrhea
9. pseud/o/cyesis
10. lact/o/genic
11. amni/o/rrhexis
12. embry/oid
13. gravid/a
14. gravid/o/puerper/al
15. multi/par/a
16. nat/al
17. neo/nat/e
18. neo/nat/o/logy
19. nulli/par/a
20. par/a
21. prim/i/gravid/a
22. post/part/um
23. prim/i/par/a
24. multi/gravid/a
25. puerper/al
26. nulli/gravid/a
27. puerper/a
28. intra/part/um
29. neo/nat/o/logist
30. post/nat/al

Exercise 26
Spelling exercise; see text, pp. 300-301.

Exercise 27

1. a	6. b
2. e	7. j
3. i	8. d
4. g	9. c
5. f	10. h

Exercise 28

1. first stool of the newborn
2. medical specialty dealing with pregnancy, childbirth, and puerperium
3. infant born before completing 37 weeks of gestation
4. vaginal discharge after childbirth
5. period after delivery until the reproductive organs return to normal
6. act of giving birth
7. physician who specializes in obstetrics
8. abnormality present at birth
9. parturition in which the buttocks, feet, or knees emerge first
10. birth of a baby through an incision in the mother's abdomen and uterus

Exercise 29
Spelling exercise; see text, p. 303.

Exercise 30

1. obstetrics
2. expected (estimated) date of delivery
3. last menstrual period

4. date of birth
5. newborn
6. multipara
7. cesarean section
8. last normal menstrual period
9. respiratory distress syndrome

Exercise 31
1. gravida
2. para
3. EDD
4. prenatal
5. gestation
6. pelvic sonography
7. fetus
8. fetal

Exercise 32
1. lungs
2. dystocia
3. amniocentesis
4. antepartum
5. has never been pregnant
6. given birth to two or more viable offspring
7. in her first pregnancy
8. parturition
9. hysterorrhexis

Exercise 33
1. *T*
2. d
3. b
4. *F*, the fetal presentation was breech.

Answers

			G	R	A	V	I	D	O		A
		F									M
	P	U	E	R	P	E	R	O			N
	E		T								I
	L		O				C				O
	V						H				N
P	R	I	M	I			O				O
S					L		R				
E				A	M	N	I	O			E
U				C		O					M
D			N	T							B
O	M	P	H	A	L	O					R
			T								Y
P	A	R	T	O			C	E	P	H	A	L	O

ANSWERS TO CHAPTER 10 EXERCISES
Exercise Figures
Exercise Figure
A. 1. blood vessel: angi/o
   2. valve: valv/o, valvul/o
   3. heart: cardi/o
   4. aorta: aort/o
   5. artery: arteri/o
   6. atrium: atri/o
   7. ventricle: ventricul/o

Exercise Figure B. ather/o/sclerosis

Exercise Figure C. end/arter/ectomy

Exercise Figure D. electr/o/cardi/o/gram

Exercise 1
1. g
2. j
3. e
4. m
5. b
6. k
7. i
8. f
9. l
10. h
11. d
12. a
13. n

Exercise 2
1. f
2. p
3. h
4. b
5. m
6. c
7. l
8. q
9. d
10. o
11. a
12. i
13. e
14. j
15. g

Exercise 3
1. heart
2. atrium
3. plasma
4. vessel
5. vein
6. aorta
7. valve
8. spleen
9. thymus gland
10. vein
11. ventricle
12. artery
13. valve
14. lymph, lymph gland

Exercise 4
1. arteri/o
2. a. phleb/o
   b. ven/o
3. cardi/o
4. atri/o
5. ventricul/o
6. lymph/o
7. aort/o
8. angi/o
9. a. valv/o
   b. valvul/o
10. splen/o
11. plasm/o
12. thym/o

Exercise 5
1. sound
2. clot
3. deficiency, blockage
4. heat
5. yellowish, fatty plaque
6. electricity, electrical activity

Exercise 6
1. thromb/o
2. ech/o
3. isch/o
4. ather/o
5. therm/o
6. electr/o

Exercise 7
1. fast, rapid
2. slow

Exercise 8
1. tachy-
2. brady-

Exercise 9
1. to separate
2. instrument used to record
3. abnormal reduction in number
4. hardening
5. pain
6. removal
7. formation
8. pertaining to

Exercise 10
1. -poiesis
2. -ac
3. -sclerosis
4. -graph
5. -penia
6. -odynia
7. -crit
8. -apheresis

Exercise 11
1. P   WR   S
   endo/card/itis
   inflammation of the inner (lining) of the heart

2. P   WR   S
   brady/card/ia
   condition of slow heart (rate)

3. WR CV   S
   cardi/o/megaly
       CF
   enlargement of the heart

4. WR CV   S
   arteri/o/sclerosis
       CF
   hardening of the arteries

5. WR CV WR   S
   cardi/o/valvul/itis
       CF
   inflammation of the valves of the heart

6. WR CV WR   S
   angi/o/card/itis
       CF
   inflammation of the blood vessels and heart

7. WR CV   S
   arteri/o/rrhexis
       CF
   rupture of an artery

8. P   WR   S
   tachy/card/ia
   abnormal state of rapid heart (rate)

9. WR CV   S
   angi/o/stenosis
       CF
   narrowing of blood vessels

10. WR   S
    thromb/us
    (blood) clot

11. WR   S
    isch/emia
    deficiency of blood (flow)

12. P   WR   S
    peri/card/itis
    inflammation of outer sac of heart

13. WR   S
    cardi/o/dynia
    pain in the heart

14. WR   S
    aort/ic stenosis
    narrowing, pertaining to the aorta

15. WR   S
    thromb/osis
    abnormal condition of a (blood) clot

16. WR CV   S
    ather/o/sclerosis
         CF
    hardening of fatty plaque (deposited
    on the arterial wall)

17. WR CV WR   S
    my/o/card/itis
       CF
    inflammation of the muscle of the
    heart

18. WR   S
    angi/oma
    tumor composed of blood vessels

19. WR   S
    thym/oma
    tumor of the thymus gland

20. WR   CV WR CV   S
    hemat/o/cyt/o/penia
         CF   CF
    abnormal reduction in the number of
    blood cells

21. WR   S
    lymph/oma
    tumor of lymphatic tissue

22. WR   WR   S
    lymph/aden/itis
    inflammation of lymph glands (nodes)

23. WR   CV   S
    splen/o/megaly
        CF
    enlargement of the spleen

24. WR   S
    hemat/oma
    tumor of blood

25. P   WR   S
    poly/arter/itis
    inflammation of many (sites in the)
    arteries

26. WR   CV WR CV   S
    cardi/o/my/o/pathy
        CF   CF
    disease of the heart muscle

27. WR CV   S
    angi/o/spasm
         CF
    spasm of the blood vessels

28. WR   WR CV   S
    lymph/aden/o/pathy
             CF
    disease of the lymph glands

29. WR   CV WR   S
    thromb/o/phleb/itis
          CF
    inflammation of a vein associated with
    a clot

30. WR   S
    phleb/itis
    inflammation of a vein

31. P   WR CV   S
    pan/cyt/o/penia
           CF
    abnormal reduction of all (blood) cells

Exercise 12

1. arteri/o/rrhexis
2. cardi/o/megaly
3. isch/emia
4. angi/o/card/itis
5. endo/card/itis
6. brady/card/ia
7. arteri/o/sclerosis
8. thromb/osis
9. cardi/odynia
10. my/o/card/itis
11. angi/o/stenosis
12. tachy/card/ia
13. ather/o/sclerosis
14. angi/oma
15. cardi/o/valvul/itis
16. aort/ic stenosis
17. peri/card/itis
18. hemat/o/cyt/o/penia
19. lymph/oma
20. thym/oma
21. splen/o/megaly
22. hemat/oma
23. lymph/aden/itis
24. cardi/o/my/o/pathy
25. poly/arter/itis
26. angi/o/spasm
27. lymph/aden/o/pathy
28. thromb/o/phleb/itis
29. phleb/itis
30. thromb/us
31. pan/cyt/o/penia

Exercise 13
Spelling exercise; see text, p. 325.

Exercise 14

1. coarctation
2. embolus
3. cardiac arrest
4. congenital
5. varicose veins
6. coronary occlusion
7. aneurysm
8. Hodgkin
9. hemorrhoids
10. angina pectoris
11. myocardial infarction
12. fibrillation
13. dysrhythmia
14. hypertensive
15. congestive heart failure
16. peripheral arterial disease
17. hemophilia
18. leukemia
19. anemia
20. sickle cell anemia
21. intermittent claudication
22. cardiac tamponade
23. mitral valve stenosis and rheumatic
    heart disease
24. deep vein thrombosis
25. rheumatic fever
26. hemochromatosis
27. acute coronary syndrome

Exercise 15

1. d		8. k	
2. c		9. g	
3. f		10. b	
4. e		11. h	
5. a		12. l	
6. j		13. n	
7. i		14. m	

Exercise 16

1. i		8. k	
2. e		9. l	
3. a		10. g	
4. h		11. c	
5. j		12. f	
6. b		13. m	
7. d			

Exercise 17
Spelling exercise; see text, p. 332.

Exercise 18

1. P   WR CV   S
   peri/cardi/o/centesis
            CF
   surgical puncture to aspirate fluid from
   (within) the outer sac of the heart

2. WR   S
   thym/ectomy
   excision of the thymus gland

3. WR CV S
 <u>angi</u>/<u>o</u>/plasty
  CF
 surgical repair of a blood vessel

4. WR CV S
 <u>splen</u>/<u>o</u>/pexy
  CF
 surgical fixation of the spleen

5. WR CV S
 <u>angi</u>/<u>o</u>/rrhaphy
  CF
 suturing of a blood vessel

6. P WR S
 end/arter/ectomy
 excision within an artery

7. WR CV S
 <u>phleb</u>/<u>o</u>/tomy
  CF
 incision into a vein

8. WR S
 splen/ectomy
 excision of the spleen

9. WR S
 phleb/ectomy
 excision of a vein

10. WR S
 ather/ectomy
 excision of yellowish, fatty plaque

Exercise 19
1. end/arter/ectomy
2. splen/o/pexy
3. angi/o/rrhaphy
4. phleb/o/tomy
5. thym/ectomy
6. peri/cardi/o/centesis
7. angi/o/plasty
8. splen/ectomy
9. phleb/ectomy
10. ather/ectomy

Exercise 20
Spelling exercise; see text, p. 335.

Exercise 21
1. hemorrhoidectomy
2. percutaneous transluminal coronary angioplasty
3. cardiac pacemaker
4. commissurotomy
5. coronary artery bypass graft
6. aneurysmectomy
7. femoropopliteal bypass
8. laser angioplasty
9. intracoronary thrombolytic
10. defibrillation
11. bone marrow transplant

12. embolectomy
13. coronary stent
14. implantable cardiac defibrillator

Exercise 22
1. h
2. o
3. k
4. l
5. d
6. m
7. a
8. c
9. e
10. i
11. b
12. j
13. g
14. f

Exercise 23
Spelling exercise; see text, p. 341.

Exercise 24

1. WR CV WR CV S
 <u>electr</u>/<u>o</u>/<u>cardi</u>/<u>o</u>/graph
  CF CF
 instrument used to record the electrical activity of the heart

2. WR CV S
 <u>ven</u>/<u>o</u>/gram
  CF
 x-ray image of the veins (after an injection of contrast medium)

3. WR CV S
 <u>angi</u>/<u>o</u>/graphy
  CF
 x-ray imaging of a blood vessel

4. WR CV WR CV S
 <u>ech</u>/<u>o</u>/<u>cardi</u>/<u>o</u>/gram
  CF CF
 record of the heart by using sound

5. WR CV S
 <u>aort</u>/<u>o</u>/gram
  CF
 x-ray image of the aorta (after an injection of contrast medium)

6. WR CV WR CV S
 <u>electr</u>/<u>o</u>/<u>cardi</u>/<u>o</u>/gram
  CF CF
 record of the electrical activity of the heart

7. WR CV S
 <u>arteri</u>/<u>o</u>/gram
  CF
 x-ray image of an artery (after an injection of contrast medium)

8. WR CV WR CV S
 <u>electr</u>/<u>o</u>/<u>cardi</u>/<u>o</u>/graphy
  CF CF
 process of recording the electrical activity of the heart

9. WR CV S
 <u>erythr</u>/<u>o</u>/cyte count
  CF
 red cell count (number of red blood cells per cubic millimeter of blood)

10. WR CV S
 <u>hemat</u>/<u>o</u>/crit
  CF
 separated blood (volume percentage of erythrocytes in whole blood)

11. WR CV S
 <u>leuk</u>/<u>o</u>/cyte count
  CF
 white cell count (number of white blood cells per cubic millimeter of blood)

12. WR WR CV S
 lymph/<u>angi</u>/<u>o</u>/graphy
  CF
 x-ray imaging of the lymphatic vessels (after an injection of the contrast medium)

13. WR CV S
 <u>angi</u>/<u>o</u>/scopy
  CF
 visual examination of a blood vessel

14. WR CV S
 <u>ven</u>/<u>o</u>/graphy
  CF
 x-ray imaging a vein

15. WR CV S
 <u>angi</u>/<u>o</u>/scope
  CF
 instrument used for visual examination of a blood vessel

Exercise 25
1. electr/o/cardi/o/graph
2. arteri/o/gram
3. ven/o/gram
4. angi/o/graphy
5. electr/o/cardi/o/gram
6. ech/o/cardi/o/gram
7. aort/o/gram
8. electr/o/cardi/o/graphy
9. hemat/o/crit
10. leuk/o/cyte
11. erythr/o/cyte
12. lymph/angi/o/graphy
13. angi/o/scopy
14. ven/o/graphy
15. angi/o/scope

Exercise 26
Spelling exercise; see text, p. 345.

Exercise 27

1. sphygmomanometer
2. coagulation time
3. complete blood count
4. Doppler ultrasound
5. stethoscope
6. bone marrow biopsy
7. prothrombin time
8. cardiac catheterization
9. hemoglobin
10. impedance plethysmography
11. thallium test
12. transesophageal echocardiogram
13. single-photon emission computed tomography
14. exercise stress test
15. digital subtraction angiography

Exercise 28

1.	d	9.	k
2.	n	10.	p
3.	h	11.	f
4.	o	12.	i
5.	g	13.	e
6.	j	14.	b
7.	c	15.	m
8.	a		

Exercise 29

Spelling exercise; see text, p. 351.

Exercise 30

1. P   WR   S
   hypo/therm/ia
   condition of (body) temperature that is below (normal)

2. WR CV S
   hemat/o/poiesis
       CF
   formation of blood (cells)

3. WR CV S
   cardi/o/logy
       CF
   study of the heart

4. WR CV S
   cardi/o/logist
       CF
   physician who studies and treats diseases of the heart

5. WR CV S
   hem/o/lysis
      CF
   dissolution of blood (cells)

6. WR CV S
   hemat/o/logist
       CF
   physician who studies and treats diseases of the blood

7. WR   S
   cardi/ac
   pertaining to the heart

8. WR CV S
   hemat/o/logy
       CF
   study of the blood

9. WR   S
   plasm/apheresis
   removal of plasma (from withdrawn blood)

10. WR CV S
    hem/o/stasis
       CF
    stoppage of bleeding

11. WR CV S
    cardi/o/genic
       CF
    originating in the heart

12. P   S(WR)
    tachy/pnea
    rapid breathing

13. WR   CV S
    thromb/o/lysis
        CF
    dissolution of a clot

14. WR CV WR   S
    atri/o/ventricul/ar
       CF
    pertaining to the atrium and ventricle

15. P   WR   S
    intra/ven/ous
    pertaining to within the vein

Exercise 31

1. cardi/o/logy
2. hemat/o/poiesis
3. hypo/therm/ia
4. hem/o/lysis
5. plasm/apheresis
6. hemat/o/logist
7. cardi/ac
8. cardi/o/logist
9. hemat/o/logy
10. hem/o/stasis
11. tachy/pnea
12. cardi/o/genic
13. thromb/o/lysis
14. atri/o/ventricul/ar
15. intra/ven/ous

Exercise 32

Spelling exercise; see text, p. 354.

Exercise 33

1. vasoconstrictor	11. hypertension
2. lumen	12. occlude
3. cardiopulmonary resuscitation	13. percussion
4. diastole	14. auscultation
5. blood pressure	15. plasma
6. hypotension	16. hemorrhage
7. extravasation	17. anticoagulant
8. venipuncture	18. serum
9. systole	19. dyscrasia
10. vasodilator	20. heart murmur
	21. extracorporeal

Exercise 34

1. space within a tubelike structure
2. escape of blood from the blood vessel into the tissues
3. pressure exerted by the blood against the vessel walls
4. puncture of a vein to remove blood, start an intravenous infusion, or instill medication
5. agent or nerve that enlarges the blood vessels
6. blood pressure that is above normal
7. emergency procedure consisting of artificial ventilation and external cardiac massage
8. phase in the cardiac cycle in which ventricles contract
9. blood pressure that is below normal
10. agent or nerve that narrows blood vessels
11. cardiac cycle phase in which ventricles relax
12. hearing of sounds within the body through a stethoscope
13. to close tightly
14. tapping of a body surface with fingers to determine the density of parts beneath
15. liquid portion of the blood without clotting factors
16. abnormal or pathologic condition of the blood
17. liquid portion of the blood in which the elements or cells are suspended and that contains the clotting factors
18. rapid flow of blood
19. agent that slows down the clotting process
20. occurring outside the body
21. humming sound of cardiac or vascular origin

Exercise 35

Spelling exercise; see text, p. 358.

Exercise 36

1. coronary artery disease; electrocardiogram; single-photon emission computed tomography; echocardiogram
2. deep vein thrombosis; impedance plethysmography
3. complete blood count; red blood count, white blood count, hemoglobin, hematocrit
4. coronary artery bypass graft; percutaneous transluminal coronary angioplasty
5. myocardial infarction; coronary care unit
6. blood pressure
7. congestive heart failure
8. cardiopulmonary resuscitation
9. hypertensive heart disease
10. prothrombin time
11. atrioventricular
12. acute coronary syndrome
13. peripheral arterial disease
14. digital subtraction angiography
15. transesophageal echocardiogram

Exercise 37

1. angina pectoris
2. thallium test
3. ischemia
4. angiography
5. stenosis
6. angioplasty
7. cardiologist
8. electrocardiography
9. cardiac catheterization
10. myocardial infarction

Exercise 38

1. atherosclerosis
2. thrombophlebitis
3. myocarditis
4. myocardial infarction
5. endarterectomy
6. hemorrhoids
7. hypothermia
8. impedance plethysmography
9. murmur
10. angioscope, angioscopy
11. thallium test

Exercise 39 Reading Exercise

Exercise 40

1. *F*, the diagnosis was made with an ultrasound procedure.
2. c
3. d
4. b

Answers

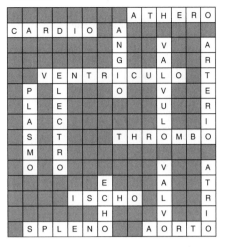

ANSWERS TO CHAPTER 11 EXERCISES

Exercise Figures

Exercise Figure

A. 1. mouth: stomat/o, or/o
2. esophagus: esophag/o
3. duodenum: duoden/o
4. ascending colon: col/o, colon/o
5. cecum: cec/o
6. anus: an/o
7. pharynx: pharyng/o
8. stomach: gastr/o
9. antrum: antr/o
10. jejunum: jejun/o
11. ileum: ile/o
12. sigmoid colon: sigmoid/o
13. rectum: proct/o, rect/o

Exercise Figure

B. 1. gums: gingiv/o
2. lips: cheil/o
3. salivary glands: sial/o
4. liver: hepat/o
5. gallbladder: chol/e (gall), cyst/o (bladder)
6. pylorus, pyloric sphincter: pylor/o
7. appendix: appendic/o
8. palate: palat/o
9. uvula: uvul/o
10. tongue: gloss/o, lingu/o
11. bile duct: cholangi/o
12. common bile duct: choledoch/o
13. pancreas: pancreat/o
14. abdomen: lapar/o, abdomin/o, celi/o

Exercise Figure C. *2*, appendic/itis

Exercise Figure D. chol/e/lith/iasis, choledoch/o/lith/iasis

Exercise Figure E. *1*, ile/o/stomy
2, col/o/stomy

Exercise Figure F. gastr/ectomy

Exercise Figure G. *2*, chol/e/cyst/o/gram

Exercise Figure H. gastr/o/scope

Exercise 1

1. alimentary canal
2. gastrointestinal tract
3. pharynx
4. esophagus
5. stomach
6. duodenum
7. jejunum
8. ileum
9. cecum
10. ascending colon
11. transverse colon
12. descending colon
13. sigmoid colon
14. rectum
15. anus

Exercise 2

1. l
2. d
3. a
4. h
5. m
6. j
7. b
8. i
9. c
10. g
11. e
12. k
13. f

Exercise 3

1. rectum
2. stomach
3. anus
4. cecum
5. ileum
6. mouth
7. duodenum
8. colon
9. mouth
10. intestines
11. rectum
12. antrum
13. esophagus
14. jejunum
15. sigmoid colon
16. colon

Exercise 4

1. cec/o
2. gastr/o
3. ile/o
4. jejun/o
5. sigmoid/o
6. esophag/o
7. a. rect/o
   b. proct/o
8. enter/o
9. duoden/o
10. a. col/o
    b. colon/o
11. a. or/o
    b. stomat/o
12. an/o
13. antr/o

Exercise 5

1. hernia
2. abdomen
3. saliva
4. gall, bile
5. diverticulum
6. gum
7. appendix
8. tongue
9. liver
10. lip
11. peritoneum
12. palate
13. pancreas
14. abdomen
15. tongue
16. common bile duct
17. pylorus, pyloric sphincter
18. uvula
19. bile duct
20. polyp, small growth
21. abdomen

Exercise 6

1. palat/o
2. sial/o
3. pancreat/o
4. peritone/o
5. a. lingu/o
   b. gloss/o
6. gingiv/o
7. pylor/o
8. hepat/o
9. chol/e
10. a. abdomin/o
    b. lapar/o
    c. celi/o
11. herni/o
12. diverticul/o
13. cheil/o
14. appendic/o
15. uvul/o
16. cholangi/o
17. choledoch/o
18. polyp/o

Exercise 7

1. digestion
2. half

Exercise 8

1. -pepsia
2. hemi-

Exercise 9

1. WR CV WR   S
   chol/e/lith/iasis
        CF
   condition of gallstones

2.   WR   S
   diverticul/osis
   abnormal condition of having
   diverticula

3. WR CV WR
   sial/o/lith
        CF
   stone in the salivary gland

4. WR   S
   hepat/oma
   tumor of the liver

5. WR   S
   uvul/itis
   inflammation of the uvula

6.   WR   S
   pancreat/itis
   inflammation of the pancreas

7. WR CV   S
   proct/o/ptosis
        CF
   prolapse of the rectum

8.   WR   S
   gingiv/itis
   inflammation of the gums

9.   WR   S
   gastr/itis
   inflammation of the stomach

10. WR CV S
   rect/o/cele
        CF
   protrusion of the rectum

11. WR   S
    palat/itis
    inflammation of the palate

12. WR   S
    hepat/itis
    inflammation of the liver

13.   WR   S
    appendic/itis
    inflammation of the appendix

14. WR CV WR   S
    chol/e/cyst/itis
         CF
    inflammation of the gallbladder

15.   WR   S
    diverticul/itis
    inflammation of a diverticulum

16. WR CV WR   S
    gastr/o/enter/itis
         CF
    inflammation of the stomach and
    intestines

17. WR CV WR CV WR   S
    gastr/o/enter/o/col/itis
         CF   CF
    inflammation of the stomach,
    intestines, and colon

18.   WR   CV WR   S
    choledoch/o/lith/iasis
              CF
    condition of stones in the common
    bile duct

19.   WR   S
    cholangi/oma
    tumor of the bile duct

20.   WR   S
    polyp/osis
    abnormal condition of (multiple)
    polyps

21.   WR   S
    esophag/itis
    inflammation of the esophagus

22.   WR   S
    periton/itis
    inflammation of the peritoneum

Exercise 10

1. hepat/oma
2. gastr/itis
3. sial/o/lith
4. appendic/itis
5. diverticul/itis
6. chol/e/cyst/itis
7. diverticul/osis
8. gastr/o/enter/itis
9. proct/o/ptosis

10. rect/o/cele
11. uvul/itis
12. gingiv/itis
13. hepat/itis
14. palat/itis
15. chol/e/lith/iasis
16. gastr/o/enter/o/col/itis
17. pancreat/itis
18. cholangi/oma
19. esophag/itis
20. choledoch/o/lith/iasis
21. polyp/osis
22. periton/itis

Exercise 11

Spelling exercise; see text, p. 385.

Exercise 12

1. f
2. b
3. e
4. n
5. d
6. g
7. a
8. k
9. h
10. j
11. m
12. i
13. c
14. l
15. o
16. p

Exercise 13

1. another name for gastric or duodenal
   ulcer
2. psychoneurotic disorder characterized
   by a prolonged refusal to eat
3. chronic inflammation that usually
   affects the ileum
4. twisting or kinking of the intestine
5. abnormal growing together of two
   surfaces that normally are separated
6. chronic disease of the liver with
   gradual destruction of cells
7. telescoping of segment of the intestine
8. ulcer in the stomach
9. ulcer in the duodenum
10. inflammation of the colon with the
    formation of ulcers
11. eating disorder involving gorging food
    followed by induced vomiting
12. tumorlike growth extending out from
    a mucous membrane
13. disturbance of bowel function
14. obstruction of the intestine, often
    caused by failure of peristalsis
15. abnormal backward flow of the
    gastrointestinal contents into the
    esophagus
16. excess body fat

Exercise 14

Spelling exercise; see text, p. 390.

Exercise 15

1. WR   S
   gastr/ectomy
   excision of the stomach

2. WR CV WR CV S
   esophag/o/gastr/o/plasty
        CF   CF
   surgical repair of the esophagus and
   the stomach

3. WR   S
   diverticul/ectomy
   excision of a diverticulum

4. WR   S
   antr/ectomy
   excision of the antrum

5. WR CV S
   palat/o/plasty
        CF
   surgical repair of the palate

6. WR   S
   uvul/ectomy
   excision of the uvula

7. WR CV WR CV S
   gastr/o/jejun/o/stomy
        CF   CF
   creation of an artificial opening
   between the stomach and the jejunum

8. WR CV WR   S
   chol/e/cyst/ectomy
        CF
   excision of the gallbladder

9. WR   S
   col/ectomy
   excision of the colon

10. WR CV S
    col/o/stomy
         CF
    creation of an artificial opening into
    the colon

11. WR CV S
    pylor/o/plasty
         CF
    surgical repair of the pylorus

12. WR CV S
    an/o/plasty
        CF
    surgical repair of the anus

13. WR   S
    append/ectomy
    excision of the appendix

14. WR CV S
    cheil/o/rrhaphy
         CF
    suture of the lips

15. WR   S
    gingiv/ectomy
    surgical removal of gum tissue

16. WR CV S
    lapar/o/tomy
         CF
    incision into the abdomen

17. WR CV S
    ile/o/stomy
        CF
    creation of an artificial opening into
    the ileum

18. WR CV S
    gastr/o/stomy
         CF
    creation of an artificial opening into
    the stomach

19. WR CV   S
    herni/o/rrhaphy
         CF
    suturing of a hernia

20. WR CV   S
    gloss/o/rrhaphy
         CF
    suture of the tongue

21. WR   CV WR CV S
    choledoch/o/lith/o/tomy
             CF   CF
    incision into the common bile duct to
    remove a stone

22. P   WR   S
    hemi/col/ectomy
    excision of half of the colon

23. WR   S
    polyp/ectomy
    excision of a polyp

24. WR CV   S
    enter/o/rrhaphy
         CF
    suture of the intestine

25. WR   CV S
    abdomin/o/plasty
           CF
    surgical repair of the abdomen

26. WR CV WR CV S
    pylor/o/my/o/tomy
         CF   CF
    incision into the pylorus muscle

27. WR CV WR CV   WR CV S
    uvul/o/palat/o/pharyng/o/plasty
         CF   CF   CF
    surgical repair of the uvula, palate,
    and pharynx

28. WR CV S
    celi/o/tomy
         CF
    incision into the abdominal cavity

29. WR CV S
    gastr/o/plasty
         CF
    surgical repair of the stomach

Exercise 16

1. append/ectomy
2. gloss/o/rrhaphy
3. esophag/o/gastr/o/plasty
4. diverticul/ectomy
5. ile/o/stomy
6. gingiv/ectomy
7. lapar/o/tomy
8. an/o/plasty
9. antr/ectomy
10. chol/e/cyst/ectomy
11. col/ectomy
12. col/o/stomy
13. gastr/ectomy
14. gastr/o/stomy
15. gastr/o/jejun/o/stomy
16. uvul/ectomy
17. palat/o/plasty
18. pylor/o/plasty
19. herni/o/rrhaphy
20. cheil/o/rrhaphy
21. hemi/col/ectomy
22. choledoch/o/lith/o/tomy
23. polyp/ectomy
24. enter/o/rrhaphy
25. abdomin/o/plasty
26. celi/o/tomy
27. pylor/o/my/o/tomy
28. uvul/o/palat/o/pharyng/o/plasty
29. gastr/o/plasty

Exercise 17
Spelling exercise; see text, p. 398.

Exercise 18
1. vagotomy
2. anastomosis
3. abdominoperineal resection

Exercise 19
Spelling exercise; see text, p. 399.

Exercise 20

1. WR   CV S
   esophag/o/scope
          CF
   instrument used for visual
   examination of the esophagus

2. WR   CV   S
  esophag/o/scopy
      CF
  visual examination of the esophagus

3. WR   CV   S
  gastr/o/scope
      CF
  instrument used for visual
  examination of the stomach

4. WR   CV   S
  gastr/o/scopy
      CF
  visual examination of the stomach

5. WR   CV   S
  proct/o/scope
      CF
  instrument used for visual
  examination of the rectum

6. WR   CV   S
  proct/o/scopy
      CF
  visual examination of the rectum

7. P   S(WR)
  endo/scope
  instrument used for visual
  examination within a hollow organ

8. P   S(WR)
  endo/scopy
  visual examination within a hollow
  organ

9. WR   CV   S
  sigmoid/o/scope
      CF
  instrument used for visual
  examination of the sigmoid colon

10. WR   CV   S
  sigmoid/o/scopy
      CF
  visual examination of the sigmoid
  colon

11. WR CV WR CV   S
  chol/e/cyst/o/gram
      CF   CF
  x-ray image of the gallbladder

12. WR   CV   S
  cholangi/o/gram
      CF
  x-ray image of bile ducts

13. WR   CV WR   CV WR   CV   S
  esophag/o/gastr/o/duoden/o/scopy
      CF   CF   CF
  visual examination of the esophagus,
  stomach, and duodenum

14. WR   CV   S
  colon/o/scope
      CF
  instrument used for visual
  examination of the colon

15. WR   CV   S
  lapar/o/scope
      CF
  instrument used for visual
  examination of the abdominal cavity

16. WR   CV   S
  colon/o/scopy
      CF
  visual examination of the colon

17. WR   CV   S
  lapar/o/scopy
      CF
  visual examination of the abdominal
  cavity

18. WR   CV   S
  colon/o/graphy
      CF
  x-ray imaging of the colon

Exercise 21

1. endo/scopy
2. gastr/o/scope
3. proct/o/scope
4. sigmoid/o/scope
5. chol/e/cyst/o/gram
6. endo/scope
7. esophag/o/scope
8. proct/o/scopy
9. esophag/o/scopy
10. sigmoid/o/scopy
11. cholangi/o/gram
12. gastr/o/scopy
13. lapar/o/scope
14. esophag/o/gastr/o/duoden/o/scopy
15. colon/o/scopy
16. lapar/o/scopy
17. colon/o/scope
18. colon/o/scopy

Exercise 22
Spelling exercise; see text, p. 406.

Exercise 23
1. series of x-ray images taken of the
   stomach and duodenum after barium
   has been swallowed
2. series of x-ray images taken of the large
   intestine after a barium enema has been
   administered
3. x-ray examination of the bile and
   pancreatic ducts
4. an endoscope fitted with an ultrasound
   probe providing images of layers of the
   intestinal wall

5. a blood test to determine the presence
   of *Helicobacter pylori* bacteria, a cause of
   peptic ulcers
6. a test to detect fecal occult blood

Exercise 24
1. d   4. b
2. f   5. c
3. a

Exercise 25
Spelling exercise; see text, p. 408.

Exercise 26

1. P   S(WR)
  a/phagia
  without swallowing (inability to
  swallow)

2. P   S(WR)
  dys/pepsia
  difficult digestion

3. WR   S
  an/al
  pertaining to the anus

4. P   S(WR)
  dys/phagia
  difficult swallowing

5. WR   CV   S
  gloss/o/pathy
      CF
  disease of the tongue

6. WR CV WR   S
  ile/o/cec/al
      CF
  pertaining to the ileum and cecum

7. WR   S
  or/al
  pertaining to the mouth

8. WR   CV WR   S
  stomat/o/gastr/ic
      CF
  pertaining to the mouth and stomach

9. WR   CV   S
  abdomin/o/centesis
      CF
  surgical puncture to remove fluid
  from the abdominal cavity

10. WR CV   S
  gastr/o/malacia
      CF
  softening of the stomach

11. WR   S
  pancreat/ic
  pertaining to the pancreas

12. WR   S
gastr/o/dynia
pain in the stomach

13.   WR   S
peritone/al
pertaining to the peritoneum

14. P   WR   S
sub/lingu/al
pertaining to under the tongue

15. WR CV S
proct/o/logy
    CF
study of the rectum

16. WR CV WR   S
nas/o/gastr/ic
   CF
pertaining to the nose and stomach

17.   WR   S
abdomin/al
pertaining to the abdomen

18. WR CV   S
proct/o/logist
    CF
physician who studies and treats
diseases of the rectum

19. WR CV WR CV   S
gastr/o/enter/o/logy
   CF   CF
study of the stomach and intestines

20. WR CV WR CV   S
gastr/o/enter/o/logist
   CF   CF
physician who studies and treats
diseases of the stomach and intestines

21. WR CV WR   S
col/o/rect/al
   CF
pertaining to the colon and rectum

22. WR   S
rect/al
pertaining to the rectum

Exercise 27
1. gloss/o/pathy
2. a/phagia
3. sub/lingu/al
4. nas/o/gastr/ic
5. stomat/o/gastr/ic
6. an/al
7. abdomin/o/centesis
8. peritone/al
9. abdomin/al
10. dys/phagia
11. ile/o/cec/al
12. gastr/o/malacia
13. gastr/o/dynia

14. proct/o/logist
15. dys/pepsia
16. pancreat/ic
17. proct/o/logy
18. or/al
19. gastr/o/enter/o/logist
20. gastr/o/enter/o/logy
21. col/o/rect/al
22. rect/al

Exercise 28
Spelling exercise; see text, p. 412.

Exercise 29
1. m		8. a
2. e		9. d
3. f		10. h
4. c		11. b
5. l		12. j
6. i		13. g
7. k		

Exercise 30
1. abnormal collection of fluid in the peritoneal cavity
2. process of feeding a person through a nasogastric tube
3. washing out of the stomach
4. waste from the digestive tract expelled through the rectum
5. urge to vomit
6. matter expelled from the stomach through the mouth
7. disorder that involves inflammation of the intestine
8. frequent discharge of liquid stool
9. gas expelled through the anus
10. abnormal backward flow
11. vomiting of blood
12. involuntary wavelike contractions that propel food along the digestive tract
13. black, tarry stools that contain digested blood

Exercise 31
Spelling exercise; see text, p. 415.

Exercise 32
1. endoscopic retrograde cholangiopancreatography
2. endoscopic ultrasound
3. nausea and vomiting
4. irritable bowel syndrome
5. percutaneous endoscopic gastrostomy
6. upper gastrointestinal
7. uvulopalatopharyngoplasty
8. gastroesophageal reflux disease
9. gastrointestinal
10. *Helicobacter pylori*
11. barium enema

12. esophagogastroduodenoscopy
13. abdominoperineal resection

Exercise 33
1. endoscopy
2. nausea
3. dyspepsia
4. hematemesis
5. melena
6. esophagogastroduodenoscopy
7. gastroscope
8. reflux
9. *H. pylori*
10. ulcers
11. gastritis
12. duodenal ulcers

Exercise 34
1. cholelithiasis
2. cholecystectomy
3. ulcerative colitis
4. proctoptosis
5. adhesion
6. gastrectomy, pyloroplasty, vagotomy
7. dyspepsia
8. gavage
9. abdominal perineal resection and colostomy
10. colonoscopy
11. ileus
12. fecal occult blood test

Exercise 35 Reading Exercise

Exercise 36
1. c
2. *T*
3. *T*
4. *F*, vomiting blood is not a warning sign of colorectal cancer.

Answers
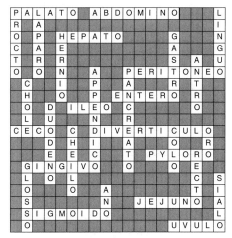

ANSWERS TO CHAPTER 12 EXERCISES

Exercise Figures

Exercise Figure

A. 1. eye: ocul/o, ophthalm/o
2. eyelid: blephar/o
3. lacrimal sac: dacry/o, lacrim/o
4. pupil: cor/o, core/o, pupill/o
5. sclera: scler/o
6. iris: irid/o, iri/o
7. conjunctiva: conjunctiv/o
8. cornea: corne/o, kerat/o
9. retina: retin/o

Exercise Figure B. blephar/itis

Exercise Figure C. blephar/o/ptosis

Exercise Figure D. dacry/o/cyst/itis

Exercise 1

1. d
2. c
3. f
4. h
5. b
6. e
7. a

Exercise 2

1. d
2. f
3. h
4. e
5. b
6. a
7. c

Exercise 3

1. eye
2. eyelid
3. cornea
4. tear, tear duct
5. retina
6. pupil
7. sclera
8. iris
9. conjunctiva
10. pupil
11. eye
12. cornea
13. iris
14. pupil
15. vision
16. tear, tear duct

Exercise 4

1. a. ocul/o
   b. ophthalm/o
2. a. corne/o
   b. kerat/o
3. conjunctiv/o
4. a. lacrim/o
   b. dacry/o
5. blephar/o
6. a. cor/o
   b. core/o
   c. pupill/o
7. scler/o
8. retin/o
9. a. iri/o
   b. irid/o
10. opt/o

Exercise 5

1. tension, pressure
2. light
3. cold
4. two, double

Exercise 6

1. cry/o
2. ton/o
3. dipl/o
4. phot/o

Exercise 7

1. vision (condition)
2. two
3. paralysis
4. abnormal fear of or aversion to specific things
5. two

Exercise 8

1. −plegia
2. a. bi-
   b. bin-
3. -phobia
4. -opia

Exercise 9

1. WR CV WR S
   scler/o/kerat/itis
   CF
   inflammation of the sclera and the cornea

2. WR S
   ophthalm/algia
   pain in the eye

3. WR CV S
   blephar/o/ptosis
   CF
   drooping of the eyelid

4. WR S
   dipl/opia
   double vision

5. WR S
   conjunctiv/itis
   inflammation of the conjunctiva

6. WR CV WR S
   leuk/o/cor/ia
   CF
   condition of white pupil

7. WR CV S
   irid/o/plegia
   CF
   paralysis of the iris

8. WR CV S
   scler/o/malacia
   CF
   softening of the sclera

9. WR CV S
   phot/o/phobia
   CF
   abnormal fear of (sensitivity to) light

10. WR S
    blephar/itis
    inflammation of the eyelid

11. WR CV WR S
    ocul/o/myc/osis
    CF
    abnormal condition of the eye caused by a fungus

12. WR CV WR S
    dacry/o/cyst/itis
    CF
    inflammation of the tear (lacrimal) sac

13. P WR S
    end/ophthalm/itis
    inflammation within the eye

14. WR S
    ir/itis
    inflammation of the iris

15. WR CV WR S
    retin/o/blast/oma
    CF
    tumor arising from a developing retinal cell

16. WR S
    kerat/itis
    inflammation of the cornea

17. WR CV S
    ophthalm/o/plegia
    CF
    paralysis of the eye (muscles)

Exercise 10

1. conjunctiv/itis
2. ocul/o/myc/osis
3. ophthalm/algia
4. dipl/opia
5. blephar/itis
6. leuk/o/cor/ia
7. irid/o/plegia
8. blephar/o/ptosis
9. ir/itis
10. retin/o/blast/oma
11. scler/o/malacia
12. dacry/o/cyst/itis
13. scler/o/kerat/itis
14. phot/o/phobia
15. kerat/itis
16. end/ophthalm/itis
17. ophthalm/o/plegia

Exercise 11

Spelling exercise; see text, p. 434.

Exercise 12

1. myopia
2. presbyopia
3. strabismus
4. chalazion
5. astigmatism
6. nystagmus
7. cataract
8. sty, or stye (hordeolum)
9. glaucoma
10. detached retina
11. hyperopia
12. emmetropia

13. retinitis pigmentosa
14. nyctalopia
15. pterygium
16. macular degeneration

Exercise 13

1. f	9. e
2. h	10. c
3. k	11. a
4. n	12. l
5. m	13. i
6. j	14. o
7. d	15. g
8. p	16. b

Exercise 14

Spelling exercise; see text, pp. 438-439.

Exercise 15

1. WR CV S
   kerat/o/plasty
      CF
   surgical repair of the cornea

2. WR CV S
   scler/o/tomy
      CF
   incision into the sclera

3. WR CV WR CV S
   dacry/o/cyst/o/tomy
      CF   CF
   incision into the tear sac

4. WR CV WR CV S
   cry/o/retin/o/pexy
      CF   CF
   surgical fixation of the retina by
   extreme cold

5. WR CV S
   blephar/o/plasty
      CF
   surgical repair of the eyelid

6. WR S
   irid/ectomy
   excision of part of the iris

7. WR CV WR CV WR CV S
   dacry/o/cyst/o/rhin/o/stomy
      CF   CF   CF
   creation of an artificial opening
   between the tear (lacrimal) sac and the
   nose

Exercise 16

1. dacry/o/cyst/o/rhin/o/stomy
2. irid/ectomy
3. kerat/o/plasty
4. scler/o/tomy
5. blephar/o/plasty
6. cry/o/retin/o/pexy
7. dacry/o/cyst/o/tomy

Exercise 17

Spelling exercise; see text, p. 440.

Exercise 18

1. retinal photocoagulation
2. enucleation
3. phacoemulsification
4. LASIK
5. trabeculectomy
6. scleral buckling
7. vitrectomy
8. PRK

Exercise 19

1. e	5. d
2. f	6. i
3. b	7. g
4. a	8. c

Exercise 20

Spelling exercise; see text, p. 444.

Exercise 21

1. WR CV S
   pupill/o/scope
      CF
   instrument for visual examination of
   the pupil

2. WR CV S
   opt/o/metry
      CF
   measurement of vision (visual acuity
   and the prescribing of corrective lenses)

3. WR CV S
   ophthalm/o/scope
      CF
   instrument used for visual examination
   of the eye (interior)

4. WR CV S
   ton/o/metry
      CF
   measurement of pressure (within the eye)

5. WR CV S
   pupill/o/meter
      CF
   instrument used to measure the pupil
   (diameter)

6. WR CV S
   ton/o/meter
      CF
   instrument used to measure pressure
   (within the eye)

7. WR CV S
   kerat/o/meter
      CF
   instrument used to measure (the
   curvature of) the cornea

8. WR CV S
   ophthalm/o/scopy
      CF
   visual examination of the eye

9. WR CV S
   angi/o/graphy
      CF
   process of recording blood vessels (of
   the eye with fluorescing dye)

Exercise 22

1. ton/o/metry
2. pupill/o/meter
3. kerat/o/meter
4. opt/o/metry
5. ophthalm/o/scope
6. ton/o/meter
7. pupill/o/scope
8. ophthalm/o/scopy
9. fluorescein angi/o/graphy

Exercise 23

Spelling exercise; see text, p. 446.

Exercise 24

1. WR CV S
   ophthalm/o/logy
      CF
   study of the eye

2. P WR S
   bin/ocul/ar
   pertaining to two or both eyes

3. WR S
   lacrim/al
   pertaining to tears or tear ducts

4. WR S
   pupill/ary
   pertaining to the pupil of the eye

5. WR CV S
   retin/o/pathy
      CF
   (any noninflammatory) disease of the
   retina

6. WR CV S
   ophthalm/o/logist
      CF
   physician who studies and treats
   diseases of the eye

7. WR S
   corne/al
   pertaining to the cornea

8. WR S
   ophthalm/ic
   pertaining to the eye

9. WR CV WR   S
   <u>nas/o</u>/lacrim/al
     CF
   pertaining to the nose and tear ducts

10. WR S
    opt/ic
    pertaining to vision

11. P   WR   S
    intra/ocul/ar
    pertaining to within the eye

12. WR   S
    retin/al
    pertaining to the retina

13.   WR   CV   S
    <u>ophthalm/o</u>/pathy
      CF
    (any) disease of the eye

Exercise 25
1. ophthalm/o/logy
2. bin/ocul/ar
3. retin/al
4. intra/ocul/ar
5. ophthalm/o/logist
6. lacrim/al
7. opt/ic
8. retin/o/pathy
9. corne/al
10. nas/o/lacrim/al
11. ophthalm/o/pathy
12. pupill/ary

Exercise 26
Spelling exercise; see text, p. 449.

Exercise 27
1. left eye
2. a health professional who prescribes corrective lenses and/or eye exercises
3. agent that dilates the pupil
4. each eye
5. sharpness of vision
6. agent that constricts the pupil
7. right eye
8. a specialist who fills prescriptions for lenses

Exercise 28
1. oculus sinister
2. mydriatic
3. oculus uterque
4. miotic
5. oculus dexter
6. optometrist
7. visual acuity
8. optician

Exercise 29
Spelling exercise; see text, p. 450.

Exercise 30
1. visual acuity
2. astigmatism
3. right eye
4. left eye
5. each eye
6. emmetropia
7. ophthalmology
8. age-related macular degeneration

Exercise 31
1. ophthalmology
2. glaucoma
3. pterygium
4. blepharoptosis
5. astigmatism
6. presbyopia
7. retinopathy
8. cataract

Exercise 32
1. mydriatic
2. astigmatism
3. cataract
4. tonometer
5. hyperopia
6. chalazion
7. nystagmus
8. trabeculectomy
9. fluorescein angiography

Exercise 33 Reading Exercise

Exercise 34
1. *T*
2. b
3. c
4. *F,* scleral buckling was used to correct a detached retina and not a cataract.

ANSWERS TO CHAPTER 13 EXERCISES
Exercise Figures
Exercise Figure
A. 1. ear: aur/i, aur/o, ot/o
   2. labyrinth: labyrinth/o
   3. stapes: staped/o
   4. tympanic membrane: tympan/o, myring/o
   5. mastoid bone: mastoid/o

Exercise Figure B. myring/o/tomy

Exercise Figure C. audi/o/metry

Exercise 1
1. g
2. j
3. b
4. f
5. h
6. k
7. d
8. e
9. a
10. c

Exercise 2
1. stapes
2. mastoid bone
3. hearing
4. ear
5. tympanic membrane (eardrum), middle ear
6. hearing
7. labyrinth
8. tympanic membrane

Exercise 3
1. a. aur/o
   b. aur/i
   c. ot/o
2. mastoid/o
3. staped/o
4. tympan/o
5. labyrinth/o
6. a. acou/o
   b. audi/o
7. myring/o

Exercise 4
1. WR CV WR S
   <u>ot/o</u>/myc/osis
     CF
   abnormal condition of fungus in the ear

2.   WR   S
    tympan/itis
    inflammation of the middle ear

3. WR CV WR   S
   <u>ot/o</u>/mastoid/itis
     CF
   inflammation of the ear and the mastoid bone

4. WR   S
   ot /algia
   pain in the ear

5.   WR   S
    labyrinth/itis
    inflammation of the labyrinth

6.   WR   S
    myring/itis
    inflammation of the tympanic membrane

7. WR CV   S
   <u>ot/o</u>/sclerosis
     CF
   hardening of the ear (stapes) (caused by irregular bone development)

8.   WR   S
    mastoid/itis
    inflammation of the mastoid bone

9. WR CV WR CV S
   <u>ot/o</u>/<u>py/o</u>/rrhea
     CF   CF
   discharge of pus from the ear

Exercise 5
1. myring/itis
2. ot/o/py/o/rrhea
3. mastoid/itis
4. ot/algia
5. ot/o/sclerosis
6. ot/o/myc/osis
7. ot/o/mastoid/itis
8. labyrinth/itis
9. tympan/itis

Exercise 6
Spelling exercise; see text, p. 464.

Exercise 7
1. vertigo; tinnitus
2. Ménière
3. otitis media
4. ceruminoma
5. otitis externa
6. acoustic neuroma
7. presbycusis

Exercise 8
1. e
2. b
3. g
4. c
5. h
6. d
7. a
8. i

Exercise 9
Spelling exercise; see text, p. 466.

Exercise 10
1. WR S
   mastoid/ectomy
   excision of the mastoid bone

2. WR CV S
   myring/o/tomy
   CF
   incision into the tympanic membrane

3. WR S
   labyrinth/ectomy
   excision of the labyrinth

4. WR CV S
   mastoid/o/tomy
   CF
   incision into the mastoid bone

5. WR CV S
   tympan/o/plasty
   CF
   surgical repair of the middle ear

6. WR CV S
   myring/o/plasty
   CF
   surgical repair of the tympanic membrane

7. WR S
   staped/ectomy
   excision of the stapes

Exercise 11
1. mastoid/o/tomy
2. labyrinth/ectomy
3. tympan/o/plasty
4. mastoid/ectomy
5. myring/o/tomy
6. myring/o/plasty
7. staped/ectomy

Exercise 12
Spelling exercise; see text, p. 468.

Exercise 13
1. WR CV S
   ot/o/scope
   CF
   instrument used for the visual examination of the ear

2. WR CV S
   audi/o/metry
   CF
   measurement of hearing

3. WR CV S
   audi/o/gram
   CF
   (graphic) record of hearing

4. WR CV S
   ot/o/scopy
   CF
   visual examination of the ear

5. WR CV S
   audi/o/meter
   CF
   instrument used to measure hearing

6. WR CV S
   tympan/o/metry
   CF
   measurement (of movement) of the tympanic membrane

7. WR S
   acou/meter
   instrument used to measure (acuteness of) hearing

8. WR CV S
   tympan/o/meter
   CF
   instrument used to measure middle ear (function)

Exercise 14
1. tympan/o/metry
2. audi/o/meter
3. ot/o/scopy
4. audi/o/gram
5. ot/o/scope
6. audi/o/metry
7. acou/meter
8. tympan/o/meter

Exercise 15
Spelling exercise; see text, pp. 469-470.

Exercise 16
1. WR CV S
   ot/o/logy
   CF
   study of the ear

2. WR CV S
   audi/o/logist
   CF
   one who studies and specializes in hearing

3. WR CV WR CV WR CV S
   ot/o/rhin/o/laryng/o/logist
   CF CF CF
   physician who studies and treats diseases of the ear, nose, and larynx (throat)

4. WR CV S
   audi/o/logy
   CF
   study of hearing

5. WR CV S
   ot/o/logist
   CF
   physician who studies and treats diseases of the ear

6. WR S
   aur/al
   pertaining to the ear

Exercise 17
1. audi/o/logy
2. ot/o/rhin/o/laryng/o/logist
3. ot/o/logy
4. audi/o/logist
5. ot/o/logist
6. aur/al

Exercise 18
Spelling exercise; see text, p. 471.

Exercise 19
1. ears, nose, throat
2. eyes, ears, nose, and throat
3. otitis media
4. acute otitis media

Exercise 20
1. thrombi
2. staphylococci
3. streptococci
4. alveoli
5. glomeruli
6. testes
7. ova
8. diagnoses
9. bacteria
10. nuclei
11. pharynges
12. sarcomata
13. carcinomata
14. anastomoses
15. prostheses
16. emboli
17. prognoses
18. spermatozoa
19. fimbriae
20. thoraces
21. appendices

Exercise 21
1. diverticula
2. bronchus
3. testes
4. melanoma
5. thrombi
6. diagnoses
7. metastases

Exercise 22
1. ENT
2. tinnitus
3. vertigo
4. otoscopy
5. otitis media
6. presbycusis
7. audiologist
8. audiometry

Exercise 23
1. myringitis
2. tinnitus
3. otologist
4. myringotomy

Exercise 24 Reading Exercise

Exercise 25
1. F, inflammation of the middle ear (otitis media) is the most common pediatric infection.

2. *T*

3. *F*, myringotomy, incision into the tympanic membrane would be performed.

Answers

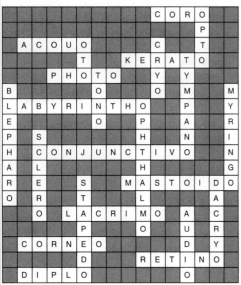

ANSWERS TO CHAPTER 14 EXERCISES

Exercise Figures

Exercise Figure

A.
1. mandible: mandibul/o
2. sternum: stern/o
3. phalanges: phalang/o
4. patella: patell/o
5. tarsals: tars/o
6. phalanges: phalang/o
7. cranium: crani/o
8. maxilla: maxill/o
9. clavicle: clavic/o, clavicul/o
10. ribs: cost/o
11. femur: femor/o
12. fibula: fibul/o
13. tibia: tibi/o

Exercise Figure

B.
1. a. vertebral column, spine: rachi/o
   b. vertebra: spondyl/o, vertebr/o
2. scapula: scapul/o
3. humerus: humer/o
4. ulna: uln/o
5. radius: radi/o
6. carpals: carp/o
7. ilium: ili/o
8. pubis: pub/o
9. ischium: ischi/o

Exercise Figure

C.
1. synovial membrane: synovi/o
2. joint: arthr/o
3. meniscus: menisc/o
4. tendon: ten/o, tend/o, tendin/o

5. cartilage: chondr/o
6. bursa: burs/o

Exercise Figure

D. 1, kyph/osis
2, scoli/osis
3, lord/osis

Exercise Figure E. arthr/o/scopy

Exercise 1
1. d
2. i
3. h
4. k
5. j
6. g
7. b
8. f
9. a
10. c

Exercise 2
1. scapula
2. sternum
3. mandible
4. clavicle
5. humerus
6. a. ulna
   b. radius
7. tarsals
8. phalanges
9. metatarsals
10. metacarpals
11. femur
12. a. fibula
    b. tibia
13. patella
14. cervical vertebrae
15. lumbar
16. pubis
17. sacrum
18. ischium
19. coccyx
20. ilium
21. carpals

Exercise 3
1. m
2. c
3. e
4. a
5. l
6. d
7. h
8. i
9. k
10. b
11. f
12. g

Exercise 4
1. movement of drawing away from the middle
2. movement that turns the palm down
3. movement that turns the palm up
4. turning around its own axis
5. movement in which a limb is placed in a straight position
6. turning outward
7. movement of drawing toward the middle
8. movement in which a limb is bent
9. turning inward

Exercise 5
1. h
2. d
3. i
4. j
5. c
6. a
7. g
8. f
9. b

Exercise 6
1. clavicle
2. rib
3. cranium (skull)
4. femur
5. clavicle
6. humerus
7. ilium
8. ischium
9. carpals
10. fibula
11. mandible
12. loin, lumbar region
13. pelvis, pelvic bone

Exercise 7
1. a. clavicul/o
   b. clavic/o
2. cost/o
3. crani/o
4. femor/o
5. humer/o
6. carp/o
7. ischi/o
8. fibul/o
9. ili/o
10. mandibul/o
11. lumb/o
12. a. pelv/i
    b. pelv/o

Exercise 8
1. vertebral column, spine
2. patella
3. vertebra
4. maxilla
5. phalanges
6. ulna
7. radius
8. tibia
9. pubis
10. tarsals
11. scapula
12. sternum
13. vertebra
14. sacrum

Exercise 9
1. maxill/o
2. uln/o
3. radi/o
4. tibi/o
5. pub/o
6. tars/o
7. a. vertebr/o
   b. spondyl/o
8. stern/o
9. scapul/o
10. patell/o
11. phalang/o
12. sacr/o
13. rachi/o

Exercise 10
1. joint
2. aponeurosis
3. meniscus
4. tendon
5. cartilage
6. tendon
7. bursa
8. tendon
9. synovia, synovial membrane
10. intervertebral disk

Exercise 11
1. menisc/o
2. aponeur/o
3. arthr/o
4. chondr/o
5. a. tendin/o
   b. ten/o
   c. tend/o
6. burs/o
7. synovi/o
8. disk/o

Exercise 12
1. muscle
2. stone
3. movement, motion
4. bone
5. lamina
6. bone marrow
7. hump
8. crooked, stiff, bent
9. crooked, curved
10. muscle
11. bent forward

Exercise 13
1. a. my/o
   b. myos/o
2. petr/o
3. kinesi/o
4. oste/o
5. lamin/o
6. myel/o
7. kyph/o
8. ankyl/o
9. scoli/o
10. lord/o

Exercise 14
1. above
2. together, joined
3. between

Exercise 15
1. a. syn-
   b. sym-
2. inter-
3. supra-

Exercise 16
1. growth
2. break
3. fusion, surgical fixation
4. break
5. fissure, split
6. break
7. weakness

Exercise 17
1. -physis
2. -asthenia
3. a. -clasis
   b. -clast
   c. -clasia
4. -desis
5. -schisis

Exercise 18
1. WR S
   oste/itis
   inflammation of the bone

2. WR CV WR S
   oste/o/myel/itis
      CF
   inflammation of the bone and bone marrow

3. WR CV WR S
   oste/o/petr/osis
      CF
   abnormal condition of stonelike bones (marblelike bones)

4. WR CV S
   oste/o/malacia
      CF
   softening of bones

5. WR CV WR S
   oste/o/carcin/oma
      CF
   cancerous tumor of the bone

6. WR CV WR S
   oste/o/chondr/itis
      CF
   inflammation of the bone and cartilage

7. WR CV WR S
   oste/o/fibr/oma
      CF
   tumor of the bone and fibrous tissue

8. WR S
   arthr/itis
   inflammation of a joint

9. WR CV WR S
   arthr/o/chondr/itis
      CF
   inflammation of the joint cartilage

10. WR S
    myel/oma
    tumor of the bone marrow

11. WR S
    tendin/itis
    inflammation of a tendon

12. WR S
    ten/odynia
    pain in a tendon

13. WR CV S
    carp/o/ptosis
       CF
    drooping wrist (wrist drop)

14. WR S
    burs/itis
    inflammation of the bursa

15. WR WR S
    spondyl/arthr/itis
    inflammation of the vertebral joints

16. WR S
    ankyl/osis
    abnormal condition of stiffness

17. WR S
    kyph/osis
    abnormal condition of a hump (of the thoracic spine)

18. WR S
    scoli/osis
    abnormal (lateral) curve (of the spine)

19. WR CV S
    crani/o/schisis
       CF
    fissure of the skull

20. WR S
    maxill/itis
    inflammation of the maxilla

21. WR S
    menisc/itis
    inflammation of the meniscus

22. WR S
    rachi/schisis
    fissure of the vertebral column

23. WR CV WR
    burs/o/lith
       CF
    stone in the bursa

24. WR S
    my/asthenia
    muscle weakness

25. WR CV S
    oste/o/sarcoma
       CF
    malignant tumor of the bone

26. WR CV S
    chondr/o/malacia
       CF
    softening of cartilage

27. WR CV S
    synovi/o/sarcoma
       CF
    a malignant tumor of the synovial membrane

28. WR CV WR S
    ten/o/synov/itis
       CF
    inflammation of the tendon and synovial membrane

29. P WR S
    poly/myos/itis
    inflammation of many muscles

30. WR S
    disk/itis
    inflammation of an intervertebral disk

31. WR S
    lord/osis
    abnormal condition of bending forward

32. WR CV WR S
    oste/o/arthr/itis
       CF
    inflammation of bone and joint

33. WR CV WR S
    fibr/o/my/algia
       CF
    pain in the fibrous tissues and muscles

Exercise 19

1. oste/o/carcin/oma
2. oste/o/chondr/itis
3. oste/o/fibr/oma
4. arthr/itis
5. arthr/o/chondr/itis
6. myel/oma
7. tendin/itis
8. ten/odynia
9. carp/o/ptosis
10. burs/itis
11. spondyl/arthr/itis
12. ankyl/osis
13. kyph/osis
14. scoli/osis
15. crani/o/schisis
16. maxill/itis
17. menisc/itis
18. rachi/schisis
19. burs/o/lith
20. my/asthenia
21. oste/itis
22. oste/o/myel/itis
23. oste/o/petr/osis
24. oste/o/malacia
25. ten/o/synov/itis
26. synovi/o/sarcoma
27. oste/o/sarcoma
28. chondr/o/malacia
29. disk/itis
30. poly/myos/itis
31. lord/osis
32. oste/o/arthr/itis
33. fibr/o/my/algia

Exercise 20

Spelling exercise; see text, p. 508.

Exercise 21

1. exostosis
2. muscular dystrophy
3. myasthenia gravis
4. bunion
5. ankylosing spondylitis
6. gout
7. a. herniated disk
   b. slipped disk
   c. ruptured disk
   d. herniated nucleus pulposus
8. fracture
9. osteoporosis
10. carpal tunnel syndrome
11. Colles fracture
12. rheumatoid arthritis

Exercise 22

1. abnormal benign growth on the surface of a bone
2. group of hereditary diseases characterized by degeneration of muscle and weakness

3. chronic disease characterized by muscle weakness and thought to be caused by a defect in the transmission of impulses from nerve to muscle cell
4. abnormal enlargement of the joint at the base of the great toe
5. form of arthritis that first affects the spine and adjacent structures
6. abnormal loss of bone density
7. disease in which an excessive amount of uric acid in the blood causes sodium urate crystals (tophi) to be deposited in the joints
8. rupture of the intervertebral disk cartilage, which allows the contents to protrude through it, putting pressure on the spinal nerve roots
9. broken bone
10. a disorder of the wrist caused by compression of the nerve
11. a type of fractured wrist
12. a chronic systemic disease characterized by inflammatory changes in the connective tissue throughout the body

Exercise 23

Spelling exercise; see text, p. 514.

Exercise 24

1. WR CV   S
    oste/o/clasis
        CF
    (surgical) breaking of a bone

2. WR   S
    ost/ectomy
    excision of bone

3. WR CV   S
    arthr/o/clasia
         CF
    (surgical) breaking of a (stiff) joint

4. WR CV   S
    arthr/o/desis
         CF
    surgical fixation of a joint

5. WR CV   S
    arthr/o/plasty
         CF
    surgical repair of a joint

6. WR   S
    chondr/ectomy
    excision of a cartilage

7. WR   CV   S
    chondr/o/plasty
          CF
    surgical repair of a cartilage

8. WR CV   S
    my/o/rrhaphy
       CF
    suture of a muscle

9. WR CV WR CV   S
    ten/o/my/o/plasty
       CF   CF
    surgical repair of the tendon and muscle

10. WR CV   S
    ten/o/rrhaphy
       CF
    suture of a tendon

11. WR   S
    cost/ectomy
    excision of a rib

12. WR   S
    patell/ectomy
    excision of the patella

13.   WR   CV   S
    aponeur/o/rrhaphy
           CF
    suture of an aponeurosis

14. WR   S
    carp/ectomy
    excision of a carpal bone

15. WR   S
    phalang/ectomy
    excision of a finger or toe bone

16. WR   S
    menisc/ectomy
    excision of the meniscus

17. WR   CV P   S
    spondyl/o/syn/desis
           CF
    fusing together of the vertebrae

18. WR   S
    lamin/ectomy
    excision of the lamina

19. WR   S
    burs/ectomy
    excision of a bursa

20. WR CV   S
    crani/o/tomy
         CF
    incision into the skull

21. WR CV   S
    crani/o/plasty
         CF
    surgical repair of the skull

22. WR   S
    maxill/ectomy
    excision of the maxilla

23. WR CV S
rachi/o/tomy
  CF
incision into the vertebral column

24. WR   S
tars/ectomy
excision of (one or more) tarsal bones

25. WR   S
synov/ectomy
excision of the synovial membrane

26. WR   S
disk/ectomy
excision of an intervertebral disk

27. WR CV S
vertebr/o/plasty
  CF
surgical repair of a vertebra

Exercise 25
1. oste/o/clasis
2. ost/ectomy
3. arthr/o/clasia
4. arthr/o/desis
5. arthr/o/plasty
6. chondr/ectomy
7. chondr/o/plasty
8. my/o/rrhaphy
9. ten/o/my/o/plasty
10. ten/o/rrhaphy
11. cost/ectomy
12. patell/ectomy
13. aponeur/o/rrhaphy
14. carp/ectomy
15. phalang/ectomy
16. menisc/ectomy
17. spondyl/o/syn/desis
18. lamin/ectomy
19. burs/ectomy
20. crani/o/tomy
21. crani/o/plasty
22. maxill/ectomy
23. rachi/o/tomy
24. tars/ectomy
25. synov/ectomy
26. disk/ectomy
27. vertebr/o/plasty

Exercise 26
Spelling exercise; see text, p. 520.

Exercise 27
1. WR CV WR CV S
electr/o/my/o/gram
  CF   CF
record of the electrical activity in a
muscle

2. WR CV S
arthr/o/graphy
  CF
x-ray imaging a joint

3. WR CV S
arthr/o/scopy
  CF
visual examination of a joint

4. WR CV   S
arthr/o/centesis
  CF
surgical puncture of a joint to aspirate
fluid

Exercise 28
1. arthr/o/gram   3. arthr/o/centesis
2. arthr/o/scopy 4. electr/o/my/o/gram

Exercise 29
Spelling exercise; see text, p. 522.

Exercise 30
1. P   S(WR)
sym/physis
growing together

2. WR   S
femor/al
pertaining to the femur

3. WR   S
humer/al
pertaining to the humerus

4. P   WR   S
inter/vertebr/al
pertaining to between the vertebrae

5. P   WR   S
hyper/kinesi/a
excessive movement (overactivity)

6. P   WR   S
dys/kinesi/a
difficult movement

7. P   WR   S
brady/kinesi/a
slow movement

8. P   WR   S
intra/crani/al
pertaining to within the cranium

9. WR CV WR   S
stern/o/clavicul/ar
  CF
pertaining to the sternum and clavicle

10. WR CV WR   S
ili/o/femor/al
  CF
pertaining to the ilium and femur

11. WR CV WR S
ischi/o/fibul/ar
  CF
pertaining to the ischium and fibula

12. P   WR   S
sub/maxill/ary
pertaining to below the maxilla

13. WR CV WR S
ischi/o/pub/ic
  CF
pertaining to the ischium and pubis

14. P   WR   S
sub/mandibul/ar
pertaining to below the mandible

15. WR CV WR S
pub/o/femor/al
  CF
pertaining to the pubis and femur

16. P   WR   S
supra/scapul/ar
pertaining to above the scapula

17. P   WR   S
sub/cost/al
pertaining to below the rib

18. WR CV WR S
vertebr/o/cost/al
  CF
pertaining to the vertebrae and ribs

19. P   WR   S
sub/scapul/ar
pertaining to below the scapula

20. WR CV WR
oste/o/blast
  CF
developing bone cell

21. WR CV S
oste/o/cyte
  CF
bone cell

22. WR CV WR S
oste/o/necr/osis
  CF
abnormal death of bone (tissues)

23. WR   S
stern/oid
resembling the sternum

24. WR   S
arthr/algia
pain in the joint

25. WR   S
carp/al
pertaining to the wrist

26. WR   S
    lumb/ar
    pertaining to the loins

27. WR CV WR S
    lumb/o/cost/al
       CF
    pertaining to the loins and to the ribs

28. WR CV WR S
    lumb/o/sacr/al
       CF
    pertaining to the lumbar region (loin)
    and the sacrum

29. WR S
    sacr/al
    pertaining to the sacrum

30. WR CV WR   S
    sacr/o/vertebr/al
        CF
    pertaining to the sacrum and
    vertebrae

31. P   WR S
    sub/stern/al
    pertaining to below the sternum

32. P   WR S
    supra/patell/ar
    pertaining to above the patella

33. P   S(WR)
    dys/trophy
    abnormal development

34. P   S(WR)
    a/trophy
    without development

35. P   S(WR)
    hyper/trophy
    excessive development

36. P   WR S
    inter/cost/al
    pertaining to between the ribs

37. WR   S
    crani/al
    pertaining to the cranium

38. WR S
    pelv/ic
    pertaining to the pelvis

39. WR CV WR S
    pelv/i/sacr/al
        CF
    pertaining to the pelvis and sacrum

Exercise 31
1. sym/physis
2. femor/al
3. humer/al

4. inter/vertebr/al
5. hyper/kinesi/a
6. dys/kinesi/a
7. brady/kinesi/a
8. intra/crani/al
9. stern/o/clavicul/ar
10. ili/o/femor/al
11. ischi/o/fibul/ar
12. sub/maxill/ary
13. ischi/o/pub/ic
14. sub/mandibul/ar
15. pub/o/femor/al
16. supra/scapul/ar
17. sub/cost/al
18. vertebr/o/cost/al
19. sub/scapul/ar
20. oste/o/blast
21. oste/o/cyte
22. oste/o/necr/osis
23. stern/oid
24. arthr/algia
25. carp/al
26. sacr/al
27. lumb/ar
28. sacr/o/vertebr/al
29. lumb/o/sacr/al
30. lumb/o/cost/al
31. sub/stern/al
32. supra/patell/ar
33. dys/trophy
34. a/trophy
35. hyper/trophy
36. crani/al
37. inter/cost/al
38. pelv/ic
39. pelv/i/sacr/al

Exercise 32
Spelling exercise; see text, p. 529.

Exercise 33
1. c   6. b
2. f   7. e
3. d   8. i
4. a, h   9. k
5. j

Exercise 34
1. specialist in chiropractic
2. system of therapy that consists of
   manipulation of the vertebral column
3. branch of medicine dealing with the
   study and treatment of diseases and
   abnormalities of the musculoskeletal
   system
4. physician who specializes in
   orthopedics
5. specialist in treating and diagnosing
   foot diseases and disorders

6. specialist in treating and diagnosing
   diseases and disorders of the foot
7. physician who specializes in osteopathy
8. system of medicine in which emphasis
   is on the relation between body organs
   and the musculoskeletal system
9. making and fitting of orthopedic
   appliances
10. an artificial substitute for a missing
    body part
11. a person who is skilled in orthotics

Exercise 35
Spelling exercise; see text, p. 532.

Exercise 36
1. cervical vertebrae; thoracic vertebrae;
   lumbar vertebrae
2. rheumatoid arthritis
3. osteoarthritis
4. myasthenia gravis
5. electromyogram
6. carpal tunnel syndrome
7. muscular dystrophy
8. herniated nucleus pulposus

Exercise 37
1. orthopedic   5. suprapatellar
2. arthroscopy   6. chondromalacia
3. arthritis   7. pathology
4. medial

Exercise 38
1. kyphosis   6. subcostal
2. chondrectomy   7. symphysis
3. dyskinesia   8. orthopedist
4. softening of   9. osteoporosis
   bones   10. carpal tunnel
5. osteoclasis   syndrome

Exercise 39 Reading Exercise

Exercise 40
1. *F*, an orthopedist and not a podiatrist is
   treating Mr. Jones.
2. b
3. d

Exercise 41
1. epiphyses   4. prosthesis
2. phalanx   5. bursae
3. vertebrae

Answers

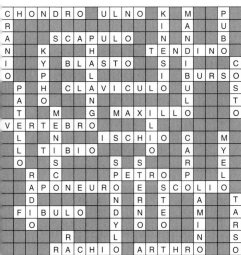

ANSWERS TO CHAPTER 15 EXERCISES

Exercise Figures

Exercise Figure

A. 1. brain: encephal/o
2. spinal cord: myel/o
3. cerebrum: cerebr/o
4. cerebellum: cerebell/o
5. meninges: mening/i, mening/o

Exercise Figure

B. 1. dura mater: dur/o
2. ganglion: gangli/o, ganglion/o
3. nerve root: radic/o, radicul/o, rhiz/o

Exercise Figure C. mening/o/myel/o/cele

Exercise Figure D. rhiz/o/tomy or
radic/o/tomy

Exercise Figure E. myel/o/graphy

Exercise Figure F. *1,* hemi/plegia
3, quadr/i/plegia or
tetra/plegia

Exercise 1

1. meninges
2. dura mater
3. arachnoid
4. pia mater
5. subarachnoid space
6. cerebrospinal fluid

Exercise 2

1. d
2. f
3. g
4. e
5. a
6. h
7. b
8. c

Exercise 3

1. cerebellum
2. nerve
3. spinal cord
4. meninges
5. brain
6. cerebrum, brain
7. nerve root
8. ganglion
9. nerve root
10. hard, dura mater
11. ganglion
12. nerve root

Exercise 4

1. cerebell/o
2. neur/o
3. myel/o
4. a. mening/o
   b. mening/i
5. encephal/o
6. cerebr/o
7. a. radicul/o
   b. radic/o
   c. rhiz/o
8. dur/o
9. a. gangli/o
   b. ganglion/o

Exercise 5

1. one
2. mind
3. four
4. mind
5. speech
6. sensation, sensitivity, feeling
7. mind
8. gray matter

Exercise 6

1. quadr/i
2. mon/o
3. a. phren/o
   b. psych/o
   c. ment/o
4. phas/o
5. poli/o
6. esthesi/o

Exercise 7

1. slight paralysis
2. specialty, treatment
3. seizure, attack
4. specialist, physician
5. four

Exercise 8

1. -paresis
2. -iatry
3. -ictal
4. -iatrist
5. tetra-

Exercise 9

1.   WR   S
   neur/itis
   inflammation of a nerve

2.   WR   S
   neur/oma
   tumor made up of nerve (cells)

3.   WR   S
   neur/algia
   pain in a nerve

4.   WR CV WR CV   S
   neur/o/arthr/o/pathy
      CF   CF
   disease of nerves and joints

5.   WR CV WR
   neur/o/blast
      CF
   developing nerve cell

6.   WR   S
   neur/asthenia
   nerve weakness (nervous exhaustion, fatigue, and weakness)

7.   WR   CV   S
   encephal/o/malacia
        CF
   softening of the brain

8.   WR   S
   encephal/itis
   inflammation of the brain

9.   WR   CV WR CV WR   S
   encephal/o/myel/o/radicul/itis
        CF   CF
   inflammation of the brain, spinal cord, and nerve roots

10.   WR   S
   mening/itis
   inflammation of the meninges

11.   WR   CV   S
   mening/o/cele
        CF
   protrusion of the meninges

12.   WR   CV WR CV S
   mening/o/myel/o/cele
        CF   CF
   protrusion of the meninges and spinal cord

13.   WR   S
   radicul/itis
   inflammation of the nerve roots

14.   WR   S
   cerebell/itis
   inflammation of the cerebellum

15.   WR   S
   gangli/itis
   inflammation of a ganglion

16.   WR   S
   dur/itis
   inflammation of the dura mater

17.   P   WR   S
   poly/neur/itis
   inflammation of many nerves

18.   WR CV WR   S
   poli/o/myel/itis
        CF
   inflammation of the gray matter of the spinal cord

19.   WR   S   WR   S
   cerebr/al thromb/osis
   abnormal condition of a clot (in) pertaining to the cerebrum

20. P   WR S   WR   S
sub/dur/al hemat/oma
blood tumor (mass) pertaining to
below the dura mater

21. WR CV   WR   CV WR   S
rhiz/o/mening/o/myel/itis
   CF   CF
inflammation of the nerve root,
meninges, and spinal cord

Exercise 10
1. neur/itis
2. neur/oma
3. neur/algia
4. neur/o/arthr/o/pathy
5. neur/o/blast
6. neur/asthenia
7. encephal/o/malacia
8. encephal/itis
9. encephal/o/myel/o/radicul/itis
10. mening/itis
11. mening/o/cele
12. mening/o/myel/o/cele
13. radicul/itis
14. cerebell/itis
15. gangli/itis
16. dur/itis
17. poly/neur/itis
18. poli/o/myel/itis
19. cerebr/al thromb/osis
20. sub/dur/al hemat/oma
21. rhiz/o/mening/o/myel/itis

Exercise 11
Spelling exercise; see text, p. 555.

Exercise 12
1. cerebrum (brain)   5. head
2. mind   6. nerve
3. upon   7. cerebrum (brain)
4. hardening

Exercise 13
1. b   9. i
2. a   10. m
3. n   11. q
4. j   12. d
5. l   13. h
6. p   14. o
7. e   15. c
8. g   16. f

Exercise 14
Spelling exercise; see text, pp. 559-560.

Exercise 15
1. WR CV S
radic/o/tomy
   CF
incision into a nerve root

2. WR   S
neur/ectomy
excision of a nerve

3. WR CV   S
neur/o/rrhaphy
   CF
suture of a nerve

4.   WR   S
ganglion/ectomy
excision of a ganglion

5. WR CV   S
neur/o/tomy
   CF
incision into a nerve

6. WR CV S
neur/o/lysis
   CF
separating a nerve (from adhesions)

7. WR CV   S
neur/o/plasty
   CF
surgical repair of a nerve

8. WR CV   S
rhiz/o/tomy
   CF
incision into a nerve root

Exercise 16
1. a. radic/o/tomy   4. ganglion/ectomy
   b. rhiz/o/tomy   5. neur/o/tomy
2. neur/ectomy   6. neur/o/lysis
3. neur/o/rrhaphy   7. neur/o/plasty

Exercise 17
Spelling exercise; see text, p. 562.

Exercise 18
1. WR CV   WR   CV S
electr/o/encephal/o/gram
   CF   CF
record of the electrical impulses of the
brain

2. WR CV   WR   CV S
electr/o/encephal/o/graph
   CF   CF
instrument used to record the electrical
impulses of the brain

3. WR CV   WR   CV S
electr/o/encephal/o/graphy
   CF   CF
process of recording the electrical
impulses of the brain

4. WR CV WR   CV   S
ech/o/encephal/o/graphy
   CF   CF
process of recording the brain
(structures) by use of sound

5. WR CV   S
myel/o/graphy
   CF
process of recording (scan) the spinal
cord

6. WR   S WR CV   S
cerebr/al angi/o/graphy
              CF
x-ray imaging of the blood vessels in
the brain

Exercise 19
1. ech/o/encephal/o/graphy
2. electr/o/encephal/o/gram
3. electr/o/encephal/o/graph
4. electr/o/encephal/o/graphy
5. myel/o/graphy
6. cerebr/al angi/o/graphy

Exercise 20
Spelling exercise; see text, p. 564.

Exercise 21
1. computed tomography
2. lumbar puncture
3. positron emission tomography
4. magnetic resonance imaging
5. evoked potential studies

Exercise 22
1. insertion of a needle into the
   subarachnoid space
2. process that includes the use of a
   computer to produce a series of images
   of the brain tissues at any desired
   depth
3. produces cross-sectional images of the
   brain by magnetic waves
4. a technique that permits viewing of a
   slice of the brain to examine blood flow
   and metabolic activity
5. a group of diagnostic tests that measure
   changes and responses in brain waves
   from stimuli

Exercise 23
Spelling exercise; see text, p. 567.

Exercise 24
1.   P   S(WR)
hemi/plegia
paralysis of half (left or right side of
the body)

2.   P   S(WR)
tetra/plegia
paralysis of four (limbs)

3.   WR CV S
neur/o/logist
   CF
physician who studies and treats
diseases of the nerves (nervous
system)

4.   WR CV S
neur/o/logy
   CF
study of nerves (branch of medicine
dealing with diseases of the nervous
system)

5.   WR   S
neur/oid
resembling a nerve

6.   WR CV S
quadr/i/plegia
   CF
paralysis of four (limbs)

7.   WR   S
cerebr/al
pertaining to the cerebrum

8.   WR CV S
mon/o/plegia
   CF
paralysis of one (limb)

9. P WR S
a/phas/ia
condition of without speaking (loss or
impairment of the ability to speak)

10. P WR S
dys/phas/ia
condition of difficulty speaking

11.   P   S(WR)
hemi/paresis
slight paralysis of half (right or left
side of the body)

12. P   WR   S
an/esthesi/a
without (loss of) feeling or sensation

13.   P   WR   S
hyper/esthesi/a
excessive sensitivity (to stimuli)

14. P WR S
sub/dur/al
pertaining to below the dura mater

15.   WR   S
cephal/algia
pain in the head (headache)

16.   WR CV WR   S
psych/o/somat/ic
      CF
pertaining to the mind and body

17.   WR CV   S
psych/o/pathy
      CF
(any) disease of the mind

18.   WR CV   S
psych/o/logy
      CF
study of the mind (mental processes
and behavior)

19.   WR   S
psych/iatry
specialty of the mind (branch of
medicine that deals with the
treatment of mental disorders)

20.   WR CV   S
psych/o/logist
      CF
specialist of the mind

21.   WR CV   S
psych/o/genic
      CF
originating in the mind

22.   WR   S
phren/ic
pertaining to the mind

23.   WR CV   S
phren/o/pathy
      CF
disease of the mind

24.   WR CV WR   S
crani/o/cerebr/al
      CF
pertaining to the cranium and
cerebrum

25.   WR CV   S
myel/o/malacia
      CF
softening of the spinal cord

26.   WR CV   S
encephal/o/sclerosis
         CF
hardening of the brain

27.   P   S(WR)
post/ictal
(occurring) after a seizure or attack

28.   P   S(WR)
pan/plegia
total paralysis

29.   P   S(WR)
inter/ictal
(occurring) between seizures or
attacks

30.   WR CV   S
mon/o/paresis
      CF
slight paralysis of one (limb)

31.   P   S(WR)
pre/ictal
(occurring) before a seizure or attack

32.   WR   S
psych/iatrist
a physician who studies and treats
disorders of the mind

33.   P   WR   S
intra/cerebr/al
pertaining to within the cerebrum

Exercise 25
1. hemi/paresis
2. an/esthesi/a
3. hyper/esthesi/a
4. sub/dur/al
5. cephal/algia
6. psych/o/somat/ic
7. psych/o/pathy
8. psych/o/logy
9. psych/iatry
10. psych/o/logist
11. psych/o/genic
12. phren/ic
13. phren/o/pathy
14. crani/o/cerebr/al
15. myel/o/malacia
16. encephal/o/sclerosis
17. hemi/plegia
18. tetra/plegia
19. neur/o/logist
20. neur/o/logy
21. neur/oid
22. quadr/i/plegia
23. cerebr/al
24. mon/o/plegia
25. a/phas/ia
26. dys/phas/ia
27. pre/ictal
28. mon/o/paresis
29. post/ictal
30. pan/plegia
31. inter/ictal
32. psych/iatrist
33. intra/cerebr/al

Exercise 26
Spelling exercise; see text, pp. 572-573.

Exercise 27

1. concussion	10. ataxia
2. unconsciousness	11. gait
3. conscious	12. dementia
4. seizure	13. incoherent
5. convulsion	14. disorientation
6. shunt	15. cognitive
7. paraplegia	16. afferent
8. coma	17. efferent
9. syncope	

Exercise 28

1. tube implanted in the body to redirect the flow of a fluid
2. paralysis from the waist down caused by damage to the lower level of the spinal cord
3. state of profound unconsciousness
4. jarring or shaking that results in injury
5. state of being unaware of surroundings and incapable of responding to stimuli as a result of injury, shock, or illness
6. awake, alert, aware of one's surroundings
7. sudden attack
8. sudden involuntary contraction of a group of muscles
9. fainting, or sudden loss of consciousness
10. lack of muscle coordination
11. lack of cognitive abilities
12. a manner or style of walking
13. pertaining to the mental processes of comprehension, judgment, memory, and reasoning
14. a state of mental confusion regarding time, place, and identity
15. unable to express one's thoughts or ideas in an orderly, intelligible manner
16. conveying away from the center
17. conveying toward the center

Exercise 29

Spelling exercise; see text, p. 576.

Exercise 30

1. i	8. d
2. m	9. h
3. b	10. f
4. c	11. e
5. j	12. l
6. a	13. k
7. g	

Exercise 31

Spelling exercise; see text, p. 579.

Exercise 32

1. echoencephalography, electroencephalogram, magnetic resonance imaging, positron emission tomography, evoked potential, lumbar puncture, multiple sclerosis

2. Alzheimer disease, amyotrophic lateral sclerosis, cerebral palsy, multiple sclerosis, Parkinson disease
3. cerebrovascular accident; transient ischemic attack
4. cerebrospinal fluid
5. posttraumatic stress disorder, obsessive-compulsive disorder, attention deficit hyperactivity disorder
6. central nervous system, peripheral nervous system

Exercise 33

1. disorientation
2. cognitive
3. aphasia
4. conscious
5. neurology
6. magnetic resonance imaging
7. encephalitis
8. electroencephalogram
9. seizure
10. incoherent

Exercise 34

1. quadriplegia
2. aphasia
3. unconscious
4. meningocele
5. psychiatry
6. hardened patches along brain and spinal cord
7. electroencephalography
8. blood clot
9. positron emission tomography
10. ganglia

Exercise 35 Reading Exercise

Exercise 36

1. b		3. a
2. *T*		

Answers

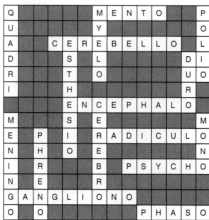

Exercise Figures

Exercise Figure

A. 1. parathyroid glands: parathyroid/o
    2. adrenal glands: adren/o, adrenal/o
    3. thyroid gland: thyroid/o, thyr/o

Exercise Figure B. cortex: cortic/o

Exercise Figure C. acr/o/megaly

Exercise 1

1. b	5. a
2. g	6. c
3. d	7. e
4. h	

Exercise 2

1. d	4. b
2. a	5. g
3. e	6. c

Exercise 3

1. cortex	5. adrenal gland
2. adrenal gland	6. thyroid gland
3. parathyroid gland	7. endocrine
4. thyroid gland	8. gland

Exercise 4

1. a. adren/o	3. endocrin/o
b. adrenal/o	4. cortic/o
2. a. thyroid/o	5. parathyroid/o
b. thyr/o	6. aden/o

Exercise 5

1. thirst	4. extremities, height
2. potassium	
3. calcium	5. sodium

Exercise 6

1. acr/o	4. kal/i
2. calc/i	5. natr/o
3. dips/o	

Exercise 7

1. run, running

Exercise 8

1. -drome

Exercise 9

1.   WR   S
   adrenal/itis
   inflammation of an adrenal gland

2.   P WR   S
   hypo/calc/emia
   deficient level of calcium in the blood

3. P   WR   S
    hyper/thyroid/ism
    state of excessive thyroid gland
    activity

4. P   WR   S
    hyper/kal/emia
    excessive potassium in the blood

5. P   WR   S
    hyper/glyc/emia
    excessive sugar in the blood

6. WR CV   S
    adren/o/megaly
        CF
    enlargement of the adrenal gland

7. WR CV   S
    aden/o/megaly
        CF
    enlargement of a gland

8. P   WR   S
    hypo/thyroid/ism
    state of deficient thyroid gland
    activity

9. P   WR   S
    hypo/kal/emia
    deficient level of potassium in the
    blood

10. WR   S
    aden/itis
    inflammation of a gland

11.   WR   S
    parathyroid/oma
    tumor of a parathyroid gland

12. WR CV   S
    acr/o/megaly
        CF
    enlargement of the extremities (and
    facial bones)

13. WR   S
    aden/odynia
    pain in a gland

14. P   WR   S
    hypo/glyc/emia
    deficient level of sugar in the blood

15. P   WR   S
    hyper/calc/emia
    excessive calcium in the blood

16. WR CV   S
    aden/o/malacia
        CF
    abnormal softening of a gland

17. P   WR   S
    hypo/natr/emia
    deficient level of sodium in the blood

18. WR   S
    aden/osis
    abnormal condition of a gland

19. WR   S
    thyroid/itis
    inflammation of the thyroid gland

Exercise 10
1. adren/o/megaly
2. hypo/thyroid/ism
3. acr/o/megaly
4. hypo/glyc/emia
5. hyper/kal/emia
6. hypo/calc/emia
7. hyper/thyroid/ism
8. aden/o/malacia
9. hyper/calc/emia
10. aden/odynia
11. parathyroid/oma
12. hyper/glyc/emia
13. aden/osis
14. hypo/kal/emia
15. adrenal/itis
16. aden/o/megaly
17. hypo/natr/emia
18. aden/itis
19. thyroid/itis

Exercise 11
Spelling exercise; see text, pp. 599-600.

Exercise 12
1. d	8. e
2. a	9. k
3. j	10. i
4. b	11. f
5. h	12. g
6. c	13. n
7. l	

Exercise 13
1. thyroid
2. parathyroid
3. islets of Langerhans (pancreas)
4. pituitary
5. thyroid
6. adrenal
7. islets of Langerhans (pancreas)
8. thyroid
9. islets of Langerhans (pancreas)
10. adrenal
11. pituitary
12. thyroid gland
13. thyroid gland

Exercise 14
Spelling exercise; see text, p. 604.

Exercise 15
1. WR CV   S
    thyroid/o/tomy
        CF
    incision of the thyroid gland

2. WR   S
    adrenal/ectomy
    excision of the adrenal gland

3. WR CV   WR   S
    thyr/o/parathyroid/ectomy
        CF
    excision of the thyroid and parathyroid
    glands

4. WR   S
    thyroid/ectomy
    excision of the thyroid gland

5.   WR   S
    parathyroid/ectomy
    excision of the parathyroid gland

6. WR   S
    aden/ectomy
    excision of a gland

Exercise 16
1. thyroid/ectomy
2. thyr/o/parathyroid/ectomy
3. adrenal/ectomy
4. parathyroid/ectomy
5. thyroid/o/tomy
6. aden/ectomy

Exercise 17
Spelling exercise; see text, p. 605.

Exercise 18
1. b	4. d
2. a	5. e
3. f	

Exercise 19
1. radioactive iodine uptake
2. fasting blood sugar
3. thyroid-stimulating hormone
4. thyroxine level
5. thyroid scan

Exercise 20
Spelling exercise; see text, p. 607.

Exercise 21
1. WR   S
    cortic/oid
    resembling the cortex

2. P   S(WR)
    syn/drome
    (set of symptoms that) run together

3. WR CV S
adren/o/pathy
    CF
disease of the adrenal gland

4. WR CV S
endocrin/o/logist
     CF
a physician who studies and treats
diseases of the endocrine system

5. P WR S
poly/dips/ia
abnormal state of much thirst

6. WR CV S
calc/i/penia
  CF
deficiency of calcium

7. WR CV S
endocrin/o/pathy
    CF
any disease of the endocrine system

8. WR CV WR CV P S(WR)
adren/o/cortic/o/hyper/plasia
   CF   CF
excessive development of the adrenal
cortex

9. P WR S
eu/thyr/oid
resembling normal (functioning)
thyroid gland

10. WR S
cortic/al
pertaining to the cortex

11. WR CV S
endocrin/o/logy
   CF
study of the endocrine system

Exercise 22

1. endocrin/o/pathy
2. cortic/oid
3. syn/drome
4. adren/o/cortic/o/hyper/plasia
5. endocrin/o/logy
6. poly/dips/ia
7. adren/o/pathy
8. calc/i/penia
9. eu/thyr/oid
10. cortic/al
11. endocrin/o/logist

Exercise 23
Spelling exercise; see text, p. 609.

Exercise 24
1. metabolism   3. isthmus
2. hormone   4. exophthalmos

Exercise 25
1. narrow strip of tissue connecting large
parts in the body
2. total of all chemical processes that take
place in living organisms
3. a chemical substance secreted by an
endocrine gland
4. abnormal protrusion of the eye

Exercise 26
Spelling exercise; see text, p. 611.

Exercise 27
1. radioactive iodine uptake
2. fasting blood sugar
3. diabetes mellitus
4. diabetes insipidus
5. thyroxine level

Exercise 28
1. polyuria   5. diabetes mellitus
2. polydipsia   6. cyanosis
3. hematemesis   7. ketosis
4. cerebrovascular   8. endocrinology
   accident

Exercise 29
1. goiter   5. overactivity
2. ketosis   6. cretinism
3. adrenal   7. adenodynia
4. antidiuretic
   hormone

Exercise 30 Reading Exercise

Exercise 31
1. a   3. c
2. b   4. d

Answers

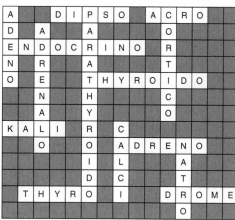

2004 Conn's current therapy, Philadelphia, 2004, WB Saunders.

Age-related macular degeneration, *Women's Healthsource Mayo Clinic,* 4(3), 2000.

Alternative medicine, Payallup, Wash, 1994, Future Medicine Publishing.

Applegate EJ: *The anatomy and physiology learning system,* ed 2, St Louis, 2000, Mosby.

Back surgery, *Mayo Clinic Health Letter,* 8(6), 2000.

Ballinger PW, Frank ED: *Merrill's atlas of radiographic positions and radiologic procedures,* ed 10, St Louis, 2003, Mosby.

Bontrager KL: *Textbook of radiographic positioning and related anatomy,* ed 6, St Louis, 2005, Mosby.

Chabner D: *The language of medicine,* ed 7, Philadelphia, 2004, WB Saunders.

"Definitions and quotes about music therapy," American Music Therapy Association, www.musictherapy.org. Accessed Aug 10, 2004.

Fitzpatrick JE, Aeling JL: *Dermatology secrets in color,* ed 2, Philadelphia, 2001, Hanley and Belfus.

Frazier M, Drzymkowski JW: *Essentials of human diseases and conditions,* ed 2, Philadelphia, 2000, WB Saunders.

Griffith J: Review of the sinus and lymphatic drainage therapy: application for the external cranial sinuses, *Massage Australia,* 41, 2003.

Haubrich WS: *Medical meanings: a glossary of word origins,* Philadelphia, 1997, American College of Physicians.

Henderson JW, Donatelle R: Complementary and alternative medicine used by women after completion of allopathic treatment for breast cancer, *Alternative Therapies,* 10(1), 2004.

Herlihy B, Maebius N: *The human body in health and illness,* ed 2, Philadelphia, 2003, WB Saunders.

Ignatavicius DD, et al: *Medical-surgical nursing: a nursing process approach,* ed 4, Philadelphia, 2002, WB Saunders.

Kim Y-H: Mindfulness meditation and chronic pain, *Alternative Medicine Alert* March 2004.

Kohatsu W: *Complementary and alternative medicine secrets,* Philadelphia, 2002, Hanley and Belfus.

Kurtz ME, Nolan RB, Rittinger WJ: Primary care physicians' attitudes and practices regarding complementary and alternative medicine, *JAOA* 103(12), 2003.

LaFleur Brooks M, Gillingham EA: *Health unit coordinating,* ed 5, Philadelphia, 2004, WB Saunders.

LaFleur Brooks M, LaFleur Brooks D: *Basic medical language,* ed 2, St Louis, 2004, Mosby.

Langford R, Thompson JM: *Mosby's handbook of diseases,* St Louis, 1996, Mosby.

Lewis SM, et al: *Medical-surgical nursing,* ed 6, St Louis, 2004, Mosby.

Littleton, LY, Engebretson JC: *Maternal, neonatal, and women's health nursing,* Albany, 2002, Delmar.

Managed care terms A thru Z, New York, Medicom International.

Masters RM, Gylys BA: *Medical terminology specialties,* Philadelphia, 2003, FA Davis.

Medicine in quotations, Philadelphia, 2000, American College of Physicians.

Mercier LM: *Practical orthopedics,* ed 4, St Louis, 1995, Mosby.

National Institutes of Health: *Age-related eye disease study.* www.nei.nih.gov/neitrials/static/study44.html. Accessed April 10, 2004.

Novey D: *Clinicians' complete reference to complementary and alternative medicine,* St Louis, 2000, Mosby.

Pagana KD, Pagana TJ: *Mosby's manual of diagnostic and laboratory test reference,* ed 7, St Louis, 2004, Mosby.

Potter PA, Perry AG: *Fundamentals of nursing: concepts, process, and practice,* ed 5, St Louis, 2001, Mosby.

Rakel D: *Integrative medicine,* Philadelphia, 2003, WB Saunders.

Spencer JW, Jacobs JJ: *Complementary and alternative medicine: an evidence-based approach,* St. Louis, 2003, Mosby.

Stedman's abbreviations, acronyms, and symbols, ed 3, Baltimore, 2003, Lippincott, Williams, & Wilkins.

Thibodeau GA, Patton KT: *Anatomy and physiology,* ed 4, St Louis, 2001, Mosby.

ILLUSTRATION CREDITS

Chapter 1

Figure 1-2 reprinted by permission of Tribune Media Services.

Chapter 2

Figure 2-3 from Kumar VK: *Basic pathology,* ed 7, Philadelphia, 2003, WB Saunders.

Figure 2-5 from Ballinger PW, Frank ED: *Merrill's atlas of radiographic positions and radiologic procedures,* ed 10, St Louis, 2003, Mosby.

Figure 2-6 from Damjanov I: *Pathology for health-related disease,* ed 2, St Louis, 2000, Mosby.

Exercise Figure C from (1) Mace JD: *Radiography pathology,* ed 4, St Louis, 2004, Mosby; (2) Habif TP: *Clinical dermatology,* ed 4, St Louis, 2004, Mosby; (3) Stevens A: *Pathology,* ed 2, London, 2000, Mosby; (4) Damjanov I, Linder J: *Anderson's pathology,* ed 10, St Louis, 1996, Mosby.

Chapter 3

Figures 3-1, 3-4, 3-5, 3-6, and Exercise Figure B from Bontrager KL: *Radiographic positioning and related anatomy,* ed 5, St Louis, 2002, Mosby.

Chapter 4

Figures 4-2 (A, B, D), 4-3 (A, B, C), 4-4, 4-6, 4-7, 4-8, and 4-9 (A) from Bork K, Brauninger W: *Skin diseases in clinical practice,* ed 2, Philadelphia, 1998, WB Saunders.

Figures 4-2 (C, E), 4-3 (D, E), and 4-9 (B) from Habif TP: *Clinical dermatology,* ed 4, St Louis, 2004, Mosby.

Figure 4-5 from Zitelli BJ, David HW: *Atlas of pediatric physical diagnosis,* ed 4, St Louis, 2002, Mosby.

Dermatology poem courtesy Julia Frank, MD.

Chapter 5

Figure 5-7 from Mace JD: *Radiographic pathology,* ed 4, St Louis, 2004, Mosby.

Figure 5-10 (A, B) from Gruber RP, Peck GC: *Rhinoplasty: state of the art,* St Louis, 1993, Mosby.

Figure 5-11 and Exercise Figure E from Lewis SM, et al: *Medical-surgical nursing,* ed 6, St Louis, 2004, Mosby.

Table 5-1 figures from Ruppel GL: *Manual pulmonary function testing,* ed 7, St Louis, 1998, Mosby; Siemens Medical Systems, Inc, New Jersey; Ballinger PW, Frank ED: *Merrill's atlas of radiographic positions and radiologic procedures,* ed 10, St Louis, 2003, Mosby; GE Medical Systems, Waukesha, Wis; Pagana KD, Pagana TJ: *Mosby's manual of diagnostic and laboratory test reference,* ed 7, St Louis, 2004, Mosby.

Figure 5-12 from Potter PA, Perry AG: *Fundamentals of nursing: concepts, process, and practice,* ed 5, St Louis, 2001, Mosby.

Figure 5-13 courtesy Nelcor Puritan Bennett.

Figure 5-14 from Lewis SM et al: *Medical-surgical nursing,* ed 6, St Louis, 2004, Mosby.

Chapter 6

Figures 6-7, 6-9, and Exercise Figure I from Ballinger PW, Frank ED: *Merrill's atlas of radiographic positions and radiologic procedures,* ed 10, St Louis, 2003, Mosby.

Figures 6-8 and 6-10 from Bontrager KL: *Textbook of radiographic positioning and related anatomy,* ed 6, St Louis, 2002, Mosby.

Figure 6-12 courtesy Baxter Healthcare Corp.

Exercise Figure E courtesy Dornier Medical Systems, Kennesaw, Ga.

Exercise Figure J courtesy Fisher Scientific, Pittsburgh, Pa.

Chapter 7

Figures 7-3 and 7-10 from Ignatavicius DD, et al: *Medical-surgical nursing: a nursing process approach,* ed 4, 2002, WB Saunders.

Figure 7-12 courtesy EDAP Technomed, Inc.

Exercise Figure B from Bork K, Brauninger W: *Skin diseases in clinical practice,* ed 2, Philadelphia, 1998, WB Saunders.

Chapter 8

Figure 8-9 (A, B) from Mayo Clinic Health Letter, with permission of Mayo Foundation for Medical Education and Research, Rochester, Minn.

Figure 8-12 (A) courtesy Biopsys Medical, Inc, Irvine, Calif.

Figure 8-12 (B, C) from Pagana KD, Pagana TJ: *Mosby's manual of diagnostic and laboratory test reference,* ed 7, St Louis, 2004, Mosby.

Figures 8-13 (A), 8-16 (B), and Exercise Figure H from Ballinger PW, Frank ED: *Merrill's atlas of radiographic positions and radiologic procedures*, ed 10, St Louis, 2003, Mosby.

Figure 8-13 (B) courtesy Martin K. Portnoff.

Figure 8-17 courtesy Richard Wolf Medical Instruments Corp.

Chapter 9

Figure 9-2 from Dickason EJ, Schultz MO, Silverman BL: *Maternal-infant nursing care*, ed 3, St Louis, 1998, Mosby.

Figure 9-6 and Exercise Figure C from Zitelli BJ, David HW: *Atlas of pediatric physical diagnosis*, ed 4, St Louis, 2002, Mosby.

Figure 9-9 from Ballinger PW, Frank ED: *Merrill's atlas of radiographic positions and radiologic procedures*, ed 10, St Louis, 2003, Mosby.

Figure 9-10 from Hagen-Ansert S: *Textbook of diagnostic ultrasonography*, ed 5, St Louis, 2001, Mosby.

Chapter 10

Figure 10-6 from Lewis SM et al: *Medical-surgical nursing*, ed 6, St Louis, 2004, Mosby.

Figure 10-7 (A) from Thibodeau GA, Patton KT: *Anatomy and physiology*, ed 4, St Louis, 2001, Mosby.

Figure 10-7 (B) from Bork K, Brauninger W: *Skin diseases in clinical practice*, ed 2, Philadelphia, 1998, WB Saunders.

Figures 10-9, 10-16 (B, C), 10-17, 10-18, 10-19 (A), and 10-21 (B) from Ballinger PW, Frank ED: *Merrill's atlas of radiographic positions and radiologic procedures*, ed 10, St Louis, 2003, Mosby.

Figure 10-21 (A) courtesy GE Medical Systems, Inc, Waukesha, Wis.

Figure 10-25 from Seidel H, et al: *Mosby's guide to physical examination*, ed 5, St Louis, 2003, Mosby.

Chapter 11

Figure 11-9 from Anderson KN: *Mosby's medical, nursing and allied health dictionary*, St Louis, 2003, Mosby.

Figure 11-10 from LaFleur Brooks M, LaFleur Brooks D: *Basic medical language*, ed 2, St Louis, 2004, Mosby.

Figure 11-12 copyright Mayo Foundation for Medical Education and Research. All rights reserved. Used with permission.

Figure 11-13 from White RA, Klein SR: *Endoscopic surgery*, St Louis, 1991, Mosby.

Figures 11-14, 11-15, and Exercise G (2) from Ballinger PW, Frank ED: *Merrill's atlas of radiographic*

positions and radiologic procedures, ed 10, St Louis, 2003, Mosby.

Exercise Figure G (1) from Hagen-Ansert S: *Textbook of diagnostic ultrasonography*, ed 5, St Louis, 2001, Mosby.

Exercise Figures H (1) and I (1) courtesy Pentax Corp, Englewood, Colo.

Chapter 12

Figure 12-2 and Exercise Figures B and D from Zitelli BJ, David HW: *Atlas of pediatric physical diagnosis*, ed 4, St Louis, 2002, Mosby.

Figure 12-3 (A, B) from Seidel H, et al: *Mosby's guide to physical examination*, ed 5, St Louis, 2003, Mosby.

Exercise Figure C from Stein HA, Slatt BJ, Stein RM: *The ophthalmic assistant: fundamentals and clinical practice*, ed 5, St Louis, 1998, Mosby.

Figure 12-4 from Newell FW: *Ophthalmology*, ed 7, St Louis, 1992, Mosby.

Figure 12-6 from Apple DJ, Robb MF: *Ocular pathology*, ed 5, St Louis, 1998, Mosby.

Figure 12-7 from Shiland BJ: *Mastering healthcare terminology*, St Louis, 2003, Mosby.

Figure 12-8 copyright Mayo Foundation for Medical Education and Research. All rights reserved. Used with permission.

Figure 12-9 from Bedford MA: *Ophthalmological diagnosis*, London, 1986, Wolfe.

Figure 12-10 courtesy Nidek, Inc, Fremont, Calif.

Figure 12-11 from Meeker MH, Rothrock JC: *Alexander's care of the patient in surgery*, ed 11, St Louis, 1999, Mosby.

Figure 12-12 from Thompson J, Wilson S: *Health assessment for nursing practice*, St Louis, 1996, Mosby.

Chapter 13

Figure 13-2 courtesy Richard A Buckingham, MD, University of Illinois, Chicago.

Figure 13-4 from Zitelli BJ, David HW: *Atlas of pediatric physical diagnosis*, ed 4, St Louis, 2002, Mosby.

Exercise Figure C courtesy Micro Audiometrics Corp., South Daytona, Fla.

Chapter 14

Figure 14-5 (C, D, E) from Gartner LP, Hiatt JL: *Color textbook of histology*, ed 2, Philadelphia, 2001, WB Saunders.

Figure 14-6 from Thibodeau GA, Patton KT: *Anatomy and physiology*, ed 5, St Louis, 2003, Mosby.

Figures 14-11 and 14-21 from Mercier LR: *Practical orthopedics*, ed 4, St Louis, 1995, Mosby.

Figures 14-15 to 14-17 copyright Mayo Foundation for Medical Education and Research. All rights reserved. Used with permission.

Figure 14-18 from Pagana KD, Pagana TJ: *Mosby's manual of diagnostic and laboratory test reference,* ed 7, St Louis, 2004, Mosby.

Figure 14-19 courtesy Marconi Medical Systems, Cleveland, Ohio.

Figure 14-20 from Ballinger PW, Frank ED: *Merrill's atlas of radiographic positions and radiologic procedures,* ed 10, St Louis, 2003, Mosby.

Chapter 15

Figure 15-1 from Thibodeau GA, Patton KT: *Anatomy and physiology,* ed 5, St Louis, 2003, Mosby.

Figure 15-4 from Perkin GD, Hotchberg FH, Miller D: *The atlas of clinical neurology,* St Louis, 1986, Mosby.

Figure 15-7 from Habif TP: *Clinical dermatology,* ed 4, St Louis, 2004, Mosby.

Figures 15-9, 15-10, 15-11, and Exercise Figure E from Ballinger PW, Frank ED: *Merrill's atlas of radiographic positions and radiologic procedures,* ed 10, St Louis, 2003, Mosby.

Chapter 16

Figure 16-4 from Zitelli BJ, David HW: *Atlas of pediatric physical diagnosis,* ed 4, St Louis, 2002, Mosby.

Figure 16-5 courtesy CD Forbes and WF Jackson.

Figure 16-6 from Seidel H et al: *Mosby's guide to physical examination,* ed 5, St Louis, 2003, Mosby.

Figure 16-7 courtesy Paul W. Ladenson, MD, The Johns Hopkins University and Hospital, Baltimore, Md.

Exercise Figure C from Thibodeau GA, Patton KT: *Anatomy and physiology,* ed 5, St Louis, 2003, Mosby.

INDEX

Basal cell carcinoma, 79, 80f
Baseline, 670
Basic health services, 654
BC. *see* Birth control
Behavior modification, 665
Behavioral health terms, 665-669
Bell palsy, 556
Belmont Report, 670
Benefit period, 655
Benefit schedule, 655
Benign, 28
Benign prostatic hyperplasia
  definition of, 207
  treatments for, 220
Benign prostatic hypertrophy, 208
Benzodiazepine, 648
Beta-blocker, 648
bi-, 48, 430
Bias, 670
Biceps brachii, 486f
Biceps femoris, 487f
Bicuspid valve, 310f, 311
Bilateral, 50
Bile acid sequestrant, 648
Bile ducts, 371
bin-, 430
Binocular, 446
bi/o, 71
Bioavailability, 648, 670
Bioequivalence, 670
Biofeedback, 123, 662
Biologic, 670
Biopsy
  bone marrow, 348, 348f
  definition of, 86
  sentinel lymph node, 256, 257f
  stereotactic breast, 256, 258f
Biotechnology, 670
Bipolar disorder, 577
Birth control, 648
Bisphosphonates, 648
Bladder
  definition of, 162
  fulguration of, 179, 179f
blast/o, 165
Blepharitis, 431
blephar/o, 426
Blepharoplasty, 439
Blepharoptosis, 431
Blind(ing), 670
Blister. *see* Vesicle
Blood
  complementary terms for, 355
  definition of, 312
  diagnostic terms for, 342, 348
  diseases and disorders of, 321
Blood pressure, 354
Blood urea nitrogen, 186
Blood vessels
  complementary terms for, 354-355
  diagnostic terms for, 341, 345-348
  diseases and disorders of, 320-321
  types of, 311
BMI. *see* Body mass index
Board certified, 655
Board eligible, 655
Body cavities, 13-14
Body language, 665
Body mass index, 678
Body movements, 489-490
Body organization, 11-13
Body structures
  combining forms of, 15-18
  prefixes for, 19-20
  terms for, 31-34

Boil. *see* Furuncle
Bone
  cancellous, 480
  compact, 480
  computed tomography of, 522, 523f
  magnetic resonance imaging of, 522, 523f
  radiography of, 522
  skeletal, 481-484, 482f-483f
  structure of, 480-481
Bone densitometry, 522
Bone marrow, 481
Bone marrow biopsy, 348, 348f
Bone marrow transplant, 335
Bone scan, 522
Borderline personality disorder, 665
BP. *see* Blood pressure
BPH. *see* Benign prostatic hyperplasia
Brachial plexus, 543f
brady-, 318
Bradycardia, 320
Bradykinesia, 523
Brain
  anatomy of, 542, 545f
  computed tomography of, 564, 565f
  magnetic resonance imaging of, 564, 565f
  positron emission tomography of, 564, 565f
Brain attack. *see* Cerebrovascular accident
Brainstem, 542, 545f
Brand name drug, 655
Breast cancer, 246
Breasts, 236, 236f
Breech presentation, 301, 301f
Bronchi, 106f, 108, 108f
bronch/i, 109
Bronchiectasis, 117
Bronchiole, 106f, 108, 108f
Bronchitis, 117
bronch/o, 109
Bronchoalveolar, 143
Bronchoconstrictor, 148
Bronchodilator, 148
Bronchogenic carcinoma, 117
Bronchoplasty, 129
Bronchopneumonia, 117
Bronchoscope, 134, 137f
Bronchoscopy, 134
Bronchospasm, 143
Bruise. *see* Contusion
Bulbourethral gland, 203f
Bulimia nervosa, 386, 577
BUN. *see* Blood urea nitrogen
Bunion, 508, 509f
Bursa, 484
Bursectomy, 514
Bursitis, 501
burs/o, 496
Bursolith, 501
Bx. *see* Biopsy
BZD. *see* Benzodiazepine

C

Ca. *see* Cancer
CA-125, 264
CABG. *see* Coronary artery bypass graft
CAD. *see* Coronary artery disease
Calcaneal tendon, 487f
Calcaneus, 484
calc/i, 595
Calcipenia, 607
Calcium channel blocker, 648
Calorie, 678
Cancellous bone, 480
Cancer
  breast, 246
  cervical, 246

Cancer *(Continued)*
  endometrial, 246
  ovarian, 247
  prostate, 211-212, 213f
  uterine, 246
Cancer antigen-125 tumor marker. *see* CA-125
cancer/o, 17
Cancerous, 31
Candida, 79
Candidiasis, 79
Capillaries, 312
Capitation, 655
capn/o, 112
Capnometer, 134
Capsule, 648
Carbohydrate, 678
Carbohydrate counting, 678
Carbon dioxide, 106
Carbuncle, 79
carcin/o, 17
Carcinogen, 31
Carcinogenic, 31
Carcinoma
  basal cell, 79, 80f
  bronchogenic, 117
  choriocarcinoma, 285
  definition of, 22
  osteocarcinoma, 503
  squamous cell, 80f, 82
  testicular, 211
Carcinoma in situ, 28
Cardiac, 351
Cardiac arrest, 326
Cardiac catheterization, 349
Cardiac glycoside, 648
Cardiac muscle, 485, 488f
Cardiac pacemaker, 335, 335f
Cardiac tamponade, 326
cardi/o, 315
Cardiodynia, 320
Cardiogenic, 351
Cardiologist, 351
Cardiology, 351
Cardiomegaly, 320
Cardiomyopathy, 320
Cardiopulmonary resuscitation, 354
Cardiovalvulitis, 320
Cardiovascular system. *see also* Heart
  abbreviations, 358-359
  anatomy of, 310f, 310-312
  combining forms of, 315-318
  complementary terms for, 351-355
  diagnostic terms for, 341-342, 348-349
  diseases and disorders of, 320-321, 326-328
  function of, 310
  medical terms for, 320-321, 326-328
  prefixes for, 318
  structures of, 310-312
  suffixes for, 318
  surgical terms for, 332-341
Carpal, 524
Carpal bones, 481, 482f
Carpal tunnel syndrome, 509, 509f, 516
Carpectomy, 514
carp/o, 491
Carpoptosis, 502
Cartilage
  articular, 484
  thyroid, 107
Carve out, 655
Case control study, 671
Case management, 655
Case mix, 655
Case report form, 671
Cataract, 434, 434f

ox/i, 112
-oxia, 115
Oximeter, 138
ox/o, 112
Oxygen, 112
Oxygen therapy, 664
Oxytocic hormones, 651
Oxytocin, 589

P

Pacemaker, 335, 335f
Pachyderma, 75
pachy/o, 72
PAD. *see* Peripheral arterial disease
Palate
    anatomy of, 107f, 368f
    cleft, 291
    hard, 107f, 369
    soft, 107f, 369
Palatine tonsil, 107f
Palatitis, 381
palat/o, 376
Palatoplasty, 393
Pallor, 95
pan-, 114
Pancreas, 368f, 370f, 371, 591f
Pancreatic, 409
Pancreatic duct, 370f
Pancreatitis, 381
pancreat/o, 376
Pancytopenia, 321
Panhysterectomy, 250
Panic attack, 577
Panplegia, 568
Pansinusitis, 118
Pap smear, 264, 265f, 266
Para, 297
para-, 73
Parallel study design, 674
Paranasal sinuses, 106f, 107
Paranoid disorder, 667
Paraplegia, 574
Parasympatholytic, 651
Parasympathomimetic, 651
Parathormone, 589
Parathyroid glands, 589, 591f
Parathyroidectomy, 604
parathyroid/o, 593
Parathyroidoma, 597
Parenteral, 651
Parenteral nutrition, 678
-paresis, 551
Parietal pericardium, 311
Parkinson disease, 557
par/o, 281
Paronychia, 76
Parotid gland, 588
Parotid salivary gland, 368f
Paroxysm, 148
Participant, 674
Participating physician, 658
part/o, 281
-partum, 284
Parturition, 301
Patella, 482f, 484
Patellar tendon, 486f
Patellectomy, 515
patell/o, 492
Patent, 148
path/o, 17
Pathogenic, 33
Pathologist, 33
Pathology, 33
-pathy, 20

PCP. *see Pneumocystis carinii* pneumonia;
    Primary care physician
PD. *see* Parkinson disease
PE. *see* Pulmonary embolism
Pectoralis major, 486f
Pediculicide, 651
Pediculosis, 81
Peer review, 674
PEG. *see* Percutaneous endoscopic
    gastrostomy
pelv/i, 492
Pelvic, 524
Pelvic bone, 481
Pelvic cavity, 14
Pelvic inflammatory disease, 247, 247f
Pelvic sonography, 293, 294f
Pelvisacral, 524
pelv/o, 492
-penia, 318
Penile implant, 218, 219f
Penis, 202
-pepsia, 380
Peptic ulcers, 387f, 388
per-, 73
Percussion, 355, 355f
Percutaneous, 89
Percutaneous diskectomy, 516
Percutaneous endoscopic gastrostomy, 392,
    393f
Percutaneous transluminal coronary angioplasty,
    338, 339f
Percutaneous vertebroplasty, 516
peri-, 241
Pericardial fluid, 310f, 311
Pericardial sac, 311
Pericardiocentesis, 333, 333f
Pericarditis, 321
Pericardium, 310f, 311
Perimetritis, 242
Perimetrium, 234
perine/o, 239
Perineorrhaphy, 250
Perineotomy. *see* Episiotomy
Perineum, 236
Periosteum, 480, 480f
Peripheral arterial disease, 328
Peripheral nervous system
    description of, 542
    organs of, 544
Peristalsis, 413
Peritoneal, 409
Peritoneal dialysis, 191, 192f
peritone/o, 376
Peritoneum, 371
Peritonitis, 382
Peroneal nerve, 543f
Peroneus brevis, 486f, 487f
Peroneus longus, 486f, 487f
Personality disorder, 667
Pertussis, 124
PET. *see* Positron emission tomography
Petechia, 95
petr/o, 498
-pexy, 115
PFTs. *see* Pulmonary function tests
Phacoemulsification, 441
-phagia, 74
Phalangectomy, 515
Phalanges, 481, 482f
phalang/o, 492
Pharmaceutical, 651
Pharmacist, 651
Pharmacodynamics, 651
Pharmacoeconomics, 674
Pharmacogenetics, 674

Pharmacogenomics, 651
Pharmacokinetics, 651, 674
Pharmacology
    definition of, 651
    terms associated with, 646-653
Pharmacy, 651
Pharyngitis, 118
pharyng/o, 109
Pharynx, 106f, 107, 368f, 369
Phase I trials, 675
Phase II trials, 675
Phase III trials, 675
Phase IV trials, 675
phas/o, 549
Phimosis, 211, 212f
Phlebectomy
    ambulatory, 328
    definition of, 333
Phlebitis, 321
phleb/o, 315
Phlebotomy, 333
PHO. *see* Physician-hospital organization
Phobia, 577
-phobia, 430
-phonia, 115
Phosphodiesterase inhibitor, 651
phot/o, 429
Photophobia, 432
Photorefractive keratectomy. *see* PRK
Phrenic, 568
phren/o, 549
Phrenopathy, 568
Physician assistant, 659
Physician extender, 659
Physician-hospital organization, 659
Physicians Current Procedural Terminology, 659
Physician's Desk Reference, 659
-physis, 500
Phytochemical, 678
Phytotherapeutics, 664
Pia mater, 544
Pica, 577, 678
PID. *see* Pelvic inflammatory disease
Pilot study, 675
Pimple. *see* Papule
Pinna, 458f, 459
Pituitary gland, 589, 590f
Placebo, 651, 675
Placebo effect, 675
Placebo-controlled study, 675
Placenta, 278, 279f
Placenta previa, 288, 288f
-plasia, 20
-plasm, 20
Plasma, 312, 355
Plasmapheresis, 352
plasm/o, 315
-plasty, 74
Platelets, 312
-plegia, 430
Pleura, 106f, 108
Pleural effusion, 124
Pleurisy. *see* Pleuritis
Pleuritis, 118
pleur/o, 109
Pleuropexy, 130
PMS. *see* Premenstrual syndrome
-pnea, 115
pneumat/o, 109
Pneumatocele, 118
pneum/o, 109
Pneumobronchotomy, 130
Pneumoconiosis, 118
Pneumocystis carinii pneumonia, 124, 126f
Pneumonectomy, 129f, 130